1,001
MEDICAL
FACTS
for every home

1,001 MEDICAL FACTS

for every home

Raymond Barr

INTRODUCTION BY
David S. Brown, M.D.

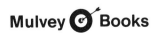 Mulvey Books

Published by
William Mulvey Inc.
72 Park Street
New Canaan, Conn. 06840

Cover design: Clark Robinson
Interior design: Angela Foote

Library of Congress Cataloging-in-Publication Data

1,001 Medical Facts
for Every Home
"A Mulvey Book"

I. Medicine, Popular — Dictionaries. I. Barr, Raymond.
II. Title: One thousand one medical facts for every home.
III. Title: One thousand and one medical facts for every
home.

RC81.A2A15   1988   610'.3'21   88–42808

ISBN 0–934791–13–9

Printed in the United States of America
First Edition

*This book is dedicated to those
who made it possible—the talented
people of the National Institutes of
Health, the Food and Drug Administration
and the American Cancer Society.*

Contents

Foreword

Seen from nearly 40 years of active medical practice, the most striking thing about this book is that most families will be able to read it with understanding sufficient to be of assistance in their doctors' management of their medical problems.

The existence of this impressive general medical knowledge is an awesome achievement of our government, educational system, press, and the patience and concern of health practitioners.

Thanks to these agents of public benefit, the average American today knows more about health and disease than the most distinguished doctors of 100 years ago.

Unfortunately, that is not enough to bring much comfort to the patient whose health problems require the knowledge acquired in these last 100 years—and most of them do. Nor is it much help to the harried health worker leading his patient through the maze of modern medicine. But a book like this can go a long way toward reducing these problems.

For thousands of years there has been a steady, slow accumulation of health-related information. Growth in the last 100 years has accelerated to an exponential explosion.

This has put the forefront of medicine at such distance from patient understanding that it is difficult to bring newer knowledge into effective contact with those it could benefit. This is worrisome—both to the health workers trying to bridge the increasing gap and to their patients trying to benefit from the new knowledge.

Until this deluge of medical information began, the relatively small difference between a doctor's knowledge and his patient's could be bridged fairly easily; the patient was comforted as much by his doctor's understanding and compassion as by what could be done for his disorder. Since most illnesses recover spontaneously anyway, this gratification of our continuing anthropologic need for a caring healer yielded great satisfaction. This satisfaction accounts for the ancient and ongoing prestige and need for physicians in our cultures.

The explosion of medical knowledge has strained the relationship. And it will continue to do so unless an increase in general medical knowledge among patients keeps them—and their doctors—fairly close to the expanding forefront of medical science.

It seems likely that we will have to endure attempts to achieve short-term economies by replacing people with systems in guiding patients. Practical necessity may even force some adaptation; but trained *people* will continue to be the way most patients come to understand their health problems. This is placing an increasing burden of patient education on the shoulders of health care workers who are already burdened with the job of keeping up with new thinking and developments.

A book like this can dramatically reduce the physician's job of patient education. It can allow him to reach more quickly and effectively levels of patient understanding which will ease his patient's progress which no compendium can cover completely.

As a healthy sign of the vigor of their growing science, physicians usually have a difference of opinion as they consider a problem of patient care. But this book presents the knowledge base which most of today's physicians possess as they enter the uncharted waters of a specific patient's care. The generalities it presents may be obsolete, or at least controversial in five years, but today they would raise few complaints or challenges from medical practitioners.

The articles are skillfully written and readily understandable by a person of average intelligence who has a basic education. If used as a resource, the book can bring a patient to the point where he understands and appreciates his physician's actions in fitting newer medical knowledge to his problem. With gratifying generosity, these thoughtful authors present their work not as a substitute or alternative for the traditional patient-doctor relationship; rather it is a means of improving the relationship by helping patients through the increasing complexities of modern health care.

To this seasoned practitioner, this book is extremely welcome. It gives new, concise, and effective ways of achieving patient education. I would strongly urge its use by all of my patients as an important tool, enabling patient-doctor relationship to utilize the newest wonders of medical science.

David S. Brown, M.D.

AIDS
Facts

The Acquired Immune Deficiency Syndrome, or AIDS, was first reported in the United States in mid-1981. Since that time, the Public Health Service has received reports of more than 29,000 cases, about 56 percent of which have resulted in death. An estimated 1 million people have been infected by the virus that causes AIDS, but have no symptoms of illness.

AIDS is a public health problem that merits serious concern. It is a major priority of the Public Health Service. Researchers in the Public Health Service and in many major medical institutions have been working for five years to study AIDS and develop treatments and preventive measures.

This fact sheet provides, in question-and-answer form, accurate information about AIDS, the risk of contracting AIDS, the actions individuals can take to reduce spreading AIDS, and current research and related activities under way in the Public Health Service.

What is AIDS?

AIDS is characterized by a defect in natural immunity against disease. People who have AIDS are vulnerable to serious illnesses which would not be a threat to anyone whose immune system was functioning normally. These illnesses are referred to as "opportunistic" infections or diseases.

What causes AIDS?

AIDS is caused by a virus that infects certain cells of the immune system, and can also directly infect the brain. This virus has been given different names by different groups of investigators: human T-lymphotropic virus, type III (HTLV-III); lymphadenopathy-associated virus (LAV); or AIDS-related retrovirus (ARV). An international committee of scientists has proposed the name, human immunodeficiency virus (HIV), for this virus. Infection with this virus does not always lead to AIDS. Many infected persons remain in good health. Others develop illness varying in severity from mild to extremely serious; these illnesses are designated AIDS-related complex (ARC).

How is AIDS transmitted?

The AIDS virus is spread by sexual contact, needle sharing, or less commonly, through transfused blood or its components. The virus may be transmitted also from infected mother to infant during pregnancy or birth, or shortly after birth (probably through breast milk). The risk of infection with the virus is increased by having multiple sexual partners, either homosexual or heterosexual, and sharing of needles among those using illicit drugs. The occurrence of the syndrome in hemophilia patients and persons receiving transfusions provides evidence of transmission of the virus through blood.

Who gets AIDS?

Ninety-eight percent of the AIDS cases have occurred in the following groups of people:
- Sexually active homosexual men and bisexual men (or any man who has had sex with another man since 1977), 65 percent;
- Present or past abusers of intravenous drugs, 17 percent;
- Homosexual and bisexual men who are also IV drug abusers, 8 percent;
- Persons with hemophilia or other coagulation disorders, 1 percent;
- Heterosexual contacts of someone with AIDS or at risk for AIDS, 4 percent;
- Infants born to infected mothers, 1 percent.

Some 2 percent of patients do not fall into any of these groups, but researchers believe that transmission occurred in similar ways. For example, some patients died before complete histories could be taken.

What are its symptoms?

Most individuals infected with the AIDS virus have no symptoms and feel well. Some develop symptoms which may include tiredness, fever, loss of appetite and weight, diarrhea, night sweats, and swollen glands (lymph nodes)—usually in the neck, armpits, or groin. Anyone who has these symptoms for more than two weeks should see a doctor.

How long after infection with HTLV-III does a person develop AIDS?

The time between infection with the HTLV-III virus and the onset of symptoms (the incubation period) ranges from about six months to five years or more. Infection with the virus may not always lead to AIDS.

Symptoms of illness appear in approximately 30 percent of individuals within five years of infection.

How is AIDS diagnosed?

The diagnosis of AIDS depends on the presence of opportunistic diseases that indicate the loss of immunity. Certain tests which demonstrate damage to various parts of the immune system, such as specific types of white blood cells, support the diagnosis. The presence of opportunistic diseases plus a positive test for antibodies to HTLV-III can also make possible a diagnosis of AIDS.

What is the geographic distribution of reported AIDS cases?

Thirty-two percent of the cases in the U.S. are reported from New York State and about 22 percent from California. AIDS cases have been reported from all 50 states, the District of Columbia, Puerto Rico, and more than 70 other countries.

How contagious is AIDS?

Casual contact with AIDS patients or infected persons does *not* place others at risk for getting the illness. No cases have been found where the virus has been transmitted by casual household contact with AIDS patients or infected persons. Infants with AIDS or HTLV-III infection have not transmitted the infection to family members living in the same household, although one possible transmission between siblings by a bite has been reported.

Emergency medical personnel, police, and firefighters who have assisted AIDS patients have not become ill. Nurses, doctors, and health care personnel have not developed AIDS from caring for AIDS patients. Two health care workers in the U.S. have developed antibodies to HTLV-III following needlestick injuries.

Health care and laboratory workers should follow standard safety procedures carefully when handling any blood and tissue samples from patients with potentially transmissible diseases, including AIDS. Special care should be taken to avoid needlestick injuries.

Is there a danger of contracting AIDS from donating blood?

No. Blood banks and other blood collection centers use sterile equipment and disposable needles. The need for blood is great, and people who are not at increased risk for getting AIDS are urged to continue to donate blood as they have in the past.

Is there danger of a child's contracting AIDS from friends or schoolmates?

No. AIDS is difficult to catch, even among people at highest risk for the disease. The risk of transmitting AIDS from daily contact at work, school, or at home is extremely rare or nonexistent. In virtually all cases, direct sexual contact, sharing of IV drug needles, transfusion of infected blood or blood products, or perinatal transmission (from infected mother to unborn or newborn baby) has led to the illness.

How is AIDS treated?

Currently, there are no antiviral drugs available anywhere that have been proven to cure AIDS, although the search for such a drug is being pursued vigorously. Some drugs have been found that inhibit the AIDS virus. One of these, azidothymidine (AZT), has shown some promise in limited, short-term clinical trials with a select group of patients. Though no treatment has yet been successful in restoring the immune system of an AIDS patient, doctors have had some success in using drugs, radiation, and surgery to treat the various illnesses of AIDS patients. Therapeutic agents are needed for all stages of AIDS infections, to block action of the virus once infection has occurred, and to restore full function in patients whose immune systems have been damaged.

Eventually, a combination of therapies to combat the virus and restore the immune system may be the most effective treatment.

Can AIDS be prevented?

Yes. Cases of AIDS related to medical use of blood or blood products are being prevented by use of HTLV-III antibody screening tests at blood donor sites and by members of high-risk groups voluntarily not donating blood. Heat treatment of Factor VIII and other blood products helps prevent AIDS in patients with hemophilia and other clotting disorders. There is no vaccine for AIDS itself. However, individuals can reduce their risk of contracting AIDS by following existing recommendations. Communities can help prevent AIDS by vigorous efforts to educate and inform their populations about the illness, with special emphasis on educational activities for members of high-risk groups. Meanwhile, the effort to produce vaccines and drugs against AIDS continues.

Recommendations for the general public

The U.S. Public Health Service recommends the following steps to reduce the chances of contracting infection with HTLV-III—the virus that causes AIDS.

- Don't have sex with multiple partners, or with persons who have had multiple partners (including prostitutes). The more partners you have, the greater your risk of infection.
- Obviously, avoiding sex with persons with AIDS, members of the risk groups,* or persons who have had a positive result on the HTLV-III antibody test would eliminate the risk of sexually transmitted infection by the virus. However, if you do have sex with a person you think is infected, protect yourself by taking appropriate precautions to prevent contact with the person's body fluids. ("Body fluids" includes blood, semen, urine, feces, saliva, and women's genital secretions.)

    Use condoms, which will reduce the possibility of transmitting the virus.

    Avoid practices that may injure body tissues (for example, anal intercourse).

    Avoid oral-genital contact.

    Avoid open-mouthed, intimate kissing.
- Don't use intravenous drugs. If you do, don't share needles or syringes. (If you believe that you may be at increased risk for HTLV-III infection, consult your physician for counseling. Consider asking to take the HTLV-III antibody test, which would enable you to know your status and take appropriate actions.)

Recommendations for persons at increased risk of infection with HTLV-III

The U.S. Public Health Service recommends the following precautions for persons at increased risk of infection by HTLV-III, the virus that causes AIDS. These recommendations are based on the fact that it is possible to carry the virus without knowing it, and thus transmit it to others.

---

* Persons at increased risk of HTLV-III infection include: homosexual and bisexual men; present or past intravenous drug users; persons with clinical or laboratory evidence of infection such as signs or symptoms compatible with AIDS or AIDS-related illnesses; persons born in countries where heterosexual transmission is thought to play a major role in the spread of HTLV-III (for example, Haiti and Central African countries); male or female prostitutes and their sex partners; sex partners of infected persons or persons at increased risk; persons with hemophilia who have received clotting factor products; and newborn infants of high-risk or infected mothers.

- Consult your physician for counseling. Consider asking to take the HTLV-III antibody test, which would enable you to know your status and take appropriate actions.
- Don't have sex with multiple partners, or with persons who have had multiple partners (including prostitutes). The more partners you have, the greater your risk of contracting AIDS.
- Don't use intravenous drugs. If you do, don't share needles or syringes.
- During sexual activity:
    Use condoms, which reduce the possibility of transmitting the virus. Avoid practices that may injure body tissues (for example, anal intercourse).
    Avoid oral-genital contact.
    Avoid open-mouthed, intimate kissing.
    Protect your partner from contact with your body fluids. ("Body fluids" includes blood, semen, urine, feces, saliva, and women's genital secretions.)
- Don't donate blood, plasma, body organs, other body tissue or sperm.
- If you are a woman at increased risk, consider the risk to your baby before becoming pregnant. (AIDS can be transmitted from infected mother to infant.) Before becoming pregnant, you should take the HTLV-III antibody test. If you choose to become pregnant, you should be tested during pregnancy.

Recommendations for persons with a positive HTLV-III antibody test

The U.S. Public Health Service recommends the following steps for persons with positive results on the blood test for antibodies to HTLV-III, the virus that causes AIDS.

- Seek regular medical evaluation and follow-up.
- Either avoid sexual activity or inform your prospective partner of your antibody test results and protect him or her from contact with your body fluids during sex. ("Body fluids" includes blood, semen, urine, feces, saliva, and women's genital secretions.) Use a condom, and avoid practices that may injure body tissues (for example, anal intercourse). Avoid oral-genital contact and open-mouthed, intimate kissing.
- Inform your present and previous sex partners, and any persons with whom needles may have been shared, of their potential exposure to HTLV-III and encourage them to seek counseling and antibody testing from their physicians or at appropriate health clinics.
- Don't share toothbrushes, razors, or other items that could become contaminated with blood.

- If you use drugs, enroll in a drug treatment program. Needles and other drug equipment must never be shared.
- Don't donate blood, plasma, body organs, other body tissue, or sperm.
- Clean blood or other body fluid spills on household or other surfaces with freshly diluted household bleach—1 part bleach to 10 parts water. (Don't use bleach on wounds.)
- Inform your doctor, dentist, and eye doctor of your positive HTLV-III status so that proper precautions can be taken to protect you and others.
- Women with a positive antibody test should avoid pregnancy until more is known about the risks of transmitting HTLV-III from mother to infant.

Further information about AIDS may be obtained from your local or State health department or your physician. The Public Health Service AIDS hotline number is 1-800-342-AIDS. New York City area callers should dial the same number.

For further information on drug abuse treatment call 1-800-662-HELP. For information on AZT, call 1-800-843-9388.

U.S. Department of Health and Human Services, Public Health Services, Winter 1987.

Allergy
On Surviving
The Sneezin' Season

"In the spring," wrote Alfred Lord Tennyson, *"a young man's fancy lightly turns to thoughts of love." But for millions of Americans, spring fever has quite a different meaning, as Nature's new greenery brings on bouts of sneezing, sniffling, coughing, and wheezing. And spring may not be the only season of discontent, nor outdoor greenery the only cause, for allergy sufferers, as this article explains.*

Most of us welcome the coming of spring as an end to the yearly bouts of runny noses, sore throats, and headaches from winter colds and flu. But millions of Americans scarcely have time to wring out their handkerchiefs and take a breath of fresh air before they encounter a second round of misery, for hay fever season is on the way.

"Hay fever" is really a misnomer, for the seasonal allergies that afflict more than 15 million Americans do not produce fever and are hardly ever caused by hay. The most common instigator are microscopic grains of pollen spewed by the millions into the spring, summer, and fall air by grasses, trees, and weeds. The usual symptoms are a runny or stuffed-up nose, watery or itchy eyes, violent sneezing (a fit of sneezing, as many as 50 times in a row, can rack the body). Sometimes an itching nose, throat, roof of the mouth, and ear canals round out the misery.

Although those conditions are enough to spoil anyone's picnic, it's not unusual for seasonal allergy sufferers also to experience fatigue, irritability, loss of appetite, difficulty in concentrating, sore throat, cough, malaise, and even depression. Some hay fever sufferers develop asthma, a serious affliction of the bronchial tubes and lungs that claims between 2,000 and 4,000 lives a year in the United States.

Allergies of one type or another afflict an estimated 35 million Americans, according to the National Institute of Allergy and Infectious Diseases (NIAID), a part of the National Institutes of Health. Simply put, an allergy is an individual's unusual sensitivity to a substance in the environment that does not bother most other people. Allergic individuals can have abnormal reactions not only to pollen but also to foods, drugs, cosmetics, insect venom, animals, mold spores, and even common house dust.

It is the allergic reaction to certain pollens and mold spores that we think of as hay fever, or seasonal allergies. Trees generally produce pollen in the spring, grasses turn it out in the early summer, and most weeds shed it in the late summer and early fall.

Often newspapers and radio and television stations will report a locale's daily pollen count. This is the number of grains of a certain kind of pollen found in the air during the previous 24 hours. Pollen counts can help alert hay fever sufferers to stay indoors to avoid these airborne assaults on high-pollen days. The counts also help allergists (physicians specializing in treating allergies) to diagnose correctly an allergy by correlating the pollen counts with the onset and severity of a patient's symptoms.

Although pollen counts are useful, allergic persons should be wary of comparing the counts of one locale with those from another. The techniques for collecting and measuring pollens are not standardized, and the variety of methods in use can make comparisons meaningless.

Airborne spores from molds are a common cause of allergies because of their many possible hiding and growing places inside and outside the house. These include areas of deep shade or heavy vegetation, damp basements, refrigerator drip trays, garbage cans, air conditioning systems, bathrooms, humidifiers, piles of leaves or logs, even old foam rubber pillows and mattresses.

In warm climates where molds and plants grow all year long, the molds- or pollen-allergic person may have no season of relief. Other such year-round, or perennial, allergies are caused by feathers and saliva, urine, and scales of skin shed from pets. Common house dust can bring on virtually inescapable allergies for persons sensitive to one or more of the components of dust. These include specks of fiber from rugs, drapes, furniture coverings, and mattress stuffings; food particles; pollen; mold spores; plant particles; and even tiny spider-like mites.

Scientists are not certain why some individuals are sensitive to certain airborne substances and most others are not. It is known that allergic reactions involve the body's immune system. When a virus, bacterium, or other microorganism invades the body, special proteins, called antibodies, are formed in the blood to help protect against future attacks by the same kind of bug. This antibody response helps explain why a person can be immunized against certain diseases. A polio vaccination, for example, consists of an injection of polio viruses that have been weakened or killed to render them harmless. The body recognizes this antigen as something foreign and produces the specific antibodies that will protect against any real attacks by healthy polio viruses in the future.

An allergic response works in much the same way, but the results are adverse instead of beneficial. Instead of providing protection, the body produces antibodies that render the person sensitive to a particular antigen. In the case of hay fever-type allergies with cold-like symptoms, the major sensitizing antibody is known as Immunoglobulin E (IgE). IgE antibodies are formed during first encounters with an antigen, or allergen, such as ragweed pollen. This first encounter is the sensitization process by which a person becomes allergic to a particular substance. From that time on, the IgE antibodies are present in the blood, ready to set off an allergic reaction whenever the individual is again exposed to the allergen. When such a subsequent exposure occurs, the IgE antibodies attach themselves to certain cells that are particularly abundant in the respiratory and gastrointestinal tracts, the skin, and the blood. These cells are like landmines, with the antibodies that cover their surfaces acting as detonators. When a particular antigen, such as ragweed, contacts an IgE antibody specifically sensitive to it, the landmine "explodes." The explosions release powerful chemicals, such as histamine, that increase the activity of the mucous glands and dilate the small blood vessels. Fluid leaking through the stretched blood vessel walls causes swelling of the tissues. If these "explosions" occur in the nose and eyes, hay fever results; in the chest they produce asthma; in the skin, hives and itching; in the gastrointestinal tract, vomiting and cramps.

These "exploding" cells are present in normal, nonallergic people, too, but the particular antibodies that "detonate" the cells are not. A predisposition to become easily sensitized to an allergen and to produce IgE antibodies can be inherited; thus allergies often run in families. But scientists generally believe that other, nongenetic properties are factors in determining who will sneeze and sniffle with allergies.

There is no "typical" case of hay fever-type allergy. Symptoms can show up at any age, although most commonly they appear before the age of 40. The symptoms may be so mild as to be mistaken for a light summer cold. Or they can be so severe that they seriously interrupt work and leisure activities for weeks at a time. The severity may vary from year to year for particular individuals, depending on the amount of allergens inhaled, the weather, and other factors. Sometimes the allergy will disappear but usually, especially if untreated, it persists for years, growing gradually worse until it reaches a plateau.

Complications can add to the suffering. Blocked sinuses can bring on severe headaches and sinus infections. The eustachian tubes, which help the ear drums function normally, can also be affected, causing inflammation of the middle ear and hearing problems. Nasal polyps—chronically swollen nasal tissue—may produce nasal blockage with loss of smell and taste. Some patients with hay fever-type allergies develop asthma, with its sometimes life-threatening attacks of wheezing and difficult breathing.

Because the symptoms are similar, a mild seasonal allergy may be mistaken for a common cold. But the two, though often of comparable degrees of misery, are not identical conditions. Sneezing, runny nose, and itchy eyes, nose, and throat are more characteristic of hay fever, while sore throat and fever are more often signs of a cold. Allergy symptoms will fluctuate from day to day as the pollen count varies and may also be worse outdoors or in the country or on windy days. Of course, if the condition reappears every year as predictably as the birds and the bees, or if it continues for several weeks, it's a good bet that it's an allergy.

Allergists use a number of tools to help in diagnosis. The patient may be instructed to keep a diary of the severity and duration of symptoms, the amount of medication needed to get relief, and other pertinent factors. By comparing the diary with the time and amount of pollination for the suspected substances in the area, the patient's medical history, and the results of "skin tests" or other procedures, the physicians can usually find the probable source of the trouble.

Skin testing consists of pricking the patient's arm or back after a tiny drop of the suspected allergen has been placed on the skin (the puncture test) or injecting it under the skin (the more sensitive intracutaneous test). A positive reaction—in the form of a bump surrounded by redness—appears, usually in about 15 to 20 minutes if the patient has specific IgE antibodies to that allergen. Usually the physician will administer more than one allergen at a time, but the choice of substances should be based on knowledge of the local environment and the patient's history, not on a predetermined "package" of tests as sometimes supplied by manufacturers.

Very rarely, an extract used in skin testing can cause an adverse reaction in an extremely allergic person. To avoid this physicians use as little of the allergen as possible for the tests. FDA, through its Bureau of Biologics, regulates the extracts used in skin testing, as well as those used in "allergy shots." There are at present, however, no standards of potency to help physicians make a better estimate of the proper amount of allergen to be used to diagnose or treat a particular patient. The bureau's Allergenic Products Branch is supporting and conducting research that should help standardize extracts and assist in the development of guidelines for use of extracts in both skin tests and allergy shots.

Besides skin tests another method has been developed to aid in diagnosing allergies. For example, very young children or patients with very sensitive skin can avoid the multiple punctures or injections through use of the radioallergosorbent technique (RAST) test. The RAST test uses a blood sample to determine the amount of specific IgE antibodies circulating in the blood. Although these blood tests are useful in special situations, they are not as sensitive as skin testing and cost four to five times more.

The 12th century physician Maimonides, when asked to treat the asthmatic son of Saladin, sultan of Egypt, candidly admitted, "I have no magic cure." Eight centuries later, scientists are still seeking a cure for asthma and other allergic diseases, including hay fever. Nor has a means been found to prevent allergies from developing in susceptible individuals.

There are, however, a number of ways to ease the misery of allergies. The first and most obvious is for the sufferer to avoid the cause of the affliction. This is most easily done when the allergen is found in a specific item, say a pillow containing feathers, that can be switched for one made of synthetic materials. Sometimes the companionship of a pet must be sacrificed to end allergic symptoms caused by the animal's proximity.

Because most allergens cannot be avoided, the allergic person may, out of frustration, consider escaping to another locale. But moving is generally not recommended. Airborne allergens are widespread—only the west coast of the United States is free of ragweed pollens, for example. And a person with specific sensitivity may in time become allergic to a different substance in a new location.

Allergy sufferers can at least partially avoid troublesome allergens without moving. Thorough housecleaning can reduce dust. Central air conditioning can help reduce the amount of pollen infiltrating the home. (But central heating with poor filtering systems can trap dust and other allergens, circulating them over and over again.) Dehumidifiers can help reduce mold growth.

Special air filters are available for room or whole-house use. But beware of exaggerated sales claims for "air purification" devices! Some such products, sold as negative ion generators, have been promoted for treating or even curing allergies, asthma, and other respiratory conditions. FDA has seen no scientific evidence that they are effective for such uses and has taken legal action against a number of promoters.

Besides trying to avoid their particular allergens, allergy sufferers should steer clear of insect sprays, fresh paint, tobacco smoke, and other substances that when inhaled can further irritate already inflamed membranes. Alcohol, because it dilates blood vessels, can also make allergy symptoms worse.

When an allergen cannot be avoided, medications may help ease the symptoms. Antihistamines, so named because they inhibit the symptoms produced by histamine, can help dry up a runny nose and relieve itchy or watery eyes. Oral decongestants may help relieve nasal congestion. Many antihistamines are available without a prescription, either as single-ingredient medications or as combinations with decongestants. Because such tablet medications can produce a variety of side effects, such as drowsiness, blurred vision, dry mouth, and rapid heartbeat, label directions should be followed precisely.

Nose sprays or drops are generally not recommended for relief of nasal congestion because use for more than a few days may cause a "rebound effect" that brings back the symptoms worse than before.

For more severe allergy symptoms, stronger medications are available by prescription. Powerful anti-inflammatory drugs called corticosteroids are of great help to some patients but can produce serious side effects after prolonged use.

For the many allergy sufferers who cannot find satisfactory relief by avoiding the harmful allergens or by use of medications, desensitization therapy—"allergy shots"—are often helpful. The patient is injected with diluted extracts of the troublesome allergen, beginning with small doses once or twice a week, and building up to higher doses repeated less frequently over time.

The shots are believed to work by causing the body to produce special "blocking antibodies" called Immunoglobulin G, or IgG. Unlike IgE, IgG antibodies are not attached to "exploding" cells. When IgG antibodies combine with an inhaled allergen they prevent it from reacting with

IgE antibodies, so there is no "explosion" and no release of histamine and other symptom-causing chemicals.

Allergy shots do not help all allergy sufferers. However, clinical studies and other reports indicate some degree of improvement in up to 80 percent of pollen hay fever patients. Some allergy experts believe that desensitization shots not only help relieve the usual symptoms of hay fever but also can prevent asthma from developing. There is, however, a lack of scientific information on the effectiveness of allergy shots for this purpose. A NIAID Task Force on Asthma and Other Allergic Diseases recommended in 1979 that long-term studies be done to determine the risk of allergy patients developing asthma and the value of allergy shots in preventing it.

When the shots are successful, they eventually build up an adequate degree of protection in the body and can be discontinued after several years of good results. Often, however, the protection will "wear off" after a number of years, and the regimen must begin again. This varies from patient to patient, but there is generally no need to continue hay fever-type allergy shots indefinitely.

As with the extracts used in skin testing, on rare occasions patients can experience adverse reactions to the shots. Emergency treatment with adrenalin or antihistamines may then be required. The most severe reaction usually occurs within the first few minutes after the injection. That is why physicians ask patients to remain 15 to 30 minutes after getting their shot, as a safety precaution.

While allergy shots can be effective in relieving the symptoms of hay fever-type allergies, they are time-consuming, costly, and carry the risk of adverse reaction. Current research is aimed at developing extracts that are safer and can provide good results with fewer injections. Work is being done to purify extracts that will contain only the part of the allergen responsible for the allergy-causing activity. Other researchers are developing chemical modifications of the actual allergens so that the extracts maintain the ability to desensitize allergy sufferers but seem to carry less risk of adverse reactions. Further studies are aimed at better understanding the role IgE plays in allergic disease; such work may someday turn up a way to prevent allergic reactions from developing, possibly by inhibiting the production of IgE.

For now, hay fever and other allergy sufferers should discuss with their physicians the best course of treatment, whether it is avoiding the source of the allergy or the proper use of medications or allergy shots. In most instances, proper treatment can reduce an allergy sufferer's misery to just an occasional sneeze or sniffle.

Bill Rados, *FDA Consumer*, Vol. 15, No. 3, April 1981.

Drug Allergy

For thousands of years, people have been treating their illnesses with various drugs. At first these were natural substances such as herbs and the juices or saps from plants that were eaten or applied to the skin. Doctors still use some of these natural products—for example, quinine obtained from the bark of the cinchona tree and digitalis prepared from the dried leaf of the foxglove plant. Today, however, most drugs available to the doctor are man-made chemicals designed to combat specific diseases or sets of symptoms.

As more drugs become available and are used, the number of adverse reactions to them increases. The World Health Organization's definition of an "adverse drug reaction" is any response to a drug that is harmful and not intended and that occurs at doses given to individuals for prevention, diagnosis, or treatment of disease.

One of the major public health problems today is drug-induced illness. Between 3 and 5 percent of medical hospital admissions are due to adverse drug effects, and 10 to 20 percent of patients hospitalized for other reasons have an adverse response to a drug prescribed while they are hospitalized. The Department of Health and Human Services has estimated that the annual cost of *treating* adverse drug reactions in U.S. hospitals is approximately $3 billion. Thus, in addition to the individual suffering and even death in rare cases, adverse drug reactions have become a costly problem indeed. Some of these adverse reactions to drugs are recognized as allergies.

What is an allergy?

An exaggerated sensitivity to a substance that causes no problem for most people is termed an "allergy" when it involves the body's immune system. Many substances can cause an allergic reaction. The most common ones are airborne pollens, molds, house dust, and animal danders; certain foods; insect venoms; and drugs. The symptoms may be mild, such as a stuffy nose or tearing eyes, or they may be generalized, severe, and even life-threatening, such as vascular collapse (anaphylactic shock) and airway obstruction.

One can encounter an allergy-provoking substance by several routes including inhalation, injection, ingestion, and skin contact. When an allergy-prone person is first exposed to such substances by any of these routes, the immune system, which is the body's defense mechanism against foreign invaders, responds in a number of ways.

One type of allergic reaction involves the immune mechanism that stimulates specialized kinds of white blood cells called lymphocytes to mature into plasma cells. It is these plasma cells that make immunoglobulin antibodies in response to their first exposure to foreign invaders (called antigens), such as viruses, bacteria, pollens, and some drugs. Usually, immunoglobulins have a protective role. However, in this case immunoglobulins of the IgE class are produced, which can "sensitize" or "prime" the affected person for a future allergic response.

Many kinds of antibodies protect the body by helping to fight off and destroy bacteria and viruses. Yet IgE antibodies, which are responsible for most allergies, have other properties that are often harmful to the allergic patient. These IgE antibodies in allergy-prone people attach themselves to certain cells in the body known as mast cells and basophils. Mast cells are found in body tissues, especially the respiratory and digestive tracts and in the skin; basophils are found in the blood.

The next time that a sensitized person encounters the specific foreign antigen, the IgE antibodies are lying in wait for it on the surfaces of the mast cells and basophils. These antigens bind to their corresponding IgE antibodies, causing the mast cells and basophils to release into the surrounding tissue certain irritating chemicals that produce the symptoms of allergy, such as sneezing, watery eyes, hives, abdominal pain, diarrhea, and skin rashes. One of these chemicals is histamine, a name familiar to many allergy sufferers. It brings on allergies by producing inflammation, which results from expansion of blood vessels and leakage of fluids through the stretched walls. A massive activation of the IgE system results in severe symptoms and possibly even fatal shock.

Interestingly, each antibody will react only to the specific antigen against which it was made. For example, an IgE antibody that is produced by plasma cells against house dust will not react to ragweed pollen. Thus a person who is allergic only to house dust will not have allergic symptoms when exposed to ragweed pollen. Similarly, a person allergic only to ragweed pollen will not have allergic symptoms when exposed to house dust.

This IgE antibody-antigen reaction is only one way that the body's immune system deals with foreign invaders. In another type of allergic response, antibodies of the IgG class are produced, enter the circulation, and attach to the surfaces of and destroy cells containing the corresponding antigen.

Such an event results from a transfusion in which mismatched blood is used. This type of reaction may also occur in unusual instances when a person's own blood cells become the target of attack by IgG if the cells are made to appear foreign by being coated with a drug. Such red blood cell destruction can lead to a drug-induced anemia.

These first two types of allergic reactions can occur quickly. A third type of reaction occurs several hours or days after exposure to an antigen and results when other types of harmful IgG antibodies and antigen combine into complexes which are then deposited in the walls of blood vessels, in the skin, or in the kidneys. Horse serum, formerly used in immunization injections against tetanus, was a common cause of this type of allergic reaction, called serum sickness. Some allergic reactions to penicillin are caused by an identical mechanism.

The allergic response known as "delayed hypersensitivity" reaches its peak two or three days after exposure of an allergic person to the offending antigen. This response is also known as "cell-mediated" immunity because certain kinds of sensitized lymphocytes themselves (rather than their antibody products) bring about the inflammatory reaction. Classic examples of this reaction are the skin test for tubercle bacilli (TB) and skin rashes caused by poison ivy. Only after 24 hours or more does the skin show a response to the test.

What is drug allergy?

When the body's immune system reacts against a drug, the adverse response that may sometimes result is known as an "allergic reaction." General reactions such as anaphylaxis, serum sickness, and asthma are typical of the unusual responses of the body's immune system to antigens; thus the occurrence of these symptoms in an adverse drug reaction is indicative of an allergic response. Other reactions to drugs are classified as allergic only on the basis of their clinical features and response to treatment. Because it is often very difficult to diagnose positively an allergy to a drug, the exact number of such reactions that occur each year cannot be counted.

How does drug allergy develop?

There are three steps in the development of drug allergy. First, a susceptible person must be *exposed* to the drug. Next, the body's immune system must be made *allergic* to the drug by the build-up of sensitized lymphocytes or antibodies produced by plasma cells. Third, the person must be *reexposed* to the same drug. Usually only after this second or later exposure will the symptoms of the allergy appear. Allergic responses to drugs differ widely, but a person's own pattern of reaction to a particular drug generally does not vary.

However, some people will occasionally tolerate a certain drug for months or even years, then they will suddenly suffer a severe allergic reaction to it. After that, even a tiny amount of the drug will cause symptoms.

The response of the body to a drug depends on such factors as the dosage, frequency and route of administration of the drug, and a person's own makeup. For example, intermittent (on-and-off) doses of a drug are more likely to lead to an allergic reaction than is long continuous use. Usually, most drugs are less likely to lead to an allergic reaction if given by mouth than by injection. A number of drugs (e.g., antihistamines) applied directly to the skin may sensitize, but they will have less allergic effect when given by injection or by mouth.

Generally, whether a person is a male or a female makes little difference in drug reactions. Age, however, is important. Children and elderly people are less likely than others to have drug reactions. This is perhaps because the immune system is immature in babies and tends to be less reactive in the elderly. It is unclear whether a person who is allergic to one drug is predisposed to allergic reactions to a new drug. Certainly, one should avoid further exposure to drugs having the same chemical makeup as the drug that first provoked the allergic response. Exposure to the sun sometimes increases the chance of an allergic reaction to certain drugs applied to the skin and even to some taken by mouth. When the intestines, kidneys, or liver are damaged and malfunction, the risk of allergy is greater because of the resulting inability of these organs to metabolize and excrete drugs.

The breakdown products of a drug that are formed as the body uses the drug occasionally may be the culprits rather than the drug itself in causing the reaction. In some cases, the body's allergic response is caused not by the drug or its breakdown products but by other chemicals added to the drug to preserve it (e.g., benzoic acid, methylparabens) or to improve its flavor or odor (e.g., terpenes).

Which drug reactions are nonallergic?

More than half of the adverse drug reactions reported by doctors are not allergic by definition. Such reactions may be classified as overdosage, idiosyncracy, side effects, paradoxical response, or drug interactions. All drugs, even over-the-counter ones, can cause these responses. Great variations occur in the symptoms, their frequency, and their severity among different patients.

Symptoms of overdosage may obviously result from too large an amount of medication taken. For example, an overdose of aspirin may cause a "ringing" in the ears. Yet overdosage may also be caused by the unexpected accumulation of a drug in a patient whose impaired or inadequate body function is unable to break it down or excrete it at a normal rate.

Many abnormal or unexpected reactions to drugs are termed "idiosyncratic." Examples include an unexpected response to an ordinary dose of a drug (e.g., reduced production of blood cells with use of the antibiotic chloramphenicol); a toxic response to a low dose of a drug (e.g., "ringing" in the ears with use of quinine, sometimes prescribed to relieve muscle cramps); or an unusual resistance to a large dose of a drug. Some idiosyncratic reactions are now known to have a genetic basis.

Side effects of drugs—undesirable yet unavoidable actions of medications and not related to the desired effect—are frequently encountered. Sleepiness after taking antihistamines and diarrhea that sometimes accompanies use of antibiotics are common examples. Patients may sometimes find it necessary to tolerate annoying yet harmless side effects of a medication in order to experience its curing effects.

Paradoxical responses are ones that vary from the reactions usually expected after a drug is administered and result in the opposite effect. One example is a case of the "jitters" after taking a sedative.

The interaction of one or more drugs being taken by a patient at the same time may also cause adverse reactions. These interactions occur when one drug alters the body's ability to use another drug or when a combination of two or more drugs modifies the effects of each drug. The interaction of two common drugs—alcohol and tranquilizers—can cause reactions that range from drowsiness to death.

Thus it is probable that a person may experience an adverse reaction to a drug without being allergic to it. The symptoms of nonallergic and allergic reactions to medication are sometimes very similar.

What are the symptoms of drug allergy?

Because drugs may affect several organs in the body, it is sometimes hard to decide whether a patient's symptoms result from the illness itself or from an allergic reaction to a drug. For example, a rash may appear during or after some streptococcal infections. Yet a rash may also be a symptom of an allergy to penicillin, an antibiotic used to treat the same streptococcal infections.

The symptoms that will appear in those who develop allergic reactions to drugs are impossible to predict ahead of time. A drug allergy may affect a single organ and a localized area of the body or it may affect many organs and many sites at the same time. Reactions on the skin are obvious and common. Reactions in other parts of the body may be difficult to detect; these are probably more frequent than people may think. The most common allergic responses of various parts of the body are reviewed here.

Skin Reactions An estimated 15 percent of all visits to dermatologists are concerned with adverse reactions to drugs. In fact, skin reactions are the most common symptoms of drug allergy and include hives, several other types of rashes, and itching. These symptoms may occur anywhere on the body and result from drugs taken by mouth or injection or from direct contact with a drug applied to the skin. Exfoliative dermatitis is an especially severe allergic reaction in which much of the skin of the body becomes red and peels off.

Contact dermatitis, which produces swelling, reddening, itching, or eruptions on the skin at the site of contact with a drug, often develops in nurses or druggists who handle drugs. Patients may also develop contact dermatitis from medications applied directly to the skin. Allergic reactions may be provoked by soap and antibiotic creams as well as by local anesthetics used to numb pain. Examples are procaine (Novocain), which dulls the pain of dental work, and many over-the-counter sprays containing benzocaine that are applied to the skin to numb the pain of sunburn, minor cuts, and insect bites.

Symptoms of contact dermatitis may appear within several hours or as long as 48 hours after the medicine is applied to the skin. If the person stops using the offending drug promptly, the reaction usually will end in a few days.

Another type of drug allergy that affects the skin is a "photosensitivity" reaction. Reddenings and eruptions appear on areas of the skin exposed to sunlight after a person has taken a sensitizing drug by mouth or injection or has applied it to the skin. For example, some people who venture out into the sun after taking griseofulvin (an antifungal agent), sulfa drugs and tetracyclines (antibiotics), chlordiazepoxide (a sedative), or thiazides (diuretics) may get a rash that looks like a sunburn.

Lung Reactions   The lung is involved in a number of allergic reactions to drugs. Certain drugs may cause a sudden onset of bronchial asthma; other drugs, such as para-aminosalicylic acid (used to treat TB), sulfa drugs, and penicillin may induce pneumonia. Still others, such as hydralazine (used to lower blood pressure), produce symptoms that mimic a disease known as lupus by causing inflammation of the membrane (pleura) that lines the lung. Usually damage to the lungs is not permanent, and after treatment is stopped the lung function becomes normal.

Reactions of Other Organs   Sometimes portions of the liver, kidneys, and blood vessels will become inflamed in response to long-term or high-dose treatment with drugs.

These allergic reactions (hepatitis, nephritis, and vasculitis) usually take weeks or months to develop. If the offending drug is discontinued when the symptoms first appear, the harmful effects may be reversed. Continued use of the drug may cause the symptoms to persist or get worse.

Certain drugs may cause an allergic reaction in which large numbers of red blood cells are destroyed; this condition is known as hemolytic anemia. Other drugs may attack blood platelets, which promote clot formation, and abnormal bleeding may result; still others may attack a type of white blood cells called granulocytes, which are active in fighting germs, and resistance to infection may be impaired.

General Systemic Reactions Such reactions as drug fever, serum sickness, angioedema, and anaphylactic shock affect many different tissues of the body. Drug fever generally will appear about a week after medication has been started. Such a fever will often subside within a day or two after the drug is withdrawn. Sometimes drug-induced fevers are not diagnosed because it is difficult to decide whether the fever is caused by the disease or by an allergic reaction to the drug being used.

Serum sickness occurs when animal serum must be injected into humans. However, conditions similar to serum sickness may also be noted after continual use of certain drugs such as penicillin, sulfa compounds, and phenytoin (an anticonvulsant). An allergic patient will develop a fever, rash, hives, swollen lymph glands, facial swelling, and painful joints. These symptoms depend on antibody formation and thus appear as early as 10 days after the first dose or two to three weeks after the last dose, but they will subside after the serum or drug and its antibodies have been cleared from the body.

Angioedema or giant hives is the sudden appearance of massive swollen areas of the skin, mucous membranes, and occasionally, internal organs. Angioedema in the throat causes the airway to become blocked and makes breathing difficult. Such cases may be life-threatening and need emergency medical treatment. The symptoms of swelling in areas other than the throat may be unpleasant but are not usually life-threatening.

Anaphylactic shock is less common than other allergic reactions to drugs. Often severe anaphylactic shock is preceded by the sudden onset of violent itching, especially on the soles of the feet and palms of the hands, and by reddening of the skin as if it were sunburned, particularly around the ears. Hives may occur, and the face may become distorted with swelling. The patient may suddenly have trouble breathing and may feel faint and anxious. The blood pressure becomes dangerously low. Convulsions, shock, and unconsciousness may occur, and occasionally the outcome may be fatal.

The typical anaphylactic reaction to drugs develops rapidly and becomes most severe within 5 to 30 minutes. The symptoms can usually be reversed if epinephrine (Adrenalin) is given quickly; however, emergency medical treatment is essential for a severe reaction.

Which drugs are the major culprits?

Antibiotics The numbers of antibiotics available today that may cause allergic reactions are too numerous to record here. This section deals with only a few.

Penicillin is probably the most common cause of drug allergy, with some type of allergic response occurring in one of every 50 persons who take this antibiotic. About 76 percent of these responses are skin reactions (hives, rashes, contact dermatitis) and about 22 percent are systemic (serum sickness, drug fever, vasculitis, angioedema, wheezing); only 2 percent of the reactions to penicillin involve anaphylactic shock.

Neomycin, an antibiotic that may be an ingredient of eye drops, often causes allergic contact conjunctivitis (pink eye). As an ingredient of ointments, neomycin may produce symptoms similar to allergic contact dermatitis.

Allergic responses to streptomycin may range from mild reactions of the skin to drug fever and even to anaphylactic shock.

Chloramphenicol, used in the treatment of Rocky Mountain spotted fever, typhoid fever, and certain types of meningitis, may affect the production of blood cells. An especially severe reaction to this antibiotic is aplastic anemia, a blood disorder in which the body's bone marrow fails to produce enough blood cells.

The new sulfonamides (sulfa drugs) now on the market produce fewer allergic reactions than did the sulfa compounds produced many years ago. However, the long-acting sulfa drugs may cause allergic responses such as hives, angioedema, skin rashes, fever, blood disorders, hepatitis, inflammation of the lungs and blood vessels, or a form of pneumonia. Included in this category of long-acting sulfas are those used as diuretics (drugs to counter fluid retention) as well as antibiotics.

Insulin Allergic reactions to insulin are common. The symptoms range from pain and swelling at the site of injection to hives all over the body and severe reactions such as shock.

Insulin is prepared from both pork and beef pancreas, and because it is an animal protein, it can cause allergic reactions. The main factors that appear to be related to insulin allergy are the type of insulin used when treatment is begun and the genetic makeup of the patient. Most patients with insulin allergy have only delayed local reactions at the injection site; these last just a short time, and the patients are able to continue treatment without further problems. (Whether these are truly allergic responses is questionable.)

Although most insulin reactions are due to the hormone itself or to the animal protein, other reactions are due to incidental components. For example, some of the allergic skin reactions to insulin are now thought to be caused by zinc, which is used in commercial preparations of insulin. Zinc-free insulin, which is now available, has not produced any allergic responses in zinc-sensitive people.

Other Drugs Some of the common drugs that may also cause allergic reactions include antituberculosis medications and other antibiotics not discussed above, anticonvulsants, barbiturates, local anesthetics, heavy metals, organ extracts, vaccines, tranquilizers and sleeping pills, laxatives, and drugs used to treat hyperthyroidism and heart disorders.

Which drugs provoke pseudoallergic responses?

Some reactions to drugs have all the symptoms of an allergic response. However, laboratory tests have failed to show evidence that the body's immune system is involved, so these reactions are termed "pseudoallergic." The most common symptoms are hives and/or angioedema, skin rashes, spasms of the airway passages, and shock.

Among the drugs known to induce pseudoallergic reactions are aspirin, tartrazine (yellow food dye No. 5), contrast dyes used in some X-ray studies, and ampicillin.

Aspirin About one million Americans have pseudoallergic reactions to aspirin. Although many otherwise nonallergic people (nearly 1 percent) react to aspirin, persons who have allergy-related problems are more susceptible to this condition. For example, a recent report by a task force of the National Institute of Allergy and Infectious Diseases (NIAID) revealed that those who suffer from chronic hives, asthma, and/or hay fever are more likely to have adverse reactions to aspirin than are those without these conditions.

Aspirin is an ingredient of many over-the-counter drugs, such as headache remedies, pain-killers, and cold medicines. It has also been found that people who have pseudoallergic reactions to aspirin may also have the same response to other drugs such as arthritis remedies (indomethacin, phenylbutazone).

Tartrazine (Yellow Food Dye No. 5) Between 15 and 25 percent of Americans with an intolerance to aspirin may also react adversely to this dye. However, pseudoallergic responses to tartrazine can occur in people who have no intolerance to aspirin. Tartrazine is common in many artificially colored foods, candies, and beverages; in the yellow coatings on some prescription pills (even some pills prescribed for asthma); and in liquid medicine colored yellow.

Contrast Dyes Sometimes dyes that contain organic iodine are injected into a patient's blood vessels during special kinds of X-ray tests. These dyes are used because they help to outline specific organs (e.g., kidneys, heart, blood vessels, gallbladder) in the X-ray picture. In about 3 percent of patients, injections of these dyes cause reactions such as hives, itching, rashes, angioedema, asthmatic attacks, or even shock.

Ampicillin This frequently prescribed antibiotic may cause a nonallergic skin rash that may be mistaken for allergic dermatitis. The rash occurs in about 9 percent of people treated with ampicillin and in as many as half of the patients with infectious mononucleosis who take the drug.

How is drug allergy diagnosed?

The diagnosis of drug allergy is usually made on the basis of the patient's medical history. Often the patient is the one who first notices the symptoms. Skin rashes, hives, swelling, fever, cough, and asthma may be signs of an allergic reaction to a drug and should be reported to the doctor, even if the reaction is slight. The doctor relies strongly on information that the patient supplies about the drug taken—when, how much, the length of time before symptoms appear, and what other medicine is being taken at the same time. Too often patients fail to report use of laxatives, nose drops, tonics, cold and cough remedies, antihistamines, vitamins, ointments, birth control pills and creams, douches, suppositories, aspirin and other pain killers, headache remedies, and antacids because they do not consider these compounds to be "drugs."

If the doctor suspects that an allergic reaction to a drug has occurred and if the symptoms generally begin to subside within 24 to 48 hours after the drug has been removed, it is likely that the drug has indeed caused the reaction. Occasionally, however, especially severe symptoms may continue or become worse for a week after a drug is stopped. A long-lasting drug may even cause allergic reactions for weeks or months after a patient has stopped taking it.

Depending on the patient's symptoms and the length of time before they subside, the doctor may again prescribe small amounts of the same medication to confirm the diagnosis. Such a rechallenge can be very dangerous, especially if the patient has had a previous life-threatening allergic reaction. The doctor's decision to reuse the drug must be based on the need to know whether the patient has a drug allergy, the severity of the allergic reaction, the seriousness of the disease, and the availability of acceptable drug substitutes.

Although skin tests are used to detect allergies to pollens, molds, dust, animal danders, and food substances, most attempts to diagnose sensitivity to a drug by using the drug itself for skin testing are usually unsuccessful. This is because the exact derivative or breakdown product of the drug that acts as the antigen is not known. The patch test, if applied carefully, may help to diagnose contact dermatitis caused by drugs or chemicals. However, useful diagnostic tests generally do not exist to tell whether a drug reaction was allergic, which drug caused it, or whether a patient will suffer an allergic response to a drug that the doctor wants to prescribe.

Thus the diagnosis of drug allergy at present relies heavily on circumstantial evidence—the medical history, present symptoms, and time lapse between use of the drug and appearance of the symptoms. Careful diagnosis is important because it may affect not only the person's current therapy but also medication in the future.

How is drug allergy treated?

Like other allergies, no simple cure exists for drug allergy. Sometimes it disappears by itself within a matter of months or years.

The first step in treating drug allergy is identification of the offending drug. The second step is its removal. Often this action is all that is needed. Mild symptoms will disappear without treatment in a few days or weeks after a patient stops taking the drug. Severe skin reactions require local or systemic treatment. Local treatment includes soothing baths, lotions, and steroid creams. (However, creams containing methyl-parabens should be used with caution, for such creams may themselves provoke contact dermatitis.) If secondary bacterial infections develop, antibiotics may be used unless a patient has shown an allergic reaction to a specific antibiotic. For severe systemic reactions, fluids or diuretics may help to eliminate the drug from the body and hasten recovery. Life-threatening anaphylactic reactions require the prompt use of epineph-rine (Adrenalin), assurance that the airway passages are open, and admin-istration of oxygen and intravenous fluids.

When reactions to a drug are similar to serum sickness, the symptoms usually disappear after the drug clears the body. Sometimes, however, antihistamines are given to control hives and aspirin is used to ease joint pain (if the patient is not sensitive to aspirin). Corticosteroids are used for severe symptoms of the skin and joints and for treatment of blood vessel inflammation and involvement of internal organs as a result of an allergic response.

Patients who are intolerant to insulin during the early stages of treatment of their diabetes usually are able to tolerate it with continued administra-tion. In some cases, however, the allergy persists. The administration of antihistamines or corticosteroids or a change in the animal source and/or purity of the insulin may give relief. When other methods are not successful, severe systemic reactions to insulin can be treated by desensitization. The patient at first receives small doses, which are in-creased gradually under the supervision of a doctor as tolerance is achieved.

If skin tests show that the patient is actually allergic to the zinc compo-nent of the insulin preparation, zinc-free insulin is recommended. Purified human insulins manufactured by new procedures are undergoing clinical trials and are expected to be of great value in the treatment of diabetes and insulin allergy.

When prompt preventive treatment for tetanus is required by patients who have not previously been immunized for tetanus, human hyperim-mune tetanus gamma globulin should be used rather than horse tetanus antitoxin. The best preventive treatment, however, is for the patient to maintain the active tetanus immunization with a booster injection once every 10 years.

Substances chemically related to an allergy-causing drug often produce similar adverse reactions. In aspirin-sensitive people, however, drugs that are *not* chemically related to aspirin (such as tartrazine) may provoke similar reactions. Such reactions are not predictable.

Substitute medications are usually available for persons with sensitivity to a particular drug. Aspirin can be replaced by acetaminophen. Tests can be conducted to find which antibiotic other than penicillin is effective against a bacterial infection.

Subacute bacterial endocarditis, an infection of the inner lining of the heart, is perhaps one of the few infections that calls for immediate treatment with penicillin, even if the patient is allergic to this antibiotic. Such patients are desensitized by being given small doses of penicillin at frequent intervals, with the amount increased gradually until the therapeutic dose is tolerated. Of course, the patient is hospitalized during this treatment and a doctor is constantly in attendance, with all emergency measures available. Unfortunately the desensitization, which allows penicillin to be tolerated, may last only for the duration of the immediate treatment, and the allergy may return after a period of time.

The best way to prevent recurrence of allergic reactions to a drug is to avoid use of the drug. The patient should be aware of hidden sources of the drug, such as ingredients of over-the-counter medications. Treatment with several drugs in combination should be avoided if possible. Patients with asthma and nasal polyps should be very careful in their use of aspirin. The allergic patient should learn both the generic name and the trade name of the offending drug and should inform other doctors who will provide care in the future. A special identification card should be carried, or a Medic Alert* tag or bracelet should be worn in case of an accident.

How can research help?

Although many of the body mechanisms involved in allergic reactions to drugs are now understood, many gaps in our knowledge of this field still exist. Further research should result in improved tests for diagnosing and even predicting allergies to specific drugs. Better methods need to be developed for preparing patients for treatment with the drugs to which they are allergic.

Throughout the United States, research supported by NIAID is helping

---

* Medic Alert tags and bracelets can be ordered from the Medic Alert Foundation, Box 1009, Turlock, California 95380.

scientists to study the various features of drug allergy in order to provide solutions to questions still unanswered.

Clinical testing of penicillin products is being coordinated currently at six university medical centers. The objective is to find out whether skin testing will predict immediate hypersensitivity reactions to penicillin. The patients are hospitalized adults who may or may not have a history of penicillin sensitivity but require treatment with penicillin. Penicillin itself and its breakdown products are used, and the tests are done very carefully.

Testing begins with the prick test. A small needle is used to puncture the skin on which the test substance has been placed. If the patient has no reaction to the prick test, the intradermal test is used to inject tiny amounts of the penicillin antigen under the skin. If the intradermal test produces no reaction, a final small test dose is injected under the skin before the penicillin is administered at full-strength levels.

When the skin test results are positive and no other drug can be substituted for penicillin, the patient must undergo desensitization with small, frequent doses increased gradually to the therapeutic level.

Clinicians at The Johns Hopkins University School of Medicine are also gathering evidence that supports the value of skin testing to predict tolerance to penicillin. They report that patients whose skin tests are negative have fewer reactions than patients not tested. They confirm previous observations that when penicillin is injected into muscle, the numbers of allergic reactions are greater than when it is taken by mouth.

At Massachusetts General Hospital, NIAID-supported scientists are studying allergy to penicillin and cephalosporins (structurally similar antibiotics) to determine if cross-reactivity occurs in allergic patients. They are also studying whether certain types of drug rashes indicate permanent hypersensitivity to these antibiotics.

Investigations on reactions to contrast dyes used for certain X-ray tests are being carried out at the University of Michigan through funding by NIAID. Blood tests of people who develop chronic hives, angioedema, and even anaphylaxis-like reactions to contrast dyes may reveal whether a tendency for this allergic-like response can be predicted and what the body mechanisms may be.

Scientists at the NIAID Asthma and Allergic Disease Centers at the Scripps Institute in La Jolla, California, and at Northwestern University in Chicago, Illinois, have also been studying reactions to contrast dyes for several years. Both groups report that it is very difficult to predict who will have a tendency to react to contrast dyes. Skin tests have been shown to be poor indicators of both sensitivity and insensitivity. However, investigators at Northwestern University report that, for a special group of high-risk patients who have a medical need for these

X-rays, the administration of antihistamines and prednisone before a scheduled X-ray significantly decreases the incidence and severity of the reactions.

The NIAID is presently funding a study of patients with insulin allergy at The Johns Hopkins University School of Medicine. Investigators there hope that observations on variations in the amounts of antibodies in patients who have been desensitized to insulin will shed light on the role of antibodies in acquiring tolerance to injections not only of insulin but also of other foreign proteins.

NIAID-supported researchers at the Scripps Institute have been successful in desensitizing aspirin-sensitive asthmatic patients by cautiously giving them small and then increasingly larger oral doses of this medication. Desensitization to aspirin may allow such patients to reduce or even discontinue their asthma medications such as corticosteroids.

What about the future?

The need to be able to predict, diagnose, and treat drug allergies is obvious. Studies such as those described, in combination with general research that is continually expanding in the basic science of immunology, will hasten and improve our ability to handle the problems of drug allergy.

Because the array of drugs available to the physician is growing annually, new potential allergens will be continually encountered. After the tools and techniques for predicting, diagnosing, and treating drug allergy are developed by scientists, new drug problems can be more readily met as they emerge.

Prepared by the Office of Research, Reporting and Public Response, National Institute of Allergy and Infectious Diseases, National Institutes of Health, Bethesda, Maryland 20205. U.S. Department of Health and Human Services, Public Health Service, National Institutes of Health; NIH Publication No. 82–703, January 1982.

Dust Allergy

House dust—a nuisance to the conscientious housekeeper—is also the source of misery for an unknown number of allergic persons who occasionally, or even continuously, are bothered by sneezing and a runny nose or by wheezing and shortness of breath.

What is an allergy?

The person with an allergy shares with an estimated 35 million Americans an unusual sensitivity to some substance, known as an allergen, that has little or no effect on most people. Sensitization to this substance may be inhaled, injected, rubbed on the skin, or taken by mouth. House dust, foods, pollens, animal dander, molds, medicines, cosmetics, and insect venoms are among the most common allergens. The symptoms they produce may be mild, such as a stuffy nose or itchy eyes, or more severe, such as obstruction of the airways. In some persons, allergic reactions can be serious, even life-threatening.

No one knows exactly why some persons have allergies while others do not, but evidence shows that heredity is an important factor in their development. When an allergy-prone individual is first exposed to a particular allergen, he or she produces a protein called IgE antibody, a specific kind of antibody responsible for allergies. (Other antibodies protect the body by helping to fight off and destroy foreign invaders, such as bacteria and viruses.) The IgE antibodies attach to the surfaces of two types of cells known as mast cells and basophils. Mast cells are found primarily in the respiratory and digestive tracts and the skin. Basophils are found in the blood.

When an allergic person again encounters the allergen, it binds to the IgE antibodies that are already sitting on the cell's surface. However, each antibody will react only with the specific allergen against which it was made. The combining of the allergen with its antibody is a signal to these cells to release irritating chemicals, known as mediators, that cause the various allergic symptoms, such as wheezing, sneezing, hives, and abdominal pain. One of these chemicals, histamine, causes blood vessels to expand and to leak fluids. This leads to swelling and, if leakage is not checked, to a drop in blood pressure and to shock. A sudden, severe allergic reaction is called "anaphylaxis."

What is house dust allergy?

An allergy to house dust usually produces sneezing, runny or stuffy nose, and watery, itching eyes. These symptoms, often called allergic rhinitis, are identical to those associated with seasonal allergy to pollen, or hay fever. However, because house dust is so widespread, an allergic reaction to this substance knows no season. In fact, an allergy to house dust is perhaps the most common cause of allergic rhinitis occurring the year round.

House dust can cause other forms of allergic disease, too. One of these is asthma—a noncontagious disease of the lungs characterized by a constriction of the bronchial airways. This constriction brings on the wheezing, coughing, and shortness of breath characteristic of an asthma attack.

What is house dust?

Rather than a single substance, house dust is a varied mixture of potentially allergenic materials. It may contain fibers from different types of fabrics; cotton linters, feathers, and other stuffing materials; bacteria; mold and fungus spores (especially in damp areas); food particles; human dander; bits of plants and insects; and other allergens peculiar to an individual home, such as hair and danders from pets.

Other important components of house dust may be disintegrated stuffing materials from pillows, mattresses, toys, and furniture, as well as disintegrated fibers from draperies, furniture coverings, blankets, and carpets. The breakdown of these materials, from use and aging, seems to enhance their ability to sensitize susceptible persons.

Geography may also play a part in the content of house dust and, thus, in the reactions to it. Samples of house dust taken in one locality may display many similarities while samples taken from different geographic areas may exhibit rather striking differences. Although the reason for these differences in make-up is not yet understood, it may be partly due to climatic conditions, heating systems, and factors such as the availability and use of certain types of furnishings.

What is the allergen?

Despite differences among samples of house dusts, scientists believe there might be a common factor in all of them. This active substance (or substances)—the actual portion of house dust that is responsible for initiating allergic reactions—is not certain. Investigators have shown that, in some instances, the allergenicity of house dust is related to mites—microscopic spider-like insects found in many house dust samples from various parts of the world.

Mites were identified in house dust as early as 1694. In recent years, investigators in the Netherlands, Japan, England, Germany, Switzerland, and the United States have found several species of mites, usually of the genus *Dermatophagoides,* in samples they studied. However, they have not been able to determine whether the hard, outer shell of the mite itself is allergenic or whether these creatures secrete or excrete an allergenic substance.

Both live and dead mites appear to contribute to allergic reactions, although dead mites may be more aggravating. Mites flourish during the summer, but symptoms of allergic patients are often worse in the colder months. This may be because after the summer the mites die and disintegrate into fragments, which can reach the respiratory tract more easily than intact mites.

Are diagnostic tests available?

When someone suspects that he or she has developed an allergy, the family physician or an allergist (a doctor specializing in allergies) should be consulted to determine the specific cause and recommend the best treatment. The physician will examine the patient and take a careful medical history, looking for clues to the cause of the patient's symptoms. If the problem is an allergy, the patient's history will probably indicate that he or she is sensitive to one or more of several possible allergens. If the physician suspects that house dust is the allergen, a commercially prepared stock extract of house dust can be used for a skin test.

One of three different types of skin tests may be done to verify the diagnosis. For both the prick (or puncture) test and the scratch test, the physician applies a drop of extract to the skin. A sharp needle is then used to prick or scratch the skin lightly. Or the physician may choose to do an intracutaneous skin test, in which a small amount of extract is injected into the superficial layers of the skin. In all types of skin tests, the results are usually evident within 15 to 20 minutes. A bump (wheal) surrounded by a reddened area (flare) on the portion of skin exposed to the allergen indicates a positive reaction.

Occasionally, and usually for research purposes, blood tests are used to diagnose dust allergy. One of these is called the RAST (radioallergosorbent test). It determines how much of a specific kind of IgE antibody is in the patient's blood. This is done by measuring how the blood reacts with a disc coated with a specific suspected allergen. Another test, less frequently used, is called the histamine-release test. It is based on the principle that certain blood cells of an allergic patient will release the chemical mediator, histamine, when these cells are mixed with an allergen that triggers the patient's response. Therefore, measuring the amount of histamine released will give some idea of how allergic the patient is. Neither blood test is as sensitive as skin testing in detecting allergies, but they may be useful in the rare patient who can not or should not be skin tested.

How is dust allergy treated?

Three types of treatment are available to relieve the symptoms of dust allergy. At present, no permanent cure is known. By far the most effective treatment for this, as well as for several other allergic conditions, is to avoid exposure to the allergen. Although complete avoidance of dust is not possible, a carefully maintained anti-dust program in the home can minimize exposure and often reduce the patient's symptoms. The anti-dust program should be given a fair trial, generally for four to six weeks.

The second aspect of treatment includes medications that are recommended or prescribed by the physician. These generally work in one of three ways: (1) to inhibit the response to histamine (antihistaminic drugs); (2) to block the release of chemical mediators by the mast cells; or (3) to counteract the effects of the mediators once they are released.

Antihistamines are the most common treatment for the symptoms of dust allergy. There are different types of antihistamines and wide variations in the ways patients react to them, which accounts in part for the large number of these preparations on the market. They do help stop nasal discharge in most patients and produce only minor side effects, usually drowsiness. Antihistamines are more effective when given prophylactically or at the first sign of symptoms, than they are after symptoms are fully developed.

Cromolyn sodium is a drug that blocks the release of chemical mediators. Asthma patients have used it for several years to prevent asthma attacks. Experimental studies with patients who have allergic rhinitis have shown that cromolyn used in a nasal spray reduces sneezing, nasal discharge, nasal congestion, and eye irritation.

Drugs that counteract the effects of the chemical mediators include those that mimic the sympathetic (adrenergic) nervous system (sympathomimetics or adrenergic agents), drugs that counteract the parasympathetic (cholinergic) nervous system (anticholinergic agents), and anti-inflammatory drugs.

Sympathomimetic agents are commonly used as decongestants, both systemically, sometimes combined with antihistamines, and topically in nose drops and nasal sprays. Prolonged topical use of these agents can cause a "rebound effect." In other words, symptoms are at first relieved, but then grow worse. Side effects of these drugs include rapid heart rate and increased blood pressure.

Anticholinergic agents were once popular medications for rhinitis, but they are seldom used today because of their side effects, such as dryness of the mouth and enlargement of the pupils of the eyes.

When traditional drugs fail or their side effects are intolerable, powerful anti-inflammatory agents called corticosteroids are very useful in some patients. Dexamethasone dipropionate was the first of these drugs to be marketed as a nasal spray, and two other corticosteroid aerosols have since become available—beclomethasone dipropionate and flunisolide. These drugs are safe and effective when used in the recommended dosages.

Oral or injected steroids can also be used on a short-term basis for severe symptoms. But all steroids should be used cautiously since they can suppress the adrenal gland activity as well as cause other systemic reactions.

One or more of these medications, accompanied by an anti-dust program, usually will control the patient's symptoms. If not, injection treatments (or allergy shots) may be used in addition.

Injection treatments can be effective for allergies to inhalants such as dust and pollen. This treatment program, which consists of injections of a diluted extract similar to the one used in skin testing, helps the body build resistance to the effects of the allergen. Initially the injections are given frequently until a maintenance level is reached and some relief is obtained. Then the schedule is changed so that fixed concentrations are administered with longer intervals between injections. When the allergic person is symptom-free for some time, the physician may modify the schedule or discontinue the therapy on a trial basis.

What is an anti-dust program?

Reducing the amount of dust in a home may require new cleaning techniques as well as some changes in furnishings to eliminate dust collectors. Water is often the secret to effective dust removal. Washable items should be washed often. Dusting with a damp cloth or oiled mop should be done frequently.

If the allergic person does the cleaning, he or she should wear a disposable surgical mask that covers the nose and mouth. It will reduce the amount of dust inhaled. Leaving the house for a while immediately after cleaning is also advisable to avoid stirred up dust.

Anti-dust measures can be carried out throughout the home. However, the most practical program is to make at least one room as dust free as possible. Since most adults spend at least one-third of their time in the bedroom, and children spend one-half, dust proofing should start there. In bedroom furnishings, avoid using ornate and upholstered furniture, carpeting, Venetian blinds, bookshelves filled with books or nicknacks, stuffed animals and wall hangings. Instead, simple metal or wood furniture should be used with washable cotton or synthetic shades, and cotton or fiberglass curtains. Scatter rugs may be used if washed weekly. Walls should be painted or covered with washable wallpaper. Closet doors should be kept closed.

Beds can be prime sources of dust. Bunk beds and canopy beds, in particular, should not be used. Mattresses, box springs, and pillows should be completely enclosed with allergen-proof coverings. Dacron or synthetic pillows are recommended rather than ones made of kapok or feathers. Blankets and bedspreads should be cotton or synthetic—not fuzzy wools or chenille.

To keep the room dust free, it should be wet dusted daily; the floor, damp mopped; and the baseboards, oil mopped. The complete bedroom, including walls, ceiling, closet, and backs of furniture, should be cleaned thoroughly once a week. Vacuum cleaners redistribute dust, so if one is used, it should be a tank type. The tank should be left outside the room during vacuuming or another hose can be attached to the air outlet and vented outside the room.

Dust seal compounds are available for application to furniture and fabrics, but the usefulness of these products is limited. They should not be relied upon as a principal means of dust control. Because such compounds sometimes damage fabrics, they should be used cautiously.

What about dust in the air?

The ideal air control system for an allergic person is one that centrally heats, humidifies, cools, and filters the air in the home. A central humidifier to add moisture to the air during the heating season will prevent nose and throat mucous membranes from becoming dry and irritated. Central air conditioning can filter out pollens, molds, and some dust from the entire home if windows and doors are kept closed.

Various types of air purifiers can be attached to the central air return to decrease still further the amount of dust in the air. An electrostatic precipitator, also called an electronic air cleaner, pulls in dust particles with a fan, gives them an electrical charge, then collects them on plates that have a reverse charge. The plates must be cleaned frequently to ensure efficient operation. The use of an activated charcoal filter effectively decreases the output of ozone, a potentially harmful by-product of the precipitator.

Another type of air cleaner is the High Efficiency Particulate Arresting (HEPA) filter. The HEPA unit works by mechanical filtration and is constructed in such a way that efficiency is actually initially increased as the unit is used. It removes 99 percent of particles larger than 6 microns from air flowing through it. Maintenance is minimal, and the HEPA unit does not produce ozone.

The dust circulated by a hot air heating system can be reduced in other ways if central air filtering is not feasible. Whenever possible, particularly in the bedroom, the hot air registers should be closed. Filters, which should be changed frequently, should be placed on the registers. The air ducts themselves should be cleaned periodically.

If the home does not have central climate control, an air conditioning unit may be beneficial in the allergic person's bedroom. It will reduce the amount of allergens in the air if the outside air vent is closed and the doors and windows are kept closed. It can be used for dust control even without cooling. Portable electrostatic precipitators and HEPA units are also available in varying sizes to suit the size of the bedroom. If they are used properly, with the doors and windows of the room closed, they can provide an oasis of clean air for the allergic patient. Often these units can be rented on a trial basis for a month or two to determine the extent of relief they give.

Beware of exaggerated claims for appliances that are being sold for air purification. Even ordinary vacuum cleaners have been promoted for preventing or treating respiratory ailments. Although some air cleaners are capable of removing dust and pollen from the air in varying degrees, no air purifier can truthfully be promoted for treating viral or bacterial diseases such as colds, influenza, pneumonia, or tuberculosis. Air treatment devices are also being promoted as "negative ion generators," but it has not been established that negative ions are of any value for preventing or treating respiratory disease.

Besides carrying out a dust avoidance program, individuals allergic to dust should try to avoid contact with such inhalants as insect sprays, fresh paint, tobacco smoke, and fresh tar. These substances have irritating effects on already inflamed membranes. High concentrations of air pollutants can also cause discomfort in persons with dust allergy.

How can research help?

A great deal remains to be learned about all allergies, including dust allergy. Scientists are studying the components that make dust allergenic in order to develop improved extracts for skin tests and injection treatments. They are also interested in perfecting a blood test or some other laboratory test to replace traditional skin testing. The RAST and the histamine-release test are useful as research tools in the search for more sensitive diagnostic tests.

Basic research is providing information about what happens in the body during an allergic reaction. Chemicals other than histamines are involved in producing allergic symptoms. More information about these and yet-to-be discovered chemical mediators, and their exact roles in the body, may lead to the production of better medications. Scientists are also trying to develop more effective steroids, nasal sprays, and better antihistamines with fewer undesirable side effects.

The National Institute of Allergy and Infectious Diseases (NIAID), part of the National Institutes of Health (NIH), supports a network of Asthma and Allergic Disease Research Centers throughout the United States. These Centers, located in biomedical institutions, encourage collaboration between basic research scientists and clinical investigators who treat allergic individuals primarily on an outpatient basis. Through this program, research results are spread quickly to scientists, community health care providers, and to those suffering with allergies.

What about the future?

The science of immunology—the study of how the body defends itself against foreign substances—has captured the interest of scientists throughout the world in recent years. Research results from this rapidly expanding field can be applied in many areas of medicine, but particularly allergic diseases.

For the present, sufferers of allergy to house dust can best alleviate their allergic symptoms by closely following the recommendations of their physicians. In the future, when new information in basic immunology can be applied to the patient, it will provide new means for preventing, as well as treating, the distressing symptoms of all allergies.

Prepared by the Office of Research, Reporting and Public Response, National Institute of Allergy and Infectious Diseases, National Institutes of Health, Bethesda, Maryland 20205. For sale by the Superintendent of Documents, U.S. Government Printing Office, Washington, D.C. 20402. U.S. Department of Health and Human Services, Public Health Service, National Institutes of Health. NIH Publication No. 83–490, revised November 1982.

Insect Allergy

As early as 2621 B.C., hieroglyphics on the walls of King Menes' tomb in Egypt recorded his death from a hornet or wasp sting. No one knows for sure how common insect sting allergy may be today, but it is estimated that at least 4 of every 1,000 people are affected. It is known that every year 50 to 100 people in this country die from reactions to stings. The number may be even higher because many summer deaths attributed to heart attacks or drownings, for example, may actually be due to an allergic reaction to an insect sting. In fact, more people are killed in this country each year by a group of insects classified as Hymenoptera— bees, wasps, hornets, yellow jackets, and fire ants—than by any other venomous creatures, even rattlesnakes.

What is an allergy?

Some people are sensitive and their bodies overreact to a substance that has little or no effect on most people. For sensitive persons, that substance is an allergen, and they are said to have an "allergy." Many substances can cause an allergic reaction. Foods, pollens, house dust, animal hairs, molds, medicines, cosmetics, and insects are the most common allergens. Symptoms may be mild, such as stuffiness in the nose or itching of the eyes, or they may be more severe, such as obstruction of the airways. In some people, the reactions can be serious, even life-threatening.

It is possible for allergens to be inhaled, injected, rubbed on the skin, or taken by mouth. In insect allergy, all of these routes are used, although the usual exposure is by a sting or bite, during which the allergen is injected into the victim by the offending insect.

An estimated 35 million Americans have allergies. No one knows exactly why some people have allergies while others do not, but evidence shows that heredity is an important factor in their development. When an allergy-prone individual is first exposed to a particular allergen, he or she produces a protein called IgE antibody, a specific kind of antibody responsible for allergies. (Other antibodies protect the body by helping to fight off and destroy foreign invaders, such as bacteria and viruses.) The IgE antibodies attach to the surfaces of two types of cells known as mast cells and basophils. Mast cells are found primarily in the respiratory and digestive tracts and the skin. Basophils are found in the blood.

When an allergic person again encounters the allergen, it binds to the IgE antibodies that are already sitting on the cell's surface. However, each antibody will react only with the specific allergen against which it was made. The combining of the allergen with its antibody is a signal to these cells to release irritating chemicals that cause the various allergic symptoms, such as wheezing, sneezing, hives, and abdominal pain. One of these chemicals, histamine, causes blood vessels to expand and to leak fluids. This leads to swelling and, if leakage is not checked, to a drop in blood pressure and to shock. Sudden, severe allergic reactions are called "anaphylaxis."

What is an insect allergy?

Insect allergy simply means that exposure to an insect brings about an overreaction of the immune system in a sensitive person. Most often, exposure involves a sting or bite. In most cases, insect allergy might be called more correctly insect *sting* allergy or insect venom allergy, since the allergic reaction is usually not caused by the whole insect but by the venom that it injects.

The Committee on Insect Allergy of the American Academy of Allergy has described some of the characteristics of people with insect allergy. First, allergy to insects is present as often in people who have no other allergies as in those who do. Second, severe reactions occur most often after the age of 30, although they have been found in people of all ages. Third, a person's previous reaction to an insect sting may be a warning of a future severe reaction. However, about one-half the victims of stings may have an entirely normal response on one occasion but suffer a serious allergic reaction to the next sting.

Insect sting reactions are most common during the summer months when insects are abundant and most active. Also, during those months people are out-of-doors and thus encounter insects more often.

Which insects cause allergy?

The salivary secretions of biting insects (such as mosquitoes, flies, lice, and fleas) or the irritating substances left on the skin by some crawling insects may lead to sensitivity, but it is the stinging insects that are generally the most dangerous.

The Hymenoptera or "membrane-winged" insects are the only insects that sting, and only a few of the stinging Hymenoptera—honey bees, wasps, hornets, yellow jackets, and ants—cause serious allergic reactions in man. Of these five, reactions to the yellow jacket and the bee are the most common.

In the Hymenoptera, the stinger, a modified egg depositor, works like a hypodermic needle. Found only in the female, the stinger has small venom-filled sacs located at its base. The venom is injected through a hollow tube in the center of the stinger.

Most stinging Hymenoptera can remove the stinger and use it again and again, but the stinger of the honey bee is barbed. When the honey bee tries to remove its stinger from human skin, both stinger and venom sacs are torn off and left in the victim as the injured bee flies away and dies.

Some Hymenoptera stingers may be contaminated with bacteria and occasionally cause infections in man. Curiously, infections occur less commonly with honey bee stings, even though the honey bee leaves its stinger in the victim's skin.

The venoms of different stinging Hymenoptera vary in their makeup, although some components are the same. Toxic components cause the irritating local reactions experienced by most people. In addition, the venoms contain chemicals, such as histamine, that are similar to those released by the body during an allergic reaction. The venom also contains certain proteins known as allergens, which are the agents responsible for allergic reactions. Honey bee venom has been studied the most, and four allergens have been identified thus far.

What is the behavior of stinging insects?

Bees feed their young (larvae) honey and pollen, so they sting only to protect themselves or their hives. Yellow jackets, wasps, and hornets, however, sting in order to kill smaller insects that are used as food for their young, and thus they tend to be more aggressive than bees.

There are two behavioral types of bees: solitary and social. The solitary bees—the carpenter, miner, mason, and cuckoo—do not form colonies, and their stings are usually quite mild.

Of the two kinds of social bees—the bumblebee and the honey bee—the bumblbee is less vicious and less organized, and it nests in the ground. Large colonies of honey bees may be either wild or domesticated. All members of a colony depend on one another. The queen lays the eggs, the males or drones fertilize the queen, and the workers gather food and care for the young. Honey bees not only produce honey but also fertilize crops.

Wasps may also be solitary or social. The most common wasp threats to man—hornets, yellow jackets, and the *Polistes* wasps (also known as "paper wasps")—fall in the social group and are very protective of their nests. Usually dark blue, yellow, or reddish brown, wasps can be identified by their narrow "waists" (the "wasp waist"). Although these three types of wasps prefer to feed on other insects, they are also attracted to nectars and overripe fruit. Some wasps nest underground, but others build their nests in the open, in trees (hornets) or under eaves (paper wasps).

Colonies of hardworking ants with their highly structured societies are found almost everywhere, but only two kinds are believed to cause allergic reactions in man. These are harvester, or agricultural, ants and fire ants. The aggressive harvester ant lives in warm, dry, sandy areas and builds mounds that are easily recognized and avoided. The fire ant, especially the imported fire ant, is becoming common in the southeastern United States. It also constructs large mounds, but these are harder to avoid since they are low and sometimes naturally camouflaged.

The ant's stinger is much like that of the bee, but it does not have barbs. Ants seem to sting because of what they see or hear and sometimes what they smell. The fire ant attaches itself to its victim by biting the skin before it stings, but probably only the sting—when venom is released—is significant for allergy sufferers.

Do other insects cause allergy?

Some biting insects cause allergic reactions, but fewer people seem to be bothered by these insects than by stinging insects, and reactions are generally less severe.

Mosquitoes, for example, bite humans to obtain blood for food. Usually, the allergic reaction to their bites consists of hives or an eczema-like rash with red, itchy lesions that become moist and then encrusted when scratched. This allergy is diagnosed by the location of the reaction, medical history, and the circumstances surrounding the bites. Avoiding exposure to mosquitoes is the best way to prevent these reactions.

Some flies, but not the house fly, bite and may cause allergic reactions. These include black flies, biting midges, deer flies, and stable flies. Bites from these cause pain, swelling, severe itching, and on rare occasions, anaphylactic shock. Local reactions can be treated by antihistamines given by mouth or by steroid creams applied to the area of skin affected. Systemic (throughout the body) reactions should be treated like those resulting from Hymenoptera stings.

Fleas usually cause only a local rash consisting of grouped, itchy, raised lesions. Antihistamines and applied medications will relieve itching due to flea bites. The best prevention is to treat the environment and household pets with appropriate insecticides.

Kissing bugs bite at night and cause a full range of reactions from local itching to extensive swelling and shock. Antihistamines, injections of epinephrine, or corticosteroids are the proper treatment, depending on the type and severity of the symptoms. Desensitization shots (immunotherapy) may be used in selected cases.

Some caterpillars (the wormlike larvae of moths and butterflies) are covered for their protection by tiny hairs that contain an irritating substance. If one of these larvae crawls on the skin of a sensitive person, the resulting symptoms may range from a local rash to a severe systemic reaction. These reactions may also occur if the hairs are swallowed or inhaled. The puss caterpillar is the worst offender. Diagnosis is relatively simple because the rash follows the gridlike track of the insect on the skin. If a sticky tape is applied to the skin as soon as possible, some of the hairs can be removed. Ice packs and antihistamines given by mouth are used to treat local reactions.

Some insects cause allergic reactions when they are inhaled or accidentally swallowed. For example, small insects like the mayfly and caddis fly are abundant near bodies of water in late spring and summer. There they can easily be inhaled. Also insect parts, such as scales, wings, bits of the hard outer body covering, and dried secretions, may be blown around by the wind. Such materials, along with the minute house-dust mite (an arachnid, not an insect) and the cockroach, can be components of house dust allergy.

These creatures cause symptoms resembling those of hay fever (allergic rhinitis) or asthma, and when no other cause can be found for seasonal respiratory allergy, insects might be suspected. Skin testing can give positive indication of this allergy.

Regardless of the precautions taken, insects are common wherever there is food, especially grains or cereals. The insect may come from the field where the food is grown, enter at any step in the food processing, or appear after the food is brought into the home. Such pests most commonly found are the cockroach, weevil, moth, beetle, mite, and silverfish. There is some reason to suspect that insects contaminating food may actually cause some cases of "food" allergy.

What are the symptoms?

Insect stings can cause a variety of reactions, depending on the type of insect, the amount of venom injected, the presence or absence of a specific type of allergy in the person attacked, and the site of the sting. In general, reactions fall into three main groups.

Normal reactions to stings involve pain, redness, swelling, itching, and warmth at the site of the sting. These symptoms, lasting for a few hours, may be quite severe, but as long as they are confined to the area of the sting, they are considered normal inflammatory responses and pose no danger. They are the result of direct action on body tissues by toxins or irritating chemicals in the venom.

Toxic reactions are the result of multiple stings. Five hundred stings within a short time are considered enough to kill because of the effects of extremely large amounts of venom injected into one person. Fewer stings, but usually at least 10, closely spaced over time, can cause serious illness and discomfort. Muscle cramps, headache, fever, and drowsiness are the most common symptoms of a toxic reaction.

Allergic reactions, the third type, produce some of the same symptoms as those of toxic reactions, but allergic reactions differ in that they can be triggered by only one sting or a minute amount of venom. Any reaction to a single sting involving extensive swelling of a large area beyond the site of the sting probably should be considered allergic until proved otherwise.

Allergic reactions to insect stings have been classified by the American Academy of Allergy as local or systemic, and both of these types may vary in severity. *Local allergic reactions* involve swelling at the site of the sting, accompanied by severe itching and sometimes a few hives near the sting. Any amount of swelling, even if it involves the entire limb, is considered local if it is continuous with the sting area and if no additional symptoms are apparent in other parts of the body. *Systemic allergic reactions* are those which affect any part of the body in addition to the portion that is stung. A *slight systemic reaction* involves the spread of hives to areas of the skin distant from the sting in addition to itching and a feeling of being "under par" and filled with anxiety. A victim with a *moderate systemic reaction* has the symptoms described above plus at least two of the following complaints: edema (swelling) of areas distant from the sting site, sneezing, chest constriction, abdominal pain, dizziness, and nausea. A *severe systemic reaction* may be recognized by the above symptoms plus two of the following: difficulty in swallowing, labored breathing, hoarseness and thickened speech, weakness, confusion, and feelings of impending disaster. The most serious reaction to a sting is closing of the airways or shock (anaphylaxis), in which the patient suffers not only from the above symptoms but also turns blue (cyanosis) or shows evidence of a drop in blood pressure, collapse, or unconsciousness. These reactions may develop within minutes or hours after a sting, and the patient may die if treatment is not given promptly.

The onset of allergic reactions can be immediate or delayed. In most cases, the shorter the time between the sting and the start of symptoms, the more severe the reaction will probably be. Most systemic allergic reactions begin 10 to 20 minutes after the sting.

A delayed reaction, occurring several hours to two weeks after a sting, is similar to a drug reaction known as serum sickness. In this situation painful joints, fever, hives or other skin rashes, and swollen lymph glands may develop. Both immediate and delayed reactions can occur in the same person following a sting, although immediate reactions are more common in the allergic person.

Most ant stings cause very little pain or itching. Stings of the imported fire ant, however, can produce severe local or systemic allergic reactions. In the local reaction, pain and a small raised area at the site of the sting are followed in a few hours by several fluid-filled blisters that eventually break or dry up. After the first day, the sting site itself becomes red and filled with pus. Days later, this spot crusts over and scar tissue forms. A systemic allergic reaction involves progressively larger local reactions, and future stings may even cause symptoms of anaphylactic shock.

Are diagnostic tests available?

Most people who have a local reaction to a single sting do not feel the need to consult a physician. However, when stings lead to more severe reactions, expert help should be sought.

A complete medical history and exact identification of the insect are the doctor's best tools for diagnosing a possible insect allergy. Careful questioning may reveal other less severe allergic reactions to previous stings. If the insect is not available, the doctor may be able to identify the culprit by asking about its appearance, its ability to fly or crawl, and the circumstances of the sting or bite (for example, the time of day and the place where the attack occurred).

The sting or bite may provide other clues to the insect's identity. Some insects leave mouthparts or a stinger at the site, and others produce characteristic symptoms or patterns of multiple bites. The location of the bite on the body may suggest a certain insect. Identification of the insect, whenever possible, is important for the doctor to be able to make a diagnosis and determine the required treatment.

Many allergies—such as those to pollen—can be diagnosed by a skin test. In this procedure a small, diluted, specially treated amount of the substance believed to be responsible for the allergy is applied to a scratch or prick on the skin (scratch or prick test) or injected into the top layer of skin (intracutaneous test). If a small area of redness and swelling develops at the site of the test within about 20 minutes, the person is suspected of being allergic to that substance.

For many years skin tests have been used to diagnose insect allergy. The arm is often used for insect allergy tests because a tourniquet can be applied to impede absorption if the person reacts too strongly to the test material. Also, in suspected severe insect allergy, the scratch or prick test is often tried first because it is less likely to cause an allergic reaction than the intracutaneous method. However, it is a less sensitive technique, and the results are not always clear-cut.

Recently, medical scientists working in the field of allergy have developed improved testing procedures based upon evidence that what most people are allergic to is the insect's venom, not its body, and that testing with venom alone will provide more accurate test results. These tests with venom can be performed by the skin test methods described above or by a blood test called the RAST (radioallergosorbent test). In this method, a blood sample from the person is exposed to specially prepared venom from the suspected insect. The RAST reveals whether the victim is producing IgE antibody in response to the venom.

Until recently, both the RAST and the use of venom were considered experimental procedures. Now venoms from honey bees, yellow jackets, hornets, and wasps are commercially available and can be used routinely for skin testing.

Because the skin will often not respond to test materials until perhaps two weeks after a sting, diagnostic studies should be delayed for at least that long. The skin needs time to replenish its supply of skin-sensitizing antibodies (IgE) used up during the allergic reaction.

People who have had an allergic reaction to insect parts that they have inhaled are presumably allergic to a component of the insect body. Such allergies can be diagnosed by the technique of skin testing with extract of the insect's whole body.

How are nonallergic reactions treated?

Following any insect sting, the stinger with the attached venom sac, if left behind, should be removed immediately by gently flicking it up and out with a fingernail or tweezers. The honey bee's venom sac continues to contract for some time after being torn from the insect, so prompt removal may prevent additional venom from being injected. Care must be taken not to squeeze or press on the venom sac when removing the stinger. The affected area should be washed thoroughly after the stinger has been taken out.

In a normal reaction, ice (*not* heat) applied to the spot may help to lessen the pain and swelling. Antihistamines taken by mouth and a calamine solution applied to the skin may help to control the itching, and aspirin or codeine (by prescription) may lessen pain.

A toxic reaction to an insect sting is treated in this same manner, but other medication may be needed to combat symptoms. Antibiotics to control secondary infections may also be necessary. A tetanus toxoid booster is advisable if one is due.

How are allergic reactions treated?

When a person is presumed to be allergic to an insect sting, three general approaches may be considered: 1) avoidance of the causative substance, 2) treatment and medication to lessen the symptoms of the allergic reaction, and 3) measures to reduce the person's sensitivity to the allergenic substance.

Avoidance Keeping away from the allergen, a major approach to treating any allergy, is vital in the prevention of allergic reactions to insect stings, and steps can be taken to reduce the chances of being stung.

Some people seem to attract insects more than others, but there are ways to make oneself less appealing and vulnerable. Close-fitting clothes will prevent the insect from getting between the material and the skin. Dark-colored clothing such as brown or black may provoke an attack; white or light khaki color is least attractive to bees. A flowered print may cause bees to come near to investigate but will not incite them to sting.

Scented soaps, perfumes, suntan lotions, and other cosmetics should be avoided, as should shiny buckles or jewelry. The amount of skin exposed out-of-doors should be minimized by wearing long-sleeved shirts, slacks, hats, socks, and shoes (not sandals). Some Hymenoptera nest in the ground, and others are attracted to low-growing plants; such insects may attack unprotected feet. Honey bees are often found close to the ground in grass and clover and are provoked to sting when trapped in sandals or loose clothing. Wasps are attracted to food and drink, and people are frequently stung at picnics and swimming pools. There are no effective repellents for the stinging Hymenoptera.

In the out-of-doors, any article that someone with an insect allergy may touch should be checked first for the presence of the insect. The feeding areas of Hymenoptera—flower beds, clover fields, garbage cans, and ripe fruit—must be avoided. As much as possible, car windows should be kept closed. An insecticide spray carried in the glove compartment can be helpful if an insect does get into the car. A piece of gauze or cheesecloth kept in the car can be used to catch the intruder.

In and around the house, screens or windows and doors should be checked for holes. Garbage cans should be kept clean, sprayed with an insecticide if necessary, and closed tightly. Nests under eaves, in trees, or in the ground should be removed by a professional exterminator. Pamphlets giving advice on this subject are available from the U.S. Department of Agriculture.

Weather can affect the temperament of Hymenoptera. For example, a rain may wash pollen from the flowers and thus anger bees. At such times an allergic person must take care to avoid attack. If that is impossible, he should move away slowly or lie on the ground, always protecting the face with the arms. Wild motion of the arms or frantic running will only anger and further provoke an insect to attack.

Preventing attack by ants involves taking special care to keep food stored properly, covering arms and legs, and locating and eliminating any nests indoors (between the floor and subfloor, under cracked basement floors, or in decaying wood). Entrances to the home as well as suspicious areas in the yard can be treated with appropriate chemicals—dimpylate, lindane, malathion, and propoxur.

Treatment and Medication Allergic sting reactions may require special attention. When stung, an allergic person should try to keep the amount of venom in the blood low by carefully removing any stinger as soon as possible and by placing a tourniquet above the sting site if it is on an arm or leg. The tourniquet should be loosened every 10 minutes so that circulation is not impaired. If possible, a cold pack should be applied.

A serious allergic reaction to a sting should be treated as an emergency. Epinephrine (adrenalin) is given by injection as soon as possible, and such an injection may have to be repeated if symptoms do not improve. Antihistamines given by injection or by mouth reduce later appearing symptoms but are not an effective emergency treatment.

Adrenal steroids (cortisones), which act more slowly than epinephrine or even antihistamines, may be given for persistent symptoms such as severe itching, swelling, and hives. Intravenous fluids, oxygen, and a tracheotomy (which provides an opening in the trachea, or windpipe, to maintain breathing) may also be necessary in acute shock or airway closure.

Antihistamines and steroids given by mouth are administered for several days for a delayed allergic reaction to a sting.

Prompt treatment is vital for any person with a history of allergic reactions to insect stings. Unfortunately, most stings occur at some distance from a doctor's office or a hospital—in parks, at the beach, on the golf course, or at the swimming pool. Therefore, anyone who has had an allergic reaction to a sting should take two steps:

First, he should wear a Medic Alert* identification bracelet or tag and/or carry information on a card in his wallet which states that he is allergic to specific insects and needs definitive treatment. Such knowledge can be lifesaving if the wearer should faint and is unable to explain what is wrong.

Second, he should always have emergency insect sting treatment at hand, such as epinephrine in a syringe ready for injection or a kit containing epinephrine in a syringe, antihistamine tablets, a tourniquet, and alcohol swabs for cleansing the injection site.

Such kits are available only with a doctor's prescription. When a doctor prescribes one, he will also instruct the allergic person on techniques for self-injection. The instructions in the kit are simple and easy to follow. The fluid in the syringe should be checked periodically, and if it has turned brown, the fluid is ineffective and should be replaced.

This kit should be carried at all times. The emergency treatment will provide the precious time needed to get the allergic person to a physician or a hospital for complete professional care. The kit is not intended to replace medical help.

A consensus development conference on the emergency treatment of insect sting allergy was held at the National Institutes of Health in September 1978. The experts in this field agreed that, to the maximum extent allowed by law, permission and encouragement should be given to all those who are properly trained to administer emergency treatment for stings at the site of the emergency. Such persons would include lifeguards, forest rangers, scout leaders, and school nurses.

Measures To Reduce Sensitivity Traditionally, allergy "shots"— injection treatments known as immunotherapy or desensitization—have been used to reduce or prevent future symptoms of allergy. In this proce-

---

* Medic Alert tags can be ordered from the Medic Alert Foundation, Box 1009, Turlock, California 95380. Identification tags may also be obtained by writing to EMI, c/o the American Medical Association, 535 North Dearborn Street, Chicago, Illinois 60610.

dure, injections of small diluted amounts of the allergen are given once or twice a week. As the person's tolerance builds up, the injections are given less often and contain increasing amounts of the allergen. Usually the shots are given by a doctor or by a nurse under the doctor's direction, and the patient remains in the office for 15 to 30 minutes to make sure that no side effect of treatment occurs.

This form of immunotherapy is believed to increase the body's supply of protective or blocking antibody, called immunoglobulin G (IgG). This is thought to combine with the allergen before it can attach to IgE, the allergy antibody on the cell's surface. Thus IgE is not stimulated to trigger the chain of events that result in the allergic reaction.

What is new in treatment?

In July 1978, investigators at the Johns Hopkins University School of Medicine, at the Good Samaritan Hospital in Baltimore, published results of the first controlled clinical trial in which whole body extracts (the only preparation then available to physicians) were compared with insect venoms for the treatment of patients with insect allergy. This study, supported by the National Institute of Allergy and Infectious Diseases (NIAID), clearly established that venoms were superior for this purpose.

As a result of this study and others, the Food and Drug Administration in March 1979 licensed five insect venoms for use in the treatment of patients who have previously had a potentially life-threatening reaction to an insect sting. These venoms are from the honey bee, the yellow jacket, the yellow hornet, the white-faced (or bald-faced) hornet, and the wasp. A preparation of mixed venoms was also licensed containing equal amounts of venom proteins from yellow jackets and yellow and white-faced hornets. These materials are now available to doctors for the treatment of patients with proven allergies to these venoms.

When a patient undergoes venom therapy, the protective IgG antibodies are built up by gradually increasing the amount and strength of the venom injection, so that over a period of time the patient progresses to full-strength venom in amounts equal to that of an insect sting. To some extent, the success of this therapy may be judged by measuring the protective IgG antibodies in the blood. Thus far at Johns Hopkins, hundreds of patients have been tested and found to have sufficient IgG antibodies after venom therapy, so that they have not shown a severe reaction to challenge stings performed in an intensive care unit.

Similar success with venom therapy has been noted at the University of Texas at Galveston, the State University of New York at Buffalo, and the Mayo Clinic and Foundation at Rochester, Minnesota.

After the strongest tolerated maintenance dose of venom is reached, this dose must be repeated regularly (for example, once a month). Such treatment does not cure the allergy but is simply protective. The allergic antibodies are still present in the body, and if treatment is stopped, the protection will wear off and leave the person in danger of an allergic reaction if he is stung again. If skin tests and blood tests show that the IgE antibodies have disappeared, then treatment may be safely stopped. Otherwise, it seems most prudent to continue the injections for an indefinite period of time. Future research may provide a better understanding of just how long therapy must be continued.

Insect allergy is unlike pollen allergy, for the pollen "season" returns annually and serves as a test of the effectiveness of therapy. Except under special circumstances, someone allergic to an insect will not want to run the risk of a severe reaction by allowing himself to be deliberately stung. Thus it is difficult to test the effectiveness of therapy except in the case of an accidental sting.

How can medical research help?

Nearly two million Americans each year have systemic allergic reactions to insect stings. The new methods of diagnosis and treatment with venoms have been proved to be highly effective, but the costs in dollars and time to treat such large numbers of patients could be staggering. The burden is especially great when booster shots have to be given for an indefinite length of time.

As a result, research workers are looking for improved ways to determine which patients should be advised to have therapy. NIAID is supporting research on these and other problems related to insect allergies.

What factors determine who will benefit from venom treatment? Scientists believe that a person who suffers large local reactions to stings should be tested for venom-specific IgE antibodies. Anyone whose skin tests show antibodies to venom should be observed closely after being restung. Preliminary data show that such persons may not need venom therapy, but they may be at risk for further large local reactions. On the other hand, some victims lose their sensitivity to insect stings over a period of time.

An ongoing study at the Johns Hopkins University School of Medicine involves children through age 16 who have a history of at least one mild systemic reaction, such as hives, to an insect sting. The children are placed into two groups, one of which receives venom therapy while the other does not. The IgE and IgG antibodies of both groups are tested regularly and skin tests are given. Results of this study should show whether children with a history of mild systemic reactions to stings will be helped more by venom injections than by use of emergency self-treatment kits alone. It is already evident that researchers will need long periods of observation to decide whether antibody testing and/or skin testing will help detect children who need venom treatment to prevent more severe reactions.

At the State University of New York (SUNY) at Buffalo and at Johns Hopkins, scientists are determining the best dosage schedules for venom treatment. They found that the patient gives a better IgG antibody response to the "rush regimen" and has fewer local and systemic side effects than when he is placed on the traditional treatment schedule. The rush regimen at Johns Hopkins involves a six-week course of injections with a higher dose of venom than is used in the traditional treatment. The interval between maintenance doses has been increased from four weeks to six weeks, yet 95 percent of the patients still receive full protection from further stings. Scientists at SUNY have had good success with a similar rush regimen.

At present, an eight-week interval between maintenance doses is being tested. These new injection schedules will not only save money but will be more convenient for both the patient and the doctor.

In another aspect of research into insect allergy, scientists at Johns Hopkins are studying the chemical makeup of venoms of different insects in order to find out which components in the venoms are similar. They already know that patients allergic to honey bee venom may not be allergic to the venom of wasps, hornets, and yellow jackets. They also know that a common sensitivity appears to exist for the venoms of the twelve known yellow jacket species. It seems likely, too, that a cross-reactivity exists between yellow hornet and white-faced hornet venoms and perhaps paper wasp (*Polistes*) venoms. When the *purified* allergens in venom become available, researchers will be able to detect such cross-reactivity. Until then, patients are being treated with each venom that causes a positive skin test.

Allergists suggest that at least 80 percent of people who have positive skin tests to yellow jackets, hornets, and paper wasps show cross-reactions and may really be allergic only to yellow jackets. This idea is being tested in clinical trials in which only yellow jacket venom is given. If such a premise is proved to be valid, it will decrease the amount of antigen the patient receives and will prevent him from being sensitized to allergens to which he did not react before. Laboratory tests are being developed to identify persons who need only one venom instead of several.

At Cornell University, NIAID-supported workers are trying to culture yellow jackets on a year-round basis in the laboratory by building artificial nesting sites and providing ideal living conditions and food sources. In this way, they hope to learn more about the stinging behavior of yellow jackets. In addition, these permanent colonies may be used as a constant source of pure venom.

At the present time, the entire venom gland is used for desensitization therapy. However, besides the venom proteins that cause the allergic reactions, the gland contains other proteins whose activity is unknown. If the proteins responsible only for these reactions could be synthesized, the costs of such therapy might be reduced.

Research on these diverse aspects of insect allergy is moving forward. Further answers will be provided by scientists as they continue to perfect the treatment, prevention, and management of this problem.

What about the future?

Altering our environment is usually not a practical solution to an allergic problem. Pollens, molds, and insects are all vital to the ecology of this planet. Thus allergies to these things must be controlled in the individual, rather than by attempts—probably futile, in any case—to eradicate a particular allergen.

In the past, insect allergy has been one of the less successfully treated allergies. However, NIAID-supported research has recently made venom therapy available to doctors. The increasingly active field of immunology is providing hope that people may be able to live free of their fear of insects and enjoy nature and the environment during all seasons.

Prepared by the National Institute of Allergy and Infectious Diseases, National Institutes of Health, Bethesda, Maryland 20205. U.S. Department of Health and Human Services, Public Health Service, National Institutes of Health, NIH Publication No. 82–1046, revised October 1981.

Pollen Allergy

Millions of Americans suffer from sneezing, coughing, itching, runny noses, and watering eyes when the pollen starts to fly. Each spring, summer, and fall tiny particles are released from trees, weeds, and grasses. These particles, known as pollen, hitch rides on currents of air. Although their mission is to fertilize parts of other plants, many never reach their targets. Instead, they make unscheduled detours into human noses and throats. At these sites, the pollen can trigger the allergic reaction that doctors call pollen allergy, or seasonal allergic rhinitis, and that many people know as hay fever or rose fever (depending on the season in which the symptoms occur).

Of all the things that can cause an allergy, pollen is one of the most pervasive. Many of the foods, drugs, or animals that cause allergies can be avoided to a great extent; even insects and household dust are not inescapable. However, short of staying indoors when the pollen count is high—and even that may not help—there is no easy way to evade windborne pollen. Yet there ARE some ways to ease the symptoms of hay fever—and scientists are working to find more and better approaches to allergy treatment.

The National Institute of Allergy and Infectious Diseases, a part of the National Institutes of Health, conducts and supports research on allergic diseases. The goals of this research are to provide a better understanding of the causes of allergy, to improve the methods for diagnosing and treating allergic reactions, and eventually to prevent them.

What is an allergy?

An allergy is a sensitivity to a normally harmless substance, one that does not bother most people. The allergen (the foreign substance that provokes a reaction) can be a food, dust particles, a drug, insect venom, or mold spores, as well as pollen. Allergic people often have a sensitivity to more than one substance.

Why Are Some People Allergic to These Substances While Others Are Not?

Scientists think that people inherit a tendency to be allergic, although not to any specific allergen. Children of allergic parents are much more likely to develop allergies than other children. Even if only one parent has allergies, a child has a one in four chance of being allergic. Another factor in the development of allergies seems to be exposure to allergens at certain times when the body's defenses are lowered or weakened, such as after a viral infection, during puberty, or during pregnancy. (However, some women find that during pregnancy their hay fever symptoms diminish.)

People with pollen allergies often develop sensitivities to other troublemakers that are present all year, such as dust and mold. Year-round allergens like these cause perennial allergic rhinitis, as distinguished from seasonal allergic rhinitis or hay fever.

What is an allergic reaction?

Normally, the immune system functions as the body's defense against invading agents (bacteria and viruses, for instance). In most allergic reactions, however, the immune system is responding to a false alarm. When allergic persons first come into contact with an allergen, their immune systems treat the allergen as an invader and mobilize to attack.

The immune system does this by generating large amounts of a type of antibody (a protein) called immunoglobulin E, or IgE. (Only small amounts of IgE are produced in nonallergic people.) Each IgE antibody is specific for one particular allergen. In the case of pollen allergy, the antibody is specific for each type of pollen: one antibody may be produced to react against oak pollen and another against ragweed pollen, for example.

These IgE molecules attach themselves to the body's mast cells, which are tissue cells, and to basophils, which are cells in the blood. When the enemy allergen next encounters the IgE, the allergen attaches to the antibody like a key fitting into a lock, signalling the cell to which the IgE is attached to release (and in some cases to produce) powerful inflammatory chemicals like histamines, prostaglandins, leukotrienes, and others. The effects of these chemicals on various parts of the body cause the symptoms of allergy.

What is pollen?

Plants produce the microscopic round or oval grains called pollen in order to reproduce. In some species, the plant uses the pollen from its own flowers to fertilize itself. Other types must be cross-pollinated; that is, in order for fertilization to take place and seeds to form, pollen must be transferred from the flower of one plant to that of another plant of the same species. Insects do this job for certain flowering plants, while other plants rely on wind transport.

The types of pollen that most commonly cause allergic reactions are produced by the plain-looking plants (trees, grasses, and weeds) that do not have showy flowers. These plants manufacture small, light, dry pollen granules that are custom-made for wind transport; for example, samples of ragweed pollen have been collected 400 miles out at sea and two miles high in the air. Because airborne pollen is carried for long distances, it does little good to rid an area of an offending plant— the pollen can drift in from many miles away.

In addition, most allergenic (allergy-producing) pollen comes from plants that produce it in huge quantities—a single ragweed plant can generate a million grains of pollen a day.

The chemical makeup of pollen is the basic factor that determines whether a particular type is likely to cause hay fever. For example, pine tree pollen is produced in large amounts by a common tree, which would make it a good candidate for causing allergy. However, the chemical composition of pine pollen appears to make it less allergenic than other types. Moreover, because pine pollen tends to fall straight down and is not widely scattered, it rarely reaches human noses.

Among North American plants, weeds are the most prolific producers

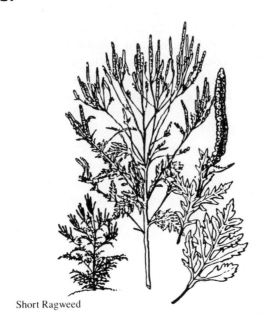

Short Ragweed

of allergenic pollen. Ragweed is the major culprit, but others of importance are sagebrush, redroot pigweed, lamb's quarters, Russian thistle (tumbleweed), and English plantain.

Grasses and trees, too, are important sources of allergenic pollens. Although there are more than 1,000 species of grass in North America, only a few produce highly allergenic pollen. These include timothy grass, Kentucky bluegrass, Johnson grass, Bermuda grass, redtop grass, orchard grass, and sweet vernal grass. Trees that produce allergenic pollen include oak, ash, elm, hickory, pecan, box elder, and mountain cedar.

It is common to hear people say that they are allergic to colorful or scented flowers like roses. In fact, only florists, gardeners, and others who have close contact with flowers are likely to become sensitized to pollen from these plants. Most people have little contact with the large, heavy, waxy pollen grains of many flowering plants because this type of pollen is not carried by wind but by insects such as butterflies and bees.

When do plants make pollen?

One of the most obvious features of pollen allergy is its seasonal nature—people experience its symptoms only when the pollen grains to which they are allergic are in the air. Each plant has a pollinating period that

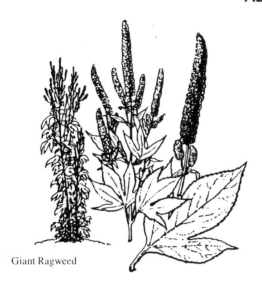

Giant Ragweed

is more or less the same from year to year. Exactly when a plant starts to pollinate seems to depend on the relative length of night and day—and therefore on geographical location—rather than on the weather. (On the other hand, weather conditions during pollination can affect the amount of pollen produced and distributed in a specific year.) Thus, the farther north you go, the later the pollinating period and the later the allergy season.

A pollen count—familiar to many people from local weather reports—is a measure of how much pollen is in the air. This count represents the concentration of all the pollen (or of one particular type, like ragweed) in the air in a certain area at a specific time. It is expressed in grains of pollen per square meter of air collected over 24 hours. A pollen count is an approximate and fluctuating measure, but it is useful as a general guide.

Pollen counts tend to be highest on warm, dry, breezy days and lowest during chilly, wet periods. Moreover, the pollen concentration in an area can be changed by population growth, land use, tree plantings and cutting, industrialization, and pollution.

What is pollen allergy?

The signs and symptoms of pollen allergy are familiar to many:
• Sneezing, the most common, may be accompanied by a runny or clogged nose

- Itching eyes, nose, and throat
- Allergic shiners (dark circles under the eyes caused by restricted blood flow near the sinuses)
- The "allergic salute" (in a child, persistent upward rubbing of the nose that causes a crease mark on the nose)
- Watering eyes
- Conjunctivitis (an inflammation of the membrane that lines the eyelids, causing red-rimmed eyes).

In people who are not allergic to pollen, the mucus in the nasal passages simply moves these foreign particles to the throat, where they are swallowed or coughed out. But something different happens to a pollen-sensitive person.

As soon as the allergy-causing pollen lands on the mucous membranes of the nose, a chain reaction occurs that leads the mast cells in these tissues to release histamine. This powerful chemical dilates the many small blood vessels in the nose. Fluids escape through these expanded vessel walls, which causes the nasal passages to swell and results in nasal congestion.

Histamine can also cause itching, irritation, and excess mucus production. Other chemicals, including prostaglandins and leukotrienes, also contribute to allergic symptoms.

Some people with pollen allergy develop asthma, a serious respiratory condition. While asthma may recur each year during pollen season, it can eventually become chronic. The symptoms of asthma include cough-

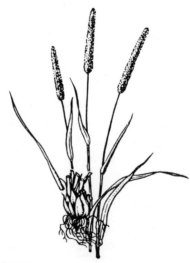

Timothy grass

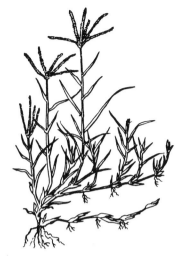

Bermuda grass

ing, wheezing, shortness of breath due to a narrowing of the bronchial passages, and excess mucus production. Asthma can be disabling and can sometimes be fatal. If wheezing and shortness of breath accompany the hay fever symptoms, it is a signal that the bronchial tubes also have become involved, indicating the need for medical attention.

How is pollen allergy diagnosed?

People with a pollen allergy may at first suspect they have a summer cold—but the "cold" lingers on. For any respiratory illness that lasts longer than a week or two, it is important to see a doctor.

When it appears that the symptoms are caused by an allergy, the patient should see a physician who understands the diagnosis and treatment of allergies. If the patient's medical history indicates that the symptoms recur at the same time each year, the physician will work under the hypothesis that a seasonal allergen like pollen is involved. The doctor will also examine the nasal mucous membranes, which in persons with allergic conditions often appear swollen and pale or bluish.

Skin Tests

To find out which types of pollen are responsible, skin testing may be recommended using pollens commonly found in the local area. A diluted extract of each kind of pollen is applied to a scratch or puncture made on the patient's arm or back or injected under the patient's skin.

With a positive reaction, a small, raised, reddened area with a surrounding flush (called a wheal and flare) will appear at the test site. The size of the wheal can provide the physician with an important diagnostic clue, but a positive reaction does not prove that a particular pollen is the cause of a patient's symptoms. Although such a reaction indicates that IgE antibody to a specific pollen is present in the skin, respiratory symptoms do not necessarily result.

Blood Tests

Skin testing is not advisable in some patients, such as those with certain skin conditions. Diagnostic tests can be done using a blood sample from the patient to detect levels of IgE antibody to a particular allergen. One such blood test is called the RAST (radioallergosorbent test). Although the RAST offers some advantages over skin testing, it is expensive to perform, takes several weeks to yield results, and is somewhat less sensitive. Skin testing remains the most sensitive and least costly diagnostic tool.

How is pollen allergy treated?

There are three general approaches to the treatment of pollen allergy: avoidance of the allergen, medication to relieve symptoms, and immunotherapy or injection treatments (commonly called allergy shots). Although no cure for pollen allergy has yet been found, one of these strategies or a combination of them can provide various degrees of relief from allergy symptoms.

Avoidance

Complete avoidance of allergenic pollen means moving to a place where the offending plant does not grow and where its pollen is not present in the air. But even this extreme solution may offer only temporary relief, since a person who is sensitive to one specific weed, tree, or grass pollen may often develop allergies to others after repeated exposure. Thus, persons allergic to ragweed may leave their ragweed-ridden communities and relocate to areas where ragweed does not grow, only to develop allergies to other weeds or even to grasses and trees in their new surroundings. Because relocating is not a reliable solution, allergy specialists strongly discourage this approach.

There are other ways to evade the offending pollen: remaining indoors in the morning, for example, when the outdoor pollen levels are highest. Sunny, windy days can be especially troublesome. If persons with pollen allergy must work outdoors, they can wear face masks designed to filter pollen out of the air reaching their nasal passages. As another approach, some people take their vacations at the height of the expected pollinating period and choose a location where such exposure would be minimal. The seashore, for example, may be an effective retreat for many with pollen allergies.

Air Conditioners and Filters   Use of air conditioners inside the home or in a car can be quite helpful in reducing pollen levels. Also effective are various types of air-filtering devices made with fiberglass or electrically charged plates. These can be added to the heating and cooling systems in the home. In addition, there are portable devices that can be used in individual rooms.

An allergy specialist can suggest which kind of filter is best for the home of a particular patient. Before buying a filtering device, it is wise to rent one and use it in a closed room (the bedroom, for instance) for a month or two to see whether allergy symptoms diminish. The air flow should be sufficient to exchange the air in the room five or six times per hour; therefore, the size and efficiency of the filtering device should be determined in part by the size of the room.

Devices That May Not Work   Persons with allergies should be wary of exaggerated claims for appliances that cannot really clean the air. Very small air cleaners cannot remove dust and pollen—and no air purifier can prevent viral or bacterial diseases such as influenza, pneumonia, or tuberculosis. Buyers of electrostatic precipitators should compare the machine's ozone output with Federal standards. Ozone can irritate the nose and airways of persons with allergies, especially asthmatics, and can increase the allergy symptoms. Other kinds of air filters such as HEPA (high efficiency particulate air) filters do not release ozone into the air.

Avoiding Irritants   During periods of high pollen levels, people with pollen allergy should try to avoid unnecessary exposure to irritants such as dust, insect sprays, tobacco smoke, air pollution, and fresh tar or paint. Any of these can aggravate the symptoms of pollen allergy.

Medication

For people with seasonal allergies who find they cannot avoid pollen, the symptoms can often be controlled with medications available by prescription or over the counter.

Effective medications that can be prescribed by a physician include antihistamines, corticosteroids, and cromolyn sodium—any of which can be used alone or in combination. There are also many effective antihistamines and decongestants that are available without a prescription.

Antihistamines   As the name indicates, an antihistamine counters the effects of histamine, which, as described before, is released by the mast cells in the body's tissues and contributes to the allergy symptoms.

For many years, antihistamines have proven useful in relieving sneezing and itching in the nose, throat, and eyes and in reducing nasal swelling and drainage.

But many people who take antihistamines experience some distressing side effects: drowsiness and loss of alertness and coordination. In children such reactions can be misinterpreted as behavior problems. Several new types of antihistamines that cause fewer of these side effects are now being developed and marketed.

Nasal Decongestants   Over-the-counter products containing decongestants can be helpful in relieving blocked nasal passages. These drugs constrict the blood vessels in nasal tissue, lessening swelling and mucus production. Nasal decongestants, although available as nasal sprays, may be taken orally; these include compounds such as ephedrine, phenylpropanolamine hydrochloride, and pseudoephedrine hydrochloride. Because these drugs can raise blood pressure, increase the heart rate, and cause nervousness in some people, persons with allergies should check with their doctors before using decongestants.

People with allergic rhinitis should avoid using decongestant nasal sprays because frequent or prolonged use can lead to a "rebound phenomenon," in which the initial effect of shrinking the nasal passages is followed by increased swelling and congestion. When this occurs, a person often will use the spray in higher doses, or more frequently, in an attempt to get relief from congestion. Instead of improving nasal congestion, however, such use of nasal sprays only intensifies the problem.

Corticosteroids   Until recently, corticosteroids, although very effective in controlling allergic disorders, were not widely used for pollen allergy because their prolonged use can result in serious side effects. Corticosteroids relieve the symptoms of pollen allergy by reducing nasal inflammation and inhibiting mucus production. Locally active steroids that penetrate the nasal membrane are now available as nasal sprays in measured-dose spray bottles. When used in this way, the drug affects only the nasal passages rather than the entire body. The side effects, which are minimal when the spray is used in recommended doses, can include nasal burning and dryness and a sore throat.

Cromolyn Sodium   Another effective agent that is available by prescription as a nasal solution is cromolyn sodium. Unlike antihistamines or steroids, cromolyn sodium is believed to control allergic symptoms by preventing the mast cells from releasing histamine. In clinical trials, cromolyn sodium has been proven safe and effective and, in contrast to some other allergy medications, appears to cause no drowsiness. Unlike antihistamines and decongestants, corticosteroid nasal sprays and cromolyn sodium nasal solutions must be used for several days to weeks before there is any noticeable reduction in symptoms.

Combination Therapy   Sometimes antihistamines, cromolyn sodium, or nasal corticosteroids are not effective when used alone. But, when prescribed in combination, these agents can often provide significant, if not total, relief from hay fever.

Immunotherapy

If environmental control methods and medication prove to be inadequate to control a person's symptoms, a physician may recommend immunotherapy (commonly called allergy shots). The aim of this treatment is to increase the patient's tolerance to the particular pollen to which he or she is allergic.

Diluted extracts of the pollen are injected under the patient's skin. The patient receives small doses once or twice a week, working up to larger doses that are given less often. The size of the largest dose depends on the patient's tolerance and the treatment's effect on the patient's allergy symptoms. Since it takes time to build up tolerance, prolonged treatment may be needed before the patient's symptoms are relieved.

Immunotherapy is not without problems. It can be expensive, and may require months before improvement is apparent. Further, it does not work well for some people and, if the size of the dose or frequency of shots is not carefully monitored, the injections can cause allergic reactions. These reactions can be quite mild—redness and swelling at the site of injection—or potentially serious systemic reactions such as hives, generalized swelling, or shock. Immunotherapy is therefore only one part of a physician's overall treatment plan for an allergic patient.

What if pollen allergy is not treated?

As anyone with allergies knows, allergic symptoms are annoying and, in severe cases, debilitating. As a rule, however, an allergy to pollen does not progress to serious pulmonary or other disease. Occasionally, when pollen allergy is not treated, complications may occur. These include swelling of the nasal passages and eustachian tubes leading to the ears, which may prevent proper drainage and airflow and lead to secondary infection of the sinuses or to middle ear problems.

How can medical research help?

Research on hay fever is proceeding on several fronts. Scientists are conducting research aimed at understanding what happens to the body in allergic disease. By knowing how this process works, they can devise ways to prevent sensitization to allergens or to prevent allergic symptoms. Meanwhile, clinical researchers are seeking better immunotherapy materials and methods as well as more effective drugs with fewer side effects.

To speed the process of applying the findings from laboratory research to the treatment of allergy patients, the National Institute of Allergy and Infectious Diseases (NIAID) supports a network of Asthma and Allergic Disease Centers throughout the United States. At the centers, laboratory scientists work closely with clinical allergy specialists to expand our knowledge of allergic disease.

Regulating IgE Antibody

A basic approach to the treatment of allergy is to prevent the immune system cells from making significant amounts of IgE antibody. NIAID-supported investigators are studying a number of naturally occurring factors that may control this process. By inhibiting the production of IgE, we could prevent allergic reactions and eliminate the need for drugs to control symptoms.

A possible new approach to regulating the production of IgE is by taking advantage of the complex feedback network of the immune system. Each molecule of IgE antibody contains a unique sequence of amino acids located on its surface near where the foreign substance or antigen attaches. This unique sequence is called an idiotype, and it enables the antibody to recognize a specific antigen. Because the body recognizes the idiotype as a foreign substance itself, another antibody is produced in response to the idiotype, which is called an anti-idiotype or antibody against an antibody. An anti-idiotype antibody can suppress the production of IgE by providing a turn-off signal to the cells that produce it. In experimental work in animals, anti-idiotype antibodies have been somewhat successful in controlling the IgE response to specific types of pollen. Such antibodies, while promising, need further development and testing.

Stimulating IgG Production

Scientists believe that immunotherapy works in part by stimulating the body to manufacture IgG, which is an antibody that blocks the effects of the allergen. By competing with IgE in combining with the allergen, these IgG antibodies apparently interfere with IgE's ability to react with pollen. A goal of immunotherapy research is to find more efficient ways to trigger the production of IgG while minimizing allergic reactions to the treatment.

Modifying Pollen Extracts

Among the most promising innovations is the development of modified pollen extracts that appear to reduce allergic reactions to the material used in immunotherapy. In addition, because the patient would be able to tolerate larger doses of the extracts, fewer injections would be needed to induce the needed high levels of the IgG blocking antibody.

One type of modified extract called allergoids has been developed by NIAID-supported investigators. Allergoids are produced from extracts subjected to a treatment process using formaldehyde. In clinical testing, allergoids appear to reduce the incidence of allergic reactions to immunotherapy while stimulating the production of protective IgG antibodies.

Other NIAID-supported scientists have developed purified allergens modified through a process called polymerization. With the use of this method, small molecules of purified material are joined into large clusters called polymers. Studies with these polymers have also been clinically promising.

As another approach to immunotherapy with pollen extracts, molecules of polyvinyl alcohol or polyethylene glycol are combined with the allergen. In attaching to the extracts, these molecules function as carriers that suppress the immune reactions. Such combined molecules are referred to as copolymers, and some are capable of activating cells (suppressor T cells) that, in turn, suppress the production of IgE. Other copolymers work directly on IgE-making cells to shut off IgE synthesis. In tests with ragweed pollen linked to polyethylene glycol, the patients' responses were very encouraging.

Still other methods of modifying pollen extracts are being developed and tested. As immunotherapy is improved, those who suffer from pollen allergy will benefit from safer, more effective treatment.

Local Nasal Immunotherapy

A different approach to the treatment of hay fever is the use of local nasal immunotherapy (LNIT). This procedure also utilizes pollen extract, but it avoids systemic side effects by acting only on nasal tissue. LNIT has been studied over the last several years by NIAID-supported researchers to determine whether it is safe and effective.

In the LNIT testing thus far, water-based extracts and allergoids have not proven to be effective in small doses. Higher doses used in testing have produced allergic symptoms and therefore are not effective. In current studies, investigators are using high doses of polymerized extracts, which appear to be effective and cause minimal side effects. Further testing is needed to determine the usefulness of this approach.

What about the future?

Because allergies result from a disorder of the immune system, scientists studying allergic diseases are benefiting from exciting new developments in immunology. The revolution taking place in molecular biology has led to significant advances in understanding how the immune system works, with applications to nearly every medical field. These advances offer the promise of better diagnosis and treatment of pollen allergy—and the hope that one day allergies will be preventable as well.

For more information:

The American Academy of Allergy and Immunology
611 East Wells Street
Milwaukee, WI 53202

The Asthma and Allergy Foundation of America
1717 Massachusetts Ave., N.W. (Suite 305)
Washington, DC 20036

Consumer Inquiries
Code HFN-10
Food and Drug Administration
5600 Fishers Lane
Rockville, MD 20857

Prepared by the National Institute of Allergy and Infectious Diseases, National Institutes of Health, Bethesda, Maryland 20892. U.S. Department of Health and Human Services, Public Health Service, National Institutes of Health, NIH Publication No. 87–493, revised August 1986.

Alzheimer's Disease

What is Alzheimer's disease?

Alzheimer's disease (pronounced altz'hi-merz) is a little-known but surprisingly common disorder that affects the cells of the brain. It is a disease that produces *intellectual impairment* in some 2.5 million American adults. While experts formerly believed that Alzheimer's disease occurred most often in persons under age 65, this disorder is now recognized as the most common cause of severe intellectual impairment in older individuals.

The changes most commonly associated with Alzheimer's disease occur in the *proteins* of the *nerve cells* in the cerebral cortex—the outer layer of the brain—leading to an accumulation of abnormal fibers. Under the ordinary microscope these changes appear as a tangle of *filaments*. These *neurofibrillary tangles* were first described in 1906 by *Alois Alzheimer,* a German neurologist.

New and highly sophisticated instruments and techniques—such as the *electron microscope* which can magnify cells more than a hundred thousand times—have revealed other changes in the brain that are characteristic of the disease. Scattered throughout the cortex, groups of *nerve endings* degenerate and disrupt the passage of *electrochemical signals* between the cells. These areas of degeneration have a special appearance under the microscope and are called *plaques*. The larger the number of plaques and tangles, the greater the disturbance in intellectual function and memory.

What are its symptoms?

At first, the individual experiences only minor and almost imperceptible symptoms that are often attributed to emotional upsets or other physical illnesses. Gradually, however, the person becomes more forgetful, particularly about recent events. The individual may neglect to turn off the oven, may misplace things, may recheck to see if a task was done, may take longer to complete a chore that was previously routine, or may repeat already answered questions. As the disease progresses, memory loss increases and other changes, such as confusion, irritability, restlessness, and agitation, are likely to appear in personality, mood, and behavior. Judgment, concentration, orientation, and speech may also be affected. In the most severe cases, the disease may eventually render its victims totally incapable of caring for themselves.

There are many different patterns in the type, severity, and sequence of changes in *mental* and *neurological functioning* that result from Alzheimer's disease. The symptoms are progressive, but there is great variation in the rate of change from person to person. In a few cases, there may be a rapid decline, but more commonly, there may be many months with little change. Limitations in physical activity during the later stages may cause the person to have less resistance to pneumonia and other physical illnesses that may shorten remaining life expectancy by as much as one-half.

Although the person with Alzheimer's disease may deny or be unaware of the full extent of his or her limitations—especially later in the course of the illness—the inexplicable changes in essential functions are a source of deep frustration for those afflicted and for their loved ones.

How is the diagnosis made?

Before a diagnosis of Alzheimer's disease is made, other illnesses which may cause memory loss must be excluded. The condition must be differentiated from the mild and occasional forgetfulness that sometimes occurs during normal aging. Depression, which is fairly common in elderly individuals facing a variety of stressful situations, may also affect memory.

Approximately one-half of elderly men and women with severe intellectual impairment are victims of Alzheimer's disease. About another fourth of the overall group suffer from *vascular disorders,* especially multiple strokes, and the balance have a variety of other conditions; for example, brain tumors, abnormal thyroid function, infections, *pernicious anemia,* adverse drug reactions, and abnormalities in the spinal fluid system (*hydrocephalus*). The specific diagnosis is very important as some causes of mental decline, other than Alzheimer's disease, can be readily treated.

Each person suspected of having Alzheimer's disease should have thorough physical, neurological, and psychiatric evaluations. *Computerized tomography (CT scan), electroencephalography,* and occasionally special studies of the spinal fluid system are often required for accurate diagnosis. Comprehensive blood studies, including tests for detecting several *metabolic disorders,* must also be carried out as part of the evaluation.

After other diseases have been ruled out, a firm diagnosis of Alzheimer's disease can usually be made on the basis of medical history, mental status, and the course of the illness. The electroencephalogram may show a general slowing of the brain waves and may help confirm the presence of Alzheimer's disease. Periodic neurological examinations and psychological testing are useful in evaluating the progress of the disease.

What causes Alzheimer's disease?

Alzheimer's disease is a neurological illness. But why plaques and neurofibrillary tangles develop in the cortex of the brain has not been determined.

It seems clear that Alzheimer's disease is not caused by hardening of the arteries. There is no evidence that it is contagious. Although emotional upsets and stress may temporarily affect the person's mood and behavior, they do not cause the disease.

Alzheimer's disease occurs in 2 to 3 percent of the general population. The additional increase in its occurrence within the same family, up to 4 to 8 percent, may represent a slight hereditary disposition or an undetermined environmental factor.

Several scientists are applying the newest knowledge and research techniques in *histology, virology, immunology, toxicology,* and *biochemistry* to the study of human brain tissue removed at autopsy. Although there are now a number of promising clues, the determination of the actual cause of Alzheimer's disease requires further scientific investigation.

What is the treatment for Alzheimer's disease?

As yet, physicians do not know how to prevent or how to cure Alzheimer's disease. However, proper medical care can reduce many of its symptoms and sound guidance can assist the person and family in coping with its significant impact on their lives.

It is imperative that the person be under the care of a physician. The physician may be a neurologist, a psychiatrist, or a family physician or internist who can consult with a neurologist. Most important, the physician selected must be willing to devote the time and interest required to closely monitor treatment, and to answer the many questions that are bound to arise during the variable course of the illness in any one individual. A physician will also be needed to treat any other physical ailments that may further complicate the course of the disease.

Drugs are not the only answer, but judicious use of tranquilizers can lessen agitation, anxiety, and unpredictable behavior. Appropriate medication can also improve sleeping patterns and can be used to treat the depression which often accompanies the illness. Proper nourishment and fluid intake are very important, particularly in the aged, but special diets or supplements are usually not necessary. Carefully guided exercise is of value, and physical therapy can help if difficulties arise in physical functioning.

Activities should be maintained at as close to a normal level as possible. A person should try to continue his or her daily routine, physical activities, and social contacts, and should be encouraged and assisted, if need be, to do a little more than he or she feels can be done. It may be helpful to provide memory aids that assist the individual in day-to-day living: a prominent calendar; lists of daily tasks; written reminders about routine safety measures; and directions to, and labeling of, frequently used items.

Although, in general, it is best to maintain an ordered environment so that a person does not have to continuously learn new things, it is important not to restrict a person from trying something new. For example, an individual with Alzheimer's disease may do very well on a trip when accompanied by a supportive family member or friend.

During the early phases of Alzheimer's disease, the person can most often be cared for by the family at home. When the condition becomes more severe, however, a special setting with professional staff and full-time care may be required. If needed, such an arrangement can be in the best interests of both the individual and the family.

Understandably, the person afflicted with Alzheimer's disease finds it difficult to comprehend the changes taking place in thinking and behavior. Family and friends will want to know how they can help. There will be questions about the activities the person can engage in with safety, how much encouragement should be given to carry out a familiar activity that has become painfully frustrating, and how to explain the memory loss to neighbors. Such questions can only be answered individually, depending on the person and the particular phase of his or her illness. The physician or an associate—a psychologist, nurse or social worker—can be helpful in meeting this need. Family members may also benefit by sharing their experiences with other families who are facing the same problems through one of several supportive groups which are just now being established across the country.

What is being done to learn more about Alzheimer's disease?

Physicians' attitudes towards an illness are shaped by whether or not they believe the illness is widespread, and whether its course can be arrested or reversed. Until recently, Alzheimer's disease was believed to be a rare occurrence, but new studies have demonstrated a higher prevalence of the disease. Theories are now being formed about its cause—theories that may ultimately contribute to the knowledge needed to halt or even reverse the illness. For example, scientists have recently identified a striking reduction—as much as 90 percent—in a particular *brain enzyme* (*choline acetyltransferase*) that is involved in the passage of nerve signals. If a deficient chemical process, rather than the destruction of cells themselves, proves to be involved, then health professionals may ultimately employ restoratives to lessen the symptoms of Alzheimer's disease in much the same way as *Parkinson's disease* is treated with *L-dopa*.

Alzheimer's disease is a very specific and major disease whose cause must be determined before it can be treated and prevented. Recent dramatic advances in medical instrumentation and technology have generated further interest in the diagnosis, treatment, and prevention of Alzheimer's disease. To stimulate new research on Alzheimer's disease, the National Institute on Aging, the National Institute of Neurological and Communicative Disorders and Stroke, and the National Institute of Mental Health have co-sponsored a series of workshop-conferences. In response to this expanding interest, studies are now underway or in the planning stages on a large variety of possible risk factors and on biological abnormalities in the brains of those with Alzheimer's disease. There is still much misinformation and lack of understanding about Alzheimer's disease, however. You can help by learning more about it and sharing the knowledge with others.

GLOSSARY

Alzheimer, Alois (1864–1915) a German physician who studied the relationship of changes in the structure of the nervous system to disease, and who first described the changes in the disease that carries his name.

Biochemistry the science that deals with the chemistry of living things.

Brain Enzyme a protein that accelerates a specific chemical reaction in the brain.

Choline Acetyltransferase an enzyme that stimulates the production of acetylcholine, a chemical compound active in the transmission of nerve impulses.

Computerized Tomography (CT or CAT scan) a new diagnostic technique using a computer and X-rays to obtain a highly detailed image of the section of the body being studied.

Electrochemical Signal the transmission of a nerve impulse by electrical and chemical changes.

Electroencephalography (EEG) the recording of the electric activities of the brain by means of wires placed painlessly on the scalp; useful in detecting tumors, epilepsy, and brain damage.

Electron Microscope one in which an electron beam, instead of light, produces a greatly magnified image.

Filament a delicate fiber or thread of protein found in the brain cells.

Histology the branch of anatomy that deals with the minute structure of cells, tissues, and organs in relation to their function.

Hydrocephalus a condition characterized by the excessive accumulation of fluid in the cavities of the brain, causing a thinning of the brain; may be present at birth or occur later in life.

Immunology a science that deals with the processes through which individuals are able to resist, or become sensitive to, a particular disease.

Intellectual Impairment a diminished capacity to think or understand.

L-Dopa a chemical similar to one which naturally occurs in the brain and is used as a medicine in the treatment of Parkinson's disease.

Mental Functioning the normal actions of the mind.

Metabolic Disorder a disturbance in the physical and chemical processes by which chemical compounds in the body are produced, maintained, and transformed into energy.

Nerve Cell a neuron, the basic unit of the nervous system consisting of a cell body and its threadlike extensions for receiving and transmitting impulses.

Nerve Ending   the fine branchlike terminations of the extensions that carry impulses away from or toward the body of a nerve cell.

Neurofibrillary Tangle   an accumulation of abnormal fibers in the nerve cells in the cerebral cortex.

Neurological Functioning   the normal activities of the nervous system.

Parkinson's Disease   a neurological disorder characterized by rhythmical muscular tremors, rigidity of movement, stooped posture, short accelerating steps in walking, and masklike expression.

Pernicious Anemia   a blood disorder characterized by a deficiency in red cells thought to result from the failure of the stomach lining to secrete an adequate amount of the factor needed to absorb vitamin B-12; occurs most commonly in later life and may affect the nervous system.

Plaques   a localized abnormal area found in the brain of a person with Alzheimer's disease.

Protein   a chemical compound consisting of a long chain of amino acids that contain a special grouping of nitrogen and hydrogen; produced by living cells or obtained as essential components of the diet.

Toxicology   a science that deals with the action, detection, and treatment of poisonous substances.

Vascular Disorder   abnormal functioning resulting from changes in the blood vessels.

Virology   a science that deals with viruses and viral diseases.

Prepared by the Alzheimer's Disease Center, Albert Einstein College of Medicine, 1300 Morris Park Avenue, Bronx, New York 10461, and National Institute on Aging, National Institutes of Health, Bethesda, Maryland 20205. U.S. Department of Health and Human Services, Public Health Service, National Institutes of Health, NIH Publication No. 85–1646, reprinted May 1985.

Amenorrhea

No Menstruation, Pregnancy = Amenorrhea

She knew she couldn't be pregnant. But she had missed three menstrual periods and, even though she felt healthy, she was beginning to wonder if something was wrong. Then she read an article in a magazine that said amenorrhea (failure to menstruate) was common among female runners. Since she had just taken up jogging six months earlier, she decided this must be the cause of her sudden irregularity. A month later she got her period and thought no more of it.

This jogger may or may not have had the right solution. Menstruation is a finely tuned physiological process, subject to many influences, internal and external. It is not uncommon for a woman occasionally to miss a menstrual period.

It's more unusual and of more concern for a woman to stop menstruating for three months or more, or never to begin at all. This condition is called amenorrhea (a = without; men is from the Greek for month; and rhea = flow, or discharge). A girl who doesn't start menstruating in her teens (usually by 16 to 18, according to most tests) is said to have primary amenorrhea. When menstruation stops after it has begun, the condition is called secondary amenorrhea.

The menstrual cycle involves a number of the body's organs and hormones in a process that stretches the length of the body. The cue to menstruate might be said to start in the brain in an area called the hypothalamus, which at the appropriate time each month releases a hormone called GnRH (which stands for gonadotropin releasing hormone). This causes the pituitary gland, a pea-sized organ attached to the hypothalamus, to release the so-called gonadotropic hormones, LH (luteinizing hormone) and FSH (follicle stimulating hormone).

LH and FSH then stimulate one (or sometimes both) of the ovaries to mature and—in the process called ovulation—produce ova, or eggs, ready to be fertilized. LH and FSH also cause the ovaries to secrete the hormones estrogen and progesterone. The quantity and order in which these hormones are released control the development of the endometrium (the lining of the uterus), which thickens each month to provide a ''home'' for a fertilized ovum. If the ovum is not fertilized during its journey to the uterus, this build-up of endometrial material is sloughed off and flows out of the body through the cervix and vagina in the process called menstruation.

A dysfunction at any point can cause menstrual problems, including amenorrhea. For example, a girl who has no vagina will not menstruate. Although this may seem unlikely, it is a relatively common cause of primary amenorrhea. Approximately 12 percent of patients with primary amenorrhea will have this condition, in which the vagina is either absent or in a state of arrested growth.

The most common causes of primary amenorrhea are in-born defects of the uterus, ovaries or vagina that are caused by chromosomal abnormalities. One of these is testicular feminization syndrome (also called pseudohermaphroditism), in which a child who appears to be a girl actually is a boy—that is, the chromosomes are XY instead of XX. Such children have normal female genitals but only a partially developed vagina and no uterus. They also have underdeveloped testes that may go unnoticed until a close examination is made.

Another condition traced to chromosomal abnormality is Turner's syndrome, caused by complete or partial absence in the female of one of the two X chromosomes. Girls with this condition have underdeveloped ovaries incapable of developing ova—or of secreting the hormones necessary to maintain the menstrual cycle.

Although primary amenorrhea is most often caused by genetic abnormalities and the resulting defects in the sexual organs, secondary amenorrhea usually has its roots in what is known as the hypothalamic-pituitary-ovarian axis (HPO axis). The HPO axis is the brain-to-ovaries communication, carried out by the various hormones (LH, FSH, estrogen and progesterone). If something disrupts communications, a result can be failure to menstruate.

Many women who complain to their doctors of secondary amenorrhea have polycystic ovary syndrome, in which one or both ovaries enlarge and thicken. It is a consequence of persistent anovulation (failure to ovulate), which eventually manifests itself as amenorrhea. Since there are many causes of anovulation—most rooted in the hypothalamus and pituitary—there are also many types of polycystic ovaries. Other symptoms of polycystic ovary syndrome are obesity, infertility and hirsutism (abnormal growth of hair), particularly on the face.

Anovulation can be caused by tumors of the pituitary gland, called adenomas, which are responsible for about a third of all secondary amenorrhea cases. The most common is the prolactin-secreting tumor.

Prolactin, secreted by the pituitary gland, stimulates the secretion of breast milk. This hormone is released in response to suckling (as nerve signals from the breasts travel to the hypothalamus, which in turn sends its signal to the pituitary gland). Excessive prolactin can cause both amenorrhea and anovulation. That's why some 50 percent of nursing mothers do not menstruate. A prolactin-secreting pituitary tumor can cause the inappropriate release of excessive prolactin, a condition called hyperprolactinemia.

Ordinary menstrual irregularities are frequently caused by physical and mental stresses that throw the hypothalamus slightly out of adjustment, but sometimes these same stresses can also lead to amenorrhea. Located in the center of the brain, the hypothalamus might be considered as an information processing center, both receiving and sending signals vital to the body. As part of the nervous system, it is sensitive to stimuli collected through the five senses. It also stimulates release from the pituitary of hormones that control many of the body's functions (including eating, sleeping, and sexual activities).

Travel, change in climate or sleep habits, and mental distress all can affect menstrual regularity. If the stresses are great enough, the clinical condition of amenorrhea can be the result. Dr. Hilde Bruch, professor of psychiatry at Baylor College of Medicine in Houston, says in her book *Eating Disorders,* that "amenorrhea is commonly observed in women under severe stress and strain. . . . Under wartime conditions, in concentration and internment camps, incidence of amenorrhea was high. . . ." Likewise, women with mental problems such as those in mental institutions can lose their menstrual cycles.

Hypothalamic amenorrhea also can be caused by acute loss of weight, as may occur in crash dieting. Dr. Rose E. Frisch, of the Harvard Center for Population Studies, Cambridge, Mass., holds that regular menstrual periods depend on the maintenance of minimum weight to height. She says amenorrhea results from a loss of about 10 to 15 percent of body weight (about one-third of body fat).

There is some evidence that loss of body fat leads to dysfunction of the hypothalamus and subsequent reduction in FSH and LH, which in turn causes failure to ovulate. Frisch claims this is an adaptive mechanism that prevents a woman from having a baby if she hasn't enough calories to nurture the fetus; not all authorities agree with this theory.

Amenorrhea is a common symptom of anorexia nervosa, a psychiatric disease characterized by aversion to eating and extreme weight loss. Patients with this condition—usually adolescents and women in their early twenties—suffer from unrealistic concerns about gaining weight and about how they look. Even when emaciated to a point requiring hospitalization, victims frequently insist that they are "too fat."

Most medical experts say that the weight loss in anorexics causes the amenorrhea. Some claim, however, that the amenorrhea in such patients precedes the weight loss. They believe an abnormality in the hypothalamus causes both the disease and the loss of menstrual periods.

Another cause of hypothalamic amenorrhea consistent with weight loss is strenuous physical activity. Dr. Phil Price, gynecologist with FDA's Center for Drugs and Biologics, says amenorrhea is occurring more frequently now in women who run long distances, as in marathons. He notes, however, that it doesn't seem to become a problem until a woman begins running about 20 miles a week or more, and even then it won't necessarily occur.

The author of one gynecology text, Dr. Leon Speroff, says that young women who weigh less than 115 pounds and lose more than 10 pounds while exercising are most likely to develop amenorrhea. One reason, Speroff says, is the loss of body fat, female athletic competitors having about 50 percent less body fat than noncompetitors. Another reason is stress and expenditure of energy, which seem to contribute to hypothalamic dysfunction. For instance, in one study researchers found that dancers who are amenorrheic during their professional season will often resume menstruating during intervals of rest.

Speroff adds, "The magnitude of the problem of exercise and amenorrhea has changed considerably in the last decade. In the early 1970s, a woman jogger was a curiosity. Today, millions of women are running, over a million girls play soccer, and more than a third of high school athletes are female."

Some drugs can also throw the menstrual mechanism out of whack, although this adverse reaction is not commonly reported. FDA's Annual Adverse Reaction Summary Listing includes 324 cases of drug-related amenorrhea from 1969 to 1983. The drugs heading the list were antipsychotics (especially the phenothiazines) and oral contraceptives.

Antipsychotic drugs, which are used to treat schizophrenia and other psychiatric conditions, may cause hyperprolactinemia (excessive production of prolactin by the pituitary). That can lead to amenorrhea. Thioridazine (brand name Mellaril) is particularly known to cause this problem.

Medical opinion differs about the relationship of oral contraceptives to amenorrhea. Many medical texts, including *The Merck Manual* and the American Pharmaceutical Association's *Handbook of Nonprescription Drugs,* say that discontinuing use of oral contraceptives is a common cause of amenorrhea.

The American Medical Association, however, in its reference book *AMA Drug Evaluations* (5th edition) says, "Whether a causal relationship exists between use of OCs [oral contraceptives] and subsequent amenorrhea is unresolved. In most studies, this effect is reported in less than 1 percent of patients who take OCs. The incidence of spontaneous secondary amenorrhea in women who do not take OCs is similar. . . ."

Some diseases can upset the menstrual cycle. Tuberculosis can attack the ovaries or uterus. Nephritis, a chronic kidney disease whose symptoms include excessive urination, can alter the hormone balance necessary for menstruation (hormones are eliminated from the body through urine). Diseases of the thyroid gland and the adrenal glands—and subsequent over- or underproduction of hormones by these organs—can also cause amenorrhea.

In treating amenorrhea, the cause must first be identified. In most cases a doctor can do this by using hormones, such as progesterone, in a series of tests.

In primary amenorrhea, menstruation can be induced with progesterone, and hormone therapy (usually estrogens or estrogen and progesterone) can be started to aid in development of secondary sex characteristics (such as development of breasts and pubic hair).

For patients with secondary amenorrhea, treatment depends both on its cause and the patient's goals. If a woman wants to become pregnant, the doctor might prescribe drugs to restore fertility. Bromocriptine mesylate (brand name Parlodel), a prescription drug that inhibits secretion of prolactin and causes pituitary tumors to shrink, is used to correct amenorrhea and infertility resulting from hyperprolactinemia. Another prescription drug, clomiphene citrate (Clomid and Serophene), can stimulate ovulation by increasing secretion of GnRH. This raises levels of FSH and LH so they are sufficient to stimulate the ovaries.

If pregnancy is not a goal, treatment with progestin may be used to restore the menstrual cycle. This is recommended by *AMA Drug Evaluations* to prevent endometrial hyperplasia (abnormal thickening of the lining of the uterus). If untreated, endometrial hyperplasia can progress to endometrial cancer.

One woman out of 100 will get amenorrhea at some time in life; many more will skip a period or two or experience some type of menstrual irregularity. Should a woman who misses several periods simply wait for her cycle to resume, assuming that if she feels healthy nothing is wrong?

Maybe, says FDA's Dr. Price. Dr. Joan Ullyot, author of *Running Free*, advises women runners not to worry about amenorrhea. Ullyot says that menstrual irregularity, "probably the single most important concern among women runners," is common among healthy runners and does not mean that something is wrong physically.

Dr. Price says for a woman who is not a jogger and who is not pregnant or on birth control pills, amenorrhea can indeed be a warning that something in the body, such as the hormones, has gone awry. Price says such women who have missed more than two periods should be checked by their doctors.

Carol Ballentine, *FDA Consumer*, May 1984.

Anorexia

Anorexia Nervosa

Anorexia nervosa is a disorder of self-starvation which manifests itself in an extreme aversion to food and can cause psychological, endocrine, and gynecological problems. It almost exclusively affects adolescent white girls, with symptoms involving a refusal to eat, large weight loss, a bizarre preoccupation with food, hyperactivity, a distorted body image, and cessation of menstruation. Although the symptoms can be corrected if the patient is diagnosed and treated in time, about 10 to 15 percent of anorexia nervosa patients die, usually after losing at least half their normal body weight.

Anorexia nervosa patients typically come from white, middle to upper-middle class families that place heavy emphasis on high achievement, perfection, eating patterns, and physical appearance. (There has never been a documented case of anorexia nervosa in a black male or female.) A newly diagnosed patient often is described by her parents as a "model child," usually because she is obedient, compliant, and a good student. Although most teenagers experience some feelings of youthful rebellion, persons with anorexia usually do not outwardly exhibit these feelings, tending instead to be childish in their thinking, in their need for parental approval, and in their lack of independence. Psychologists theorize that the patient's desire to control her own life manifests itself in the realm of eating—the only area, in the patient's mind, where she has the ability to direct her own life.

In striving for perfection and approval, a person with anorexia may begin to diet in order to lose just a few pounds. Dieting does not stop there, however, and an abnormal concern with dieting is established. Nobody knows what triggers the disease process, but suddenly, losing five or ten pounds is not enough. The anorectic patient becomes intent on losing weight. It is not uncommon for someone who develops this disorder to starve herself until she weighs just 60 or 70 pounds. Throughout the starvation process she either denies being hungry or claims to feel full after eating just a few bites.

Another related form of anorexia nervosa is an eating disorder known as "bulimia." Patients with this illness indulge in "food binges," and then purge themselves through vomiting immediately after eating or through the use of laxatives or diuretics. While on the surface these patients may appear to be well adjusted socially, this serious disease is particularly hard to overcome because it usually has been a pattern of behavior for a long time.

Whom does it affect?

Most researchers agree that the number of patients with anorexia nervosa is increasing. Recent estimates suggest that out of every 200 American girls between the ages of 12 and 18, one will develop anorexia to some degree. Therapists find that persons with anorexia usually lack self-esteem and feel they can gain admiration by losing weight and becoming thin.

While most anorexia nervosa patients are female, about 6 percent are adolescent boys. Occasionally the disorder is found in older women and in children as young as eight years old.

Some researchers believe that certain characteristics are common to the families of persons who develop the disorder. Although this "typical" family model may not apply to all patients, it is common to many. Researchers describe these families as warm and loving on the surface. Evidently, this loving atmosphere masks a series of underlying problems in which family members are excessively involved in each other's lives and overly dependent on one another. Apparently, they often are unable to deal with conflicts within the family. Either they deny that conflicts exist, or they become so overwhelmed by numerous petty conflicts that they are unable to recognize real problems.

What are the symptoms?

Psychological symptoms such as social withdrawal, obsessive-compulsiveness, and depression often precede or accompany anorexia nervosa. The patient's distorted view of herself and the world around her are the cause of these psychological disturbances.

Distortion of body image is another prevalent symptom. While most normal females can give an accurate estimate of their body weight, anorectic patients tend to perceive themselves as markedly larger than they really are. When questioned, most feel that their emaciated state (70–80 lbs.) is either "just right" or "too fat."

Profound physical symptoms also occur in cases of extreme starvation. These include loss of head hair, growth of fine body hair, constipation, intolerance of cold temperatures, and low pulse rate.

Certain endocrine functions also become impaired. In females this results in a cessation of menstruation (amenorrhea) and the absence of ovulation. Menstruation usually will not resume until endocrine balance is restored. Ovulation is suppressed because production of certain necessary hormones decreases.

Anorexia in boys has effects similar to those in girls: severe weight loss, psycho-social problems, and interruption of normal reproductive system processes.

Many differences in symptoms are apparent between anorectics and bulimics. Anorexia nervosa patients usually are not obese before onset of their illness. Typically, they are good students who become socially withdrawn before becoming ill and often come from families who fit the anorexia prototype described earlier. Bulimics, on the other hand, usually are extroverted before their illness, are inclined to be overweight, have voracious appetites, and have episodes of binge eating. Anorexia patients often have a better chance of returning to normal weight because their eating patterns, unlike those of bulimics, have been altered for a relatively shorter time.

Causes of anorexia

While the cause of anorexia is still unknown, a combination of psychological, environmental, and physiological factors are associated with development of the disorder.

Researchers have discovered that a part of the brain called the hypothalamus begins to work improperly after the onset of anorexia. The hypothalamus controls such activities as maintenance of water balance, regulation of body temperature, secretion of the endocrine glands, and sugar and fat metabolism. In anorexia patients, this improper functioning may result in lower blood pressure and body temperature, a lack of sexual interest, and hormonal changes resulting in amenorrhea and reduced production of thyroid hormone.

Some scientists are studying the possibility that the abnormalities in certain endocrine functions may actually precede the onset of anorexia. Further studies are needed, however, to determine if anorexia patients have a biological predisposition to develop the illness.

Treatment

Treatment for anorexia nervosa is usually threefold, consisting of nutritional therapy, individual psychotherapy, and family counseling. A team made up of pediatricians, psychiatrists, social workers, and nurses often administers treatment. Some physicians hospitalize anorexia patients until they are nutritionally stable. Others prefer to work with patients in the family setting.

But no matter where therapy is started, the most urgent concern of the physician is getting the patient to eat and gain weight. This is accomplished by gradually adding calories to the patient's daily intake. If she is hospitalized, privileges are sometimes granted in return for weight gain. This is known as a behavioral contract, and privileges may include such desirable activities as leaving the hospital for an afternoon's outing.

Physicians and hospital staff make every effort to ensure that the patient does not feel overwhelmed and powerless. Instead, weight gain is encouraged in an atmosphere in which the patient feels in control of her situation, and in which she wants to gain weight.

Individual psychotherapy is necessary in the treatment of anorexia to help the patient understand the disease process and its effects. Therapy focuses on the patient's relationship with her family and friends, and the reasons she may have fallen into a pattern of self-starvation. As a patient begins to learn more about her condition, she is often more willing to try to help herself recover.

In cases of severe depression, drugs such as antidepressants are part of therapy. Behavior improvement generally occurs rapidly in these cases, and the patient is able to respond more quickly to treatment.

The third aspect of treatment, family therapy, is supportive in nature. It examines how the patient and her parents relate to each other.

Persons with anorexia often become a source of family tension because refusals to eat cause frustration in the parents. The goal of family therapy is to help family members relate more effectively to one another, to encourage more mature thinking in the anorectic patient, and to help all family members work together for the well-being of the patient and the family unit.

In treating anorexia, it is extremely important to remember that immediate success does not guarantee a permanent cure. Sometimes, even after successful hospital treatment and return to a normal weight, patients suffer relapses. Follow-up therapy lasting three to five years is recommended if the patient is to be completely cured.

Self-help groups for patients, parents, spouses, and siblings can be a useful part of the overall treatment. Information on groups, treatment centers, hospitals, clinics, and doctors specializing in anorexia can be obtained from any of the following voluntary organizations:

American Anorexia Nervosa
Association, Inc.
133 Cedar Lane
Teaneck, N.J. 07666

National Anorexic Aid
Society, Inc. (NAAS)
P.O. Box 29461
Columbus, Ohio 43229

Anorexia Nervosa and
Associated Disorders (ANAS)
Suite 2020
550 Frontage Rd.
Northfield, Ill. 60093

Current research

The National Institutes of Health is sponsoring research to determine the causes of anorexia, the best methods of treatment, and ways to identify who might have a high risk of developing the disorder.

University scientists, sponsored by the National Institute of Child Health and Human Development, are examining the various factors in society, personality, and families influencing persons who develop anorexia. Other projects are comparing weight gain in patients fed high-protein versus low-protein diets.

Researchers at the National Institute of Mental Health are studying the biological aspects and changes in brain chemistry which may control appetite. Although psychological or environmental factors may precipitate the onset of the illness, the study indicates that it may be prolonged by starvation-induced changes in body processes. Persons with anorexia are sometimes admitted for study and treatment at the Clinical Center, a research hospital located on the National Institutes of Health campus in Bethesda, Md.

The National Institutes of Health, through its Division of Research Resources, supports ten General Clinical Research Centers throughout the country in which anorexia research is underway. Topics currently under investigation include sexual maturation, endocrine evaluation, hypothalamic and pituitary aspects of anorexia nervosa, and potassium levels in persons with anorexia.

The National Institute of Arthritis, Diabetes, and Digestive and Kidney Diseases sponsors studies in the endocrine disturbances of the hypothalamic, pituitary and ovarian function in the anorectic patient.

Ms. Jody Dove, Office of Research Reporting, NICHD, NIH. U.S. Department of Health and Human Services, Public Health Service, National Institutes of Health.

Antihistamines

Antihistamines Wear Many Therapeutic Hats

Antihistamines are remarkable for their multiplicity of uses. But they also have a multiplicity of side effects, and even though they are available in both over-the-counter and prescription drug products, they should be taken with care.

There's a drug that will relieve the symptoms of hay fever, and there's one that will ease the itching of hives. There's a product that helps the traveler who is prone to motion sickness, and another to put the weary into the arms of Morpheus. And there is a drug that aids the healing of stomach ulcers.

What's remarkable is that these agents are basically the same and all belong to a class of drugs called antihistamines. Although they've never made the headlines as a miracle cure for anything, antihistamines have played an important role in medicine for 35 years.

Antihistamines do exactly what their name suggests—counteract the effect of histamine, a chemical substance found in almost all the body's tissues. When released, histamine causes some very uncomfortable reactions. It contracts some smooth muscles, such as those of the bronchi and gut. At the same time it relaxes other muscles, such as those of the fine blood vessels. The resulting dilation of the blood vessels produces a redness or erythema in the tissues. Although all the tiny blood vessels in the body are involved, the response is most noticeable in the face and upper part of the body, the so-called "flushing area."

A second effect of histamine is a localized swelling or edema, the result of plasma protein and fluids moving from the blood vessels into the extracellular space around them. This reaction is most pronounced in areas where there are many tiny blood vessels, such as the inside of the nose. Still another response to histamine is itching and pain, caused by the chemical's effect on the sensory nerve endings. The three responses—redness, swelling, and itching—are considered the classic symptoms of histamine release.

Histamine also is a powerful stimulator of gastric acid production and can stir up secretions from other exocrine glands, such as the sweat glands. Release of large amounts of histamine can lead to histamine shock. Histamine-induced dilation of blood vessels in the brain can cause headache.

Release of histamine from the tissues can be triggered by a number of bodily insults, including the antigen-antibody response (allergy, in everyday language), physical trauma, heat or radiation injury severe enough to damage the cells, and reactions to certain drugs, foods, and dyes. Snake and insect venoms also stimulate histamine release. It's not yet clear what sets off the histamine that stimulates gastric acid production, leading, in turn, to stomach ulcers.

As early as 1927 scientists were able to show that histamine is found naturally in living tissue, but no one yet knows exactly what function, if any, it has while it is stored there waiting to be released. Early efforts to diminish the effects of the chemical proved fruitless. In 1933 a breakthrough was made by French researchers who found that certain substances with a chemical similarity to histamine had a counteractive effect. Although these early products proved toxic, they did pave the way for modern antihistamines.

The first effective drugs in this class—Antergan and Neoantergan—were developed in France in 1945. First on the American scene, in 1946, were diphenhydramine hydrochloride (Benadryl) and tripelennamine hydrochloride (Pyribenzamine). Both are still widely used.

Initial hopes that antihistamines would be the answer to allergy patients' prayers were dashed when it was realized that these drugs do not stop the release of histamine. What they do is block the chemical at "receptor sites."

Receptor sites are located on the surface of tissues that react to histamine. If the chemical gets to the receptor site, the classic reaction occurs. If the antihistamine gets to the site first, it prevents the histamine from doing its dirty work. As long as an antihistamine occupies the receptor site, histamine cannot cause a reaction.

Unfortunately, not all receptor sites are equal. In the mid-1960's scientists discovered that the antihistamines then in use did not block all histamine reactions, most particularly those stimulating gastric acid secretion. This new information led to a revised terminology. Henceforth, receptor sites blocked by the conventional antihistamines were called H_1 receptor blockers, while all others were designated H_2 receptor blockers.

A major breakthrough in the treatment of duodenal ulcer came in 1972 when researchers at the Smith Kline and French laboratories in England described a series of antagonists that selectively blocked gastric secretions and other responses to histamine that the H_1 blocking drugs could not touch. Thus were developed the first H_2 blocking agents. The first drug of this type to be marketed in the United States is cimetidine (trade name Tagamet), now the No. 1 prescribed drug in this country. Its use is limited to the treatment of duodenal ulcer, since H_2 blockers do not work on H_1 receptor sites.

There are 23 basic H_1 antihistamines that are grouped in five categories according to their chemical makeup (see Table 1). They all do basically the same thing, though some are better than others for certain uses. Some are available only by prescription; others can be bought over the counter.

Antihistamines are most useful in relieving the sneezing, runny nose, nasal congestion, and watery eyes that plague the victims of hay fever, technically called allergic or seasonal rhinitis. They are somewhat effective in cases of nonseasonal rhinitis, but not much good at all for perennial vasomotor rhinitis, a condition with symptoms like those of hay fever but with no known cause.

A panel of experts who evaluated ingredients in over-the-counter (OTC)

Table 1
H₁ Histamine Blocking Agents

Chemical Type	Generic Name	Representative Trade Names
Alkylamines	Brompheniramine maleate	Dimetane, Veltane
	Chlorpheniramine maleate	Chlor-Trimeton, Histaspan, Teldrin
	Dexbrompheniramine maleate	Disophrol, Drixoral, Disomer
	Dexchlorpheniramine maleate	Polaramine
	Dimethindene maleate	Forhistal, Triten
	Triprolidine hydrochloride	Actidil, Actifed-C
Ethanolamines	Carbinoxamine maleate	Clistin, Rondec
	Dimenhydrinate	Dramamine
	Diphenydramine hydrochloride	Benadryl, Ambenyl, Rhusticon
	Diphenylpraline hydrochloride	Hispril, Diaphen
	Doxylamine succinate	Decapryn, Bendectin
Ethylenediamines	Pyrilamine maleate	Fiogesic, Histalet, Triaminic
	Tripelennamine citrate	Pyribenzamine Citrate
	Tripelennamine hydrochloride	Pyribenzamine
Piperazines	Thonzylamine hydrochloride	Anahist, Resistab
	Cyclizine hydrochloride	Marezin, Migral
	Hydroxyzine hydrochloride	Atharax, Cartrax, Marax
	Meclizine hydrochloride	Antivert, Bonine
	Buclizine hydrochloride	Bucladin-S
Phenothiazines	Methdilazine hydrochloride	Tacaryl
	Promethazine hydrochloride	Phenergan, Maxigesic
	Trimeprazine tartrate	Temaril
Other	Cyproheptadine	Periactin

cough, cold, and allergy drugs, as part of FDA's massive review of all nonprescription drugs, said that 11 antihistamines are safe and effective for the self-treatment of allergies. (Two of these ingredients, methapyrilene hydrochloride and methapyrilene fumarate, were taken off the market in 1979 when it was learned they could cause cancer in laboratory rats.) (Table 2)

Many OTC cough-cold remedies also contain antihistamines because their anticholinergic (drying) effect stops the sniffles. FDA recently approved the use of diphenhydramine hydrochloride as an OTC cough suppressant. However, these drugs are not recommended for the treatment of bronchial asthma because the drying effect of antihistamines can make it difficult to get rid of irritating secretions in the bronchial tubes.

Their tendency to cause drowsiness makes antihistamines useful as ingredients in sedatives and preoperative medications. Three of these drugs have been marketed as OTC sleep-aids: methapyrilene hydrochloride, methapyrilene fumarate, and pyrilamine. Another panel of experts studying OTC drugs for FDA felt that in order to avoid adverse reactions in patients, the manufacturers may have used too low a dose of antihistamine to produce an effective sleep-aid. The panel recommended that a higher dosage level be tested for safety and effectiveness. As already noted, two of these three antihistamines have been taken off the market. Two additional antihistamines have been approved as sleep-aid ingredients: doxylamine succinate was approved through a New Drug Application and diphenhydramine was approved during the course of an OTC review.

Antihistamines were among a number of ingredients once sold as "daytime sedatives" that were supposed to relieve "occasional simple nervous tension." FDA banned the entire class of drugs, effective Christmas Eve 1979, because the drowsiness that accompanies the taking of these drugs does nothing to relieve tension or anxiety.

Antihistamines are also used to relieve the swelling and itching that often goes along with allergic reactions to drugs, such as penicillin, or to foods and food coloring. Dermatologists may prescribe antihistamines for skin conditions such as contact dermatitis, acute urticaria (hives), or pruritis ani (itching of the anus). These drugs may also be used to take the itch out of insect bites and poison ivy.

One of the most common reasons for taking antihistamines is to prevent the queasy stomach and dizziness that comes with motion sickness. The piperazines are the category of drugs primarily used for this purpose, although Dramamine (dimenhydrinate) is the name that is probably most familiar to consumers. These same drugs are often used to counteract vertigo, a sensation that the world is turning around you (not to be confused with dizziness).

Table 2

OTC Panel Recommendations on Antihistamines for Allergies

Brompheniramine maleate	Methapyrilene hydrochloride*	Thonzylamine hydrochloride
Chlorpheniramine maleate	Phenindamine tartrate	* Withdrawn from market by FDA
Diphenhydramine hydrochloride	Pheniramine maleate	because they can cause cancer
Doxylamine succinate	Promethazine hydrochloride	
Methapyrilene fumarate*	Pyrilamine maleate	

Annabel Hecht; reprinted from September 1981 *FDA Consumer*, HHS Publication No. (FDA) 81–3121. Department of Health and Human Services, Public Health Service, Food and Drug Administration, 5600 Fishers Lane, Rockville, Md. 20857, Office of Public Affairs. U.S. Government Printing Office 1981—341–174/81

Several of the H_1 antihistamines have a local anesthetic activity and often are used in the form of creams and lotions to relieve itching. There is one problem, however. They can also cause contact dermatitis.

While there is a wide gap between a safe therapeutic dose and an unsafe, toxic dose, antihistamines can still cause adverse reactions. Drowsiness, or sedation, is the major problem an antihistamine user might encounter. Fortunately, not all antihistamines cause the same degree of sedation, which gives the physician a choice when prescribing this type of drug. If one antihistamine makes the patient too sleepy, another may provide the same relief without the side effects.

Drowsiness is most likely to occur with the ethanolamine antihistamines and least likely with the alkylamines (listed in Table 1). In between are the ethylenediamines. Drinking alcoholic beverages will increase the sedative effect of antihistamines, as will other drugs that have a depressant effect, such as minor tranquilizers or sedatives.

Dizziness, lassitude, lack of coordination, fatigue, and confusion are also reactions affecting the central nervous system.

The next most frequent side effects are those striking the digestive system: loss of appetite, vomiting, abdominal pain, constipation, or diarrhea.

Sometimes the drying action of antihistamines causes excitation that leads to insomnia, tremors, nervousness, irritability, and palpitation of the heart. Dryness of the mouth, blurred vision, or urinary retention may occur when high doses of these drugs are used. Because of these reactions, antihistamines should not be taken by people who have glaucoma except on the advice of a physician. The drying effect may be intensified if the patient is also taking MAO inhibitors, drugs used to treat hypertension and depression.

Anyone taking antihistamines and planning to get a summer tan should be sure to use a good sunscreen, or give up the idea of tanning for the duration of the medication's use. Some of these drugs can make a person especially sensitive to sunlight. For instance, diphenhydramine hydrochloride, chlorpheniramine maleate, and dimethindene maleate cause this effect.

Despite the high margin of safety enjoyed by antihistamines, acute poisoning can occur from overdoses. Cases of suicide from antihistamine overdoses have been reported. Children are especially susceptible to the adverse effects of these drugs and may become excited, nervous, and irritable rather than drowsy. Too much antihistamine may produce hallucinations or convulsions in children and an overdose can be fatal.

All of the above adverse reactions are attributable to H_1 receptor blocking agents. The H_2 blocker, cimetidine, also can cause some side effects, including mild and transient diarrhea, muscular pain, dizziness, and rash. A few cases have occurred of gynecomastia (swelling of the breast in men) and of reversible confusional states, usually in the elderly. Studies have been reported suggesting that the ulcer drug can alter the effectiveness of other drugs taken at the same time. For instance, the blood thinning effect of warfarin-type anticoagulants may be increased, and the metabolism of diazepam (Valium) and chlordiazepoxide (Librium) may be slowed down, thus prolonging the effect they have on the body.

Keeping antihistamines and other drugs out of the reach of children is a primary rule for every household. Here are some other suggestions to help consumers use antihistamines in the safest and most effective way.

- Follow your doctor's directions carefully. If you feel the drug prescribed is making you too drowsy, ask if another drug or a different dosage can be prescribed.
- If you are taking antihistamines, don't drink alcoholic beverages or take other drugs that have a depressant effect, such as minor tranquilizers or sedatives.
- Avoid driving a car, operating appliances or machinery while taking antihistamines.
- If you are using an over-the-counter drug, follow the directions on the label carefully.
- Check the list of ingredients on the OTC drug labels. Don't take two products containing antihistamines at the same time. You could risk getting an overdose.
- Don't take OTC antihistamines without checking with your doctor if you have asthma, glaucoma, or difficulty in urination due to enlargement of the prostate gland.
- Don't give an OTC antihistamine to a child under 6 except on the advice of a doctor.

Arthritis
For Treating Arthritis, Start With Aspirin

When John Milton included ''joint-racking Rheums'' (rheumatism) among the dire diseases mankind would suffer as a result of Eve's taste for apples (*Paradise Lost,* Book XI), he knew what he was writing about. The great English poet was afflicted with arthritis.

It is now known that arthritis is not a specific disease. The word itself means "joint inflammation," a symptom that can occur in over 100 conditions. In 17th-century England, the time of Milton, gout and rheumatism were the names commonly given to this painful condition that has plagued humankind since before the centuries were counted.

Milton's biographers don't say how the poet's disease was treated. If Thomas Sydenham had been his doctor, he might have been prescribed "a draught of small beer," a favorite remedy of the celebrated 17th-century English physician, himself a victim of both gout and arthritis.

What would not have been prescribed were salicylates, one form of which is aspirin. Although willow bark and leaves, the original source in nature of these compounds, had been known as fever reducers since the time of Hippocrates, salicylates were not used to treat rheumatic diseases until 200 years after Milton's death.

Today, there are a variety of drugs used to treat arthritis, including more than a dozen that can provide significant relief from the pain, inflammation, and swelling of the most common forms of arthritis. There are a number of other drugs that can slow and possibly halt the potentially crippling effects of rheumatoid arthritis, one of the most serious forms. Unfortunately, none will cure any of the arthritic conditions.

In all but the most severe or unresponsive cases, the drugs of choice for treatment of arthritis are the nonsteroidal anti-inflammatory drugs (NSAIDs). The name is significant, for it distinguishes this class of drugs from the steroids, cortisone-like compounds produced by the adrenal glands. Steroids are used only in very ill arthritis patients.

The NSAIDs are also called "prostaglandin inhibitors," since they interfere with the production of prostaglandins, unique compounds in the body's tissues that trigger inflammation.

NSAID drugs, which can relieve pain and reduce inflammation, often are the only therapy needed for patients who are able to move their joints with relative ease. Oldest of the NSAIDs is plain aspirin, still the most frequently prescribed arthritis drug. Aspirin, however, has its drawbacks. The large doses required for effective treatment—as many as 18 to 20 tablets a day—may cause stomach irritation and gastrointestinal bleeding. Ringing in the ears, temporary hearing loss, and interference with blood clotting are also common side effects. Some of aspirin's side effects can be reduced by using buffered or timed-release versions.

In addition to aspirin, known technically as acetylsalicylic acid, there are a number of other salicylates for the treatment of arthritic conditions. (See accompanying article for a description of the various types of arthritis.) Choline magnesium trisalicylate and magnesium salicylate are used for the relief of the signs and symptoms of rheumatoid arthritis, osteoarthritis, and other musculoskeletal disorders. Diflunisal may be used for osteoarthritis as well as for mild to moderate pain from any cause.

Fortunately, there are other nonsteroidal anti-inflammatory drugs that may provide relief from pain and inflammation in patients who cannot tolerate or who are not helped by aspirin. These drugs, available only by prescription, generally have fewer side effects and are more convenient, since the patient needs to take fewer tablets a day.

Eleven drug products are on the market for the treatment of osteoarthritis and rheumatoid arthritis: fenoprofen, ibuprofen, indomethacin, meclofe- namate sodium, oxyphenbutazone, phenylbutazone, piroxicam, sulindac, tolmetin, naproxen, and naproxen sodium. (See accompanying table for brand names and indications.)

Sulindac, oxyphenbutazone, phenylbutazone, indomethacin, naproxen and naproxen sodium are also effective in treating ankylosing spondylitis (spinal arthritis) and gout.

Tolmetin is the only drug with indications for the treatment of juvenile arthritis. One other drug, benoxaprofen (Oraflex), was withdrawn by the manufacturer because of an increasing number of reports of severe adverse reactions, including death from liver disease.

Effective as they are, these drugs are not totally free of side effects. Nausea, vomiting, abdominal distress, pain, diarrhea, blurred vision, dizziness, and skin rashes are among the adverse reactions variously associated with these drugs. Because blood disorders may occur in patients getting phenylbutazone and oxyphenbutazone, these drugs are used for limited periods at the lowest possible dose.

For certain rheumatoid arthritis patients, but not those with osteoarthri- tis, there are several drugs that can prove helpful when the NSAIDs fail. Called disease-modifying antirheumatic agents, these drugs can help about 70 percent of patients whose rheumatoid arthritis persists or becomes active, and whose joints continue to be swollen and inflamed after other forms of therapy have been tried.

The major disease-modifying drugs in current use are gold compounds, D-penicillamine (a distant cousin of penicillin), antimalarial drugs such as hydroxychloroquine, and immunosuppressive drugs.

Gold is one of the oldest arthritis treatments, having been used for more than 50 years. Injectable gold compounds can reduce joint swelling and morning stiffness and increase the gripping power of affected hands. It may, however, take several months of treatment before improvements are evident, and even then changes may be imperceptible from one day to the next. Gold does not cure rheumatoid arthritis, and if the treatments are stopped, there is a strong chance that the disease may recur. Kidney and bone marrow damage and skin rash are among the side effects of gold therapy.

Many of the same things can be said of D-penicillamine. It may take several months to become effective and it has serious side effects, including blood disorders, kidney problems, gastrointestinal problems, and skin rash.

The antimalarial drugs are derivatives of quinine. Toxic effects of these drugs are usually mild and include generally reversible clouding of the cornea. Because degeneration of the retina can occur, continuing even after the drug is stopped, frequent eye examinations are called for during long-term therapy.

Immunosuppressive agents, drugs that prevent the body's rejection of transplanted organs, are used only in severe, active rheumatoid arthritis that has not been relieved by rest and other drugs, including gold compounds.

Drugs called corticosteroids must also be used with caution. The most potent anti-inflammatory drugs available, corticosteroids can bring rapid relief from pain and inflammation. At the same time, they have some serious side effects, including edema (swelling), thinning of the bones, and psychoses. Because of these effects, these steroids are used in the lowest possible dose if they must be used orally. Some forms of corticosteroids can be injected directly into a joint to reduce pain and increase mobility, a technique that is less hazardous, although there is still a chance the joint may become infected.

For gout, drug treatment is aimed first at stopping acute attacks; second, at preventing recurrent attacks. Colchicine, a derivative of a type of crocus plant, is often used for the first goal. It is one of the oldest drugs around (Benjamin Franklin is said to have introduced it into this country in 1763). Colchicine is given in multiple doses with a lot of water until the initial pain subsides. Unfortunately, the price of relief may be diarrhea and cramps. As has been noted earlier, several of the nonsteroidal anti-inflammatory drugs are also helpful in reducing pain and inflammation of gout attacks.

To prevent attacks of gout and to lessen their number and severity, probenecid, allopurinol and sulfinpyrazone may be given. Such drugs must be taken daily to keep uric acid levels in check. They are not effective in treating acute attacks, however. Colchicine also may be used as a preventive measure.

The treatment for spinal arthritis—ankylosing spondylitis—includes a program of anti-inflammatory drugs such as sulindac, oxyphenbutazone, phenylbutazone, indomethacin, naproxen, and naproxen sodium, along with spinal exercises and, if necessary, deep-breathing exercises.

Some over-the-counter (OTC) drug products can provide temporary relief from minor joint pains. Called "counterirritants," these products include ingredients such as methyl salicylate, turpentine oil, histamine dihydrochloride, and capsicum. One of FDA's advisory panels reviewing ingredients in all OTC drugs recommended that label claims for counterirritant products include "for temporary relief of minor aches and pains of muscles and joints, such as simple backache, lumbago, arthritis, neuralgia, strains, bruises, and sprains." Such products do not reduce inflammation and should not be used for long-term treatment of arthritis.

Drug therapy is just one aspect of the management of arthritis. Rest when the disease flares up, programmed exercise, physical therapy, splints and other home-help devices, and a well-balanced diet all play a part in a total treatment program. In severe cases, damaged joints can even be replaced with prosthetic devices. The kind of therapy and the drugs, or combinations of drugs, that will provide the most relief must be determined on an individual basis.

What should not be included in a treatment program are quack remedies such as unusual diets, uranium-filled mittens, or Chinese herbal medicines that are not herbs at all but combinations of powerful drugs. The arthritis patient who turns to such "cures" will get only false hopes and a thin purse.

Annabel Hecht.

Commonly Prescribed Arthritis Drugs

Generic/Brand Name	Indications
Nonsteroidal Anti-inflammatory Drugs *Salicylates*	
Aspirin Bayer, Ascriptin, Anacin, Bufferin, various generics	Rheumatoid arthritis, juvenile rheumatoid arthritis, osteoarthritis
Choline magnesium trisalicylate Trilisate	Rheumatoid arthritis, osteoarthritis, and other arthritic conditions
Magnesium salicylate Magan, Arthrogesic, Durasal, Magsal	Rheumatoid arthritis, osteoarthritis, bursitis, and other musculoskeletal disorders
Diflunisal Dolobid	Osteoarthritis
Non-Salicylates	
Fenoprofen Nalfon	Rheumatoid arthritis, osteoarthritis, acute flare-ups, long-term management
Ibuprofen Motrin, Rufen	Rheumatoid arthritis, osteoarthritis
Indomethacin Indocin	Moderate to severe rheumatoid arthritis, ankylosing spondylitis, osteoarthritis, gout

Commonly Prescribed Arthritis Drugs (Continued)

Generic/Brand Name	Indications
Meclofenamate sodium Meclomen	Acute and chronic rheumatoid arthritis and osteoarthritis (not recommended as initial drug)
Oxyphenbutazone Oxalid, Tandearil	Acute gouty arthritis, active rheumatoid arthritis, ankylosing spondylitis, acute degenerative joint disease
Phenylbutazone Butazolidin, Azolid	Acute gouty arthritis, active rheumatoid arthritis, ankylosing spondylitis, acute attacks of degenerative joint disease of hips and knees
Piroxicam Feldene	Osteoarthritis, rheumatoid arthritis
Sulindac Clinoril	Osteoarthritis, rheumatoid arthritis, ankylosing spondylitis, acute shoulder pain, gout
Tolmetin Tolectin	Rheumatoid arthritis, osteoarthritis, acute and long-term management, juvenile arthritis
Naproxen Naprosyn	Rheumatoid arthritis, osteoarthritis, ankylosing spondylitis, tendinitis and bursitis, and acute gout
Naproxen sodium Anaprox	Rheumatoid arthritis, osteoarthritis, ankylosing spondylitis, tendinitis and bursitis, and acute gout

Disease-Modifying Drugs

Gold compounds Myochrysine, Solganal	Selected cases of active adult and juvenile rheumatoid arthritis
D-penicillamine Cuprimine, Depen	Severe active rheumatoid arthritis where conventional therapy has failed
Hydroxychloroquine Plaquenil Sulfate	Antimalarial for acute and chronic rheumatoid arthritis
Azathioprine Imuran	Immunosuppressive drug for severe active rheumatoid arthritis unresponsive to other therapy

Other Arthritis Drugs

Corticosteroids (Aristocort, Celestone, and others)	For short-term administration in rheumatic disorders, including rheumatoid arthritis, juvenile arthritis, acute gouty arthritis, ankylosing spondylitis

Commonly Prescribed Arthritis Drugs (Continued)

Generic/Brand Name	Indications
Additional Drugs for Gout	
Colchicine Colchicine, ColBENEMID	Acute gouty arthritis
Sulfinpyrazone Anturane	Chronic or intermittent gouty arthritis
Probenecid Benemid	Gout and gouty arthritis
Probenecid and colchicine ColBENEMID	Chronic gouty arthritis complicated by recurrent gouty attacks
Allopurinol Zyloprim, Lopurin	Primary or secondary gout, uric acid kidney disease, tophi (uric acid deposits)

What arthritis is and isn't

An estimated 30 to 40 million Americans suffer from arthritis, but that doesn't mean that they all have the same ailment. In fact, arthritis isn't a specific disease at all. The word "arthritis" simply means joint inflammation, something that can occur in over 100 conditions.

Among the most common forms of what is called arthritis are osteoarthritis, rheumatoid arthritis, gout, and ankylosing spondylitis.

Osteoarthritis is a degenerative joint disease, occurring most often in men and women over 50. It is believed to be related to the wear and tear of the hardest working joints of the body and to other uncertain and unknown factors. The cartilage that protects the ends of the bones in the joints is worn away due to weakness of the supporting structures, such as the tendons, ligaments, and muscles. The bones then grate against each other with accompanying pain and a decrease in movability.

In the beginning only one joint may be affected, but as time goes on additional joints can begin to hurt, usually one at a time. Some people with osteoarthritis don't know they have it, even though X-rays show joint damage. For those who do have trouble, the major symptoms are pain in and around joints and loss of ability to move joints easily. In advanced cases joints take on an outwardly knobby look.

Rheumatoid arthritis is potentially the most severe, crippling form of arthritis and can strike at any age, even during childhood, although it generally occurs first after the age of 25. Women are afflicted more often than men. Rheumatoid arthritis is thought to be related to a disordered immune system that causes the body to attack its own cells.

Rheumatoid arthritis affects tissues within the whole body and the victim may feel weak and listless even before the joints are affected. The disease attacks one joint or many joints at the same time. Usually, the same joint on each side of the body will be affected. Sometimes symptoms may disappear for months or years, and in a small proportion of cases they never return. Usually, however, they remain or get progressively worse unless the patient gets proper treatment.

Juvenile rheumatoid arthritis is very similar to the adult form of the disease, especially in joint involvement. It can begin in infancy or in the teens and affects girls more than boys.

Gout (gouty arthritis) is an acutely painful condition that usually attacks middle-aged men, although it can occur in women after menopause. In an attack of gout, excess uric acid in the blood forms needle-like crystals that irritate and inflame one or more joints in the body, particularly the big toe.

An inherited defect in body chemistry may be behind some cases of gout. Others develop following use of diuretic drugs, commonly prescribed for high blood pressure treatment.

Ankylosing spondylitis is an inflammatory disease of the spine. It is a hereditary ailment that usually afflicts men in young adulthood. Small joints of the spine and sacroiliac are attacked first, making pain in the lower back and legs an early symptom. Other joints, especially the hips and shoulders, also may become involved. Without treatment, the spine may become progressively stiffer until it is completely rigid. Curvature of the spine may develop, forcing the victim into a stooped position.

Revised March 1984 *FDA Consumer,* HHS Publication No. (FDA) 84–3145. Department of Health and Human Services, Public Health Service, Food and Drug Administration, 5600 Fishers Lane, Rockville, Md. 20857. U.S. Government Printing Office 1984—421–174/128.

Asthma

What is asthma?

Asthma is a chronic but reversible obstruction of the airways. Since scientists do not yet fully understand the underlying causes of asthma, the disease can be described but not truly defined.

An estimated seven million Americans have asthma. Of these, approximately two to three million are children.

The course of the disease can sometimes be predicted by the age at which it first occurs. In general, an earlier age of onset means a better prognosis except when the asthma begins under 2 years of age. A history of allergic eczema in infancy—either with or followed by hay fever—increases the likelihood that asthma will persist into adolescence or adulthood. Some children do "outgrow" the condition, being free of symptoms by the time they are 16, but the exact percentage in whom this happens is still unknown. However, the finding that half of asthmatic adults developed their disease as children emphasizes the need for an asthmatic child to receive proper medical treatment; one should not simply wait for asthma to be outgrown. If a person develops asthma as an adult, the disease is frequently severe and persistent.

Asthma is not usually fatal, although nearly 3,000 Americans die annually from this disease. When properly treated, asthma, in the absence of other associated lung diseases, does not cause permanent lung damage. However, because of its chronic and unpredictable nature, it is extremely debilitating. Although this disability cannot be measured directly, one can appreciate its impact by looking at statistics such as the days lost from school or work, the cost of medication, and the psychological problems incurred with a chronic illness.

In one recent year, it was estimated that asthma was responsible for the loss of over 10 million days from work and $435 million in wages. In that same year, Americans made more than 28 million office visits to physicians for asthma and spent over $292 million for asthma drugs and $170 million for hospital care. Asthma may also have devastating effects on children; among chronic childhood diseases, it is *the* major cause of school absenteeism.

Normal breathing

To understand what happens during an asthmatic attack, one must first know how we breathe normally. When we breathe air in through the nose or mouth, it passes into the throat and through the larynx, also known as the voice box. The larynx is at the top of the trachea, or windpipe, which branches into two tubes called bronchi, one of which enters each lung. Inside the lung, the bronchi split many times, forming a tree-like network of thousands of tiny branches known as bronchioles. At the end of each bronchiole is a cluster of tiny hollow air sacs called alveoli.

It is in these sacs that the vital processes of breathing take place. The oxygen in the air that we inhale is picked up from the air sacs by the blood and pumped throughout the entire body. At the same time, carbon dioxide, which is a waste product, is removed from the blood by the air sacs and eliminated by exhaling.

The walls of the air passages contain smooth muscles—ones over which we have no conscious control. Although we do not yet fully understand their function, we know that these muscles—by contracting and relaxing—can regulate the flow of air to the air sacs.

Normally, the airways offer little resistance to this flow. However, during an asthmatic attack, the smooth muscles tighten around the airways. The lining of the airways becomes swollen and filled with blood cells known as eosinophils. In addition, respiratory mucous glands produce too much mucus, which further plugs the airways. As a result of the muscle tightening, swelling, and congestion with cells and mucus, the airways become quite narrow and forced breathing becomes necessary. The rush of air through the narrowed passageways and the vibration of mucus produce the wheezing sounds that are typical of asthma.

Although air flow obstruction is always found in asthma, it cannot account for all the difficulties an asthmatic experiences. One striking feature of an asthma attack is overinflation of the lungs. Air is trapped behind the narrowed airways so that, after exhaling as hard as possible, air remains in the lungs. This air is stale and prevents the exchange of fresh air. The lungs do not get enough oxygen, and carbon dioxide builds up in the body. If the carbon dioxide level rises too sharply, this indicates the respiratory system is under severe stress and the patient's life is endangered.

An asthma attack also puts a strain on the cardiovascular system. For example, the increased air pressure in the lungs can collapse the tiny blood vessels (capillaries) in the air sacs. To prevent this from happening, the blood pressure in these small vessels must be increased. Thus, the heart must pump harder to achieve this vital balancing of pressures.

Triggers of asthma

Scientists do not yet know the basic abnormalities that underlie asthma. However, many factors are known to trigger or induce an asthmatic attack in a susceptible individual. Because each patient's reactions grow out of his or her own make-up and environment, the physician must determine which factors play a role in each case and plan the treatment accordingly.

Extrinsic asthma—asthma triggered by an outside factor—is a term frequently used to refer to allergic asthma. Most children with asthma are allergic. While only half of adult asthmatics (over 30 years old) are allergic, it is not unusual for people in their fifties, sixties, or seventies to develop extrinsic asthma. Over the last decade, research sponsored by the National Institute of Allergy and Infectious Diseases (NIAID) has resulted in an enormous expansion of our understanding of allergies. This progress has made it possible to describe the events which underlie allergic asthma.

The tendency to develop an allergy is inherited. Patients with allergic diseases almost always have a close relative with some type of allergic problem. The first step in developing an allergy is exposure to certain environmental substances such as pollens, house dust, animal danders and feathers, wool, cosmetic powders, molds, foods, or organic dusts.

The body reacts or becomes allergic to these substances—allergens— by producing a protein known as IgE antibody. IgE antibody is specific for the allergen against which it is made. For example, an IgE antibody made against oak pollen will react only with another grain of oak pollen.

In the allergic individual, IgE antibodies attach to the surface of either basophils (a type of white blood cell) or mast cells (tissue cells found primarily in the linings of the respiratory tract, the gastrointestinal tract, and the skin). When an allergic person again encounters the allergen— such as oak pollen—the pollen binds to the IgE antibodies already sitting on the surface of the mast cells. This combination of allergen and antibody is a signal to these cells to release from their interiors little packets of irritating chemicals. It is the release of these chemicals, known as media- tors, into the surrounding tissues that is responsible for the allergy symp- toms. For example, the release of mediators in the nose, eyes, and sinuses of an individual with allergic rhinitis (hay fever) results in sneez- ing, a runny nose, and itchy eyes; mediators released in the skin produce the swelling and redness characteristic of urticaria (hives). A person with food allergies may have vomiting or diarrhea as a result of mediators released in the tissues of the gastrointestinal tract.

When chemical mediators are liberated in lung tissue, they cause the changes that are recognized as asthma: swelling of the lining of the airways, attraction of certain types of cells into the airways, the overpro- duction of mucus, and powerful tightening of the muscles in the airways.

In addition to allergies, there are many other triggers of asthma, includ- ing respiratory infections, aspirin and other anti-inflammatory drugs, and exercise.

Exercise-induced asthma is quite common. It can occur alone or as a complication of other types of asthma. The exact mechanisms responsible for this form of the disease have not yet been conclusively identified, but loss of moisture due to exercising may be an important factor. Swim- ming has been found to be the best kind of exercise for individuals with this problem.

Respiratory infections play a major role in causing asthma, particularly in children. Studies of infants born to allergic parents indicate that allergy and asthma may occur in these children following respiratory infections.

Several viral infections of the respiratory tract were found to be capable of inducing wheezing directly in small infants or predisposing them to the development of asthma in later life. Other investigations have shown that viral infections can cause profound changes in certain responses of white blood cells. These changes may lead to an increased release of chemical mediators from basophils or mast cells.

For those asthmatics in whom environmental allergies are known to play a role, moving may be considered. However, relocating often results in only temporary, if any, improvement and should not be undertaken without expert advice. Many patients feel that another environmental factor, air pollution, adversely affects their asthma. This association, however, has been difficult to prove.

In a significant number of asthmatics, aspirin will set off an attack. Interestingly, this reaction is not a true allergy to the drug. Such persons are usually advised to avoid other types of anti-inflammatory medications including phenylbutazone and indomethacin, as well as the yellow food dye No. 5—tartrazine yellow—since these substances may also be harmful to them. Asthmatics who are sensitive to these drugs usually have nasal polyps. The combination of these three conditions is a syndrome called triad asthma. Such individuals frequently suffer from sinusitis and are prone to serious asthma attacks.

Another condition that occurs in asthmatics is associated with heavy brownish sputum production, bronchiectasis (chronic dilation of the bronchi), and fungal infection. Individuals with this problem—allergic bronchopulmonary aspergillosis—require close medical supervision to prevent lung damage.

Emotional stresses can also trigger attacks in many children and adults with asthma. However, emotions do not cause this disease. There is a complex interaction between parts of the nervous system and airway obstruction, which may explain why some individuals with asthma worsen at times of emotional stress. The importance of emotional factors cannot be ignored; the mental suffering and loss of initiative and confidence that result from repeated asthma attacks can hinder the normal development of children.

Treatment

In the long-term treatment of asthma, the best results are usually obtained by identifying the causes, avoiding them where possible, and directing specific therapy toward those factors that cannot be avoided.

There are irritants in the environment such as cigarette smoke, cooking odors, and aerosol sprays that can adversely affect a person with asthma.

These should be avoided as much as possible. An asthmatic should not smoke nor be active outdoors for prolonged periods of time during air pollution alerts.

In allergic asthma, attacks can often be prevented if the source of the allergy—that is, the responsible allergen—is removed. Therefore, the physician must obtain a good history of the patient's responses to his environment, including pollens, foods, organic dusts, and animals, if the offending agent is to be identified and eliminated. For example, if the dander from a pet dog is the culprit allergen, a new home for the dog may have to be found. Often items in the bedroom—where adults spend about one-third of their time, and children spend as much as one-half of theirs—are to blame. Air conditioning units, whose filters are changed frequently, permit windows and doors to be kept closed, thus preventing airborne allergens, as well as some irritants, from entering the home.

Often allergens such as pollen or mold cannot be eliminated from the patient's environment. In these cases, the physician may try immuno-therapy—the standard allergy treatment also known as hyposensitization, injection therapy, or "allergy shots." Evidence suggests that immunother-apy has a useful role in managing the allergic component of asthma. Such injections, however, cannot be expected to cure the underlying disease nor replace appropriate drug therapy in allergic asthmatics. Immu-notherapy is also not effective in treating those asthmatics who do not have allergies.

Patients who produce large amounts of lung secretions may find a technique known as postural drainage—in which the head and trunk are placed downward—helpful in coughing up the mucus. They should also drink plenty of liquids to help keep the secretions loose, thus prevent-ing them from clogging up the airways. Expectorants (cough medicines) are also widely used but they have not been definitely proven to enhance the clearance of mucus.

The various drugs used to relax the muscles in the airways (bronchodila-tors) act by several different mechanisms. Thus, if one of these drugs fails to work, in many cases, a physician can substitute or add another.

Among the oldest and most useful bronchodilators for many asthma patients are the xanthines. Two members of this class, theophylline and aminophylline, can be given in various forms—orally, rectally, or in hospitalized patients, intravenously. The dosage of theophylline must be tailored for each individual and closely monitored by the physician. This is important not only to obtain the most benefit from the drug but also to avoid side effects, some of which can be serious.

Another group of bronchodilators is the beta$_2$ adrenergic agents. These relax the smooth muscles and inhibit the release of chemical mediators from mast cells while minimizing the unwanted side effects on the heart and circulatory system, which result from the use of other types of adrenergic drugs. Metaproterenol and terbutaline are beta$_2$ agents.

Among the drugs used to reduce inflammation is disodium cromogylcate (DSC). It is believed to act by blocking the release of chemical mediators from mast cells. DSC appears to be useful in the *prevention* of acute attacks, mainly in those with allergic or exercise-induced asthma.

Although their action is not completely understood, steroids are extremely effective for all types of asthmatics. However, their use is restricted to patients with severe or moderately severe asthma that cannot be controlled by other drugs. In addition, prolonged use of steroids can result in serious side effects, such as growth inhibition, diabetes, or suppression of the adrenal glands. If steroids must be taken, efforts should be made to maintain an every-other-day schedule. Recently, a steroid inhaled in aerosol form—beclomethasone dipropionate—has been licensed. This method of delivering the drug directly to the airways appears to be quite useful and carries less risk of side effects than steroids given orally.

None of these drugs, however, cures asthma—they relieve the symptoms. Because these medications can have side effects, they should never be used except under the careful supervision of a physician. Self-medication without a physician's advice can be dangerous.

Exercise and physical fitness are as essential for individuals with asthma as they are for everyone else. Having this disorder should certainly not constitute an automatic excuse from physical education classes. Although some exercises—such as swimming—seem to produce less bronchospasm than others, asthmatics, and particularly those who are children, should be encouraged to the extent of their capabilities to participate in any sport they wish. With appropriate premedication, nearly all asthmatics can exercise.

Research

Why some people develop asthma and others do not is still a medical mystery. Only recently have scientists begun to understand some of the underlying complex mechanisms of allergy and asthma. To help translate laboratory findings into improved diagnosis and treatment of patients with these disorders, NIAID has established a network of Asthma and Allergic Disease Centers (AADC's).

Scientists at these centers have played leading roles in the identification of IgE antibody, its interaction with mast cells and basophils, and the consequent release of chemical mediators that cause the symptoms of allergy. Presently, much effort is being concentrated on controlling the release of these mediators.

The use of $beta_2$ adrenergic agents in the treatment of asthma has already been mentioned. The development of these useful drugs has come from research directed at unraveling the complex interactions between parts of the nervous system and airway obstruction. There are two main nervous systems—the sympathetic (or adrenergic), and the parasympathetic (or cholinergic). The first system is divided into alpha and beta. The beta is further divided into $beta_1$ and $beta_2$.

It has been found that agents which stimulate the $beta_2$ adrenergic system benefit asthmatics. Conversely, stimulation of the other branches of the adrenergic and/or cholinergic system can be detrimental to these patients. NIAID-sponsored research has demonstrated that many asthmatic individuals have diminished beta adrenergic function and increased cholinergic and alpha adrenergic responses. This combination predisposes individuals to asthma. Identification of this pattern of responses enables physicians to treat patients with asthma more effectively.

Some forms of asthma are thought to be caused by a blockade of certain structures (receptors) on bronchial cells that normally interact with the beta adrenergic agents. To test this hypothesis, NIAID-supported scientists at Creighton University in Omaha administered, to normal individuals and those with asthma, drugs that stimulate these receptors. Their results support the concept that agents that stimulate the beta receptors protect against bronchial asthma. The search is on to find drugs that will selectively stimulate beta receptors without producing undesirable side effects. Scientists are also studying the role that blockade of alpha adrenergic receptors may play in causing asthma.

Other research may also help explain the biochemical basis of emotional factors in an asthma attack. It appears that the chemical mediators released from the mast cells make bronchial smooth muscles very sensitive to the effects of the hormones released from nerves. Consequently, an emotional state that stimulates nerves to release these chemicals could aggravate an asthma attack already in progress.

Investigations into occupational exposures that cause bronchial asthma are being conducted at the AADC at Tulane University in New Orleans. One such substance is toluene diisocyanate (TDI), a chemical used in the manufacture of plastics. Scientists there have found that TDI causes bronchial constriction by means of a druglike mechanism that alters beta adrenergic function. This effect is related to the amount of TDI inhaled. In another occupational area, these researchers have shown that a blood test (RAST) can be used to diagnose asthma caused by inhalation of coffee dust by workers in this industry and as a predictive tool in screening prospective workers.

Outlook

Many questions remain to be answered about asthma, especially identification of the basic abnormalities that cause it. However, NIAID-supported researchers are rapidly expanding our knowledge of this disease. With increased comprehension, scientists should be able to develop new and sophisticated techniques for diagnosing asthma, as well as more effective agents for treating the disease and, perhaps, preventing it.

U.S. Department of Health and Human Services, Public Health Service, National Institutes of Health. Prepared by the National Institute of Allergy and Infectious Diseases, Bethesda, Md. 20205. NIH Publication No. 83–525, July 1983.

Back Pain
Ubiquitous, Controversial

A drug that can serve as an alternative to back surgery was approved by FDA a short time ago. Hailed by some as a breakthrough drug, chymopapain (Chymodiactin) is useful in those cases of back pain involving a herniated disc in the lower back that has not responded to more conservative treatment over an extended period.

But most back pain does not fit into this category and before assuming that a back problem can be helped by this new therapy, a person should try to determine what is causing the pain and what can be done about it.

The answers may be far from clear-cut. Experts often disagree on some of the causes and treatments of back pain.

Although theories vary as to what causes backs to hurt, most experts would agree that the most common causes are gradual wear and tear, stress (emotional and physical), and lack of proper exercise. Most back experts agree that the key to a pain-free back is strong muscles, particularly abdominal muscles.

In the opinion of Leon Root, M.D., in *Oh, My Aching Back* (Signet, 1975), many vague back maladies are due to disc problems that are not developed enough to be diagnosed as such. "Most severe disc problems," Dr. Root says, "got that way because they were neglected in the early stages." Dr. Root recommends a program of stretching and strengthening exercises for back problems. He says it is likely that "if you suffer from back pain your condition is caused not by organic disease, but by muscles that are weak, tense, fatigued, or all three.''

Alexander Mellerby, in *The Y's Way to a Healthy Back* (New Century Publishers, 1982), maintains that 80 percent of lower back pain is caused by weak or tense muscles, not by more serious problems. Mellerby claims that in the YMCA's nationwide program of exercise, which emphasizes relaxation, flexibility and strengthening, 80 percent of those enrolled experience some improvement. Pain is completely eliminated for 31 percent, Mellerby says.

Hatha Yoga is another physical regimen for which both preventive and recuperative benefits have been claimed. The two most important focuses in this ancient discipline are breathing and the spine and, as in the Y program, relaxation is combined with increasing flexibility and strength. Many postures that originated in Hatha Yoga, such as ''The Cat'' and ''The Bridge,'' have been incorporated into other back exercise programs.

Hamilton Hall, M.D., author of *The Back Doctor* (McGraw Hill, 1980), says that the most common sources of lower back problems are worn facet joints, herniated discs, and pinched nerves.

Dr. Hall explains that a person with a worn facet joint, one aspect of osteoarthritis of the spine, experiences worsening of pain when arching the back and lessening of pain when bending forward. He says the opposite is true of someone with a herniated disc.

A worn facet joint may result in misalignment of vertebrae due to loss of thickness in the disc separating them. The result is that vertebrae grind against one another. The joints wear down and in some cases bone spurs grow from the vertebrae, causing pain. Almost everyone eventually has a certain degree of osteoarthritis since it is an inevitable part of the aging process. The principal symptoms of osteoarthritis are pain, stiffness, and limitation of motion, particularly upon arising.

A herniated disc, or what is referred to in a misnomer as a ''slipped disc,'' occurs when a disc flattens out and the gelatin-like material within bulges or protrudes, sometimes also pressing on a nerve. A herniated disc also may be referred to as a ruptured or protruding disc.

It is not uncommon for a person to have both worn facet joints and a ruptured disc. In addition, a pinched nerve frequently occurs when a disc protrudes and presses on a nerve. This may cause leg pain that sometimes may be even more severe than the back pain a person is experiencing.

Middle-aged people are more prone to disc problems, and women in their late 50s are the most vulnerable of all. Back problems become rarer as people reach their 60s and beyond because the vertebrae stabilize.

Other causes of back pain include rheumatoid arthritis, gouty arthritis, some metabolic diseases, circulatory problems, osteoporosis (thinning of the bones), kidney infections, stomach ulcers, viral pneumonia, tipped uterus, and infections of ovaries and Fallopian tubes. Back pain can also be a symptom of cancer, even if the back is not the site of the cancer. However, this is not the usual cause of back pain.

Because there are so many possible causes of back pain, anyone who suffers from it should consult a physician for a diagnosis before embarking on any treatment or exercise program.

A number of peculiar problems arise in the diagnosis and treatment of back pain. One is that the extent of the physically apparent damage does not necessarily correspond to the amount of pain felt by the patient. Another is that disc abnormalities may not show up on X-rays because of their location. A third idiosyncrasy of back pain is the high placebo effect encountered in treatments. When double-blind tests (that is, tests in which neither physician nor patient knows which patient is receiving a real medication and which one is getting a placebo or inert substance) are conducted with various types of treatments, it is not unusual for the placebo to be reported as effective in relieving pain in 30 percent of the patients. The placebo effect in double-blind clinical trials of chymopapain was particularly high, with placebo being effective in 45 percent of the cases and chymopapain in 75 percent of the cases. One theory to explain this phenomenon is that when a person believes he or she is receiving a pain-relieving drug, the body releases endorphins, naturally occurring chemicals known to act as painkillers. However, this theory has not been scientifically proven, and why the placebo rate should be higher with back pain than with other types of pain remains unexplained.

The initial treatment prescribed by most medical doctors for back pain is limiting activity and, in severe cases, complete bed rest. Sometimes a physician will also prescribe aspirin and other painkilling drugs, nonsteroidal anti-inflammatory drugs (such as naproxen, ibuprofen, phenylbutazone or indomethacin), or muscle-relaxing drugs. Other treatments included in the term ''conservative treatment'' when talking about back pain may be one or more of the following: hot or cold packs, ointment rubs, back braces, traction, physical therapy, and exercise programs.

Because these measures may take a long time to be effective and require persistence, some physicians and patients try newer, less proven treatments such as manipulation, acupuncture, and TENS (Transcutaneous Electric Nerve Stimulation).

Chiropractors believe that manipulating the back or spine can provide relief from backache and cure various back problems. Their treatments are often similar to those provided by physical therapists; however, the physical therapist's manipulation is usually just one part of a program recommended by a physician. Often the results from manipulative therapy in terms of pain relief are rapid and dramatic. However, whether a cure can be effected solely by these methods alone is a matter of controversy.

The theory of acupuncture, the ancient Chinese healing art, is that needles inserted at certain points of the body can affect physical functioning, and back pain is one problem acupuncturists claim they can treat.

In Transcutaneous Electric Nerve Stimulation (TENS), a mild electric current is applied to certain sites on the body and purportedly relieves pain in another body area such as the back.

When treatments tried have not been successful, a physician and patient may want to consider surgery or treatment with chymopapain.

Before proceeding, however, the physician will want to make as definitive a diagnosis as possible to assure that the problem is one that can be treated by either of these.

Because disc problems often do not show up on conventional X-rays, other methods of imaging the spine must be used. Several procedures combine X-rays and an injected radiopaque solution.

In a discogram, the patient is put under anesthesia and the radiopaque liquid is injected directly into a disc. A normal disc retains the liquid, but if the disc is ruptured, the liquid leaks out.

A more frequently performed procedure is the myelogram, in which the radiopaque material is injected into the subdural space surrounding the spinal cord and nerve roots. In this procedure, the abnormality that the disc produces may be revealed but the disc itself is not seen. Side effects of this procedure sometimes include headache and irritation of the dural sac.

Other more recently developed procedures are the epiduralgram, epidural venogram, and CAT scan.

In an epiduralgram, the radiopaque liquid is injected outside the dural sac and an X-ray is taken to outline the bulging disc.

In the epidural venogram, the radiopaque fluid is injected into veins in the groin and flows into the back. If a disc is protruding enough to compress a nerve root, it will also probably compress a vein, a compression that may be revealed on the X-ray. This procedure produces the least discomfort of all the tests mentioned so far.

Additional ways to define nerve and joint involvement are by nerve root injection and joint injection. In both, a solution is made with radiopaque fluid and an anesthetic. If pain ceases when the solution is injected around a specific nerve root or facet joint, this gives the physician a pretty good clue as to the pain's origin, although it may not be totally accurate because nerves are so close to each other.

By far the least invasive, least painful, and usually the most accurate of procedures is Computed Axial Tomography (CAT). During a CAT scan, the patient lies motionless while the CAT scanner takes multiple X-ray exposures that are combined by a computer into one picture showing both soft tissue and bones. However, this is an expensive technology, not available everywhere.

When a person needs surgery for a severe and persistent herniated disc, a laminectomy is performed. During the operation, the protruding portion of the disc is removed and the surgeon makes certain that the disc no longer presses on nerves. The success rate for disc surgery has been estimated at 50 to 95 percent. The recuperation period is usually long, and the surgery and hospital stay make it an expensive option.

Chemonucleolysis, the technical name for the procedure in which chymopapain is used, is a procedure that must be performed in a hospital. However, it does not involve major surgery and the recuperative period is usually shorter than for back surgery. However, it does carry certain risks.

A relatively new procedure, chemonucleolysis requires specially trained physicians. Orthopedic and neurologic surgeons have been taught how to perform this procedure in courses sponsored jointly by the American Academy of Orthopedic Surgeons and the American Association of Neurologic Surgeons.

Chymopapain is a papaya-derived enzyme, very much like one of the active ingredients in meat tenderizer. In the chemonucleolysis procedure, after the patient is anesthetized, the physician—guided by fluoroscope—inserts a needle. The physician then checks the position of the needle and status of the herniated disc by performing a discogram. Then, into the disc the physician injects the chymopapain, which dissolves the mucoprotein portion of the protruding material to correct the herniation. The procedure is usually completed in less than an hour. The patient generally stays in the hospital 24 to 48 hours after the procedure.

According to some estimates, about half of the 200,000 persons who are candidates for disc surgery in the United States each year might benefit from treatment with chymopapain.

The most serious possible side effect with chymopapain treatment is anaphylaxis, an acute allergic reaction which, if not treated promptly, can be fatal. About 1 percent of patients treated with chymopapain can be expected to have such a reaction, and people who have had allergic reactions to papaya or meat tenderizers should not receive the drug. In clinical trials of chymopapain, anaphylaxis led to two deaths in approximately 1,400 patients, for a death rate similar to that of lumbar disc surgery.

Other common side effects with chymopapain are back pain, stiffness, soreness or muscle spasm. These usually disappear several days after treatment, although sometimes minor stiffness or soreness persists for several months.

For those who suffer from back pain of disc origin, then, a new option has been added to the treatments available. However, the number of patients for whom this option is appropriate is vastly outnumbered by those back pain sufferers who can be helped by less extreme measures. Persons with backaches should consult their physicians and explore with them the full range of possibilities for relief from this all too common ailment.

Judith Willis, reprinted from November 1983, FDA Consumer, HHS Publication No. (FDA) 84–3147. Department of Health and Human Services, Public Health Service, Food and Drug Administration, 5600 Fishers Lane, Rockville, Md. 20857. U.S. Government Printing Office 1987—181–341/40082.

Biofeedback
Plain Talk

What is biofeedback?

Biofeedback is a treatment technique in which people are trained to improve their health by using signals from their own bodies. Physical therapists use biofeedback to help stroke victims regain movement in paralyzed muscles. Psychologists use it to help tense and anxious clients learn to relax. Specialists in many different fields use biofeedback to help their patients cope with pain.

Chances are you have used biofeedback yourself. You've used it if you have ever taken your temperature or stepped on a scale. The thermometer tells you whether you're running a fever, the scale whether you've gained weight. Both devices "feed back" information about your body's condition. Armed with this information, you can take steps you've learned to improve the condition. When you're running a fever, you go to bed and drink plenty of fluids. When you've gained weight, you resolve to eat less and sometimes you do.

Clinicians rely on complicated biofeedback machines in somewhat the same way that you rely on your scale or thermometer. Their machines can detect a person's internal bodily functions with far greater sensitivity and precision than a person can alone. This information may be valuable. Both patients and therapists use it to gauge and direct the progress of treatment.

For patients, the biofeedback machine acts as a kind of sixth sense which allows them to "see" or "hear" activity inside their bodies. One commonly used type of machine, for example, picks up electrical signals in the muscles. It translates these signals into a form that patients can detect: It triggers a flashing light bulb, perhaps, or activates a beeper every time muscles grow more tense. If patients want to relax tense muscles, they try to slow down the flashing or beeping.

Like a pitcher learning to throw a ball across homeplate, the biofeedback trainee, in an attempt to improve a skill, monitors performance. When a pitch is off the mark, the ballplayer adjusts the delivery so that he performs better the next time he tries. When the light flashes or the beeper beeps too often, the biofeedback trainee makes internal adjustments which alter the signals. The biofeedback therapist acts as a coach, standing at the sidelines setting goals and limits on what to expect and giving hints on how to improve performance.

The beginnings of biofeedback

The biofeedback techniques used to treat patients were developed only recently. The word "biofeedback" is itself so new that it can't be found in most dictionaries. It was coined in the late 1960s to describe laboratory procedures then being used to train experimental research subjects to alter brain activity, blood pressure, heart rate, and other bodily functions that normally are not controlled voluntarily.

At the time, many scientists looked forward to the day when biofeedback would give us a major degree of control over our bodies. They thought, for instance, that we might be able to "will" ourselves to be more creative by changing the patterns of our brainwaves. Some believed that biofeedback would one day make it possible to do away with drug treatments that often cause uncomfortable side effects in patients with high blood pressure and other serious conditions.

Today, most scientists agree that such high hopes were not realistic. Research has demonstrated that biofeedback can help in the treatment of many diseases and painful conditions. It has shown that we have more control over so-called involuntary bodily functions than we once thought possible. But it has also shown that nature limits the extent of such control. Scientists are now trying to determine just how much voluntary control we can exert.

How is biofeedback used today?

Clinical biofeedback techniques that grew out of the early laboratory procedures are now widely used to treat an ever-lengthening list of conditions. These include:

- Migraine headaches, tension headaches, and many other types of pain
- Disorders of the digestive system
- High blood pressure and its opposite, low blood pressure
- Cardiac arrhythmias (abnormalities, sometimes dangerous, in the rhythm of the heartbeat)
- Raynaud's disease (a circulatory disorder that causes uncomfortably cold hands)
- Epilepsy
- Paralysis and other movement disorders

Specialists who provide biofeedback training range from psychiatrists and psychologists to dentists, internists, nurses, and physical therapists. Most rely on many other techniques in addition to biofeedback. Patients usually are taught some form of relaxation exercise. Some learn to identify the circumstances that trigger their symptoms. They may also be taught how to avoid or cope with these stressful events. Most are encouraged to change their habits, and some are trained in special techniques for gaining such self-control. Biofeedback is not magic. It cannot cure disease or, by itself, make a person healthy. It is a tool, one of many available to health care professionals. It reminds physicians that behavior, thoughts, and feelings profoundly influence physical health. And it helps both patients and doctors understand that they must work together as a team.

Patients' responsibilities

Biofeedback places unusual demands on patients. They must examine their day-to-day lives to learn if they may be contributing to their own distress. They must recognize that they can, by their own efforts, remedy some physical ailments. They must commit themselves to practicing biofeedback or relaxation exercises every day. They must change bad habits, even ease up on some good ones. Most important, they must accept much of the responsibility for maintaining their own health.

How does biofeedback work?

Scientists cannot yet explain how biofeedback works. Most patients who benefit from biofeedback are trained to relax and modify their behavior. Most scientists believe that relaxation is a key component in biofeedback treatment of many disorders, particularly those brought on or made worse by stress.

Their reasoning is based on what is known about the effect of stress on the body. In brief, the argument goes like this: Stressful events produce strong emotions, which arouse certain physical responses. Many of these responses are controlled by the sympathetic nervous system, the network of nerve tissue that helps prepare the body to meet emergencies by "flight or fight."

The typical pattern of response to emergencies probably emerged during the time when all humans faced mostly physical threats. Although the "threats" we now live with are seldom physical, the body reacts as if they were: The pupils dilate to let in more light. Sweat pours out, reducing the chance of skin cuts. Blood vessels near the skin contract to reduce bleeding, while those in the brain and muscles dilate to increase the oxygen supply. The gastrointestinal tract, including the stomach and intestines, slows down to reduce the energy expended in digestion. The heart beats faster, and blood pressure rises.

Normally, people calm down when a stressful event is over—especially if they have done something to cope with it. For instance, imagine your own reactions if you're walking down a dark street and hear someone running toward you. You get scared. Your body prepares you to ward off an attacker or run fast enough to get away. When you do escape, you gradually relax.

If you get angry at your boss, it's a different matter. Your body may prepare to fight. But since you want to keep your job, you try to ignore the angry feelings. Similarly, if on the way home you get stalled in traffic, there's nothing you can do to get away. These situations can literally make you sick. Your body has prepared for action, but you cannot act.

Individuals differ in the way they respond to stress. In some, one function, such as blood pressure, becomes more active while others remain normal. Many experts believe that these individual physical responses to stress can become habitual. When the body is repeatedly aroused, one or more functions may become permanently overactive. Actual damage to bodily tissues may eventually result.

Biofeedback is often aimed at changing habitual reactions to stress that can cause pain or disease. Many clinicians believe that some of their patients and clients have forgotten how to relax. Feedback of physical responses such as skin temperature and muscle tension provides information to help patients recognize a relaxed state. The feedback signal may also act as a kind of reward for reducing tension. It's like a piano teacher whose frown turns to a smile when a young musician finally plays the tune properly.

The value of a feedback signal as information and reward may be even greater in the treatment of patients with paralyzed or spastic muscles. With these patients, biofeedback seems to be primarily a form of skill training—like learning to pitch a ball. Instead of watching the ball, the patient watches the machine, which monitors activity in the affected muscle. Stroke victims with paralyzed arms and legs, for example, see that some part of their affected limbs remains active. The signal from the biofeedback machine proves it. This signal can guide the exercises that help patients regain use of their limbs. Perhaps just as important, the feedback convinces patients that the limbs are still alive. This reassurance often encourages them to continue their efforts.

Should you try biofeedback?

If you think you might benefit from biofeedback training, you should discuss it with your physician or other health care professional, who may wish to conduct tests to make certain that your condition does not require conventional medical treatment first. Responsible biofeedback therapists will not treat you for headaches, hypertension, or most disorders until you have had a thorough physical examination. Some require neurological tests as well.

How do you find a biofeedback therapist? First, ask your doctor or dentists, or contact the nearest community mental health center, medical society, or State biofeedback society for a referral. The psychology or psychiatry departments at nearby universities may also be able to help you. Most experts recommend that you consult only a health care professional—a physician, psychologist, psychiatrist, nurse, social worker, dentist, physical therapist, mental health counselor, for example—who has been trained to use biofeedback.

Professional associations

The Biofeedback Society of America, 4301 Owens Street, Wheat Ridge, CO 80033, (303) 422–8436. The Biofeedback Society has established application guidelines for biofeedback practitioners. It also maintains a network of State societies.

The Biofeedback Certification Institute of America, 4301 Owens Street, Wheat Ridge, CO 80033, (303) 420–2902. The BCIA was established as an independent agency to provide national certification for biofeedback providers. The BCIA holds membership in the National Commission for Health Certifying Agencies.

American Association of Biofeedback Clinicians, 2424 Dempster Avenue, Des Plains, IL 60016.

Bette Runck, Division of Communications and Education, National Institute of Mental Health; Plain Talk about Biofeedback, DHHS Pub. No. (ADM) 85–1273, National Institute of Mental Health, 1983, 1985.

Bloodclots
The Story Behind the Scab

Our bloodstream—the circulatory, or vascular, system—serves many functions. It is a food and sewage conduit, a pipeline for defense supplies, and a communications system. It is also continually answering its own version of the question with which Hamlet grappled so fiercely: "To be or not to be?" But for the blood, the crucial, constant question is: "To clot or not to clot?"

Blood is under considerable pressure as it races out from the pumphouse of the heart to the arteries, to the smaller tributaries called arterioles, to the gossamer mesh of the capillaries, and then via venules through the gauntlet of one-way valves in our veins back to the heart. This pressure means that any break in a vessel wall is potentially life-threatening.

To contend with this ever-present threat, whenever a vessel ruptures—no matter how tiny the tear—almost instantly, at the exact point of break, a remarkable process transforms a portion of the swiftly moving liquid into a solid clot that seals and mends, and thus maintains life. The process involves an interplay among the vessel wall, certain cell fragments called platelets, and clotting agents in the blood plasma.

The platelets, which are constantly circulating within the bloodstream, are manufactured by very large cells, appropriately called Giant Cells, in the bone marrow. The platelets are actually fragments of these cells, shed into the blood. The word "fragment" usually connotes something partial and comparatively unimportant, but that connotation scarcely applies to platelets. Without these fragments life would be impossible, for they play a key role in the silent, internal drama surrounding that "to clot or not" question.

A blood specialist (hematologist) compared the platelet (so-called because of its plate-like shape) to a sponge ". . . loaded with diverse and biologically active compounds, some of which it can soak up during its voyage through the circulation and all of which it can discharge where . . . needed." These platelet/sponges, so tiny that 250,000 are needed to seal a pinhole, move with the flow of blood until they encounter a break in the lining of the blood vessel. That encounter triggers a remarkable sequence of events, called the hemostatic mechanism.

The sequence begins with the vascular phase, when various signals cause blood vessels to contract to reduce the flow of blood to the injury. The second—the platelet—phase is absolutely critical. The platelets make contact with collagen, a fibrous substance exposed by the break in the vessel wall. This contact triggers release of a chemical "signal" called adenosine diphosphate (ADP). The signal recruits more platelets to stick to the vessel wall, forming a loose, temporary plug at the point of injury. Meanwhile, the platelets release various chemicals that start the third—the coagulation—phase.

Coagulation—creation of a clot to replace the temporary plug—involves a cascade of chemical reactions involving more than a dozen different proteins (usually found in the plasma), as well as components such as phospholipids (fats) released by the activated platelets. The result is a mesh of tough, fibrous strands—fibrin—formed in and around the platelet plug, where it captures the bricks and mortar needed to build the clot: red and white blood cells as they pass, as well as more platelets and plasma. Within minutes, the clot begins to contract, squeezing out fluid and, if exposed to air, becomes a rough, hard lump.

Without this intricate system of vascular self-defense, a pinprick on the skin or a microscopic fissure in the smallest capillary deep within the body would be as fatal as a sword thrust through the heart. (Major breaks in a blood vessel set off additional mechanisms; some, such as a severed artery, are under such pressure that they cannot self-seal but require medical assistance.)

Truly, as the Devil said in Goethe's *Faust,* the "blood is a wonderful juice." But the workings of this wonderful juice can be disrupted in a number of ways, all injurious to health, some fatally so. Failure of the clotting mechanism, for example, can occur from hereditary defects. (Hemophilia from lack of a clotting agent known as Factor VIII is the best-known example.) The mechanism can also be disturbed by defects in the blood vessels themselves (such as hereditary hemorrhagic telangiectasia) or a deficiency in the number or function of the platelets (as in idiopathic thrombocytopenic purpura).

Clotting deficiencies can also result from destruction of bone marrow, the manufacturing site of platelets, caused by toxic chemicals (such as benzene), radiation or cancer (especially leukemia). Deficiencies can also result from liver disease, such as acute hepatitis and cirrhosis (caused by excessive alcohol consumption). Other clotting troubles result from the use of certain drugs, such as heparin, aspirin, phenylbutazone, dextran, indomethacin and warfarin; from scurvy (a lack of vitamin C, which is needed to maintain blood vessel integrity); a shortage of vitamin K, needed by the liver to produce substances required for coagulation; and infection and allergies.

Clotting deficiencies can even result from medical treatment, including use of antibiotics that destroy intestinal bacteria that produce vitamin K. Clotting deficiencies also are associated with massive blood transfusions (storing blood results in platelets and clotting agents of poor quality).

Balancing the delicate clotting mechanism, the body also possesses an equally precise system for clot elimination. This system (called fibrinolysis, or simply lysis) is so finely tuned that normally a clot is removed neither too soon, which would cause resumed bleeding, nor too late, which would needlessly block circulation. Fibrinolysis involves substances to keep blood from turning solid and processes to clean up the fragments when parts of it do turn solid. The liver, bone marrow, spleen, white blood cells, and various enzymes are all involved in the cleanup process. The liver, bone marrow and spleen continually filter small clots from the blood; white blood cells devour any fragments they encounter; and a family of enzymes called plasminogen activators triggers a process that produces plasmin, which consumes any stray fibrin threads it finds in the bloodstream.

Unfortunately, the blood sometimes responds to its Hamlet-like question by deciding to clot when it should not. In terms of overall health impact, this problem is a far greater risk to overfed, underexercised humans than clotting deficiencies. Deaths caused by thrombosis—the inappropriate or unnecessary appearance of clots in blood vessels—far exceed the toll from cancer.

Inappropriate clots—thrombi (plural of thrombus, the Greek word for "clot")—have a multitude of causes, ranging from long periods of immobility when blood flow is sluggish to a blood disease such as polycythemia, in which the bone marrow produces an excessive number of blood cells.

In the arteries, clot formation is associated with atherosclerosis, a gradual narrowing of the blood vessels due to an accumulation of cholesterol and other substances in the form of plaque. This plaque provides a surface to which blood components can stick, eventually resulting in the formation of clots.

When a thrombus remains in one place in a vein, accompanied by inflammation of the vessel wall, the condition is called thrombophlebitis, or just phlebitis. Superficial phlebitis occurs in veins close to the skin (usually in the forearm). In a deep vein surrounded by muscles (usually in the thigh or pelvis), it is called deep-vein thrombosis, a much more serious problem. The blocked vein in superficial phlebitis reveals itself by the visible presence of a tender, inflamed area extending along the course of the vein. Deep-vein phlebitis is far more difficult to diagnose. Symptoms may include pain, often accompanied by swelling, and a feeling of weakness together with fever, chills and loss of appetite. While these symptoms are distressing enough, the real danger is that the offending clot, or a portion of it, may break off and be carried along in a vein or an artery, transforming phlebitis—even the superficial variety—into a potentially fatal affliction.

A clot that moves is called an embolus. From a vein, an embolus can move through the bloodstream, pass through the heart, and on into the artery connecting the heart and the lungs (the pulmonary artery). There it can block some of the blood supply to one of the lungs, reducing the volume of oxygen-rich blood that eventually reaches the rest of the body. It is estimated that there are over 600,000 pulmonary embolism cases in the United States each year, with the death rate about one in 400.

An embolism can also start in an artery. Since blood moves from the heart through arteries that gradually divide into ever narrower vessels, at some point an embolus can move no farther, creating an internal dam. Unless there are other blood vessels—collaterals—that can maintain circulation to the affected area, tissues denied oxygen and nutrients are damaged and usually die. Such tissue destruction is called an infarction.

Among the most dramatic examples of infarction are stroke from an embolus lodging in one of the arteries of the brain (cerebral embolism) and heart attack (myocardial infarction), where it blocks one of the coronary arteries that supply blood to the heart muscle itself.

If the tissue destruction of a myocardial infarction continues, it will eventually cripple the heart, with a possibly fatal outcome. However, this sequence is not inevitable. If the clot can be removed within about six hours of onset of the chest pain that signals a heart attack, the affected portion of the heart can be saved; afterward the damage is usually irreversible. That there is hope if a heart attack victim gets to a hospital on time is due not only to a greater understanding of the role played by clots (together with platelet buildup and spasms in the vessel wall) in triggering heart attacks, but also to new surgical techniques and the availability of various drugs. These advances have caused a revolution in treating persons at risk from or undergoing a heart attack.

Certain drugs (aspirin, dipyridamole, sulfinpyrazone) can be administered to prevent platelet buildup where an artery is narrowed as the result of plaque formation. Enzymes called thrombolytic agents (streptokinase, derived from bacteria, and urokinase, derived from human urine) can be used to break down the thrombus blocking a coronary artery. Some drugs (nitroglycerin and calcium channel blockers such as verapamil, nifedipine and diltiazem) relax the wall of the coronary artery, while others (calcium channel blockers—again—and the beta blockers metoprolol and propranolol) decrease the workload and oxygen demands being made on the heart muscle.

Much is still to be learned about how best to orchestrate these therapies and avoid complications. Tests are currently under way at the National Heart, Lung, and Blood Institute to assess the effectiveness of various combinations of these drugs in clearing out (lysing) coronary clots.

There are many preventive practices that can reduce the risk of clotting problems. Smoking, drinking alcohol to excess, poor nutrition, high blood pressure, and stress have been associated with recurrence of thrombosis and embolisms. This is particularly important regarding heart attacks, where, in about one-quarter of the patients, the first sign that a problem exists is also the last—sudden death.

A recent report by an expert team assembled by the National Institutes of Health strongly urged Americans to follow a low-fat diet in order to lower individual levels of cholesterol, which is largely responsible for the plaque buildup to which platelets and thrombi adhere. Exercise and not sitting too long in one position are also very important in preventing thrombosis. The understanding of the importance of exercise in preventing circulatory problems has produced a new approach toward hospitalized persons. Physicians now realize that patients should move around as much as their condition will permit. For heart attack victims, exercise plays a triple role: It strengthens the heart, it helps restore confidence, and it helps prevent new clots from forming.

However, it is not possible to prevent all clotting problems by lifestyle changes. Some problems stem from congenital conditions such as deficiencies in anti-clotting agents. Others are related to an event such as an operation, injury, childbirth, illness, an unavoidable prolonged period of bed rest, or use of contraceptives or other drugs containing estrogen.

There are two primary and related ways of contending with inappropriate clotting: removing the cause and making the blood less subject to coagulation. For example, for thrombophlebitis, the physician will consider antibiotics to fight the infection that has inflamed the blood vessel wall, as well as methods to speed up blood return to the affected vein. Deep-vein thrombosis poses a more difficult problem, and the physician may, after necessary tests, prescribe anticoagulant drugs or even surgery.

Anticoagulant drugs, such as those used to treat heart attack victims, fall into three classes: those that impede fibrin formation (for example, heparin, which interferes with active clotting factors, and dicumarol, which inhibits production of certain clotting factors); those that keep platelets from sticking together (aspirin); and those that consume the fibrin clot (urokinase and streptokinase). Before considering use of such medicines, the physician needs to know whether the patient has any condition—such as recent surgery or ulcers—in which bleeding might constitute a significant hazard or be hard to manage because of its location.

In addition to drugs already approved by the Food and Drug Administration and on the market, a genetically engineered blood clot dissolver is currently being tested. Made from tissue plasminogen activator, or TPA (one of the substances found in the body in minute quantities as part of the normal clot-removal process), it is being produced in large quantities by splicing the TPA gene into bacteria. TPA is still experimental and has not yet been submitted to FDA for marketing approval. But it may offer a significant advantage over both streptokinase and urokinase in that, while these enzymes work throughout the body and thus can lead to unwanted bleeding, TPA seeks out the clot and activates the clot-removing mechanism only in that immediate area. If studies prove it safe and effective, it could join the front rank of drugs that help the body's circulatory system correctly decide just where and when "to clot or not to clot."

Tim Larkin, *FDA Consumer*, March 1985.

Brain Tumors
Hope Through Research

She was 20, an attractive English major at a Boston college, engaged to be married. Then she was diagnosed as having a brain tumor of a particularly advanced and malignant type that was invading the right frontal lobe of her brain. Marriage was definitely out, she decided, but she wasn't giving up. The surgeons removed the bulk of the tumor and followed up with radiation and chemotherapy. Now, seven years later, there is no sign of cancer. She still rules out marriage, but she's back in college.

A 45-year-old minister and biblical scholar recently underwent his fourth operation for a meningioma, a tumor of the outer coverings of the brain. Usually a meningioma is a slow-growing tumor, often completely removable by surgery. In the minister's case, however, the tumor recurred, first after a year or so, then after only months. This time the brain surgeons planned to follow up with a new anticancer drug.

Usually. Slow-growing. Removable. Malignant. Invasive. Advanced. The words are the common jargon of the cancer expert. The words are familiar to nonexperts as well, for who among us has not been touched by the death of friend or relative who has succumbed to cancer?

When it comes to brain tumors, however, the familiar words take on new meanings. The brain is a special organ, special in the cells that compose it, in its position in the head, and in its relation to the rest of the body. When a tumor grows in the brain, doctors have to consider not only the nature of the tumor, but its relation to the brain's distinctive features.

The nature of the brain

First and foremost among those features is that the brain is the organ of thought, emotion, and behavior. The idea that a mass of abnormal tissue could encroach on that domain, undermining the mental faculties that make us human and ultimately threatening life itself, is what terrifies most people when they hear the words *brain tumor*. Yet some brain tumors can be removed completely at surgery leaving no neurological damage. Even advanced cancers growing deep inside the brain are being tackled today by new treatments that have saved or at least prolonged lives, while preserving the integrity of those lives.

Experts can also point to other features of the brain that offer some reason for hope. Tumors are generally classified as benign—if the tumor cells look much like ordinary cells and the tumor is confined to one place—or malignant, if the tumor cells look very disordered and the tumor can spread (metastasize) to other parts of the body. (Strictly speaking, the word *cancer* applies only to malignant growths.) Tumors that originate in the brain—primary brain tumors—may be either benign or malignant. Surprisingly, while malignant brain tumor cells can spread throughout the brain, only rarely do they spread to other parts of the body. That means that once you destroy a brain cancer, you need not worry that some cells may have escaped to seed tumors elsewhere in the body.

Another fact that startles many people is that brain tumor tissue almost never consists of the fundamental working cells of the brain—the nerve cells (neurons). Once mature, these complex nerve cells no longer divide and multiply. Instead, it is the surrounding and supporting cells of the brain that occasionally get out of control. Thus a brain tumor that is diagnosed and treated early may do little or no damage to essential brain matter—the neurons and their circuits that underlie every act of mental life and behavior.

Confusing symptoms

There are "if's." Brain tumors are not always easy to diagnose. The symptoms can vary widely according to the brain area affected. If a tumor grows in the temporal lobe on the left side of the brain, for example, it may affect speech and memory, or alter mood and emotional state. Such symptoms might suggest mental illness or psychological problems, rather than a brain tumor. If a tumor lies near the cerebellum, an area at the back of the brain important in the control of movement, there may be early symptoms of dizziness and lack of coordination. Tumors growing on or around the major nerves supplying the ears or eyes may lead to symptoms of hearing loss, headaches, or visual problems, diverting attention from the brain as the source of trouble.

On the other hand, some brain tumors may produce few symptoms. Parts of the frontal lobes, for example, are presumed to play a role in thinking and other higher mental activities. Yet tumors can sometimes cause considerable tissue damage in these areas with little effect on a person's behavior.

Once a tumor is found, still another "if" centers on its location in relation to surrounding tissue. The brain is one of the most protected organs in the body. It is wrapped in the tough outer coverings of the meninges, bathed in shock-absorbing and nutrient liquid—the cerebrospinal fluid—and armored by the strong bones of the skull.

If a tumor lies near the skull bones or close to major blood vessels or channels circulating cerebrospinal fluid, it need not grow very large before it blocks blood or cerebrospinal fluid circulation and causes increased pressure inside the skull. Or, if the tumor is discovered deep inside the brain, surgery to remove it may be risky, with too great a chance of damaging vital brain centers. Ironically, the distinction between benign and malignant blurs in such cases. If a benign tumor is inaccessible it can be fatal. On the other hand, the young woman with the malignant tumor invading her frontal lobe had a major portion of the lobe removed and is alive and well today.

Neurosurgeons who treat brain tumor patients are well aware of the ironies of the condition. They can all tell stories of exceptional survivals as well as tragic deaths. Scientists who have made research on brain tumors their specialty are particularly concerned that the public understand the complex problems posed by brain tumors as well as the growing efforts to solve those problems.

Those investigators include scientists supported by the National Institute of Neurological and Communicative Disorders and Stroke (NINCDS)— the leading Federal agency supporting research on the brain—the National Cancer Institute, and other Federal health agencies. One major group effort is the clinical research program carried out by NINCDS neurosurgeons working at the Clinical Center, the research hospital of the National Institutes of Health in Bethesda, Md.

11,000 cases a year

The chances of developing a primary malignant brain tumor are relatively rare—about 1 in 22,000. Such cancers account for less than 2 percent of all cancers diagnosed in the United States every year. That is still an impressively large number—11,000 brain cancers annually. At least twice as many patients have secondary brain cancers, the result of cancer metastasizing to the brain from other sites in the body, principally the breast, lung, or kidney.

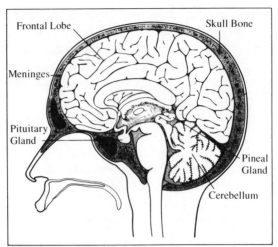

The brain, wrapped in its meningeal coverings, fits snugly against the bones of the skull.

Brain tumors affect children as well as adults. Indeed, primary tumors of the brain or spinal cord (the central nervous system) are the most common tumors of childhood after the leukemias. The peak for brain tumors in children is between the ages of 6 and 9. Childhood brain tumors generally differ in location and cellular makeup from adult tumors, differences thought to reflect a still growing and developing nervous system. Adult brain tumors are most common between the ages of 40 and 60, with men affected slightly more than women.

Why primary brain tumors occur remains a mystery. Tumor sleuths have considered the vast array of environmental and genetic factors that have been linked to cancers in other parts of the body, but in the case of brain tumors there are no clear-cut associations. The recent finding of a slightly higher than normal occurrence of brain tumors in workers at certain petrochemical plants is interesting, but the cases are too few for scientists to come to firm conclusions. There are also a few families in the United States where cancer, including brain cancer, occurs frequently. Some genetic factor could possibly account for these families' high cancer prevalence—perhaps some defect in the body's immune system. Again, more detailed genetic and biochemical studies are needed.

Diagnosing brain tumors today

Clearly not every headache, dizzy spell, or visual disturbance is a sign of brain tumor. And while symptoms can vary widely, specialists pay particular attention to certain signs:

- *Progressive unrelenting symptoms.* Whatever they may be, the symptoms never let up and they get worse over time.
- *Headache.* Given the tight confines of the head, a growing tumor sooner or later will create pressure or swelling that affects tissues in the head, producing severe headache. Often the patient reports that the headache is worse upon first waking in the morning. Interestingly, brain tissue itself is normally insensitive to pain. But the meningeal layers, blood vessel walls, and the tissues lining the cavities of the brain and skull are rich in nerve endings sensitive to pain.
- *Visual complaints.* Double vision, blurring, or other visual symptoms may occur as a result of increased pressure on the optic nerve or the blood vessels supplying the retina.
- *Motor signs.* Some patients report weakness or numbness in their arms and legs. Sometimes reflexes (like the familiar knee jerk reflex) are very strong. In the case of spinal cord tumors, patients may experience a growing loss of sensation below a certain level in the trunk, or increasing difficulty in moving limbs.
- *Seizures.* The onset of seizures or convulsions in a patient who has not been in an accident, been ill with fever, or suffered some other injury or illness is "presumptive evidence of a brain tumor until proven otherwise," says one leading authority.

To confirm the diagnosis, neurologists and neurosurgeons can conduct a battery of tests including simple X-rays of the head, standard brainwave recordings (the electroencephalogram or EEG), analysis of cerebrospinal fluid, and so on. Their principal diagnostic aid today, however, is the CT scan, the technique that produces a computerized three-dimensional X-ray image of the brain. The CT scan is highly accurate, detecting the presence of a tumor mass in 90 to 95 percent of cases—even when that mass is no larger than half an inch across.

The CT scan can not only indicate the presence of a tumor, but will pin down its location in the brain. At this point the specialist may call for an arteriogram: an X-ray that will outline the arteries supplying blood to the tumor. Some tumors are richly endowed with blood vessels; others are less so. Thus the arteriogram provides another clue to the kind of brain tumor.

The next step

Surgery is the first line of attack against brain tumors. How extensive the operation will be depends on the tumor size and location and whether the tumor cells are concentrated in a mass or spread throughout the brain. "Each patient's tumor is different," notes the chief of the NINCDS

Surgical Neurology Branch in the NIH Clinical Center. "It is different pathologically, it behaves differently, and it grows differently."

For that reason, some of the tissue removed at brain surgery is always reserved for pathological analysis. Studies of this "biopsy" material indicate whether the tumor is benign or malignant. Malignant tumor tissue removed at surgery is also being used in promising research studies aimed at improving treatment—even predicting which treatments will be successful.

Observers examining samples of brain tissue microscopically can tell what kinds of cells make up a tumor, and whether the cells are benign or malignant. Benign cells resemble normal cells of the tissue in question. Malignant cells lose more and more of their distinctive trademarks and acquire the classic characteristics of cancer: large or multiple nuclei, abnormal numbers of chromosomes, and changes in the cell's surface membrane. These changes seem to help very malignant cells to invade and take root in other tissues more easily. The extent of these changes permits classifying tumor cells by degree of malignancy from Grade I, benign, to Grade IV, the most advanced stage of malignancy.

Tumor varieties

Most brain tumors are *gliomas,* derived from the glial cells that support the neurons of the brain. Gliomas can be either benign or malignant. Unfortunately, one of the most malignant gliomas—the *glioblastoma multiforme*—is also the most common brain tumor. In all, gliomas account for 43 percent of primary brain cancers. Glial tumors are further described in terms of the type of glial cell they contain:

- *Astrocytomas.* Star-shaped cells called astrocytes are the cells affected in a large subgroup of gliomas. Benign cerebellar astrocytomas are common childhood tumors. With today's tools and techniques, these tumors are often completely removable surgically. They are one of the recent success stories in tumor treatment. On the other hand, the young woman college student's frontal lobe tumor was a malignant astrocytoma. What makes her story so impressive is that it was a Grade IV malignancy—an aggressive, rapidly growing tumor that is usually fatal in a year or so.
- *Medulloblastomas.* The root "blast" refers to a cell in an early stage of development. Medulloblasts are immature cells that may develop into either neurons or glial cells. Medulloblastomas are malignant tumors found in the rear of the brain. They typically occur in youngsters under 12 and account for a small percentage of all brain tumors.
- *Ependymomas.* The cells lining the hollow cavities of the brain—

ependymal cells—also give rise to a small percentage of brain tumors. These "ependymomas" tend to be benign.

Other gliomas are composed of other varieties of glial cells, such as those that produce the fatty insulating material (myelin) that surrounds many nerve fibers in the brain.

The second major group of primary brain tumors are those made up of covering cells:

- *Meningiomas*. Tumors of the meninges (the membrane coverings of the brain and spinal cord) are usually benign, and account for some 15 percent of all brain tumors.
- *Schwannomas*. These tumors arise from the Schwann cells that form the fatty sheath that envelops nerve fibers in the body. One such tumor develops in relation to the nerve of hearing, the acoustic nerve. Acoustic nerve tumors, called *acoustic neuromas,* are benign tumors which, if detected early, can be completely removed without loss of hearing or other nervous system damage.

The successful removal of acoustic neuromas is a good illustration of how far neurosurgeons have advanced in techniques. During the first decade of this century the mortality rate for acoustic neuroma surgery was close to 80 percent. The tumor was deep-seated and difficult to remove because of its close relation to the brain stem, a core of brain tissue that contains vital nerve centers such as those controlling breathing. By 1917, however, the doctor considered to be the father of neurosurgery, Harvey Cushing, demonstrated a new technique for acoustic neuroma removal which reduced mortality to 20 percent. With more experience Cushing was able to reduce mortality to below 10 percent. Today the mortality rate for acoustic neuroma is down to 1 percent.

Other kinds of tumor may involve cells in or near the pituitary gland at the base of the brain, or the pineal gland, deep in the center of the brain. In rare instances a brain tumor will develop from types of nerve cells.

Surgery plus . . .

In the case of a benign accessible brain tumor, surgery may be the beginning and end of treatment: The tumor is completely removed and the patient resumes activities with little likelihood of recurrence. If the tumor is malignant, it may not be possible to remove it completely. In that case, or if a tumor is large or difficult to reach, treatment will include radiation and chemotherapy. Radiation is sometimes used before surgery in the hope of reducing tumor size.

Today, an increasing number of tumors formerly considered inoperable can be tackled surgically. Microsurgery—the use of an operating microscope—has played an important role in that development. But often it is a combination of great technical skill and an ingenious strategy for getting at the tumor that has led to surgical success.

A few neurosurgeons are currently using high frequency sound waves (ultrasound) and laser beams to destroy brain tumors. In one laser technique, for example, the surgeon uses an operating microscope and aims the laser beam at the center of the tumor, using the high intensity rays to burn out the tissue. The exact position of the tumor is calculated by a computer that translates CT scan images into a set of coordinates referable to a framework set up around the patient's head. Time will tell whether such techniques will improve the success rate for tumor treatment.

Radiation usually begins within a week or two after surgery and continues for six weeks. Among recent refinements in radiation therapy are the use of drugs that make tumor tissue more sensitive to radioactive bombardment, and new radioactive sources that provide more powerful rays or charged particles that can be sharply focused on the tumor.

Chemotherapy, the other major weapon in the attack on brain tumors, has also benefited from refinements and advances. The principal brain tumor-killing drugs in use today go by the initials BCNU and CCNU, both chemically known as nitrosoureas. These drugs pass readily into the brain when given by mouth or injected into the bloodstream. Many drugs are prevented from reaching brain cells by an elaborate meshwork of fine blood vessels and cells—the blood-brain barrier—that filters blood reaching the brain.

The combined treatment of brain cancers with better drugs and radiotherapy, along with surgical techniques aimed at removing as much tumor tissue as possible, has meant longer survival times and richer lives for brain cancer patients. Further improvements in these traditional forms of treatment can be expected in the years ahead. In addition, scientists are developing new therapies based on promising laboratory studies.

The new research

If a single word could describe the aim of much current research on malignant brain tumors, it might be the word *fingerprint*. Scientists want to characterize tumor tissue in ways that make the tissue as unique to the patient as his or her fingerprints. Armed with that information, the hope is that doctors can design more effective treatments—with added confidence that those treatments will work.

The impetus for this research comes first from the need to determine what kinds of cells are found in the tumor and their degree of malignancy.

Second, there is a strong suspicion that the reason that those tumor cells are there to begin with is that the body's immune system is deficient in some way.

Normally, the immune system seeks out and destroys invading organisms or foreign tissue. These defense mechanisms are called into play because foreign tissue is studded with telltale surface proteins—antigens—that differ from the surface antigens normally found on body cells. The immune system recognizes the foreign tissue and is stimulated to make a variety of cells—scavengers, "killer" cells, and others—as well as the protein compounds called antibodies—all specifically designed to fight that particular foreign invader. When the body's *own* cells become cancerous, their surface antigens also change. They, too, should appear foreign. By rights, a person's immune system ought to attack the cancer and destroy it.

There is evidence that the immune system tries to do just that. Investigators have been able to take samples of brain tumor tissue removed during surgery and grow the cells in tissue culture. When the scientists later expose the cultured cells to blood serum from the patient who provided the cells, they find that the serum contains antibodies that attack the tumor cells. The ammunition is there; it is just not powerful enough.

Scientists at NINCDS and elsewhere are exploring ways to boost patients' immune responses so that they can successfully fight their brain tumors or any remnants of tumor tissue not removed during surgery. One way is through immune *stimulation*. The idea is to use the patient's own tumor cells as the stimulating material. The cells are grown in tissue culture and then irradiated to prevent them from reproducing. The cells still contain their surface antigens, however, and so when injected back into the patient's body, they should provoke a strong response—both cells and antibodies—from the immune system. Currently NINCDS investigators are conducting such experimental treatments in selected patients with highly malignant astrocytomas.

The ability to grow human brain cancer cells in tissue culture has paid off in other ways as well. Tumor samples from a patient can be grown on separate culture plates and subjected to a variety of tests. Some tests are used to determine the degree of malignancy of tumor cells, a necessary step in planning treatment. One way to measure malignancy is to observe how rapidly the cells multiply and fill the culture plate. Investigators can also expose the cells to a fine-holed filter and see how aggressively the cells try to penetrate the openings.

Scientists can also transplant human brain tumor cells to laboratory animals to see if the human tumor will take root in the animal's body. The animals used are mice with a hereditary defect that renders them hairless as well as lacking the thymus, an organ important in the immune system. The immune system defect makes these "nude mice" less likely than normal animals to reject foreign tissue. The ability to grow a human cancer in a living animal is in itself of great importance: Scientists can observe how the tumor behaves at all stages of growth, as well as experiment with new therapies.

Tailor-made treatments

Provided with samples of a patient's tumor cells in tissue culture, investigators can also test the effectiveness of antitumor drugs. There appears to be a correlation between the way tumor cells respond to drugs in the laboratory dish and the way they respond in the brain. Thus if the lab studies show that BCNU and CCNU have little or no effect on cells grown in culture, there is little likelihood that these drugs will benefit the patient. For these "nonresponders," investigators may try other tactics, such as the use of new antitumor drugs still in the experimental stage. (The biblical scholar will receive such an experimental drug.)

With continued experience and refinements in culturing techniques, it may be possible to custom design brain tumor treatment programs, selecting the right drug at the right dosage and initiating treatment quickly, without having to go through a lengthy trial and error period. Such tactics not only save precious time, they also spare the patient the futility of ineffective treatments and may also reduce side effects.

Tissue culture techniques may also make it easier to diagnose a brain tumor early—when physicians may suspect that a tumor is present, but nothing is detectable on a CT scan. NINCDS scientists and others have taken blood samples from patients with suspected malignancies and added the serum to established laboratory cultures of human brain tumor cells. If the patient has a brain tumor, there is a high probability that the blood serum will contain antitumor antibodies that will react with the tumor cells on the laboratory plate.

Alternative treatments

The tissue culture and immunotherapy techniques are among the most promising and exciting lines of investigation being explored in brain tumor research today. There are others as well. Radiologists continue to seek out more effective methods of irradiating tumor tissue in the brain without jeopardizing surrounding tissue. Likewise, pharmacologists search for better antitumor drugs and ways of delivering those drugs to the brain. The use of a type of sugar called mannitol, for example, can disrupt the blood-brain barrier for a brief period of time and allow chemicals access to brain tissue. However, specialists have noted that the blood-brain barrier does not appear to be as intact around tumor tissue, so the need to circumvent it may not be so crucial.

Scientists are also exploring the use of agents that can cause malignant cells to become more like normal cells again. Such a transformation may be effective in halting tumor growth or in enhancing sensitivity to other forms of treatment. The advantage of this technique—called *biological modification*—is that the substances used are nontoxic compounds that are normally produced in the body.

Professional journals as well as popular magazines and newspapers report a steady stream of promising new treatments for cancer. One reads, for example, of heat produced by microwaves being used to kill brain tumors. Some investigators are also experimenting with raising body temperature on the theory that an artificial fever will provoke the immune system into action. Another well-publicized potential cure for cancer is interferon, the substance body cells produce naturally to fight infection. These new therapies may prove to be important, but as yet there is not enough evidence to establish their roles as therapeutic agents. All new approaches to treating brain tumors must stand the test of well-designed, carefully controlled clinical tests and long-term follow-up before any conclusions can be drawn about the safety or the effectiveness of treatments.

Watching the brain in action

Aiding and abetting follow-up of new treatments for brain tumors, as well as providing a versatile research tool in many basic and clinical studies, is a new form of brain scanning called positron emission tomography (PET). PET scans of the brain show which brain cells are most active metabolically. An aggressively growing tumor, for example, might show up on a PET scan as an area lighter or brighter than surrounding tissue, indicating higher metabolic activity. A tumor that is dying, however, might be correspondingly lower in activity, and, over time, shrink in size.

The PET technique depends on the fact that metabolically active cells absorb nutrients at a high rate. The bloodstream of a patient or an experimental animal is injected with a nutrient like sugar that is labeled with a radioactive compound. As the blood circulates in the brain, the most active cells will take up more of the labeled sugar and then broadcast their location by virtue of their radioactivity. Detectors placed around the head pick up the radioactivity, and with the aid of a computer, translate the readings into a brain image. PET scans can be color-coded to make the differences in cell uptake of nutrient stand out better. PET studies are being used to compare the healthy brain with the tumorous brain and to observe changes in brain metabolism at all stages of disease.

When brain tumor strikes

It is especially important to have a clear idea of the facts, should you or someone close to you be diagnosed as having a brain tumor. The news inevitably comes as a shock, so much so that much of what the specialist may say by way of explanation may be lost in the immediate emotional reaction to the news. Most patients and their families are caught up in a turmoil of feelings which may range from disbelief to paralyzing grief at the thought of impending death. Yet it is precisely at this point that hard decisions have to be made about the course of treatment and about family affairs. During this time you may find it helpful to turn to the larger family, friends, and outside resources such as clergymen or hospital counselors. Such people may assist you with many of the practical arrangements that may have to be made, as well as provide psychological and moral support.

What you should also do is inform yourself about the tried and true treatments as well as the highly regarded clinical research and treatment programs available in major medical centers in the United States. You should also seek treatment by physicians who are experienced in tumor therapy. Because brain tumors are relatively rare, many physicians see only a few brain tumor patients a year. There are others, however, who have made brain tumors their speciality.

Psychologically, the brain tumor patient and the family need to adapt to the situation. No one says that this is easy, and it is expected that there may be stages of anger or indignation (Why me?), denial, frustration, sadness, and depression. Some parents have seen a child die from a brain tumor and have written books about their experience, as John Gunther did in *Death Be Not Proud*. Knowing that others experience grief and tragedy, reading their stories, or sharing accounts can help in working through the emotional upheaval. In this regard the Association for Brain Tumor Research, a voluntary health organization formed by individuals concerned about brain tumors—usually because of personal experience—can be a valuable source of information and help. NINCDS, the National Cancer Institute, groups like the American Cancer Society, and major treatment centers like New York's Memorial Sloan-Kettering Center for Cancer Research and Houston's M.D. Anderson Hospital and Tumor Institute are other useful sources of information.

Probably one of the most unsettling aspects of the diagnosis and treatment of brain tumors is the uncertainty with which you have to live. In some cases of secondary brain tumors or advanced primary malignancies, death may be imminent. As we have seen, however, the combination of new and improved therapies have added months or even years to life, while preserving its quality.

As more and more brain tumors come to treatment earlier, and the treatments themselves prove more effective, there will still be worrisome wait-and-see problems. Will the tumor recur? Is a minor memory lapse or mood change an omen of cancer's return? Those questions and fears are not helped when brain tumor patients experience episodes of brain swelling, fever, or headache as a result of treatment. Needless to say, checkups can allay such fears, and there are medications that can relieve brain swelling or other side effects of treatment.

In the end, how well patients, friends, and family members adapt to the experience of a brain tumor depends on their understanding of the problem and the inner resources and personality traits they bring to bear on it. For a 27-year-old college student in Boston, it has paid to be an optimist.

Voluntary health organizations

The Association for Brain Tumor Research supports research on brain tumors and provides information to the general public through brochures and newsletters.

> Association for Brain Tumor Research
> 6232 N. Pulaski Road, Suite 200
> Chicago, Ill. 60646
> (312) 286–5571

The Acoustic Neuroma Association is a new organization for patients, families, and medical personnel concerned with tumors of the acoustic nerve as well as other cranial nerves.

> Acoustic Neuroma Association
> 240 Mooreland Avenue
> Carlisle, Pa. 17013
> (717) 249–2973

The Candlelighters is an organization for parents of children with cancer. The group publishes a newsletter and promotes the establishment of self-help chapters throughout the country.

> The Candlelighters Foundation
> 2025 I Street, N.W.
> Washington, D.C. 20006
> (202) 659–5136

The American Cancer Society is a source of information on all varieties of cancer. The society has divisions in many cities in the United States and headquarters in New York.

American Cancer Society
777 3rd Avenue
New York, N.Y. 10017
(212) 371–2900

National institutes of health

For additional information on brain tumor research and clinical treatment programs contact:

Office of Scientific and Health Reports
National Institute of Neurological and Communicative Disorders and Stroke
Building 31, Room 8A06
National Institutes of Health
Bethesda, Md. 20205
(301) 496–5751

Office of Cancer Communications
National Cancer Institute
Building 31, Room 10A29
National Institutes of Health
Bethesda, Md. 20205
(301) 496–6631

U.S. Department of Health and Human Services, Public Health Service, National Institutes of Health. U.S. Government Printing Office: 1982 O—365–254.

Cancer

How cancer works

Normally, the cells that make up the body reproduce themselves in an orderly manner so that worn-out tissues are replaced, injuries are repaired, and growth of the body proceeds.

Occasionally, certain cells undergo an abnormal change and begin a process of uncontrolled growth and spread: One cell divides into two, those redivide into four, and so on. These cells may grow into masses of tissue called tumors—some benign and others malignant (cancerous).

The danger of cancer is that it invades and destroys normal tissue. In the beginning, cancer cells usually remain at their original site, and the cancer is said to be localized. Later, some cancer cells may invade neighboring organs or tissue. This occurs either by direct extension of growth or by becoming detached and carried through the lymph or blood systems to other parts of the body. This is called metastasis of a cancer.

This spread may be regional—confined to one region of the body—when cells are trapped by lymph nodes. If left untreated, however, the cancer is likely to spread throughout the body. That condition is known as advanced cancer, and usually results in death.

Because a case of cancer becomes progressively more serious with each stage, it is important to detect cancer as early as possible. Aids to early detection include cancer's Seven Warning Signals and the cancer risk factors.

Trends in diagnosis and treatment

The diagnosis and treatment of cancer has become increasingly individualized. Early detection is followed by more precise staging, and the use of more than one kind of therapy, often in combination.

Some cancers, which only a few decades ago had a very poor outlook, are today being cured: acute lymphocytic leukemia in children, Hodgkin's disease, Burkitt's lymphoma, Ewing's sarcoma (a form of bone cancer), Wilms' tumor (a kidney cancer in children), rhabdomyosarcoma (a cancer in certain muscle tissue), choriocarcinoma (placental cancer), testicular cancer, ovarian cancer and osteogenic sarcoma. Other cancers have not yet yielded to effective treatment, and are the focus of continuing research.

An outstanding example of progress is the improvement in the management of testicular cancer in young men. More precise diagnostic tools and staging allow better selection of treatment. The use of combinations of cancer drugs has resulted in remarkably improved survival. In 20 years, the five-year survival rate of testicular cancer rose from 63% to 88%.

The following developments indicate the directions of current and future research:

- A genetic fusing of cancer cells with normal cells can produce disease-fighting "monoclonal antibodies"—specific antibodies tailored to seek out chosen targets on cancer cells. The potential of monoclonal antibodies in the diagnosis and treatment of cancer is under study.
- New understanding of the causes of pain in cancer patients has increased the options for control. Regular use of oral pain medicines, infusions or injections of analgesics, procedures to interrupt pain pathways, are among the effective approaches available to control pain in cancer patients.

- Studies with agents like synthetic retinoids (cousins of Vitamin A), and other substances are being undertaken to see if recurrences of certain cancers can be prevented. Another step is to see if these agents can reduce cancer in high-risk groups. For example, studies of dietary intervention will examine the effect of low-fat diets in women at high risk of developing breast cancer.
- New approaches to drug therapy use combination chemotherapy and chemotherapy with surgery. New classes of agents are being tested for their effectiveness in treating patients resistant to drug therapies now in use.
- Many patients with primary bone cancer now are treated successfully by removing and replacing a section of bone rather than by amputating the leg or arm. Drugs and radiation therapy are being used effectively in bone cancer surgery, resulting in dramatic improvement in survival.
- New high technology diagnostic imaging techniques have replaced exploratory surgery for some cancer patients. Magnetic Resonance Imaging (MRI) is one example of such technology under study. It uses a huge electromagnet to detect tumors by sensing the vibrations of the different atoms in the body. MRI could revolutionize the diagnosis of cancer and other diseases. Computerized tomography (CT scanning) uses X-rays to examine the brain and other parts of the body. Cross-section pictures are constructed which show a tumor's shape and location more accurately than is possible with conventional X-ray techniques. For patients undergoing radiation therapy, CT scanning may enable the therapist to pinpoint the tumor more precisely to provide more accurate radiation dosage while sparing normal tissue.
- Immunotherapy holds the hope of enhancing the body's own disease-fighting systems to control cancer. Interferon, interleukin-2 and other biologic response modifiers are under study. Recently, interferon was made available as the treatment for hairy cell leukemia, a rare blood cancer of older Americans. The exciting research area of biologic response modifiers will probably require many years to find the proper role of these agents in cancer treatment.
- Many cancers are caused by a two-stage process through exposure to substances known as initiators and promoters. Research scientists are exploring ways of interrupting these processes to prevent the development of cancer.
- The transfusion of blood components is becoming increasingly available and effective as a support in cancer therapy. Platelets are used to prevent hemorrhaging, and red blood cells to combat anemia. Infections, a common complication in cancer patients, can now be better anticipated, and with new drugs and antibodies, better controlled and treated.
- New technologies have made it possible to use bone marrow transplanta-

tion as an important treatment option in selected patients with aplastic anemia and leukemia. Bone marrow transplantation for other cancers is under study. The administration of larger doses of anti-cancer drugs or radiation therapy may be tolerated by some patients if their bone marrow is stored and later transplanted to restore marrow function (autologous bone marrow transplants).

- Hyperthermia is a way to increase the heat or temperature of the entire body or a part of the body. It is known that heat can kill cancer cells. A cell temperature of 45 degrees kills cancer cells. A temperature of 42 to 43 degrees makes the cell more susceptible to damage by ionizing radiation (X-rays). Studies are underway to learn if hyperthermia can increase the effect of radiation or chemotherapy.
- With medical progress producing longer survival periods for many cancer patients, clinical concerns are expanding to include not only patients' physical well-being but also their psychosocial needs. The patient's and family's reactions to the disease, sexual concerns, employment and insurance needs, and ways to provide psychosocial support, have emerged as important areas of research and clinical care. Health professionals have become increasingly interested in quality-of-life issues for cancer patients and their families.
- Improvements in cancer treatment have made possible more conservative management of some early cancers. In early cancer of the larynx, many patients have been able to retain their larynx and their voice; in colorectal cancer, fewer permanent colostomies are needed; and the surgery required in many cases of breast cancer is often more limited.
- Prostatic ultrasound, a rectal probe using ultrasonic waves producing an image of the prostate, is currently being investigated as a potential means to increase the early detection of occult, or not clinically suspected, prostate cancer.

Cancer Facts & Figures, 1987. National Headquarters: American Cancer Society, Inc., 90 Park Avenue, New York, N.Y. 10016. 87–500M—No. 5008-LE.

Facts on Breast Cancer

Here are the facts about breast cancer—signs and symptoms, progress in diagnosis and treatment, prognosis, rehabilitation, and hope for the future.

Currently breast cancer strikes more than 112,000 American women annually. One out of 11 women will get breast cancer during her lifetime. At present the disease kills over 37,000 women annually. It is the major cancer killer of women and its main target is women over 35. In fact, breast cancer is the leading cause of all deaths in women from 40 to 44. It also strikes men, but very infrequently.

Hormonal influences play a significant role in the development of some breast cancers, but the causes are largely unknown. There is a common misconception that an injury to the breast can cause breast cancer, but there is no evidence to support this. The injury may call a woman's attention to a tumor that is already there. Most breast cancers are discovered by women themselves through the regular practice of BSE (breast self-examination) or accidentally.

All breast problems should be discussed with a physician and, when needed, in consultation with a specialist in breast diseases.

BSE and cancer-related checkups

Every woman should take the time to examine her breasts for signs of possible cancer. Once a month is often enough, and the best time is about seven to ten days after the start of the menstrual period. After the menopause, any set day, such as the first of the month, is a good time to do BSE. After a hysterectomy, she should check with her doctor for the best time. When one breast has been treated for cancer, a woman should examine the opposite breast regularly, as well as the treated breast. Changes in the breast not previously noted should be reported promptly to a physician.

In addition to monthly BSE starting at age 20, American Cancer Society guidelines for cancer-related checkups recommend that asymptomatic women 20 to 40 have a breast exam by a physician at three-year intervals and one baseline mammogram (breast X-ray) between ages 35 and 40. Women 40 and older should have a breast examination by their physician every year, followed by annual or biennial mammograms between ages 40 and 49, and annual mammograms after age 50.

The anatomy of the breast

The consistency of breast tissue varies from woman to woman. A lumpy breast may feel less so after the menstrual period when swelling and breast engorgement are less. Normally, the skin of the breast is smooth, but weight loss or advancing age may cause wrinkles. The size and shape of the nipples also vary. An inverted nipple may be normal or indicative of a disease process. The circular area (areola) which surrounds the nipple usually enlarges during pregnancy. A woman's breasts seldom match exactly—the shape is determined by heredity, weight and by the strength of supporting ligaments.

What is cancer?

Cancer is a disease characterized by uncontrolled growth and spread of abnormal cells. Normally, the cells that make up all parts of the body reproduce themselves in an orderly manner so that growth occurs, worn out tissues are replaced and injuries repaired. Occasionally, certain cells grow into a mass of tissue called a tumor. Some tumors are benign; others are malignant.

Benign tumors may interfere with body function and require surgical treatment, but they do not invade neighboring tissue and seldom threaten life. However, malignant tumors invade and destroy normal tissue. By a process called metastasis, cells break away from a malignant tumor and spread through the blood and lymphatic systems to other parts of the body where they form new colonies of cancer. Sometimes cancer grows and spreads rapidly; sometimes the process takes years.

Breast cancer occurs most often as a painless lump or thickening, frequently in the upper outer portion of the breast, although it can occur anywhere in the breast. It can spread from its site of origin to the lymph nodes in the armpit, neck, chest, and eventually to other parts of the body via the blood stream.

Breast cancer risk factors

Under age 35, the risk of breast cancer is minimal but the risk increases with age; about 75% of breast cancers occur after age 50.

Women are at higher risk if they have a personal history of breast cancer or a history of breast cancer in the immediate family—mother or sisters. Increased risk is also evident for women with onset of menstruation prior to age 12, for those with menopause after age 55, for those who have never given birth to a child or had their first child after age 30, and for those who are overweight.

Some physicians believe that women with chronic cystic mastitis (lumpy breasts) also have an increased risk of developing breast cancer.

Signs and symptoms

Besides a lump, or thickening, other changes that should be checked by a physician are swelling, puckering or dimpling, redness, or skin irritation that persists. Changes in the nipples and areolae to look for are a whitish scale, distorted shape, inverted nipple, or nipple discharge. Pain or tenderness should also be reported to the physician.

Diagnosis

The physician examines the breasts for lumps or thickenings, changes in contour or consistency, nipple abnormalities, and enlarged lymph nodes in the armpit or neck.

Mammography (X-ray examination of the breast) is a very important diagnostic tool, particularly in symptomatic and high-risk women. The newer techniques and equipment, when properly used, have permitted physicians largely to dispel the concern about X-ray exposure from mammography causing breast cancer. The known risk of breast cancer in all women over 50 and in high-risk groups between 35 and 50 is far greater than the theoretical risk for mammography. It is the only method that can find tumors before they can be felt by the most experienced physician.

Thermography, which depicts heat patterns of the skin of the breast, has been used as an adjunct in breast cancer detection. Higher temperatures can indicate the presence of cancer, but benign conditions like inflammation also show increased heat. This technique is less specific and is not a substitute for thorough physical examination or mammography.

Ultrasound (sonar) and transillumination or diaphanography (shining a bright light through the breast) are techniques currently being evaluated for effectiveness as diagnostic procedures. They have yet to be proven as good as mammography.

Biopsy is the surgical removal, for microscopic examination, of a piece of tissue from the suspected growth or, if small, the entire growth itself. This is the only way to determine if cancer cells are present. About 80 percent of all breast lumps biopsied turn out to be benign.

Treatment

Breast cancer is currently treated by several different methods. There is no one approach suited to the needs of all patients with breast cancer. The decision regarding the extent of the surgical procedure, the use of radiation therapy, chemotherapy, or hormonal manipulation is based upon the findings of the local physical examination, additional studies, the kind of cancer reported by the pathologist after microscopic examination, the age and preference of the patient and the considered judgment of the responsible physician. Each patient with breast cancer must be individualized. All women are encouraged to discuss with their physicians the options available, the details of the recommended approach, and the reasons for the specific procedure being recommended.

Women, when asked to sign a consent form for surgery, should feel free to talk with the surgeon about the possibility of a two-step procedure. The biopsy is done first and the appropriate type of surgery is determined after the final pathology report. Such a time interval offers the opportunity for further discussion, additional studies, if needed, and another consultation should the physicians and/or patient wish to have one. Again, these are matters to be resolved between the patient and her physician on an individual basis.

At the time breast cancer is diagnosed, it is extremely important for the tumor to be tested for hormone receptors. This information can be very useful in the later management of breast cancer which has recurred. A woman undergoing breast surgery for possible cancer should make a specific request of her physician to do this hormone receptor test.

When breast cancer is found, the appropriate operation may vary. As a general rule, lesser procedures which preserve the breast are usually reserved for very early breast cancer—so called Stage I—in which the cancer is small and there is no clinical evidence of spread to the axillary lymph nodes.[*] These procedures may include removal of the tumor and some adjacent breast tissue (lumpectomy, tumorectomy, partial mastectomy, tylectomy), or removal of the quadrant (25% of the breast) which contains the cancer, and partial removal of axillary lymph nodes (sampling) or complete axillary lymph node removal. The above surgical procedures are frequently followed by radiation therapy to the remaining breast tissue on the same side.

Surgical procedures which remove the breast nodes include:[*]

1) Simple or total mastectomy—removal of the breast only.
2) Modified radical mastectomy—removal of the breast and the axillary lymph nodes.
3) Radical mastectomy—removal of the breast, underlying muscles and axillary lymph nodes.

When the breast is removed, every attempt is made to obtain the best cosmetic and functional result to facilitate possible reconstruction.

If the microscopic examination of the lymph nodes shows the presence of cancer, chemotherapy may be recommended after radiation therapy or any of the mentioned surgical procedures.

Chemical and hormonal therapies are important in the management

---

[*]Lymph nodes are removed as noted above to see if there is microscopic evidence of spread and to better evaluate the type of surgery, radiation therapy and chemotherapy needed by the individual patient.

of patients with cancer at all stages. Following surgery and/or radiation therapy of primary breast cancer, some women with an increased risk for recurrence may be treated with chemotherapeutic drugs to destroy residual cancer. This can definitely reduce or delay the chance of recurrence of breast cancer in selected patients.

Chemical or hormonal therapy may provide prolonged control in many patients with advanced breast cancer. Shrinkage or disappearance of the cancer may occur, and the cancer may go into remission for long periods of time.

Chemotherapy works in several different ways, but the primary mechanism is interference with cell division and growth. Rapidly growing normal or cancer cells are most vulnerable to chemotherapy. The drugs selected produce more injury to cancer cells than to normal cells. The physician maintains a delicate balance between dose and frequency by giving enough chemotherapy to kill cancer cells without permanently destroying too many normal tissues.

Most chemotherapy is given on an ambulatory basis in the doctor's office or the outpatient department of hospitals. However, for some patients short periods of hospitalization may be necessary to monitor treatment.

Before chemotherapy begins, the physician will explain the reactions that might occur during the administration of specific drugs. Additional printed materials may be supplied for the patient's information.

Individuals tolerate drugs differently. Therefore, any unexplained event should be reported to the physician. Reactions to drugs are usually temporary. When treatment is stopped, most side effects disappear; hair grows back, for example, or anemia is corrected.

Hormonal manipulation is of two types: **Additive**—the administration of appropriate hormones, or **Ablative**—suppression of function or removal of hormone-producing organs like the ovaries, adrenal gland or pituitary gland.

Rehabilitation and reconstruction

Most women resume normal productive lives within a month or two after mastectomy. Many do so with the help of the Reach to Recovery Program of the American Cancer Society. Ask your surgeon about the program in your community. This free service involves the participation of more than ten thousand ACS volunteers who have successfully adjusted to the loss of a breast. The program provides cosmetic, psychological, and physical support. These carefully selected and trained volunteers visit thousands of mastectomy patients in hospitals all over the country when requested to do so by the responsible surgeon. The Reach to Recovery volunteer talks with the patient on a woman-to-woman, person-to-person basis, as someone who has experienced the same type of surgery and who has fully recovered. The volunteer brings a temporary Dacron-filled breast form which may be worn until the patient has a more permanent prosthesis. Information is given about where to purchase a prosthesis and how to do wardrobe adjustments including bathing suits, if needed. With the surgeon's approval, the patient is taught how to do simple exercises to maintain good arm function.

Most important, Reach to Recovery volunteers offer reassurance and support. Patients learn that although they have had major surgery, they are the same women as before, capable of loving and being loved, and living happy, normal, productive lives. Often, to the new mastectomy patient, just the sight of another attractive woman functioning well after a mastectomy is enough to relieve a feeling of depression and give hope for the future.

Rehabilitation after mastectomy should not only concern physical, but psychological matters as well. The mastectomy patient is not only confronted by the loss of her breast, but also by a diagnosis of cancer—both issues will often need attention. It is not uncommon for her to question her femininity and sexual attractiveness initially. Feelings of fear, of ''Why me?'' or ''What have I done to deserve this?'' are often experienced, accompanied by periods of anger and even mild depression. While not all women having a mastectomy will feel or act the same way, most will benefit from support and encouragement from family, friends and medical staff. She and her family should be encouraged to express feelings, to ask questions and to participate in the overall process of recovery. While it is normal to experience periods of depression, moodiness, etc., if the depression becomes disabling it should be reported to the surgeon who will evaluate the condition for further intervention or possible referral to a professional counselor. Referral to patient and family education programs such as the American Cancer Society's *I CAN COPE* program can also alleviate anxiety and answer many of the questions about cancer. This program serves only as an adjunct; the patient and family are always referred back to the surgeon or physician for specific answers to questions pertaining to the patient's condition or further care.

Although many women who have had a mastectomy are satisfied with wearing an external prosthesis, others choose breast reconstruction performed by a plastic surgeon. Surgical techniques and special prostheses not available many years ago have made it possible now for a great number of mastectomy patients to have reconstruction with good cosmetic results and an enhanced quality of life. Breast reconstruction has become an important part of treatment and rehabilitation after mastectomy.

Women who are interested in reconstruction should discuss the matter with their surgeons to be sure that the procedure is suited to their individual medical situation. A pamphlet entitled "Breast Reconstruction Following Mastectomy for Cancer—Some Questions and Answers" is available through the American Cancer Society. It was prepared by the Public Education Committee of the American Society of Plastic and Reconstructive Surgeons, Inc.

Hope for the future

The real hope for the future is in earlier detection. Cancer specialists all over the world are improving diagnostic techniques, learning more about the nature of "early" cancer, and developing more effective combinations of treatments. The public and medical profession must be alerted to the need for earlier detection by better identification of those women at higher risk of developing breast cancer.

How to help save lives from breast cancer

Make it a lifetime habit to do breast self-examination (BSE) once a month. Learn how from your doctor and the American Cancer Society. See instructions on page 15.
- If you discover a breast lump, or other changes, see your doctor promptly.
- Have regular cancer-related checkups. See ACS guidelines on page 4.
- At present, the key to saving more lives from breast cancer is earlier detection and treatment.

This publication was made possible by your contributions to the American Cancer Society. 78–(750M)—Rev, 1/84—No. 2003-LE.

Facts on Colorectal Cancer

Here are the facts about cancer of the colon and rectum—signs and symptoms, progress in diagnosis and treatment, prognosis, rehabilitation of the colostomy patient, and hope for the future.

More than 120,000 new cases of colorectal cancer (colon and rectum) are diagnosed each year, the same number as lung cancer. The only

How to examine your breasts

1 In the Shower: Examine your breasts during bath or shower; hands glide easier over wet skin. Finger flat, move gently over every part of each breast. Use right hand to examine left breast, left hand for right breast. Check for any lump, hard knot or thickening.

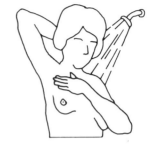

2 Before a Mirror: Inspect your breasts with arms at your sides. Next, raise your arms high overhead. Look for any changes in contour of each breast, a swelling, dimpling of skin, changes in the nipple.

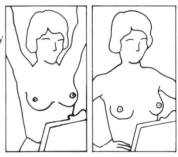

Then rest palms on hips and press down firmly to flex your chest muscles. Left and right breast will not exactly match—few women's breasts do.

3 Lying down: To examine your right breast, put a pillow or folded towel under your right shoulder. Place right hand behind your head—this distributes breast tissue more evenly on the chest. With left hand, fingers flat, press gently in small circular motions around an imaginary clock face. Begin at outermost top of your right breast for 12 o'clock, then move to one o'clock, and so on around the circle back to 12. A ridge of firm tissue in the lower curve of each breast is normal. Then move in an inch, toward the nipple; keep circling to examine *every part of your breast,* including the nipple. This requires at least three more circles. Now slowly repeat the procedure on your left breast with a pillow under your left shoulder and left hand behind your head. Notice how your breast structure feels. Finally, squeeze the nipple of each breast gently between thumb and index finger. Any discharge, clear or bloody, should be reported to your doctor immediately.

Regular inspection shows what is normal for you and will give you confidence in your examination.

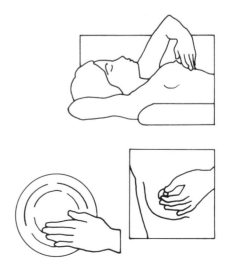

site accounting for a large number of new cases is skin cancer. Despite the high mortality rate—about 54,900 die from colorectal cancer annually—the potential for saving lives from the disease is greater than for most other types of cancer.

More than 90 percent of colorectal patients are past 40 years of age, and men and women are affected in almost equal numbers.

The functions of the colon and rectum

Their purpose is to extract liquid from the remains of digested food and to hold the solid waste matter until ready to be expelled from the body. The colon, also called the large bowel, is the lower 5 to 6 feet of intestine. The rectum is the last 5 to 6 inches at the end of the colon, leading to the outside of the body (see sketch).

What is cancer?

Cancer is a disease characterized by uncontrolled growth and spread of abnormal cells. Normally, the cells that make up all parts of the body reproduce themselves in an orderly manner so that growth occurs, worn-out tissues are replaced and injuries repaired. Occasionally, certain cells grow into a mass of tissue called a tumor. Some tumors are benign, others are malignant (cancer).

Benign tumors may interfere with body function and require surgical treatment but they do not invade neighboring tissue and seldom threaten life. However, cancers invade and destroy normal tissue. By a process called metastasis, cells break away from a malignant tumor and spread through the blood and lymphatic systems to other parts of the body where they form new cancers. Sometimes cancer grows and spreads rapidly; sometimes the process may take years.

Colorectal cancers can develop in the intestinal tract from the cecum to the anus (see sketch), with most tumors occurring in the lower one-third segment of the lower bowel.

Colorectal risk factors

Although the cause of colorectal cancer, like that of most cancers, is unknown, statistical evidence indicates a relationship between cancer of the colon and two other diseases of the digestive tract: chronic ulcerative colitis and congenital multiple polyposis. Studies have shown that patients who have had ulcerative colitis for 10 years or more have an increased risk of colon cancer. Congenital multiple polyposis is a hereditary disease

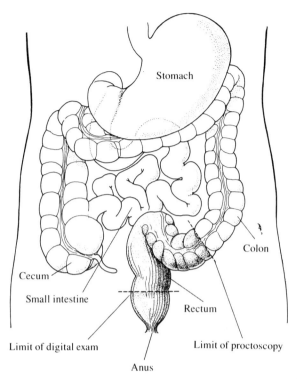

Stomach

Colon

Cecum

Small intestine

Rectum

Limit of digital exam

Limit of proctoscopy

Anus

in which numerous polyps grow in the colon and rectum. These growths have a tendency to become malignant.

Environmental Risks

Evidence has been developed in recent years suggesting that most bowel cancer is caused by environmental agents. There is a growing indication that dietary patterns play a key role, with some scientists believing that a diet high in beef and/or deficient in high fiber content may be a significant causative factor. Research in both these areas is continuing.

Signs and symptoms

Since the digested matter in the colon and rectum becomes increasingly solid as it descends, a colorectal cancer will result in obstruction. The closer the cancer is to the rectum, the more pronounced will be the signs and symptoms of obstruction: rectal bleeding, appearing in or on the stool; constipation or diarrhea, or both alternately; increase in intestinal gas, causing various degrees of abdominal discomfort.

People with hemorrhoids are apt to ignore rectal bleeding since it is a common result of the condition. This is unwise, because although hemorrhoids do not cause cancer, a person with hemorrhoids may also have cancer. Rectal bleeding can never be assumed to be the result of hemorrhoids alone; only an examination can rule out cancer.

Diagnosis of colorectal cancer

Fortunately, colorectal cancer can be detected at an early, even asymptomatic, stage with procedures and tests now available: digital rectal examination, stool blood test, proctosigmoidoscopy, fiberoptic colonoscopy and barium enema with air contrast examination.

1. Digital Rectal Examination By inserting a gloved finger into the rectum, the physician can inspect the anal area. He can feel irregular or abnormally firm areas that may be malignant. Approximately 12 to 15 percent of all colorectal cancers can be detected by digital examination.

2. Stool Blood Test The use of guaiac-impregnated slides is a simple, inexpensive method of testing the feces for blood. This is often done in the doctor's office; there is also a kit for use at home where the individual prepares stool samples on guaiac slides from three consecutive bowel movements. The reason for the multiple specimens is that bleeding may be intermittent. To increase the accuracy of the stool analysis, it is believed that a special meat-free, high-residue diet should be started at least 24 hours before the first stool specimen is collected and continued during the next three days. Vitamin C and aspirin should not be taken because they interfere with the test.

3. Proctosigmoidoscopy A lighted tube is passed into the rectum and lower colon through which the physician can inspect the wall visually for a distance of about 12 inches. If a growth is discovered, a small tissue sample is removed for microscopic examination (biopsy). Two-thirds of all colorectal cancer can be detected with the aid of this instrument.

4. Fiberoptic Colonoscopy The colonoscope is a flexible instrument with greater range than the rigid proctosigmoidoscope. It allows the physician to examine the entire length of the colon. Any suspicious growth can also be biopsied through the colonoscope for immediate microscopic examination.

5. Barium Enema with Air Contrast Examination This technique is essential for patients with signs and symptoms of colorectal cancer. The method uses a contrast medium to visualize the lower bowel. By careful X-raying of the colon, small or large lesions overlooked by palpation, proctosigmoidoscopy or colonoscopy may be detected. If a barium enema examination is negative, but suspicious signs and symptoms persist, the examination should be repeated.

Treatment

Although surgery is the most effective current method of treating colorectal cancer, radiation therapy and chemotherapy, in combination with surgery, are being used in some cases.

Surgery

Depending on the type and stage of the disease, an operation for colorectal cancer consists of removing the part of the bowel containing the tumor. The lymph nodes that drain this area may also be removed because the lymph system is one of the main routes for carrying cancer cells to other parts of the body.

When the operation involves more extensive surgery and the two ends of the bowel cannot be connected again, an opening is made in the abdominal wall through which bodily wastes can be evacuated. The surgical procedure is referred to as a colostomy and the opening is called a stoma. The colostomy may be either temporary or permanent. In the latter case, the patient, after being helped to adjust to some initial problems, can lead an otherwise normal, fully active life.

Radiation Therapy

The basic principle of radiation therapy is to bombard a cancer with rays which damage or destroy the cancer cells yet produce only minimum damage to surrounding tissue. Radiation therapy is proving effective in

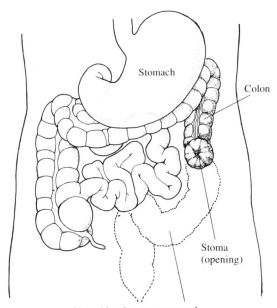

Sigmoid and rectum removed

reducing the size of some colorectal tumors, helping prevent their spread, and in relieving pain. It may be used before surgery to reduce the size of the tumor and, following surgery, to kill malignant cells not reached in the operation.

When radiation therapy is combined with surgery, it should not always be assumed that the disease is necessarily any worse than it is for patients who have surgery alone. Each case is different and requires individual treatment.

Skin reactions, nausea, vomiting, and a feeling of tiredness can be side effects of radiation. Rest and good nutrition help the body recover more quickly.

Chemotherapy

Chemotherapy may be used alone or in combination with surgery or radiation therapy to treat some cancers. The anti-cancer drugs used in chemotherapy produce more extensive injury to cancer cells than to normal cells, and the physician maintains a delicate balance between dose and frequency by giving enough chemotherapy to kill cancer cells without destroying too many healthy ones. Chemotherapeutic drugs work in several different ways, but they usually interfere with cell division or growth. Rapidly growing cells, both normal and cancer, are most vulnerable to chemotherapeutic drugs.

Chemotherapy has proved useful for patients with colorectal cancer when their disease cannot be treated surgically. A chemical known as 5-fluorouracil, or 5-FU, can reduce the size of a tumor and can relieve pain, occasionally for long periods of time.

Most chemotherapy is given in the doctor's office or the outpatient department of hospitals. For some patients, however, short periods of hospitalization may be necessary to monitor treatment.

During the treatment, certain common side effects may occur. They include nausea and vomiting; diarrhea; hair loss; anemia; reduced blood-clotting ability; susceptibility to infections, and mouth sores.

Individuals tolerate drugs differently and when treatment is stopped, side effects disappear; hair grows back, for example, or anemia is corrected. Any unexpected side effect should be reported to the physician.

Prognosis

Almost two out of three patients can be saved if the disease is found early and treated promptly. When the colorectal cancer is treated early, it is regarded as highly curable. Even when the cancer is advanced, prospects may still be good if proper surgery is done.

Because of advances in surgical techniques and nursing care, surgery is now possible for persons who were once considered too old, or whose disease was thought to be too advanced for this treatment. Approximately 70 percent of patients undergoing surgery for early colorectal cancer live at least five years after diagnosis and treatment, and many of them much longer and may be considered cured.

Rehabilitation

Thousands of people from all walks of life—businessmen, doctors, lawyers, housewives, teachers, laborers, actors, nurses—have had colostomies and have returned to normal, useful, socially acceptable lives.

Recognizing that stoma patients often find the change in body habits overwhelming at first, both physically and psychologically, many American Cancer Society Divisions sponsor students and fund schools for training enterostomal therapists—a new kind of allied health professional. Enterostomal therapists, or ETs, have a nursing or similar medical background and are given an intensive six-week course of instruction, becoming experts on every phase of stomal care. They sometimes confer with surgeons prior to the operation on the best location for the opening, and afterwards teach the patient methods of daily care.

Also through its local Units and Divisions, the ACS supports a volunteer visitation program under which an individual who has had a colostomy works with a new colostomy patient. With the approval of the attending physician, these carefully selected and trained volunteers provide invaluable help—someone for the patient to see and talk to who has successfully coped with the same surgery. These former patients demonstrate that having a colostomy does not preclude a career, marriage, sexual relations, traveling, or engaging in sports or other forms of recreation.

Hope for the future

The real hope for the future is in earlier detection. Cancer specialists all over the world are improving diagnostic techniques, learning more about the nature of "early" or "minimal" cancer, and developing more effective combinations of treatments. The public and medical profession must be alerted to the need for earlier detection by better identification of those people at high risk of developing colorectal cancer.

How to protect against colorectal cancer

A cancer-related health checkup is the first line of defense against cancer.

The American Cancer Society recommends the following guidelines for men and women *without* symptoms of colorectal cancer. TALK WITH YOUR DOCTOR—Ask how the following guidelines relate to you:

- If you are over 50, you should have a "procto" every three to five years (after you have two negative examinations a year apart.)
- If you are over 50, you should have a guaiac slide test once a year.
- If you are over 40, you should have a digital rectal examination once a year.
- If you do have a possible symptom such as abnormal bleeding, you should see your doctor.

The key to saving two out of three colorectal patients is early detection and prompt treatment.

This publication was made possible by your contributions to the American Cancer Society. 78–(1MM)—Rev. 3/84—No. 2004-LE.

Facts on Lung Cancer

The lung cancer problem

Lung cancer is now the leading cause of cancer deaths among men and women. In the last few years, the figure for estimated annual new cases of lung cancer in men has stabilized, but in women it certainly will continue to increase.

The steady increases in the rates of people developing and dying from lung cancer are the delayed effects of increased smoking by Americans from the 1920's to the 1950's. (Lung cancer can take 10 to 30 years to develop.) During recent years, however, as the dangers of smoking have become clearer, fewer people are smoking. In 1976, 42 percent of adult American males and 32 percent of adult American females smoked. By 1985, those rates had fallen to 32 percent of males and 28 percent of females. Lung cancer rates are finally levelling off and actually dropping among younger age groups. In 1986 they were 29.5 percent in males and 23.8 percent in females.

After 10 to 15 years of not smoking, the risk of lung cancer for the former smoker is about twice that of a person who never smoked, but far less than the 15 to 25 times increased risk for those who continue to smoke. The best safeguard against lung cancer is never to start to smoke, or to stop immediately.

Exposure to certain workplace chemicals and minerals, particularly asbestos, has also contributed to high lung cancer rates, though to a far lesser degree than smoking. Acting together, smoking and industrial agents can do much greater damage than would either alone.

The Healthy Lung

The air we inhale enters the lungs through tubes called bronchi. These branch into the smaller brochioles and finally into tiny air sacs, the alveoli. The average lung has more than 300 million of these air sacs, providing a combined surface area of more than 750 square feet for oxygen to be absorbed into the bloodstream and carbon dioxide to be expelled.

To some extent our breathing apparatus can clean itself. Mucus produced by some cells in the bronchi traps unfamiliar material, and the movement of the cilia, tiny hair-like structures on other cells, sweeps the mucus toward the throat, where it can be coughed out. Other impurities are carried away by the blood and lymph systems.

The Smoke-Damaged Lung

The constant assault of cigarette smoking on the cells lining the bronchi can cause mucus-secreting cells to become enlarged and to increase the production of mucus. The cilia lining the air passages become worn away and are then unable to sweep foreign particles out of the throat. This causes what is known as ''smoker's cough.''

If the smoker quits at the time of these early changes, the inner surface of the bronchi can return to normal. If the smoker continues smoking, many of the air sacs can be destroyed. Smoking beyond this stage can cause the lung cells to form abnormal growth patterns that may eventually become lung cancer.

A person who doesn't smoke, but is frequently with someone who does, can also be at higher risk for developing lung cancer. Nonsmoking wives have a 35 percent higher risk of lung cancer if their husbands smoke. Children whose parents smoke are directly threatened with respiratory infections and are more likely to develop lung disease later in life.

The Cancerous Lung

Cancer is a group of more than 100 diseases caused by the abnormal growth of cells. Normally, the body cells divide and reproduce in an orderly manner, so that we grow, replace worn-out tissue, and repair any injuries. Sometimes, however, cells divide without control and form masses known as tumors.

Tumors may invade or destroy normal tissue, interfere with body functions, and require removal by surgery. Benign tumors do not spread to other parts of the body. Cancerous or malignant tumors do. By a process known as metastasis, cells break away from the original malignant tumor and spread through the lymph and blood systems to form more malignant tumors elsewhere in the body.

This spread can occur rapidly or over a period of years. Lung cancers tend to spread more quickly than most types of cancer. This is because the lungs are richly supplied by the blood and lymph systems, the very systems that carry cells to other parts of the body.

Risk factors for lung cancer

- CIGARETTE SMOKING. An estimated 85 percent of lung cancer cases in males and 75 percent in females are caused by cigarette smoking. Less than 10 percent of lung cancers occur among nonsmokers. Risks of developing lung cancer increase with the number of years smoking, the number of cigarettes smoked each day, and the tar and nicotine contents. There are, however, no safe levels of smoking. Even smoking one half pack a day of low-tar and nicotine cigarettes is risky. There is no such thing as a safe cigarette.
- PIPE AND CIGAR SMOKING. Those who smoke pipes and cigars are more likely to get lung cancer than nonsmokers, but much less so than cigarette smokers. Pipe and cigar smokers also have a greater risk than nonsmokers of cancers of the mouth, esophagus and larynx.
- INDUSTRIAL HAZARDS. If you work around certain industrial substances, you have an increased risk of developing lung cancer. These substances include chemicals and minerals such as asbestos, nickel, chromates, coal gas, mustard gas, arsenic, vinyl chloride, and the radon by-products of uranium mining and processing. Your risk, however, may be higher if you smoke. For example, asbestos workers who also smoke increase their risks of developing lung cancer 60 times.
- INVOLUNTARY SMOKING. Also known as "passive smoking" or "secondhand smoking," involuntary smoking is the breathing in of tobacco smoke by nonsmokers. While the smoke breathed in by involuntary smokers is not as concentrated as that inhaled directly by smokers, it does contain the same harmful substances. Now that several studies have shown that nonsmoking wives of cigarette smokers have an increased risk of lung cancer, the link between involuntary smoking and lung cancer has become more apparent.

In addition to these definite risk factors, some scientists suggest that air pollution and heavy doses of radiation may also contribute to lung cancer risk. There is no proof, however, of any direct cause-and-effect relationship.

Types of lung cancer

Cancers that originate in the skin, glands, or lining of internal organs (such as the lungs), are known as carcinomas. There are four main types of carcinomas of the lungs which can be further categorize non-small or small cell cancers.

Small Cell Carcinoma

Also called oat cell carcinoma because the cells are shaped like grains of oats, this form of lung cancer accounts for 20 percent to 25 percent of lung cancers. It is the most aggressive form and the most likely to have spread by the time of diagnosis.

Non-Small Cell:

a. SQUAMOUS or EPIDERMOID. These arise from the flat, scaly cells that line the air passages. It is the most common form of lung cancer, accounting for 35 to 40 percent of all lung cancers. Squamous cell carcinoma tends to be centrally located.
b. ADENOCARCINOMA. This type of tumor can begin in the mucous membrane of both smaller or larger bronchi. It accounts for about 25 percent of all lung cancers and is the most common form of lung cancer among women. It can also be caused by smoking, but to a lesser degree than other forms of lung cancer.
c. LARGE CELL CARCINOMA. This is the least common form of lung cancer, accounting for only 10 percent of all cases. It usually develops in the bronchus and is characterized by large, round cells.

Symptoms of lung cancer

Lung cancer rarely gives an early warning of its presence. The earliest symptoms are likely to be so ordinary—coughing or wheezing—that they are often dismissed as minor irritants. This is especially true of the heavy smoker, long accustomed to smoker's cough.

The most common symptoms are persistent cough and blood in the sputum. Other symptoms include repeated bouts of pneumonia, fever, weakness, weight loss, and chest pain. More advanced disease may be signalled by hoarseness, shortness of breath, swollen lymph nodes in the neck, shoulder and arm pain, difficulty in swallowing, and drooping of the upper eyelids. In many cases, patients first notice symptoms caused by the spread of the disease, rather than the primary lung cancer. These symptoms can include headaches, blurred vision, dizziness, and bone pain.

Can Lung Cancer be Detected in Those Without Symptoms?

Several studies have been conducted to see if chest X-rays and other tests like sputum cytology could detect lung cancer in an early, curable stage in individuals without symptoms. These tests were not shown to be effective in either increasing the cure rate or reducing the death rate from lung cancer. At the present time, neither chest X-rays or sputum cytology can be recommended as an effective or practical method to detect lung cancer in individuals without symptoms.

The diagnosis of lung cancer

There are a variety of methods physicians use to confirm the presence of lung cancer and to identify the type and the extent or stage of disease. An accurate diagnosis is needed to plan the best possible treatment.

1. HISTORY AND GENERAL PHYSICAL. The physician first needs to evaluate the overall health of the patient and learn the medical history. Does the patient smoke? If so, for how many years and how many cigarettes a day? How well are the lungs functioning? Any previous lung or heart problems?

2. CHEST X-RAYS. Chest X-rays are valuable in locating suspected tumors. Lung cancer usually appears on the X-ray as a centrally located tumor.

3. TOMOGRAMS. These are X-rays that show one thin layer of the lung at a time. They may reveal a small cancer not visible on a standard X-ray.

4. CT SCANS. Computerized Tomography Scans use an X-ray beam that rotates around the body to produce a series of X-rays taken from different angles. This information is then processed by a computer to produce a complete picture of a cross-section of a selected body area. By showing the relationship of a lung tumor to other structures in the chest, the CT Scan can indicate the extent of the tumor and whether it involves other organs.

5. SPUTUM CYTOLOGY. This is the microscopic examination of cells coughed up from the lungs or bronchial tubes. In some cases, sputum cytology can reveal lung cancers in patients with normal X-rays or can determine the type of lung cancer. Because it cannot pinpoint the tumor's location, a positive sputum cytology test is usually followed up with further diagnostic procedures.

6. BRONCHOSCOPY. In this procedure, a flexible tube with lighting and magnifying devices is inserted through a nostril or the mouth and into the bronchus. The physician can then obtain samples of cells, discover the precise location of the tumor, and judge whether the tumor can be completely removed.

7. NEEDLE BIOPSY. Guided by a fluoroscope, an X-ray machine that projects the image on a fluorescent screen, a physician can insert a long, thin needle into the tumor to draw out a tissue sample.

This is particularly useful for patients who are not considered candidates for surgery, but who need a diagnosis prior to planning other treatments.

8. THORACOTOMY. An operation known as a thoracotomy may be done as an exploratory procedure if other diagnostic methods fail, but there is reason to believe cancer is present. The procedure is usually only performed when the surgeon is reasonably sure that if cancer is diagnosed, the tumor can be completely removed.

9. LYMPH NODE BIOPSY. If lymph nodes in the neck seem enlarged or otherwise abnormal, they may be removed for biopsy to see if the cancer has spread there.

10. RADIONUCLIDE SCANS. These scans can show whether cancer has spread to other areas of the body. The patient is injected with a small amount of radioactive material that can only be absorbed by cancer cells. Any cancerous tumors found are projected on a small screen.

Other tests are now being studied to see how useful they might be in detecting lung cancer and determining if and where it has spread. These include blood tests, MRI (Magnetic Resonance Imaging), and monoclonal antibodies. Like CT Scans, MRI can build composite, three-dimensional images of sections of the body, but MRI does not use radiation. Monoclonal antibodies are specially bred proteins that may be useful in seeking out cancer cells.

Treatment of lung cancer

Surgery, radiation, and chemotherapy are the primary methods of treating lung cancer. The specific treatment depends on the patient's general health, the type of cancer, and the stage of the disease.

Surgery

Surgery involves removal of part of the lung or the whole lung depending on the extent of the tumor. Five-year survival rates for patients with early stages of non-small cell carcinoma varies from 40 to 50 percent.

When a lung cancer is removed, an area surrounding the tumor is also removed and examined for cancer cells. Control of any remaining cells is carried out through additional treatment.

Patients recovering from surgery usually need to use a machine to help them breathe in the first few days after surgery. They may need to limit their physical activity somewhat, depending on the amount of lung removed and the remaining function of the lungs as well as overall health.

Radiation

Radiation may be used along with surgery to deal with any remaining tumor or distant spread of the cancer. It is used in place of surgery when that treatment is not a possibility, because it can relieve pain and other symptoms.

Side effects of radiation therapy include a general feeling of tiredness that usually leaves within a week after treatment is complete, temporary dry or sore throat, and scarring of the lungs.

Chemotherapy

Chemotherapy is becoming more important in the treatment of lung cancer, particularly in small cell lung cancer. Combined chemotherapy has helped increase survival time for about 70 percent of patients with the early stage of this lung cancer—some to the point where they can be considered cured.

For patients with other types of lung cancer, combination chemotherapy is generally used only when the cancer cannot be controlled by surgery or radiation, and the response rates tend to be lower than those seen in small cell lung cancer. Clearly newer and more effective drugs are needed. Patients with non-small cell lung cancer, when possible, are encouraged to participate in studies to develop new treatments. Side effects of chemotherapy depend on the drugs used. Some common side effects include hair loss, nausea and vomiting, changes in blood count and a feeling of tiredness.

Prognosis

Prevention of lung cancer is especially important because it is very difficult to detect early. By the time a diagnosis is made, two-thirds of lung cancer patients have disease that has passed the stage when it might be curable. Only 13 percent of lung cancer patients (all stages, whites, and blacks) live five or more years after diagnosis. The survival rate is 33 percent for cases detected in a localized stage. Therefore, the outlook for many patients is not optimistic.

Future directions

Prevention is vital to future change in patient survival. Quitting smoking or never starting is the best defense against lung cancer. However, help for chronic smokers is being evaluated. Studies are being undertaken to determine how to help high-risk populations, especially in understanding the addiction process and why smoking is so difficult to give up for some people. Cessation clinics or activities to halt the tobacco habit are part of American Cancer Society prevention plans. Young people must be convinced never to start smoking.

Research is concentrating on chemoprevention and immunotherapy which may prove to be useful as well. Meanwhile the search continues for better ways to treat patients and offer rehabilitation.

Facts on Skin Cancer

Here are the facts about cancer of the skin—signs and symptoms, progress in diagnosis and treatment, prognosis, and hope for the future.

Cancer of the skin is the most common of all cancers. With the exception of malignant melanoma, a rare form of the disease, the overall cure rate for skin cancer is higher than 90 percent. More than 300,000[*] new cases of non-melanoma skin cancer are detected each year; the annual incidence of malignant melanoma is 9,600 reported deaths from skin cancer each year, but at least two-thirds of them result from melanoma.

Functions of the skin

The skin protects the body from injury. It also receives sensory impulses, excretes waste substances, and regulates body temperature. This is done through specialized structures such as nerves, hair, nails, and various types of glands.

The skin is divided into two main layers and several sublayers. The layer nearest the surface is the epidermis; the main underlying layer of connective tissue is dermis.

It is constantly exposed to sun, wind, industrial elements and other harsh external and internal injury. Although abnormalities resulting from these conditions are usually not malignant, some can lead to cancer.

Precancerous skin conditions

Certain abnormal skin conditions have a tendency to become malignant (cancer). The most common condition is senile or actinic (sun-ray) kerato-

---

[*] This estimate is based upon data from the National Cancer Institute's Third National Cancer Survey (1969–1971).

sis, a scaly skin thickening that develops in a small area, usually the face, neck or hands. This type of keratosis most often develops in older persons whose skin has been exposed for many years to the ultraviolet rays of the sun.

What is cancer?

Cancer is a disease characterized by uncontrolled growth and spread of abnormal cells. Normally, the cells that make up all parts of the body reproduce themselves in an orderly manner so that growth occurs, worn out tissues are replaced, and injuries repaired. Occasionally, certain cells grow into a mass of tissue called a tumor. Some tumors are benign, others are malignant.

Benign tumors may interfere with body function and require surgical treatment, but they do not invade neighboring tissue and seldom threaten life. However, malignant tumors compress, invade, and destroy normal tissue. By a process called metastasis, cells break away from a malignant tumor and spread through the blood and lymphatic systems to other parts of the body where they form new cancers. Sometimes cancer grows and spreads rapidly; sometimes the process may take years.

Types of Skin Cancer

There are three main types of skin cancer, classified according to the cells involved—basal cell, squamous cell, and melanoma. More than 90 percent of all skin cancers fall into the first two classifications.

Basal cell cancer occurs more frequently, but grows more slowly. It rarely spreads, but if left untreated, it can extend to underlying bone. Squamous cell cancer occurs less often, but is a greater danger because of rapid spread.

Although these two types of skin cancer can appear on almost any area of the skin, they most commonly develop on exposed parts of the body—face, neck, forearms, and backs of hands. From outward appearance the two types are often indistinguishable. They generally show up on the skin in one of two forms—either as a pale, waxlike, pearly nodule that may eventually ulcerate and crust, or as a red, scaly, sharply outlined patch.

Malignant melanoma, though relatively uncommon, is a virulent form of skin cancer which spreads rapidly. Melanomas are usually distinguished by a dark brown or black pigmentation. They start as small, mole-like growths that increase in size, change color, become ulcerated and bleed easily from a slight injury.

Skin cancer risk factors

Repeated overexposure to the ultraviolet rays of the sun is the principal cause of skin cancer. No one is immune. Men and women who continuously seek out the sun to swim, ski, play tennis, boat, golf, fish, or simply stretch out to get a tan, need to protect themselves from the direct rays of the sun. They should use sun block preparations, and wear hats and long-sleeved shirts as often as possible.

Farmers and sailors, as well as other outdoor workers, are at high risk, especially if they live and work in such sunny regions as the southwest United States.

However, fair-skinned people, notably redheads and blonds, are the most susceptible group. Their problem is they lack sufficient quantities of melanin, the pigment substance that filters out the rays of the sun. The wide range of brown skin tones is determined by the amount of melanin in the skin; the darker brown the skin, the greater the amount of melanin.

Blacks, among whom skin cancer is rare, have sufficient melanin to protect their skin from ultraviolet rays; the albino has no melanin.

Other less common risk factors are prolonged contact with coal tar, pitch, arsenic compounds, paraffin oil, or radium. These substances no longer pose a major cancer hazard because their potential danger is recognized and their use is carefully regulated by government agencies.

Diagnosis of skin cancer

People should be alert to any unusual skin condition and have it checked by a physician. This is especially important in case of a change in the size or color of an existing mole or other darkly pigmented growth. Only the doctor can determine whether an abnormal growth is benign, precancerous, or malignant.

If there is any possibility of cancer, the doctor will order a biopsy. A biopsy is a surgical procedure in which a small piece of tissue is removed from the suspected area and examined under a microscope. This is the only way to determine if cancer cells are present.

Treatment

If the biopsy shows the growth to be cancer, or even precancerous, the doctor will decide on the most effective treatment for the particular type of cancer cells.

There are four methods of treatment—radiation (destroying cancers with rays that produce only minimal damage to surrounding normal tissues), surgery, electro desiccation (tissue destruction by heat), or cryo-surgery (tissue destruction by freezing). In non-melanoma cancer, the extent of the growth and its location will determine the method used.

For malignant melanoma, wide and deep surgical excision and removal of nearby lymph nodes is required. Advances in cosmetic surgery aid in successfully rehabilitating patients, particularly those with facial and neck areas involved.

In some cases a combination of therapies may be employed. One treatment may be sufficient; other times repeated treatments are needed. Over the last few years, application of drugs in the form of ointment or lotions, especially the drug 5-Fluorouracil, has also been effective in treating skin cancers as well as precancerous skin conditions.

Immunotherapy (stimulating the patient's immune reaction) has been used successfully for patients with a number of extensive, superficial cancers as well as for those with precancerous lesions.

Each patient must be considered individually. Success in treating skin cancer depends on the extent and stage of the cancer, the degree of malignancy, and how the abnormality responds to treatment. For basal cell and squamous cell cancers, cure is virtually assured with early detection and treatment.

Malignant melanoma metastasizes quickly. This fact accounts for the lower five-year survival rate for patients with this disease—63 percent compared with 95 percent for patients with other kinds of skin cancer.

Hope for the future

The real hope for the future is in earlier detection. Cancer specialists all over the world are improving diagnostic techniques, learning more about the nature of "early" or "minimal" cancer, and developing more effective combinations of treatments. The American public and the medical profession must be alerted to the need for earlier detection by better identification of those at risk of developing skin cancer.

How to help protect against skin cancer
- Avoid repeated over-exposure to the sun—especially between 10 A.M. and 3 P.M.
- Use a sunscreen preparation to absorb ultraviolet rays

  or
- Use a sunblock preparation that will deflect ultraviolet rays.
- Wear protective clothing, such as long-sleeved shirts, wide-brimmed hats.

- The key to saving lives from skin cancer is the early detection and prompt and adequate treatment of a skin abnormality.

This publication was made possible by your contributions to the American Cancer Society. 78–1MM—No. 2049-LE.

Facts on Uterine Cancer

Here are the facts about cancer of the uterus—signs and symptoms, progress in diagnosis and treatment, prognosis, and hope for the future.

Uterine cancer is a major site of cancer among American women. Each year about 54,000 women develop the disease. And it kills almost 10,300 women annually. Yet this is a form of cancer readily detectable and highly curable. With current medical knowledge and techniques, the death rate from uterine cancer could be dramatically reduced. The answer lies in regular medical checkups which would allow early detection and treatment.

The function of the uterus

The uterus, or womb, is a small, pear-shaped organ located in the pelvis, consisting of the cervix, or neck of the uterus, and the corpus or main body of the uterus (see sketch). The uterus is the organ in which the fertilized egg attaches itself and develops during pregnancy.

What is cancer?

All cancer is an uncontrolled growth of abnormal cells. Normally, the cells that make up all parts of the body reproduce themselves in an orderly manner so that the body grows, replaces worn out tissues, and repairs itself after injury. But occasionally certain cells grow into a mass of tissue called a tumor. Some tumors are benign, others are malignant (cancer).

Benign tumors may interfere with body function and require surgical treatment, but they do not invade neighboring tissue and seldom threaten life. Malignant tumors are always dangerous; they compress, invade and destroy normal tissue. And by a process called metastasis, cells break away from the malignant tumor and spread through the blood and lymphatic systems to other parts of the body where they form new

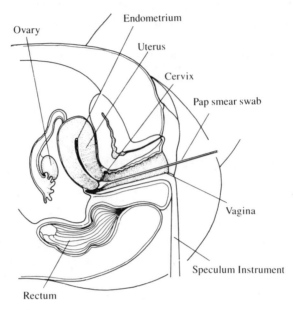

cancers. Sometimes cancer grows and spreads rapidly; sometimes the process may take years.

The two common forms of uterine cancer are cervical (from the neck of the uterus) and endometrial (from the lining of the corpus or body of the uterus). The cells covering the cervix usually go through mild to severe changes called dysplasia before becoming cancer. Similarly, tissue lining the corpus goes through mild to severe changes called hyperplasia before becoming cancer.

These precancerous conditions do not necessarily lead to cancer. It is important, however, that any woman with such a condition be treated and then examined by a physician at regular intervals.

The earliest stage of uterine cancer is called carcinoma in situ (cancer confined to its original site). If not detected and treated properly, cancer cells penetrate into deeper layers of the uterus, then spread to neighboring organs such as the vagina, bladder, or rectum, and eventually metastasize to other parts of the body.

Uterine cancer risk factors

At higher risk of *cervical cancer* are women who have unusual bleeding or vaginal discharge between periods, had frequent sex before age of 20, or sex with many partners, and women with poor genital hygiene. The highest incidence occurs in women aged 40 to 49.

Most cases of *endometrial* cancer are diagnosed in women between the ages of 50 and 64. It rarely occurs in women under 40. At higher risk are women who, during or after menopause, have unusual bleeding or discharge; have estrogen therapy during or after menopause; had a late menopause (after 55); have diabetes, high blood pressure; and an overweight problem.

Estrogen, the pill, the IUD

Estrogen, which is a hormone, is given to women during and after the menopause to make up for the decline in estrogens normally produced by the ovaries. Estrogen helps to control menopausal symptoms such as hot flushes or thinning of the vaginal lining causing painful sexual intercourse.

For older women, there are certain risks associated with such treatment, including an increased risk for endometrial cancer. However, estrogen can be given safely under careful physician control and for limited periods of time.

Oral contraceptives contain estrogen, but they also contain progesterone, and this combination of hormones in oral contraceptives has not been linked with uterine cancer. Neither do experts see any relationship between the use of the intra-uterine device (IUD) for birth control and the development of endometrial cancer.

Signs and symptoms

The earliest warning signs of cervical cancer are irregular bleeding or vaginal discharge. Warning signs of endometrial cancer include bleeding between menstrual periods, excessive bleeding during periods, and bleeding after menopause.

Any of these signs should be reported promptly to a physician.

Diagnosis of uterine cancer

Cancer of the Cervix

The Pap test is highly accurate in detecting cervical cancer at an early stage. It can also show cell changes that could develop into cancer.

The Pap test takes but a few minutes, is painless, and can be done in the physician's office. It is the examination under a microscope of cells normally shed from the body of the uterus and from the cervix. These cells collect in the vaginal fluid and can be collected, along with cells taken from the surface of the cervix, on a cotton swab or stick.

If the cell samples reveal any abnormality, additional diagnostic techniques may include:

1. COLPOSCOPY—the visual examination of the vagina and cervix with a magnifying instrument called the colposcope to check tissues for abnormality.
2. BIOPSY—the surgical removal, for microscopic examination, of a piece of tissue from a suspected area. This is the only way to determine positively if cancer cells are present.
3. CONIZATION—a surgical procedure to remove a cone-shaped specimen of tissue from the cervical canal. This provides a larger tissue sample than is removed for a biopsy.

Cancer of the Endometrium

The Pap test is only about 40 percent effective in detecting endometrial cancer. More effective diagnostic techniques are:

1. *Dilation and Curettage (D and C)*—removal of tissue samples from the body of the uterus, by a scraping technique while the patient is anesthetized. It is done in the hospital and the tissue samples can be studied microscopically for cell changes characteristic of cancer.
2. *Aspiration Curettage*—This provides samples of tissue from the walls of the body of the uterus, through suction with a small instrument inserted through the cervix. The procedure is painless and can be performed in a physician's office. The tissue samples are then studied under the microscope for abnormal cell changes.

Treatment

Uterine cancer is generally treated by surgery or radiation, or by a combination of the two. In the precancerous stages:

1. Cervical changes may be treated by *cryotherapy* which is the destruction of tissue by extreme cold, or by *electrocoagulation,* the destruction of tissue through intense heat delivered by electric current—in some very early cases, childbearing function can be maintained.
2. Endometrial changes may be treated with the hormone *progesterone*.

Surgery

Surgery is the treatment of choice when the cancer has not spread beyond its original site. The purpose is to remove all malignant tissue. The surgical procedure is hysterectomy—removal of the uterus.

Radiation Therapy

The basic principle of radiation therapy is to bombard a cancer with rays which damage or destroy the cancer yet produce only minimum damage to surrounding normal tissues.

Radiation can be used alone or in combination with surgery to help cure uterine cancer, to control tumor growth, or to alleviate pain.

Following surgery, radiation therapy may be used to kill cancer cells that could not be removed by the operation.

When radiation therapy is combined with surgery, it should not always be assumed that the disease is necessarily any worse than it is for patients who have surgery alone. Each case of uterine cancer is different and requires individual treatment.

Radiation may be beamed from an outside source such as the X-ray or cobalt machine, or it may be applied directly to the cancerous growth, through inserting in the uterus a capsule of radioactive material, such as radium. Fortunately most cancerous tissue of the uterus is more sensitive to radiation than is normal tissue.

Skin reactions, nausea, vomiting, or a feeling of tiredness can be side effects of radiation. Rest and good nutrition will help the body recover more quickly.

Chemotherapy

Drugs and hormones are used in treating some cases of advanced uterine cancer. Such treatment, termed chemotherapy, may be used either alone or in combination with surgery or radiation.

These anti-cancer drugs produce more injury to cancer cells than to normal cells, but the physician maintains a delicate balance between dose and frequency by giving enough chemotherapy to kill cancer cells without destroying too many healthy ones. Chemotherapeutic drugs work in several different ways but they usually interfere with cell division and growth. Rapidly growing cells, both normal and cancer, are most vulnerable to chemotherapeutic drugs.

Most chemotherapy is given in the doctor's office or the outpatient department of hospitals. For some patients, however, short periods of hospitalization may be necessary to monitor treatment.

Certain common side effects may occur. They include nausea and vomiting, diarrhea, hair loss, anemia, reduced bloodclotting ability, susceptibility to infections, and mouth sores.

Individuals tolerate drugs differently, and when treatment is stopped, side effects disappear; hair grows back, for example, or anemia is corrected. Any unexpected side effect should be reported to the physician.

Prognosis

If every woman had a Pap test as often as recommended, there would be virtually no deaths from cervical cancer. The overall cure rate for cancer of the endometrium is about 75 percent, but the cure rate for cases detected in the earliest stages is 80 to 90 percent.

Scientists are studying the use of hormones in treating advanced cancer of the uterus. The administration of large doses of progesterone has significantly extended lives in some patients with advanced endometrial cancer.

Hope for the future

The real hope for the future is in earlier detection. Cancer specialists all over the world are improving diagnostic techniques, learning more about the nature of "early" or "minimal" cancer, and developing more effective combinations of treatments. The public and medical profession must be alerted to the need for earlier detection by better identification of those women at higher risk of developing uterine cancer.

How to help protect against uterine cancer

A cancer-related health checkup is the first line of defense against cancer.

The American Cancer Society recommends the following guidelines for women without symptoms of uterine cancer. TALK WITH YOUR DOCTOR—ask how the following guidelines relate to you:

- If you are age 20 to 40, you should have a pelvic exam every three years; a Pap test—after two initial negative tests one year apart—*at least* every three years, includes women under 20 who are sexually active.
- If you are over 40, you should have the pelvic exam and Pap test as directed above and also an endometrial tissue sample taken at menopause if at risk (ask your doctor).
- If you do have a symptom such as abnormal bleeding, or discharge, either between periods or during or after menopause, see your doctor.

This publication was made possible by your contributions to the American Cancer Society. 78(1MM)—Rev. 1/81—No. 2006-LE. 1978, revised 1981.

Cancer Prevention

The news is getting better all the time

Before today, you may not have thought of cancer and good news together. Now, though the news about cancer is getting better—the best news is about cancer prevention.

In the past few years, scientists have identified many causes of cancer. Today it is known that about 80 percent of cancer cases are tied to the way people live their lives. For example, the foods they eat, the work they do, and whether they smoke all affect their likelihood of getting cancer.

Once you know some of the factors that increase the possibility that you might get cancer, you can take some control over them. Some are hard to control—such as your work environment; but others are easy—such as eating good foods. This booklet tells you some things you can do every day to help protect yourself from cancer.

You will find a glossary at the end of this book.

Important Questions About Cancer

1. WHAT CAUSES CANCER?

No one knows for sure how a normal cell becomes a cancer cell. But scientists agree that people get cancer mainly through repeated or long-term contact with one or more cancer-causing agents called carcinogens. The carcinogens cause body cells to change their structures and to grow out of control.

2. ARE THERE DIFFERENT KINDS OF CANCER-CAUSING AGENTS?

Yes. Scientists now believe most cancers are caused in two steps by two kinds of agents: initiators and promoters. Initiators start the damage to a cell that can lead to cancer. For example, cigarette smoking, X-rays, and certain chemicals have been shown to be initiators.

Promoters usually do not cause cancer by themselves. They change cells already damaged by an initiator from normal to cancer cells. For example, studies show that alcohol promotes the development of cancers in the mouth, throat, and possibly the liver when combined with an initiator, such as tobacco.

3. WHAT IS A CANCER RISK FACTOR?

An agent that has been linked to the cause of a particular kind of cancer is called a risk factor. Contact with that agent increases an individual's likelihood (or risk) of getting that kind of cancer. Exposure to a particular risk factor does not necessarily mean that you will get the disease, but it does mean that the possibility that you might get cancer has increased. Risk factors are described in several ways.

There are both "avoidable" and "unavoidable" risk factors. You can cut down or cut out your contact with avoidable risk factors, such as tobacco or alcohol. Unavoidable risk factors are those which you personally cannot control. For example, the risk of getting any type of cancer increases as you get older.

There are both "known" and "suspected" risk factors. A known risk factor is an agent that has been shown by either studies of human populations or by laboratory tests to be capable of producing cancer. A "suspected" risk factor is thought to produce cancer, although studies have not yet confirmed the link to cancer.

4. IS CANCER CURABLE?

Yes. Of all the chronic diseases, cancer is the most curable. Today, nearly half of all cancer patients can be cured by modern treatment methods. Great advances have been made in our ability to prevent, detect, and treat cancer.

5. IS CANCER CONTAGIOUS?

No. Cancer is not catching. It cannot be spread from person to person by sneezing, coughing, kissing, or in any other way.

6. DOES MY DIET AFFECT MY CHANCES OF GETTING CANCER?

Studies suggest that certain foods and some nutrients contained in those foods may be associated with the development of cancer.

- Findings suggest that a high intake of dietary fat is a risk factor for cancer.
- Population studies indicate that obesity increases the risk of developing certain cancers.
- Other studies suggest that some vitamins and dietary fiber may help protect you from developing some forms of cancer.

Current evidence suggests that by choosing carefully and eating a well-balanced diet, you may reduce your cancer risk. For a well-balanced diet:

- Eat a variety of foods every day. Include fresh fruits and vegetables, especially those high in vitamins A and C, such as oranges, grapefruit, nectarines, peaches, strawberries, cantaloup, and honeydew melons. Choose leafy green and yellow-orange vegetables like spinach, kale, sweet potatoes, and carrots, as well as cabbage, cauliflower, broccoli, and brussels sprouts.
- Keep your intake of all fats low, both saturated and unsaturated fats. Choose lean red meats, fish, and poultry. Trim fat from steaks, roasts, and chops, and skin poultry before cooking. Try broiling, roasting or

baking meats and fish, or simmering them in their own juices, rather than frying them. Limit your use of butter, margarine, cream, shortening, and vegetable oils. Avoid hidden fats in salad dressings and snack foods like potato chips. Choose lowfat or skim milk, low fat cheeses, and dairy desserts. Choose fruit instead of high fat desserts.

Eat foods with fiber, such as whole grain breads and cereals; a variety of raw fruits and vegetables, especially if eaten with the skin; beans, peas, and seeds.

A well-balanced diet will help keep you from being either over or underweight. You can lose weight by increasing your physical activity, eating smaller portions of food,.eating less sugar and sweets, and limiting your consumption of alcoholic drinks to one or two drinks per day.

7. DO VITAMINS CHANGE MY CANCER RISKS?

Scientists have found some relationship between a lack of certain vitamins—A and C—and cancer. For example, diets low in vitamin A have been linked to cancers of the prostate gland, cervix, skin, bladder, and colon.

On the other hand, studies indicate that vitamin A and vitamin C may help protect the body from some types of cancer. You can get all the vitamins A and C your body can use if you choose two helpings daily from the same fruits and vegetables that are in a balanced diet— dark green vegetables, yellow-orange vegetables, and yellow-orange fruits.

8. DOES DRINKING ALCOHOL CAUSE CANCER?

Excessive amounts of alcoholic beverages have been linked to a number of cancers. Heavy drinking is associated with cancers of the mouth, throat, esophagus, and liver. People who both smoke cigarettes and drink have a higher risk of getting cancers of the mouth and the esophagus.

9. DOES CIGARETTE SMOKING CAUSE CANCER?

Yes. People who smoke have a ten times greater chance of getting cancer than people who don't smoke. Overall, smoking causes 30 percent of all cancer deaths. The risk of getting lung cancer from cigarettes increases with the number you smoke, how long you have been smoking, and how deeply you inhale. Smoking also has been linked to cancers of the larynx, esophagus, pancreas, bladder, kidney, and mouth.

Although stopping is better, switching to low-tar, low-nicotine cigarettes may reduce somewhat your risk of developing lung cancer if you do not inhale more deeply, take more puffs, or smoke more cigarettes than you did before you switched.

However, switching to low-tar, low-nicotine cigarettes will not reduce your risks of developing other cancers and diseases, such as heart disease.

Animal studies also have confirmed that by-products (tar) produced by smoking marijuana can cause cancers.

Once you quit smoking, though, your risks begin to decrease at once. The only way to eliminate your cancer risks due to smoking is not to smoke at all.

10. DO ALL TOBACCO PRODUCTS INCREASE CANCER RISKS?

Yes. Although people who smoke cigars and pipes are less likely to develop lung cancer than cigarette smokers, they do risk developing cancers of the mouth, tongue, and throat. People who use snuff and chewing tobacco also risk getting cancer of the mouth.

11. WILL SUNLIGHT CAUSE SKIN CANCER?

Repeated exposure to sunlight over a long period of time has been linked to skin cancer. The sun's ultraviolet (UV) rays harm the skin. These rays are strongest from 11 A.M. to 2 P.M. during the summer, so that is when risk is greatest. Fair-skinned people are at greater risk than dark-skinned people. They have less of a pigment called melanin in their skin to block some of the sun's damaging rays. The harm done is never fully repaired, even though the suntan or burn fades away.

You can protect yourself from the sun's rays and still spend a lot of time outdoors. Wear lightweight clothing but choose long-sleeved shirts and long pants. Wear a broad-brimmed hat or a bandana. Use sunscreens. A number 15 on the label means most of the sun's UV rays will be blocked out.

12. CAN TOO MANY X-RAYS INCREASE MY RISK OF GETTING CANCER?

Yes. Large doses of radiation are known to cause cancer. Although you are exposed to very little radiation in a single X-ray, getting many X-rays over a long period does increase your cancer risk. The best practice is to discuss each X-ray with your doctor or dentist to learn if each is needed. If the X-ray is necessary, ask if X-ray shields can be used to protect other parts of your body.

13. IS THERE ANY ASSOCIATION BETWEEN ESTROGEN USE AND CANCER IN WOMEN?

Use of the hormone estrogen has been linked to cancer of the uterus. Studies have shown that women who took large doses of estrogens for menopause symptoms have a greater risk of developing uterine cancer than women who did not take estrogens. Increases in risks to other cancers have been studied, but the results have been unclear.

The association of birth control pills with cancer risk has been studied. There is no conclusive evidence that cancer is caused by any pills now sold. Study results suggest, though, that the risk of breast and cervical cancer might be higher in some groups of pill users. Also, there is some evidence that pill users may have a lower risk of cancers of the uterine lining and ovary. Pill users should examine their breasts regularly and get regular Pap tests.

Today, estrogens for menopause symptoms and for birth control can be prescribed at very low levels. If you are taking estrogens, you can help protect yourself by discussing dose levels with your doctor.

14. WILL ON-THE-JOB EXPOSURE TO CANCER-CAUSING AGENTS INCREASE THE RISK OF DEVELOPING CANCER?

Exposure to some industrial agents increases cancer risks. The kinds of workplace substances that cause cancer can be divided into three broad groups: chemicals, metals, dusts, and fibers. Only a small number of agents in these groups actually cause cancer. They do damage by acting alone or, probably more often, by acting in combination with another workplace carcinogen or with cigarette smoke. For example, studies have shown that breathing in asbestos fibers creates an especially high risk of lung disease and cancer. The risk is extremely high for workers who smoke. In fact, some scientists suggest that the main carcinogen in the workplace is the cigarette.

Regulatory agencies, industries, and organized labor have developed health and safety measures related to hazardous exposures in the workplace. Industries can take a number of steps to reduce or eliminate risks to workers. Individuals can also take steps. Health and safety rules of the workplace ought to be known and followed.

15. DO BUMPS, BRUISES, OR OTHER INJURIES CAUSE CANCER?

No. Injuries to the body cannot cause cancer. Sometimes, treatment for an injury leads the doctor to find a cancer that had existed before but had not been noticed.

16. WHAT CAN I DO TO REDUCE MY CHANCES OF GETTING CANCER?

You can reduce your cancer risks by limiting or avoiding exposure to or use of cancer-causing agents. You can help protect yourself if you:

- Don't smoke. Smoking causes cancer and increases the risk from other carcinogens.
- Vary your diet to include foods high in fiber, low in fat and low enough in calories so that you will stay trim. Include fresh fruits and vegetables and whole grain breads and cereals in your daily diet.
- Avoid too much sunlight, particularly if you are fair-skinned, by wearing protective clothing and using sunscreens.
- Don't ask for an X-ray if your doctor or dentist does not recommend

it. If you need an X-ray, ask if X-ray shields can be used to protect other parts of your body.

- Follow worksite health and safety rules. Wear protective clothing; use provided safety equipment.
- Drink alcoholic beverages only in moderation, particularly if you smoke. (One or two drinks a day is considered moderate.)
- Discuss estrogen use with your doctor; use only as long as needed.

Help Protect Yourself From Cancer

Answer the following questions to identify your own personal risks of developing cancer. If you answer **yes** to any of these questions, there is something you can do to protect yourself. Check the chart on pages 169 and 170.

1. Do you smoke?
   cigarettes _____ yes _____ no
   pipes _____ yes _____ no
   cigars _____ yes _____ no

2. Do you use smokeless tobacco products?
   chewing tobacco _____ yes _____ no
   snuff _____ yes _____ no

3. Do you often work or play in the sun?
   _____ yes _____ no

4. Are you taking estrogens?
   _____ yes _____ no

5. Do you work with or near industrial cancer-causing agents, such as asbestos, nickel, uranium, chromates, petroleum, vinyl chloride?
   _____ yes _____ no

6. Do you have X-rays taken frequently?
   _____ yes _____ no

7. Do you eat many foods that are high in fats?
   fried foods _____ yes _____ no
   whole milk/
     cheeses _____ yes _____ no
   fatty meats _____ yes _____ no
   potato chips _____ yes _____ no

8. Do you have more than two drinks of an alcoholic beverage per day?
   _____ yes _____ no

Facts on Cancer Risk Factors

Known Risk Factor	The Risk
Cigarettes, Cigars, Pipes	Increased risk of lung cancer. For cigarette smokers, 10 times that of nonsmokers.
Chewing Tobacco, Snuff	Increased risk of mouth cancer.
Estrogens (for menopause)	Long-term, high-dose use; increased risk of cancer of the uterus.
Occupation	Exposure to one or a combination of certain known cancer-causing industrial agents (nickel, chromate, uranium, asbestos, petroleum, vinyl chloride) in many cases with smoking; increased risk of several cancers.
X-rays	Overexposure (for example, a large number of X-rays over a long period of time); increased risk of many types of cancers.
Sunlight	Long exposure and no sunscreen protection; increased risk of skin cancer.
Alcohol	Heavy drinking, especially with smoking; increased risk of mouth, throat, liver, and esophagus cancer.

Action

Don't smoke. Low-tar, low-nicotine cigarettes do not eliminate risk of getting cancer.

Don't use smokeless tobacco products.

Take estrogens in the smallest possible dose, and only as long as necessary. Discuss benefits and risks with a physician.

Industries can take a number of steps to reduce or eliminate occupational hazards for their workers. Health and safety rules of your workplace should be known and followed. Don't smoke.

Avoid X-rays that aren't medically needed. Be sure X-ray shields are used to protect other parts of your body when possible.

Don't stay in the sun for more than brief periods of time without protection (hats, long sleeves, long pants, sunscreen lotions).

If you drink alcohol, do so only in moderation. (One or two drinks per day is considered moderate.)

Suspected risk factor

Diet

The Risk
A diet high in fat, and/or high in total calories that may lead to obesity; increased risk of several cancers.

Action
A generous intake of dietary fiber from whole grain breads and cereals, fruits and vegetables, peas and beans is prudent.

Vary diet to include foods low in fat (fresh fruit, vegetables, whole grain breads and cereals, low-fat dairy products, lean meat, poultry—without the skin—fish, peas, and beans). Prepare foods by baking, broiling, poaching, and simmering with little or no added fat, rather than frying. Use margarine, butter, oils, and salad dressings sparingly. Treat yourself to baked goods and desserts only on special occasions.

You can control many of the factors that cause cancer. This means that you can help protect yourself from the possibility of getting cancer. You can decide how you're going to live your life—which habits you will keep and which ones you will change.

The habits that help protect you from cancer are many of the same ones that help keep you feeling healthy and fit.

GLOSSARY

Agent   a substance that causes some changes.

Cancer   a group of diseases in which abnormal cells grow out of control and can spread throughout the body.

Carcinogen   (câr sin′ ō gĕn) any agent that is known to cause cancer either in animals or humans.

Cells   the basic structural units that make up all tissues of the body and carry on all the body's functions.

Esophagus   (ĕ sŏf′ ă gus) the tube that carries food from the throat to the stomach.

Estrogen   (ĕs′ trō gĕn) any of several female sex hormones that are secreted by the ovaries and that help regulate the functions of the uterus; man-made copies of this hormone that are used to mimic or alter natural body functions.

Hormone   a substance formed by one organ of the body, which is carried (for example, by the bloodstream) to another organ and stimulates the second organ to function.

Initiator   (ĭ nĭsh′ ē ā tôr) any agent that may start the cancer process in animals or in humans.

Menopause   (mĕn′ ō păuz) the time in a woman's life when menstruation stops, usually around age 50.

Promoter   (prō mō′ ter) an agent that advances the development of cancer, once a cell has been damaged by an initiator.

Risk factor   an agent or substance that increases an individual's possibility of getting a particular type of cancer.

Uterus   the womb.

Cancer prevention tips

Don't smoke or use tobacco in any form.

Eat foods high in fiber and low in fat.

Include fresh fruits, vegetables, and whole grain cereals in your daily diet.

Health and safety rules of your workplace should be known and followed.

Avoid unnecessary X-rays.

If you drink alcoholic beverages, do so only in moderation.

Avoid too much sunlight; wear protective clothing; use sunscreens.

Take estrogens only as long as necessary.

The role of fiber in cancer

Why Eat Fiber?

Dietary fiber is material from plant cells that is nondigestible or partially digested. Fiber helps move food quickly through the intestines and out of the body. It helps prevent constipation and promotes a healthy digestive tract. Recent studies indicate that foods high in fiber—fruits and vegetables, peas and beans, whole-grain breads and cereals—protect against some cancers, particularly colorectal. Diets high in fat, on the other hand, appear to increase risk for some cancers.

The National Cancer Institute is recommending, therefore, that Americans increase the fiber-rich foods in their diets and decrease the proportion of fats in their diets.

How Much Fiber Should I Eat?

Americans now eat about 10 to 20 grams of fiber a day. The NCI recommends that we eat foods which provide 25 to 35 grams of fiber a day (28 grams = 1 ounce).

Fiber supplements, unless they're ordered by your physician, aren't the answer, because all studies to date show protective effects are associated with fiber-rich foods.

How Can I Get More Fiber in My Diet?

As a general rule, eat several servings of fiber-rich foods, fruits, vegetables, peas and beans, and breads and cereals made from whole grains, daily. Eating much more of these fiber-rich foods, known as complex carbohydrates, won't necessarily make you gain weight, either, particularly if you're cutting down on fat. Each gram of protein and each gram of complex carbohydrates contains 5 calories. But each gram of fat contains 9 calories.

High fiber, low-fat diets are a good lifetime habit for everyone!

Choose More Often:

Whole grain products:
- Crackers, bran muffins; brown rye, oatmeal, pumpernickel, bran and corn breads; whole wheat English muffins and bagels
- Breakfast cereals such as bran cereals, shredded wheat, whole grain or whole-wheat flaked cereals, and others that list dietary fiber content
- Other foods made with whole-wheat flours, including barley, buckwheat grouts, bulgur wheat, macaroni, pancakes, pasta, and taco shells

Fruits and vegetables:
- Apples, pears, apricots, bananas, berries, cantaloupe, grapefruit, oranges, pineapples, papayas, prunes, raisins, and others
- Artichokes, carrots, broccoli, potatoes, corn, cauliflower, Brussels sprouts, cabbage, celery, green beans, parsnips, kale, spinach, other greens, yams, sweet potatoes, turnips

Dried peas and beans:
- Black, kidney, garbanzo, pinto, navy, white, and lima beans
- Lentils, split peas, and black-eyed peas.

Snacks:
- Fruits and vegetables
- Unbuttered popcorn

Choose Less Often:

Refined bakery and snack products:
- Bakery products, including refined flour bread and quickbreads, biscuits, buns, croissants, snack crackers, and chips, cookies, pastries, pies.

For more information, write for *"Diet, Nutrition and Cancer Prevention: A Guide to Food Choices"*

> National Cancer Institute
> Building 31,
> Room 10A18,
> Bethesda, MD 20205

For answers to questions you may have about cancer, including information about early detection, call the following toll-free telephone number and you will be automatically connected to the Cancer Information Service office serving your area:

1–800–4–CANCER*

* In Alaska call 1–800–638–6070; in Washington, D.C. (and suburbs in Maryland and Virginia) call 202–636–5700; in Hawaii, on Oahu call 808–524–1234 (Neighbor Islands call collect).

Spanish-speaking staff members are available to callers from the following areas (daytime hours only): California (area codes 213, 714, 619, and 805), Florida, Georgia, Illinois, Northern New Jersey, New York City, and Texas.

Department of Health and Human Services, Public Health Service, National Institutes of Health, Bethesda, Maryland 20205.

Cerebral Palsy
Hope Through Research

A child is born. And it is only natural to want that child to be normal and healthy. But complications can arise throughout pregnancy and birth. Certain infections in a mother-to-be can seriously harm her unborn child. Cigarette smoking, excessive use of alcohol, and a variety of drugs can also impair a baby's growth and development. Labor and delivery are sometimes long and difficult. Birth may be premature, or result in a full-term infant of low birth weight. Each of these possibilities is known to increase the risk of injury to the baby—a risk that is especially high for the baby's rapidly developing brain. If the injury affects the brain areas vital in the control of movement—the motor systems—the baby may develop cerebral palsy.

Cerebral refers to the two large wrinkled hemispheres that dominate any picture of the human brain. *Palsy* means paralysis, but frequently is used to refer to problems in the control of nerves and muscles that make voluntary movements difficult or impossible. The words are broad enough in meaning to allow the term *cerebral palsy* to cover a large group of movement disorders of varying symptoms and severity. A child with mild cerebral palsy may be a little awkward. A child with more severe cerebral palsy may be mentally retarded or subject to convulsions, as well as physically handicapped.

For a disorder to be classified as cerebral palsy, not only must there be a problem with movement or posture, but the problem must also occur early in development, during the time of the brain's most rapid growth. (By age 5 the brain will have reached 90 percent of its adult weight.) Doctors can't always pinpoint the precise cause of brain injury, but agree that sometimes it is the end result of a shortage of oxygen to brain cells, possibly combined with a diminished blood supply. Since the brain makes a high demand on blood-borne oxygen and nutrients, periods of deprivation can have devastating effects.

In many cases of cerebral palsy, the movement disorder may be accompanied by mental or emotional impairment, convulsive seizures (epilepsy), or losses in hearing, vision, or the other senses. Some of these associated conditions can be treated successfully, and some kinds of movement disturbance may improve in time. However, nerve cells are extremely limited in their powers of repair and regeneration, and even in cases where a child appears to recover full control over the limbs, mental or emotional deficits may remain.

On the other hand, the brain damage doesn't get worse over time: cerebral palsy is a nonprogressive disorder (although symptoms may change as a child matures). Cerebral palsy is not contagious, either, and only rarely are the symptoms associated with a hereditary disorder. Close to 90 percent of the time the brain damage happens in pregnancy, often around the time of birth (the perinatal period). The condition is then called *congenital* cerebral palsy. Head injuries, infections such as meningitis, and other forms of brain damage (including injury from child abuse) occurring in the first months or years of life are the main causes of *acquired* cerebral palsy.

The words "may" and "can" used to describe the mishaps of pregnancy and early life are important. Not every infection or trauma of pregnancy harms the unborn child (the fetus). Not every fetus is equally vulnerable: many newborns endure long complicated deliveries with no lasting effects. Some low birth weight babies—today even babies under 2 pounds—may spend months in a newborn (neonatal) intensive care unit and emerge with all systems intact. Indeed, advances in neonatal care have been so impressive that babies are surviving today for whom there would have been no hope a decade ago.

At the same time, research has progressed in identifying some of the leading causes of cerebral palsy and finding means of prevention and treatment. One of the largest, most comprehensive research projects ever undertaken was the Collaborative Perinatal Project sponsored by the National Institute of Neurological and Communicative Disorders and Stroke (NINCDS). The project entailed following 55,000 women through pregnancy and delivery, and periodically examining their offspring from birth to age 7. The results of the study, still being analyzed, have already revealed a variety of environmental factors and events in pregnancy that increase the risk that a child will develop cerebral palsy or other serious nervous system disorders, and have helped focus attention on what can be done about these problems.

Meanwhile other researchers have found ways to prevent or treat several well-known causes of cerebral palsy. There is now a vaccine for German measles (rubella), a virus disease notorious for its destructive effects on the fetal nervous system. Mothers-to-be are now urged to seek prenatal care early, eat wisely, and avoid the use of any nonessential drugs, including alcohol and nicotine. (One finding confirmed by the Collaborative Perinatal Project was that women who smoke during pregnancy tend to produce babies of lower than normal weight.)

Preventive methods as well as treatments are now available for a number of blood disorders, such as Rh incompatibility, in which antibodies in the mother's bloodstream attack fetal red blood cells—the very cells that carry oxygen and nutrients to all parts of the baby's body. Usually a mother's first child is not affected, but the first-born's red blood cells may sensitize the mother, causing her body to manufacture antibodies that will attack the fetus in the next pregnancy. A mother with Rh incompatibility can be injected with a special serum shortly after her first child's birth to prevent the unwanted antibody production. Babies born with the Rh blood disorder can be treated with exchange transfusions in which a large volume of the baby's blood is removed and replaced with normal blood.

Treatments are also available for jaundice of the newborn, a blood disorder associated with Rh incompatibility, but one that can arise independently. In this condition there is a buildup of bile pigments in the baby's bloodstream (hyperbilirubinemia) which, if unrelieved, can destroy brain cells. As a result of Collaborative Perinatal Project findings, it now appears that even moderate hyperbilirubinemia in the newborn can be toxic to the brain and should be treated accordingly. Thus some major causes of cerebral palsy can now be eliminated.

Still cerebral palsy occurs. The majority of cases (58 percent in the Collaborative Perinatal Project study) develop in babies born at full term and full weight. Exact figures for the United States population are not available because doctors are not obliged to report cases of cerebral palsy to state health boards. The estimate of the United Cerebral Palsy Associations, the major voluntary health organization concerned with this problem, is that between one and three infants out of every thousand liveborn develop cerebral palsy—about 9,000 new cases a year. At present, the association estimates there are 750,000 Americans alive with the condition. The most severely handicapped usually do not survive infancy, but most patients will reach maturity and many will attain a normal life span.

While better prenatal and obstetric care and new treatments are undoubtedly preventing some cases of cerebral palsy, it is not clear whether the number of new cases each year has significantly decreased. Moreover, the premature and very frail infants who are able to survive today, thanks to the new intensive care technology, do not always escape damage to the nervous system. Sadly, too, there are still some babies whose deliveries are uncomplicated, who appear normal at birth, yet later show signs of cerebral palsy.

Complicating the search for a cause of cerebral palsy in cases where no obvious mishap is implicated, is the fact that the brain is one of the most inaccessible organs in the body to study. Doctors cannot conveniently sample brain tissue or fluids the way they can blood or urine. This situation has improved greatly in the last decade with the development of new, safe diagnostic tools such as computerized tomography—the CT scan—which produces a computer-drawn X-ray image of the brain, and ultrasound, which uses the echoes from high-frequency sound waves to detect brain abnormalities. These methods can sometimes reveal treatable cases of brain swelling or show up a small blood clot or hemorrhage—a stroke—not otherwise evident in an infant with cerebral palsy. But many times brain abnormality eludes detection.

A delay in development

Generally the diagnosis of cerebral palsy is made on the basis of symptoms that develop over the first or second year of life. Cerebral palsy is frequently not evident at birth because newborns have very little voluntary control over their bodies. They depend on reflexes—automatic responses built into the nervous system. Reflexes serve to protect and preserve the baby. For example, if you thump the mattress sharply on either side of a newborn lying flat on its back in a crib, the baby will react by throwing its arms around in an embrace-like gesture called the Moro reflex. Or if you touch a nipple to the baby's mouth, it will automatically pucker its lips in the sucking reflex. As development unfolds, a normal infant gradually loses the more primitive reflexes (which often involve movement of major parts of the body) and gains increasingly fine control over the body's separate parts.

In contrast, an infant with cerebral palsy usually shows a delay in development. Often the primitive reflexes remain and may dominate behavior so that the child has difficulty mastering such familiar landmarks of growth as rolling over, sitting, crawling, smiling, or making speech sounds. Sometimes an infant will favor a particular side of the body or assume an unusual posture. In other instances, the major symptom may be an overall muscle weakness or decreased muscle tone (hypotonia): the baby is as floppy as a Raggedy Ann doll, and even some of the primitive reflexes may be weak or absent.

Alert parents are often the first to note signs of developmental delay or abnormality. In other cases the family doctor may be suspicious and refer the parents to a neurologist, a specialist in nervous system disorders. The neurological examination is important because it will be on the basis of the findings that the specialist will decide whether the child has cerebral palsy and will discuss treatment. Corrective measures including orthopedic surgery, drugs, the use of casts, braces, hearing aids, and other devices, as well as an overall program of education, psychological support, and rehabilitation can then be initiated. These measures are aimed at relieving symptoms and increasing the mobility, confidence, and independence of the child. At the same time they can forestall serious secondary changes in muscles, joints, and bones, such as curvature of the spine or hip dislocation, that can result from abnormal postures.

Early detection of hearing loss is especially important since the development of speech is so crucially linked to a child's ability to hear.

Many symptoms and mixed varieties

Doctors classify cerebral palsy according to the quality of the movement disturbance and the limbs affected. If the legs are primarily affected, the condition is called *diplegia.* If both the arm and leg on one side are affected, it is a case of *hemiplegia* or *hemiparesis.* If both arms and legs are affected, the term is *quadriplegia* or *quadriparesis.* (The ending "plegia" means paralysis and "paresis" means weakness; while both terms are used, "paresis" is more accurate since cerebral palsy rarely leads to total paralysis.)

Spastic Cerebral Palsy   Spastic muscles are tense and contracted, resistant to movement. When reflexes are tested, they may be very brisk, resulting in repeated contractions: clonus. If a child with spastic diplegia is supported under the arms, the legs often hang straight down, unable to flex at the knees. The lower legs may turn in and cross at the ankle. The movements of the legs are stiff and resemble the crossed blades of a pair of scissors, hence the term "scissors" gait. This condition can sometimes be corrected by surgery to release tight hip muscles. Sometimes the leg muscles are so tightly contracted the child's heels do not touch the floor, so the child walks on tiptoe. Physical therapy, plaster casts, or, if necessary, orthopedic surgery to release the heel tendons can permit more normal walking.

Spasticity is the most common abnormality in cerebral palsy. Spastic diplegia is also the characteristic form of cerebral palsy seen in either premature or low birth weight infants, as revealed in the Collaborative Perinatal Project and other studies.

Athetoid Cerebral Palsy   A second common form of cerebral palsy is characterized by involuntary writhing movements of the parts of the body affected. This incessant, slow activity is called athetosis. The hands may turn and twist, and often there is facial grimacing, tonguing, and drooling. Another form of involuntary movement, sometimes occurring with athetosis, involves abrupt flailing or jerky motions of the body, described as *chorea,* from the Greek word for dance. Many cases of athetoid or choreic cerebral palsy involve damage to motor centers only. To the uninformed, however, the unnatural movements and facial expressions of such patients are often taken as signs of mental or emotional disturbance—a tragic compounding of the patient's problems.

Ataxic Cerebral Palsy   In some cases of cerebral palsy the principal movement disturbance is a lack of balance and coordination described as ataxia. Persons with ataxic cerebral palsy may sway when standing, have trouble maintaining balance, and may walk with feet spread wide apart to avoid falling. The motor centers involved lie in the cerebellum, a large white globe of tissue at the back of the brain tucked under the cerebral hemispheres.

Mixed Cases   When several motor centers are affected, the symptoms of cerebral palsy are mixed. The doctor's lengthy description may be spastic diplegia with athetosis of the upper limbs (tense, contracted leg muscles with writhing arms); right hemiparesis with rigidity (stiff muscles in right arm and leg), diplegia with hypotonia (floppy muscles in both legs) and so on.

Other Symptoms   In addition to the major limb disturbances, cerebral palsy patients sometimes have hand tremors, making fine movements difficult. They may have problems in speaking, chewing, or swallowing, maintaining visual focus, or following a moving target. There may also be drooling, a cooler surface temperature over affected parts of the body, or the loss of bowel or bladder control.

The common associated problems of convulsive seizures, mental or emotional impairments, hearing, visual, or other sensory handicaps, such as the loss of the ability to identify objects by touch, add to the difficulties faced by many cerebral palsy patients and their families. In such complex cases it is particularly important to distinguish true intellectual deficits from problems in language, learning, and attention that may be due to severe speech and sensory handicaps.

"Will my child ever walk?"

The diagnosis of cerebral palsy is always upsetting and parents are inevitably anxious and concerned over the future. Will the child ever talk? Walk? Go to college? Be able to work? In mild cases the doctor can usually be reassuring. But often there are no simple answers. Every individual with cerebral palsy presents a unique set of symptoms along with a unique capacity and potential for coping. A lot may depend on rehabilitation and education programs; a lot on the cooperation and positive but realistic attitudes of all concerned. Some physicians generalize that if a child can sit up unsupported by the end of the second year, or stand by age 3, the chances for independent walking are good. But there are always exceptions. Sometimes orthopedic surgery may be necessary. Almost always there will be a need for a coordinated treatment program provided by a team of skilled professionals. Still, not all children may respond.

Coordinated programs are available through the physical medicine or rehabilitation departments of hospitals, state crippled children's programs, and a variety of clinics or centers for the handicapped financed by public or private agencies. Both the United Cerebral Palsy Associations, Inc., and the National Easter Seal Society, Inc., have local chapters and clinics throughout the country. In addition, special programs are available to assure that no handicapped person is denied free public education.

At the same time, it is important to maintain a stable and reassuring home environment. The presence of a handicapped child is hard on all members of the family. Parents may quarrel or feel guilty, and occasionally experience such strain that the marriage is threatened. Parents are sometimes overprotective and pampering, creating serious personality and behavioral problems for the child, and leading brothers and sisters to feel denied attention and love. In a few instances parents may be rejecting or show indifference to the handicapped child. Excellent advice comes from the mother of a child with cerebral palsy: "If the parents accept the child, the child will then accept himself." Many agencies and clinics providing treatment for individuals with cerebral palsy include social workers or psychologists skilled in family counseling, or else can refer families to appropriate professionals to guide families through the initial adjustment and as problems arise.

The combined education and rehabilitation programs currently available will enable some children to progress to excellent control over their bodies and a nearly normal life. Those with more severe handicaps may be able to move from bed to wheelchair or from wheelchair to braces or other mechanical aids. Most authorities agree that progress in overcoming handicaps is harder if there are mental impairments.

Treatments old and new

Physical Therapy An integral part of rehabilitation is physical therapy, a program of exercises and activities supervised by a professional therapist. The program is designed to make the most of the individual's potential and to recruit whatever reserves the nervous system may have for learning new skills.

Some physical therapy programs popular today follow specific principles of nervous system development. The Bobath technique, for example, pioneered by a husband-wife team in England, is based on the idea that the primitive reflexes exhibited by many children with cerebral palsy are major impediments to learning voluntary control. The reflexes also give rise to abnormal sensations: the child's muscles always feel very tense or very loose. The therapist tries to break down the reflexes by deliberately positioning the child in opposing postures. If an arm had been extended, it is now flexed, and so on. Gradually some children are able to maintain the new "reflex inhibiting postures" and begin to experience more normal muscle tone. As therapy proceeds, the child gradually is able to extend his repertoire of voluntary movements. Some therapists report that the combination of relaxation and success achieved with limb muscles helps the child with speech problems, enabling real progress in learning how to talk.

Other innovations in physical therapy make use of the psychological principles of behavior modification in which the individual is rewarded ("positively reinforced") for certain behavior. Thus a child who habitually turns his head to one side in a primitive neck reflex may learn to turn it to the opposite side if rewarded by the sight of a toy, the sound of a music box, or other pleasant surprises.

Many therapists stress the importance of providing a varied and stimulating environment for the physically handicapped child. This constitutes "treatment" that can be as valuable as more formal therapies. Children normally learn by active exploration of their world—think of the toddler crawling to reach a block or ball, or turning to listen to his mother and look at her face. All the more reason to make sure that the child who is limited in exploration is not additionally deprived the richness of sights, sounds, and other pleasurable experiences of life.

Biofeedback   One of the latest methods of treatment of cerebral palsy combines behavior modification with the techniques of biofeedback. In biofeedback an individual is supplied with information—usually in the form of vivid visual or auditory signals—about the functioning of a particular part of the body. Heart rate, for example, may be translated into a musical tone which rises and falls according to whether heart rate goes up or down. The individual is told to alter the rate—usually lower it—by concentrating on making the musical tone fall. Surprisingly, many people are able to do this, although exactly how they do it is not clear.

Now investigators whose research is supported by NINCDS have been able to train some youngsters with cerebral palsy to lower the tension of their muscles by lowering the pitch of muscle "sounds." The sounds correspond to the electrical activity generated whenever muscles contract; the greater the tension, the higher the voltage (and the musical pitch). Concentrating on one muscle at a time, and rewarding each little step in the right direction, scientists at Johns Hopkins Hospital in Baltimore have trained children to drink from a cup and to control their bowels and bladder. One 7-year-old boy with severe athetoid cerebral palsy was able to keep his arm muscles relaxed for some time even after the training sessions were over. In some cases the investigators have observed a transfer phenomenon: a child trained to relax one group of muscles is able to lower the tension in other groups.

Similar studies of the use of biofeedback to control spastic muscles are being supported by NINCDS at Emory University in Atlanta, Ga.

Further research is needed to explore what nervous system activities are involved, specify which patients are most likely to benefit, and evaluate long-term results.

Occupational Therapy   The urge for independence is universal. Occupational therapy teaches the practical skills that enable a person to say, "I can do it myself." For handicapped children occupational therapy means learning how to dress, comb hair, clean teeth, hold a cup or a pen or pencil. For older people occupational therapy may mean vocational training or learning how to shop, cook, or keep house. Today there are a growing number of safe and ingeniously designed gadgets and aids to make the handicapped more self-sufficient, ranging from shoes with laces that can be tied with one hand to elaborate voice synthesizers or pint-sized portable typewriters that enable patients with speech and hearing impairments to communicate. For children there are learning toys like illuminated pens to facilitate eye-hand coordination. A number of these devices are the by-products of engineering research supported by the United Cerebral Palsy Associations and other groups.

In discussing cerebral palsy, the focus is so often on children that it is easy to forget that children with cerebral palsy grow up to be adults with cerebral palsy. Some are bright college students who may go on to professional careers; others may learn skilled or semiskilled jobs and be financially independent; for still others, the handicaps are so extensive, so unresponsive to treatment—or the condition so neglected—that they face life in an institution.

Rehabilitation may still be possible, however, as was recently demonstrated in a group of patients long confined to state mental institutions or homes for the retarded. The patients were established in a cerebral palsy clinic, weaned off all medication, and provided with therapists who worked with individuals on a nearly one-to-one basis. Within a year or two of the start of the program some patients were able to find jobs and live in halfway houses; others were developing new social and practical skills and working in a sheltered workshop.

Drugs   Certain drugs are important in the treatment of cerebral palsy. If epilepsy is a complication, for example, anticonvulsant drugs are usually prescribed and are very effective in preventing seizures in many patients. Diazepam (Valium) and other muscle-relaxant drugs can sometimes help to relieve the tension of spastic muscles. Other nervous system drugs may also enable a child who is restless, easily distracted, or has other behavior problems to relax and concentrate in school. However, the chronic use of any drugs in children must be watched carefully. There may be unwanted side effects, and the long-term effects on the developing nervous system are largely unknown.

Surgery   Over the years there have been attempts to modify the symptoms of cerebral palsy through surgery to destroy the brain sites assumed to be responsible for involuntary movements. More recently surgery has been performed to implant electrodes in the brain. The electrodes can be activated by a transmitter to stimulate nerves important in motor coordination and control. These techniques are experimental and very controversial; they involve some risk to the patient, and the results have been mixed: some patients report improvements, others none at all.

Electrical Stimulation   An alternative technique that involves far less risk to the patient than implanting electrodes in the brain is the use of electrical stimulating devices applied locally to nerves in affected limbs. NINCDS is currently encouraging research on the development of such devices to control spasticity.

There have been no carefully controlled studies to determine if any one treatment or combination of treatments for cerebral palsy is superior to any other. Such studies require the careful matching of patient groups by age, symptoms, and so on—a requirement difficult to achieve in a disorder as varied and complex in symptoms as cerebral palsy. The studies might also entail withholding treatment from one group of patients, which would be undesirable. In addition, there have been no objective measurements or scales of motor performance in cerebral palsy patients which could be used to assess progress or change. To address that need NINCDS is currently supporting research at Rush-Presbyterian-St. Luke's Medical Center in Chicago, where an investigator is developing standard measures of spasticity in patients with cerebral palsy and other forms of brain damage.

Working toward prevention

Much of the research on cerebral palsy supported by NINCDS and other Federal agencies, such as the National Institute of Child Health and Human Development, the National Heart, Lung, and Blood Institute, and the National Institute of Allergy and Infectious Diseases, as well as by private voluntary agencies, is aimed at eliminating known risks and threats:

Breathing and Circulation Problems   The Collaborative Perinatal Project confirmed the greater risk for cerebral palsy—especially spastic diplegia—associated with premature and low birth weight infants. The risk in relation to weight was highest for babies weighing under 3.3 pounds at birth (no matter how many weeks of gestation). Very immature babies often have serious breathing and circulatory problems which constitute a threat to the brain. Current research is focusing on lung development in prematurely delivered experimental animals, with emphasis on finding ways to prevent or treat respiratory disease.

Other investigators are studying the flow of blood through the immature brain. Brain hemorrhage—especially bleeding into the fluid-filled spaces of the brain (the ventricles)—is a major cause of death or neurological handicap in low birth weight infants. But little is understood of how such intraventricular hemorrhage occurs. Possibly breathing problems lead to an oxygen shortage (hypoxia), which causes changes in blood pressure and acidity, along with other metabolic alterations. In turn, these changes may cause the very tiny blood vessels in the infant's brain to distend and rupture. Fortunately, better and safer means of measuring blood gases and careful monitoring of the brain using ultrasound or CT scanning are helping to identify the problem and evaluate complicating factors.

The NINCDS is currently supporting research at Pennsylvania State University to study the effects of hypoxia on the brains of fetal, newborn, and adult rats. In particular, the researchers are concerned with how oxygen deprivation affects the ability of nerve cells to transmit impulses from one to another.

At NINCDS, scientists have found that a partial cut-off of oxygen may cause the immature brain to swell. This sets up a vicious cycle in which the swelling compresses brain blood vessels, further limiting oxygen to brain cells, and ultimately leading to their death. Armed with this knowledge, neonatal specialists are developing better methods of monitoring circulation to prevent brain swelling; they are also developing treatments for brain swelling, should it occur.

Low Birth Weight There is also growing interest in the problem of low birth weight itself. In spite of improvements in maternal care, the number of babies born weighing under 5.5 pounds has remained stable in America at about 7½ percent of all births each year. Poor nutrition, illness, accidents, and psychological stress during pregnancy are contributing factors, certainly, and some women may also be genetically predisposed to premature labor and delivery. Scientists currently investigating the problem are particularly interested in the hormonal and other chemical changes that occur in pregnancy. In research supported by the United Cerebral Palsy Research and Education Foundation, for example, investigators are studying the role of relaxin, a hormone produced in pregnancy which may prevent premature contractions of the uterus as well as prepare the cervix for birth.

Seizures Collaborative Perinatal Project data showed that convulsive seizures in the first months of life were serious events associated with a relatively high rate of death. Seizures in the newborn—not always obvious because they may not look like seizures in older infants—were also found to be a major marker for subsequent neurological problems, including cerebral palsy. In every case the examining physician will try to determine the underlying cause of the seizures, such as infection, hemorrhage, or oxygen shortage, and correct it if possible. Control of the seizures themselves may be important because very lengthy or repeated seizures in early life may in themselves cause damage to the developing brain.

Infections While vaccines to prevent German measles have greatly reduced the hazard to the fetus from this infection, not all women have been immunized. An estimated 15 to 20 percent of women now entering childbearing age are at risk for German measles. These women, who were already in school in the late 1960's when immunization programs were begun for preschoolers, have not acquired natural immunity because there have been no epidemics in their lifetimes. It is important that all women know their immunological status and are vaccinated *before* becoming pregnant.

Several major infectious diseases for which there are no vaccines and no treatments remain serious threats to the fetus or newborn. Again, the nervous system is particularly vulnerable to these infectious agents, which, while not as well known as the rubella virus, are no less destructive.

Toxoplasmosis, a disease caused by a parasite that infects cats, other domestic animals, and food sources, produces few or no symptoms in most adults but may be highly damaging to the fetus. Infection is common in adults and increases with age: between one-third and one-half of women of childbearing age have been infected. The danger to the fetus occurs if a woman acquires toxoplasmosis while pregnant.

Also highly prevalent is cytomegalovirus, estimated to infect 3 percent of all pregnant women. The virus causes few or no symptoms in a woman, although it infects a variety of body organs, including the cervix. It is estimated that 1 out of every 100 infants born in the United States is infected with cytomegalovirus, while half of those infants exposed prenatally but not infected at birth will become infected through breast milk or handling in the first months of life. Some babies will be severely damaged and may die. Between 5 and 10 percent of those remaining will later show signs of hearing loss, especially for high tones, and have I.Q.'s less than 80. Research under way at NINCDS laboratories in Bethesda, Md., and elsewhere is aimed at developing an animal model for the human disease, a key step in evaluating vaccines and effective treatments.

Cytomegalovirus is one of the viruses of the herpes group. These agents include the virus that causes cold sores, and, of more consequence to the newborn, the type II herpes virus which infects the genital tract and is usually transmitted sexually. The infection is particularly painful in women, and often recurs after initial infection. The virus lies dormant in the nervous system but periodically may descend the genital tract to cause an acute attack. Babies can acquire infection during passage through the birth canal. Physicians attempt to prevent this infection by recognizing the disease in the mothers and delivering the child by cesarean section to avoid exposure to the virus. Investigators at NINCDS are working on new methods for the rapid viral diagnosis of genital herpes to aid physicians in selecting patients for cesarean section. As with the cytomegalovirus, research is also directed toward developing safe and effective vaccines, as well as treatment for those already infected.

A "cure" for cerebral palsy?

While research goes on to eliminate known risks and find more effective treatments for cerebral palsy, the disorder has also inspired research on the most basic questions of nervous system operation: How does the nervous system develop? Is it true that the nervous system cannot recover from major damage? Why are the motor systems so often vulnerable in pregnancy? Why should spastic diplegia be the prevalent form of cerebral palsy in low birth weight babies?

Years ago scientists lacked the tools and techniques to tackle these questions and were generally pessimistic about the potential of the nervous system for healing itself once damaged. Nowadays, not only are they more hopeful, they have also developed extraordinarily powerful methods for studying the nervous system. The result is a far more detailed picture of nerve cell behavior. Scientists know, for example, that when nerve cells fire off nerve impulses—tiny bursts of electrical energy—to neighboring cells, a minute amount of a chemical—a neurotransmitter—is usually released. That transmitter allows the nerve impulse to cross the gap between cells. Scientists know, too, that certain chemicals called growth factors are important in the development of nerve cells, guiding nerve fibers to their proper connections in the system, and playing a role in nervous system maintenance and repair.

This kind of information is leading some researchers interested in cerebral palsy to examine the chemicals involved in muscle movements. For example, one researcher at the University of Michigan is studying the neurotransmitters used by small nerve cells in the spinal cord of rats. The rat develops spasticity after its spinal cord is severed, and the investigator is studying the chemical changes that then occur in nerve cells below the level of injury. Other researchers are studying the effects of drugs on motor centers of the brain. Certain drugs injected into the brains of pregnant rabbits are able to cross the placenta and damage motor centers in the fetal brain, producing a movement disorder similar to cerebral palsy. Such neurochemical research might some day lead to new drug treatments for cerebral palsy in which the drug would restore the balance of neurotransmitters needed for normal muscle coordination and control.

A window on the living brain

Equally exciting in terms of research potential is the recent advance in brain scanning techniques: positron emission transverse tomography (PETT). Development of PETT's potential is now being supported by NINCDS at over half a dozen universities throughout the United States. When a patient or an experimental animal is supplied with a radioactive form of a natural nutrient used by the brain (like sugar) bursts of energy are generated and recorded by the equipment. The cells that are most active in taking up the radioactive substance will show the greatest concentrations of energy on the PETT scan. Thus, investigators can actually observe the living brain in action. They can note exactly which parts of the brain are working when you plan and execute a muscle movement, for example, or do a problem in mental arithmetic. With such a dynamic window into the brain scientists can determine more precisely what goes wrong in the brain of a child with cerebral palsy—and, ultimately, find out what can be done to make things go right.

National voluntary agencies

Two national voluntary agencies support research and provide services to patients. For information about their programs, and listings of their local chapters and clinics, write to:

United Cerebral Palsy Associations, Inc.
66 East 34th Street
New York, N.Y. 10016
(212) 481-6300

The National Easter Seal Society, Inc.
2023 West Ogden Avenue
Chicago, Ill. 60612
(312) 243-8400

Tissue banks

The study of brain and other tissue from persons with neurological disorders is invaluable to research, especially in disorders like cerebral palsy where the causes and associated changes in the brain are complex. NINCDS supports two national human specimens banks, one in Los Angeles, Calif., and one near Boston, Mass. For information about tissue donation and collection write:

Dr. Wallace W. Tourtellotte, Director
Human Neurospecimen Bank

VA Wadsworth Hospital Center
Los Angeles, Calif. 90073

Dr. Edward D. Bird, Director
Brain Tissue Bank
Mailman Research Center
McLean Hospital
Belmont, Mass. 02178

Prepared by the Office of Scientific and Health Reports, National Institute of Neurological and Communicative Disorders and Stroke. National Institutes of Health, Bethesda, Maryland 20205. NIH Publication No. 81–159, December 1980.

Cesarean

Facts About Cesarean Childbirth

Cesarean childbirth, an operation to deliver a baby through an incision in the abdomen, can be traced back through history to Egypt in 3000 B.C. The procedures's name comes from a set of Roman laws, *Lex Caesare,* which in 715 B.C. mandated surgical removal of an unborn fetus upon death of the mother.

Until recent decades, the operation usually had been used as a last resort because of a high rate of maternal complications and death. But with the availability of antibiotics to fight infection and the development of modern surgical techniques, the once high maternal mortality rate has dropped dramatically. As a result, the cesarean childbirth rate has increased dramatically. From 1970 to 1980, the number of cesareans in the U.S. more than tripled, increasing from 5 percent of all births to 16.5 percent. In some localities the rate is much higher.

This startling increase has become a matter of national concern. In the fall of 1980, the National Institute of Child Health and Human Development convened a panel to gather information and develop a draft report on the subject. This report formed the basis for a three-day conference held to examine the issues related to cesarean childbirth, reach general agreement and make recommendations to guide practicing physicians. This "consensus development" panel, made up of leading scientists, practicing physicians and consumers, produced a 540-page final report which is highlighted in this fact sheet.

Basically, the panel concluded that the rising cesarean birth rate can be stopped and perhaps reversed, without sacrificing continued improvements in the quality and success of pregnancy care.

What is cesarean childbirth?

A major operation, each cesarean actually involves a series of separate incisions in the mother. The skin, underlying muscles, and abdomen are opened first, and then the uterus is opened allowing removal of the infant.

There are two main types of cesarean operations, each named according to the location and direction of the uterine incision:

- *cervical*—a transverse (horizontal) or vertical incision in the lower uterus, and
- *classical*—a vertical incision in the main body of the uterus.

Today, the low *transverse cervical* incision is used almost exclusively. It has the lowest incidence of hemorrhage during surgery as well as the least chance of rupturing in later pregnancies. Sometimes, because of fetal size (very large or very small) or position problems (breech or transverse), a *low vertical* cesarean may be performed.

In the *classical* operation, a vertical incision allows a greater opening and is used for fetal size or position problems and in some emergency situations. This approach involves more bleeding in surgery and a higher risk of abdominal infection. Although any uterine incision may rupture during a subsequent labor, the classical is more likely to do so and more likely to result in death for the mother and fetus than a cervical incision.

Why have cesarean rates increased?

Many factors account for rising cesarean birth rates. By the 1960's, increasing emphasis was being placed on the health of the fetus. With

Types of Cesarean Incisions

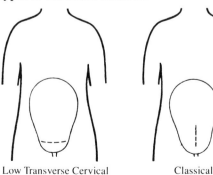

Low Transverse Cervical   Classical

declining birth rates and couples having fewer children, even greater attention was given to improving the outcome of pregnancy, and infant survival in general. The nation's infant mortality rate began to be seen as an international yardstick on the quality of health care. At the same time, advances in medical care combined to make maternal death from cesarean childbirth a rare occurrence. The safer the procedure became, the easier it was to decide to perform the operation. As a safe alternative to normal delivery, the cesarean became a practical way to try to improve the outcome of difficult pregnancies.

Studies suggesting the benefit of cesarean birth in dealing with various pregnancy complications also led to more cesareans. Obstetricians came to favor surgery in pregnancies with difficult deliveries that formerly would have required the use of forceps. The diagnosis of "dystocia," a catch-all term meaning difficult labor, was made more frequently and handled more often with the cesarean operation. Fetal distress during labor—a condition often resulting in a cesarean—was more apt to be detected with the introduction of electronic fetal monitoring. Increasingly, physicians used the cesarean method to deliver infants in the breech position prior to birth, adding still further to the rising cesarean rate.

Another important contributing factor was the rising number of repeat cesareans. As the number of women having their first cesarean increased, the long-held tenet "once a cesarean, always a cesarean" led to a rapid increase in the number of repeat cesarean births.

What is the current medical thinking about repeat cesarean deliveries?

Having had a prior cesarean delivery is one of the two major reasons women have the operation today. (The other is the diagnosis of dystocia.) The consensus development panel found that the rate of repeat cesareans is likely to increase further if present trends continue. Currently more than 98 percent of women in the U.S. who have had a cesarean undergo a repeat cesarean for subsequent pregnancies.

This practice was begun in the late 1900's to avoid the risk of uterine scar rupture and hemorrhage during labor. At that time the classical cesarean incision was most widely used and the cesarean birth rate was extremely low.

Physicians now know that the classical, low vertical and "inverted T" incisions have a higher rate of rupture than the low transverse incision now in general use. The low transverse cervical cesarean also has been shown to result in fewer cases of lasting health disorders or death among mothers and infants. Today, many women who had earlier low transverse cesareans safely deliver subsequent children vaginally.

In studying the issue, the consensus panel found that the risk of maternal death in a repeat cesarean is two times that of a vaginal delivery. In addition, the maternal mortality rate for repeat cesareans has not fallen since 1970. The group concluded that the practice of routine repeat cesarean birth is open to question, and that labor and vaginal delivery after a previous low *transverse cervical* cesarean birth are of low risk to the mother and child in properly selected cases.

The panel recommended that:

- In hospitals with appropriate facilities, services and staff for prompt emergency cesarean birth, some women who have had a previous low transverse cervical cesarean may safely be allowed a trial of labor and vaginal delivery.
- The present practice of repeat cesareans should continue for patients who have had previous cesareans with classical, inverted T or low vertical incisions, or for whom there is no record or the type of incision.
- In hospitals without appropriate facilities, services, and staff, the risk of labor for women having had a previous cesarean may exceed the risk to mother and infant from a properly timed, elective repeat cesarean birth. To allow patients to make an informed decision, they should be told in advance about the limits of the institution's capabilities and the availability of other institutions offering this service.
- More adequate information should be compiled on the risks and benefits of trying labor in patients with previous low transverse cervical incisions.
- Institutions offering labor trials following low transverse cesareans should develop guidelines for managing those labors.
- Patient education on initial and repeat cesarean birth should continue throughout pregnancy as an important part of patient participation in making decisions about the delivery.

What if the baby is in the breech position prior to birth?

There is a continuing trend to use the cesarean method to deliver a "breech baby"—a fetus positioned in the womb to be born in some way other than the normal head first manner. Nationally, the proportion of breech positioned infants delivered by cesarean rose from about 12 percent in 1970 to 60 percent in 1978.

Breech positioning involves higher risks for the mother and child, regardless of whether the delivery is vaginal or cesarean. Cesareans are being selected more often in these cases to try to improve the outcome in the face of the increased risks. But the consensus group found scientific data in this area generally inadequate to make firm conclusions about the desirability of one approach over the other.

Most clinical reviews suggest that the cesarean may involve less risk for the premature breech infant, but this may not be true for term breech babies. Several studies indicate that vaginal delivery of the uncomplicated term breech infant is preferable because an elective cesarean birth involves risk of significant complications for the mother and little or no decrease in the risk of infant death.

Deciding which method of delivery to use in these situations involves considering many factors. These include maternal pelvic size, size of the fetus, the type of breech position and the experience of the physician with vaginal breech delivery.

In general, the consensus panel concluded that the cesarean presents a lower risk to the infant than a vaginal delivery when a breech fetus is 8 pounds or larger, when a fetus is in a complete or footling breech position or when a fetus is breech with marked hyperextension of the head.

The group recommended that vaginal delivery of term breech babies should remain an acceptable choice when the following conditions exist:
• anticipated fetal weight of less than 8 pounds;
• normal pelvic dimensions and structure in the mother;
• frank breech positioning without hyperextended head; and
• delivery by a physician experienced in vaginal breech delivery.

What is the most common, single reason for performing a cesarean?

Dystocia is a catch-all medical term covering a broad range of problems which can complicate labor. The consensus group found that this diagnosis was the largest contributor to the overall rise in the cesarean rate, accounting for 30 percent of all cesareans.

Included under the dystocia, or difficult labor, diagnosis are the following three basic types of problems which may impede labor:
• abnormalities of the mother's birth canal, such as a small pelvis;
• abnormalities in the position of the fetus, including breech position or large fetal size; and
• abnormalities in the forces of labor, including infrequent or weak uterine contractions.

The first two categories are well-defined areas. The physician usually recognizes size or position problems early; guidelines for appropriate obstetrical action are available; and the effects of the various approaches for mother and infant are reasonably well known.

The consensus panel agreed that the last category—forces of labor— is most in need of scrutiny and offers an opportunity for moderating the cesarean rate. Generally, this diagnosis occurs with low-risk infants of normal weight and size. Studies have not shown that infants in this group are better off with either cesarean or vaginal deliveries, although the maternal mortality rate for dystocia in 1978 was 41.9 deaths per 100,000 cesarean births compared with 11.1 deaths per 100,000 vaginal births.

The panel concluded that in handling a difficult or slowly progressing labor without fetal distress, a physician should consider various options before performing a cesarean. These include having the patient rest or walk around, sedating the patient or stimulating labor with a drug called oxytocin.

The panel recommended that because the diagnosis of dystocia is poorly defined and so prominent in increasing the cesarean rate, practice review boards in hospitals should include dystocia cases when conducting reviews. The panel also stressed the need for more research on the factors affecting the progress of labor.

Has the use of electronic fetal monitoring led to more cesareans?

Another diagnosis accounting for the rise in cesarean birth rates is fetal distress. Occurring during labor, this problem can result in various complications, the most serious being fetal brain damage because of oxygen deprivation.

The use of electronic fetal monitoring techniques has led to an increase in the diagnosis of fetal distress but not necessarily to the increase in cesarean deliveries, according to the consensus panel.

Because current data are insufficient on the possible risks or benefits of handling this condition with either cesarean or vaginal deliveries, the panel recommended studies to gather information on the outcomes of births involving fetal distress and development of new techniques to improve the accuracy of the diagnosis. These steps, the panel said, may be expected to improve fetal outcome and lower cesarean birth rates.

Are there other medical conditions which would necessitate a cesarean?

Because of a need for early delivery, certain medical problems in either the mother or fetus can lead to cesarean birth. Examples include maternal diabetes, pregnancy-induced hypertension, vaginal herpes infection, and erythroblastosis fetalis, a blood disease related to the Rh factor in the mother. This entire group, however, contributes only a small part of the cesarean birth rate increases.

The consensus panel said that in some of these situations vaginal birth would be a safe alternative if a more effective method of stimulating labor before term was available. The panel recommended research to develop such methods.

What are the benefits of the cesarean method?

There are certain times when conditions in the mother or infant make cesarean delivery the method of first choice. By providing an alternate route of delivery, the procedure offers great benefit in situations when a vaginal delivery carries a high risk of complications and death.

A cesarean is usually used when an expectant mother has diabetes mellitus. Such women have a high risk of having stillborns late in pregnancy. In these cases, a slightly early cesarean helps prevent this occurrence.

The cesarean can also be a lifesaving procedure when the following conditions are present:
- Placenta previa—when the placenta blocks the infant from being born.
- Abruptio placentae—when the placenta prematurely separates from the uterine wall and hemorrhage occurs.
- Obstructed labor—which can occur with a fetus in the shoulder breech, or any other abnormal position.
- Ruptured uterus.
- Presence of weak uterine scars from previous surgery or cesarean.
- Fetus too large for the mother's birth canal.
- Rapid toxemia—a condition in which high blood pressure can lead to convulsions in late pregnancy.
- Vaginal herpes infection—which could infect an infant being born vaginally, and lead to its eventual death.
- Pelvic tumors—which obstruct the birth canal and weaken the uterine wall.
- Absence of effective uterine contractions after labor has begun.
- Prolapse of the umbilical cord—when the cord is pushed out ahead of the infant, compressing the cord and cutting off blood flow.

What are the maternal risks in cesarean childbirth?

The risks of any medical procedure are determined by examining the related mortality statistics showing death rates and morbidity figures showing complications, injuries or disorders linked to the event. These vary from hospital to hospital and from locale to locale.

Although maternal death during childbirth is extremely uncommon, national figures show cesarean birth carries up to four times the risk of death compared to a vaginal delivery. The maternal mortality rate for vaginal delivery in 1978 was about 10 deaths per 100,000 births. For cesareans, the rate was about 41 deaths per 100,000 births. (In some cases, maternal deaths indicated in these figures were caused by illness rather than the surgery.)

The morbidity rates associated with cesarean births are higher than with vaginal delivery. Because major surgery is involved, the chance of infection and complication is greater. The most common are endometritis (an inflammation of tissue lining the uterus) and urinary tract or incision infections.

Does cesarean childbirth require special anesthesia?

The use of anesthesia during childbirth is unique because it requires attention to the infant about to be born as well as the mother. Although rare, anesthesia-related maternal deaths continue to occur. Most, however, are potentially avoidable.

There are three major anesthetic techniques for cesarean birth. Spinal anesthesia is widely used, although the use of lumbar epidural anesthesia is increasing. Both are considered "regional" anesthesia because they deaden pain in only part of the body without putting the patient to sleep. General anesthesia, which renders the patient unconscious, is often used in an emergency situation and with women who object to the spinal or epidural approach.

The consensus panel recommended that the types of anesthesia available should be discussed among the patient, obstetrician, and anesthesiologist. Each approach has advantages and disadvantages. If possible, the report recommends, the patient should have the option of receiving regional instead of general anesthesia.

Are there risks to the infant?

Infants delivered with elective cesarean surgery, especially if it is performed before the onset of labor, appear to have a greater risk of respiratory distress syndrome (RDS). This condition, in which the infant's lungs are not fully mature, may result if an error is made in estimating the age of the developing fetus. Under these circumstances, an infant—who otherwise would have been healthy if allowed to develop fully—encounters the problems of prematurity when removed too soon by cesarean. These include RDS and other lung disorders, feeding problems and various complications which in some cases require a long hospital stay.

Measures and techniques to assess the maturity of the fetus and the degree of lung development are readily available in the United States. The consensus report stressed the need for improving physician and patient education about the safe and effective use of these techniques in planning for elective cesarean delivery. Respiratory distress is unlikely to be a problem, regardless of the type of delivery, if the infant is born at or near term.

What are the psychological effects of cesarean childbirth?

Other factors must be taken into consideration when weighing the prospects of a cesarean. Although there has been only limited research on the psychological effects on parents following a cesarean birth, it is clear that surgery is an increased psychological and physical burden compared to vaginal delivery. In limited follow-up studies of infants, there has been no evidence of an adverse psychologic effect on infants born by cesarean.

In some hospitals, family-centered maternity care has been extended to cesarean deliveries. The presence of the father in the operating room and the closer contact between the mother and newborn in this approach appear to improve the cesarean process.

The consensus panel recommended strengthening the information exchange and education of prospective parents about the overall cesarean experience. They urged hospitals to allow fathers in the operating room when possible and to avoid routinely separating the newborn from its parents immediately following delivery.

For more information

Single free copies of the following publications are available by writing to the Office of Research Reporting, NICHD, NIH, Room 2A32, Bldg. 31, 9000 Rockville Pike, Bethesda, MD 20205.

- *Cesarean Childbirth* is the 540-page final report of the consensus development task force. The report contains evidence gathered by the panel, as well as findings and recommendations. Ask for NIH Publication No. 82–2067.
- "Cesarean Childbirth Consensus Statement" is a ten-page summary of the questions examined at the three-day Consensus Development Conference held September 22–24, 1980. The summary contains the specific findings and recommendations of the panel.

Brent Jaquet, Office of Research Reporting, NICHD, NIH. U.S. Department of Health and Human Services, Public Health Service, National Institutes of Health. U.S. G.P.O. 1984–421–948:7.

Colon

The Colon Goes Up, Over, Down and Out

The colon is one organ of the body not likely to be mentioned in romantic literature. In fact, it is a part of the anatomy most people would probably rather not talk about, considering what it does.

Situated at the nether end of the digestive tract, the colon is the final loop in the journey of food through the gastrointestinal system. The colon has two primary functions: (1) the final absorption of fluids and electrolytes (sodium, potassium, chloride, and bicarbonate) from the undigestible food residues and (2) the storage of the semisolid remains, called feces or stool, until they are evacuated.

Although it is relatively short—only a fifth of the total length of the intestinal canal—the colon is the site of a surprising variety of discomforting and sometimes life-threatening disorders. Virtually no part of this organ is immune from disease, ranging from appendicitis at the point where the colon begins to hemorrhoids at the point where it ends. In between, the colon is beset by inflammatory and infectious diseases, polyps and, of course, cancer.

Here's a look at what can go wrong in the colon and what can be done about it:

Appendicitis is the most common cause of emergency abdominal surgery. The appendix literally hangs onto the cecum (see accompanying article, ''Anatomy Of The Colon'') and shares the contents of the colon. If it becomes obstructed, circulation is cut off, the appendix becomes inflamed, and appendicitis develops.

The so-called ''classic'' symptoms of appendicitis include pain, nausea or vomiting, sensitivity over the area of the appendix, and fever. However, not everyone has these symptoms. The only treatment is prompt removal of the appendix. Delay can lead to gangrene, rupture and peritonitis (inflammation in the abdomen).

Hemorrhoids are abnormally large conglomerates of blood vessels, supporting tissues, and mucous membranes in the anorectal area—that is, the anal canal and lower rectum. The human species gets hemorrhoids because of erect posture, heredity, occupation, diet, and cultural patterns. This ofttimes uncomfortable condition can be set off by constipation, diarrhea, pregnancy, anal infection, and cancer of the rectum.

A variety of nonprescription (OTC) products are available to relieve the itching, burning, pain, inflammation, irritation, swelling, and discomfort of hemorrhoids. An FDA advisory panel on OTC drugs reviewed these products and made recommendations as to their safety and effectiveness. FDA has not as yet issued the final standards for such products.

More serious symptoms—bleeding, seepage, protrusion, prolapse and thrombosis—should be treated by a physician who may decide to use one of a number of surgical procedures.

The entire colon or just parts of it can be affected by ulcerative colitis and Crohn's disease, two conditions frequently lumped together under the general term "inflammatory bowel disease."

Ulcerative colitis is a chronic disease marked by inflammation of the inner lining of the colon and rectum. In some cases the entire colon is affected; in others, only the last segment (the sigmoid colon) and rectal areas are involved. The symptoms range from a small amount of rectal bleeding to severe diarrhea that can be disabling. Other symptoms include abdominal and rectal pain, weight loss, anemia, and loss of body fluids and minerals.

Ulcerative colitis typically affects young adults, with three-quarters of the cases developing before the age of 30. Young children and the elderly may also be victims. It was once thought to be a disease limited to the United States and Europe. However, it is being seen with increasing frequency in Japan, India, Thailand, and other countries in the Far East.

In about 60 percent of the cases, the disease is mild and attacks are intermittent—that is, they come and go. Some patients may have only one attack with no symptoms again for 10 or 15 years. In the moderate form, symptoms of the disease include diarrhea and low-grade fever. For 15 percent of the victims, the disease starts suddenly and doesn't let up. One of the worst symptoms is a severe bearing-down kind of pain with an inability to have a bowel movement. Deaths from ulcerative colitis are rare but can occur among those with a markedly inflamed and/or dilated bowel.

Ulcerative colitis was first described in 1875, yet its cause remains a mystery. It was once thought to be the result of an infection, because of its inflammatory nature, but no infectious agent has been identified. Another theory is that the disease has a genetic basis, since additional cases of ulcerative colitis are frequently seen in families of victims.

The disease also has been attributed to emotional or psychological disorders, sensitivity to certain foods, or the phenomenon of "autoimmunity," in which the body's defense mechanisms attack its own tissues.

Most patients respond satisfactorily to medical treatment with no further problems. About 10 to 29 percent, however, develop complications such as hemorrhoids, pseudopolyps, and anal fissures. Major problems resulting from ulcerative colitis are toxic megacolon (acute dilation of the colon), colonic perforation, massive hemorrhage, and cancer. The risk of developing cancer increases in cases of long duration, usually 10 years or more, where most of the colon is involved.

Complications of this disease can reach outside the colon. Inflammation of the small joints of the fingers, hands, feet, ankles, knees, and of the spine and sacroiliac joints sometimes occurs. Skin complications include erythema nodosum (raised, tender swellings on the arms and legs) or the more severe pyoderma gangrenosum, which starts out looking like boils and ends up as large gangrenous lesions.

The eyes and mouth also may become involved in a small number of cases. Blockage of the pulmonary artery in the lung resulting from a clot in the leg or pelvic vein is another complication, as are some liver and kidney disorders. Children with ulcerative colitis do not grow at the normal rate.

Ulcerative colitis is usually diagnosed on the basis of the patient's medical history, examination of the stool, and direct examination of the diseased area through optical instruments called endoscopes. X-rays, blood counts, and other blood analyses may be used, although there are no specific laboratory tests for ulcerative colitis. The diagnosis can be complicated in that a number of intestinal diseases may mimic ulcerative colitis.

Treatment of this disease must be tailored to the individual patient's needs. Medical therapy is directed toward correcting malnutrition and loss of blood, fluids and electrolytes, and controlling inflammation with steroids (prednisone, hydrocortisone and others) and sulfasalazine. While such drugs offer relief from symptoms, they do have a number of undesirable side effects. And they do not cure the disease.

The only sure cure is surgical removal of the colon, an option usually reserved for high-risk patients who have not been helped by other treatments. Known as a proctocolectomy, this operation leaves the patient with a permanent ileostomy, an artificial opening to which the ileum (the last segment of the small intestine) is attached. Liquid bowel waste empties into a disposable bag attached over the new opening. Most patients who undergo this operation can lead a reasonably normal life and eat a normal diet. There are studies under way examining a new surgical procedure, called endo-rectal pull-through, which will connect the ileum to the rectum and avoid an ileostomy.

Crohn's disease, the second of the conditions that constitute inflammatory bowel disease, shares many of the features of ulcerative colitis though it is generally believed to be a separate disease. It occurs throughout the world, with the greatest frequency among Europeans. It is more common among Jews than non-Jews, and it is seen more often in whites than non-whites.

Named for the doctor who first described it in 1932, Crohn's disease is characterized by a thickening and inflammation of all layers of the intestinal wall. Diseased portions of the intestine may be separated by normal tissue, giving rise to the term "skip lesions."

Unlike ulcerative colitis, Crohn's disease can attack any part of the alimentary canal, although the ileum and the colon are the most common sites.

Like ulcerative colitis, the cause of Crohn's disease is unknown. There is a familial connection in that patients often have relatives with either of the two diseases; recent observations suggest that it may be caused by an infectious agent. There is also some speculation that the body's immune mechanisms may be involved.

Diarrhea and abdominal pain are often the earliest signs of Crohn's disease. Joint pains, lack of appetite, weight loss and fever are also common.

The course of the disease is unpredictable. Some patients' symptoms may be mild, though continuing for many years. In other cases, there may be a single attack followed by a long period without symptoms. Diagnosis may not be made until late in the course of the disease, and then it must be made by excluding infections with look-alike symptoms.

Small bowel obstruction, formation of fistulas, and mild bleeding are among the major bowel complications of Crohn's disease. (A fistula is an abnormal channel occurring between two loops of intestine or between the intestine and another structure such as the bladder, vagina, or skin.) Systemic manifestations—those outside the immediate bowel area—are very similar to those associated with ulcerative colitis.

The treatment of Crohn's disease includes supportive measures such as bed rest and replacement of fluids, electrolytes and vitamins. Patients with severe or complicated disease may be fed intravenously to allow the bowel to rest. Drug therapy is similar to that of ulcerative colitis and includes steroids and sulfasalazine. Diseased portions of the bowel are not usually removed surgically, for the disease tends to recur in the remaining intestine. Surgery may be undertaken in more complicated cases, however, especially when obstruction is present.

Two common intestinal disorders that are often confused with the inflammatory bowel diseases are diverticulosis and irritable bowel syndrome.

Diverticulosis is common in developed Western societies, affecting by some counts as much as one-third of all people over the age of 50. Diverticulosis is not a disease per se but is a condition characterized by the presence of diverticula, or saclike outpouchings of the colon. For the most part, these pouchings, which occur most often in the sigmoid colon, cause no problems. But about 15 percent of persons with those pouches will develop an inflammation known as diverticulitis. This condition is found more often in men than women.

The symptoms of diverticulitis are very like those of appendicitis—crampy or steady pain with local tenderness. Fever, loss of appetite, nausea, and vomiting may also occur. About 25 percent of patients experience bleeding.

Many attacks are mild and clear up by themselves or in response to medical treatment, such as bed rest and intravenous fluids. Complications such as intra-abdominal abscesses, fistulas, bowel obstruction, and generalized peritonitis require surgery.

There was a time when patients with diverticulosis were advised to eat a soft diet and avoid what is commonly called roughage (bran, whole grain bread, etc.). Today high-fiber diets are being recommended to prevent the development of diverticula and of diverticulitis.

Irritable bowel syndrome is not a disease, but a disorder of the intestinal contractions by which food and waste are propelled along the GI tract. One of the most common chronic abdominal problems seen by physicians, irritable bowel syndrome ranks close to the common cold as a cause of absenteeism from work. Women are twice as likely to suffer from this disorder; whites more often than non-whites.

The symptoms are variable, usually including some combination of cramping abdominal pain, constipation or diarrhea, bloating, burning, increased belching and flatulence, nausea and vomiting. An anatomic cause has not yet been found. What is observed is an abnormal pattern of muscular contractions including excessive intestinal spasms.

Patients often note that they first experienced a change in bowel movements in adolescence or early adult life. Their symptoms, often appearing after or during periods of stress, follow a constant pattern, though they may vary in severity.

As there is often an emotional factor causing or resulting from this syndrome, reassurance and psychological support play important roles in treatment. Dietary changes may be helpful, along with drugs for temporary relief of symptoms.

Cancer, that most feared of all diseases, attacks the colon with a vengeance. Colon and rectal cancer is the fourth most common form of cancer among Americans, ranking behind skin, lung, and breast cancer. An estimated 113,000 new cases will be diagnosed this year. And 59,400 Americans will die from colon and rectal cancer; that's second only to lung cancer.

Most prevalent in people over the age of 40, colon and rectal cancer (or colorectal cancer, as it's called) strikes men and women equally.

There appears to be little difference in incidence rates among blacks and whites. Survival rates are higher when the disease is found before it has spread beyond the wall of the colon.

Symptoms of this type of cancer are blood in the stool (either bright red or black), changes in bowel habits (such as constipation or diarrhea), abdominal discomfort, and pain.

Diagnosis involves a number of procedures, including digital examination of the rectum, direct viewing of the rectum and sigmoid colon with instruments called the proctoscope and sigmoidoscope, X-ray examination, and, thanks to fiberoptics, examination of the entire colon with a flexible colonoscope. This instrument not only permits the identification of colon cancers at an early stage but is equipped with a wire loop to "ensnare," cauterize, and remove precancerous polyps or other suspicious growths.

Surgical removal is the primary treatment for colon and rectal cancers. A colostomy may be necessary following surgery, depending on the location and extent of the cancer. Like the ileostomy described previously, a colostomy provides an opening between the colon and the abdominal wall, to permit elimination of body wastes.

Until recently, radiation therapy played a minor role in the treatment of colorectal cancer. However, new research suggests that irradiation before surgery can slow the growth of cancer cells and reduce the risk of the cancer spreading. The use of combinations of anti-cancer drugs (chemotherapy) has been explored in patients with advanced colorectal cancer. New studies are under way using anti-cancer drugs alone or in combination with radiation soon after surgery to reduce the risk of recurrence of the disease.

There is strong evidence that environmental factors have a role in the development of colorectal cancer. The disease is common in Western industrialized countries, rare in underdeveloped countries. Studies of migrant populations have shown that people who leave areas where there is little colorectal cancer eventually exhibit incidence rates similar to those found in their new homeland.

In view of these findings it has been suggested that diet, particularly one that is high in fat, protein, and beef and low in dietary fiber, is a major factor in the development of colorectal cancer. One theory is that the higher the fiber, the less time it takes for the undigested material to move through the colon. Thus, cancer-causing agents have less contact with the bowel lining.

Intestinal polyps, or growths in the colon, are believed to be precursors of colorectal cancer. The most common type is adenomatous polyps (those having glandular cell structures), which occur in 2 to 15 percent of adults in the United States. Found most often in the rectum and the sigmoid colon, these polyps are usually removed surgically as a preventive measure.

If all these assaults on the colon aren't enough, there are other conditions, such as radiation enteritis, which occurs in 5 to 15 percent of patients receiving large doses of radiation for pelvic disorders.

Another is a severe, sometimes fatal, gastrointestinal disease with the fearsome name "pseudomembraneous enterocolitis." This condition is characterized by the formation of oozing plaques attached to the mucosa of the small bowel, colon, or both. In the majority of cases, this condition results from exposure to antibiotics, particularly clindamycin, ampicillin, and the cephalosporins. Use of these antibiotics alters the microbial balance in the gut, allowing the overgrowth of an organism called *Clostridium difficile*. The toxin produced by this organism causes the colitis, which is marked by severe, persistent diarrhea and abdominal cramps and the passage of blood and mucus. Mild cases may clear up when the offending drug is discontinued. More severe cases usually can be treated successfully with the drug vancomycin.

Annabel Hecht.

Anatomy of the colon

The convulted tube called the intestines measures up to 25 feet in an adult. About 20 feet constitute the small intestine, while the remaining five belong to the colon. The diameter of the colon is greater than that of the small intestine, hence its alternative names—large intestine or large bowel. A trip through the colon goes up, over, down and out.

Unlike the small intestine with its many loops and folds, the colon is relatively fixed in position. It consists of four sections. It begins at the cecum, a dilated pouch connecting the small and large intestines. The first section, called the ascending colon, lies in the right side of the abdomen. Making a sharp turn at the liver, the tube becomes the transverse colon, the longest of the four sections. A turn downward at the spleen is the beginning of the descending colon. (We're now on the left side of the abdomen.) This passes into the pelvic area and forms a curving loop called the sigmoid colon. At the very end is the rectum, which is 8 to 10 inches long. The final few inches of the rectum is called the anal region or anus.

The appendix is a long, narrow, worm-shaped tube attached to the cecum. Averaging about three inches in length, this appendage serves no known useful purpose.

The external muscles of the colon are three bands running from the tip of the cecum to the rectum and converging at the base of the appendix.

These muscle bands are actually shorter than the colon itself and tend to draw it into sacs. Separated by folds, the size and shape of the sacs are determined by the contractions of the circular muscles as they move the contents of the intestines along.

The primary functions of the intestines are to extract essential nutrients, fluids, and electrolytes (sodium, potassium, chloride, and bicarbonate) from food and to dispose of waste residues from the digestive process.

One to two liters of fluid pass through the colon every day. The fluids are absorbed in the ascending and transverse colon. Unabsorbed food substances are reduced to a semisolid substance called feces or stool, which is stored in the descending colon until it is time for defecation. A normal bowel movement begins with the stimulation of receptors in the rectum by the feces. Wave-like muscular contractions propel the stool to the anal canal, from whence it is evacuated.

Aiding in the breakdown of waste products are billions of microorganisms that are the normal residents of the colon. The majority are anaerobic organisms (living without oxygen) that are harmless to their human host. Organisms that can cause disease, such as *Escherichia coli,* hemolytic *Streptococci, Clostridia,* and yeast, are also found in the colon, but are far outnumbered and are held in check by the anaerobic microbes— that is, unless some outside influence such as diet, a change in bowel acidity, gastrointestinal disease, or drugs (antibiotics) changes the balance of these populations. If harmful bacteria are allowed to grow without control, serious complications can develop.

Reprinted from June 1984, FDA Consumer, HHS Publication No. (FDA) 84–1111. Department of Health and Human Services, Public Health Service, Food and Drug Administration, 5600 Fishers Lane, Rockville, Md. 20857. U.S. Government Printing Office 1985—461–367/20061.

Contraceptives

Comparing Contraceptives

Contraception is a very individual matter. There are many options today for a couple who do not want more children or who want to delay childbearing. The choices range from over-the-counter (OTC) products, such as condoms, vaginal spermicides and the contraceptive sponge, to doctor-prescribed items such as birth control pills, intrauterine (IUD) devices, and diaphragms. There is also natural family planning, and for those sure they want no more children there is voluntary sterilization. Each of these methods has risks and benefits that need to be considered before making a choice, keeping in mind that what's best for one person may not suit someone else.

To help consumers weigh the pros and cons of various types of contraception, here is a brief discussion of each, along with a comparison chart. The percentages for effectiveness are based on the proportion of women who would be expected to become pregnant in the first year while using that method. Thus, a rate of 85 percent means that during the first year of use, 15 of 100 women would be expected to become pregnant. Many factors, such as motivation and correct use of the method, are considered when estimating effectiveness. Therefore, effectiveness of some methods will vary with individual use. For this reason, when appropriate, ranges of effectiveness are given.

As with all health matters, questions about risks and effectiveness of contraceptives are best resolved with the help of a doctor.

Condom

The condom (also called ''prophylactic,'' ''rubber,'' and ''safe'') is the only temporary male contraceptive. A thin sheath, usually made of latex rubber or lamb cecum (commonly referred to as lamb skin, it actually comes from the intestine), the condom is fitted over the erect penis before intercourse. When the man ejaculates, the sperm are trapped inside the condom.

The effectiveness of the condom in actual use can vary from 64 to 97 percent. Condoms are also useful in protecting against sexually transmitted diseases such as syphilis and gonorrhea. They may also protect against herpes and AIDS (acquired immunodeficiency syndrome), although their effectiveness against these viral diseases is unproven.

A few manufacturers have added the spermicide (sperm-killing chemical) nonoxynol-9 to some condoms, on the theory that it will inactivate any sperm that may accidentally spill from the condom. However, the spermicide's effectiveness in the condom for this purpose, or for additional disease protection, has not yet been proven.

About the only health drawback to the condom is that on rare occasions a person may be allergic to the rubber material. This problem can often be solved by using a natural material (such as lamb cecum) instead.

Vaginal spermicides alone

Contraceptive foams, creams, jellies, gels, and suppositories are not as effective as condoms. The active ingredient in these spermicides is nonoxynol-9 or, in the case of one product, octoxynol. Although effectiveness has been variously estimated, recent data submitted to FDA shows effectiveness may be as low as 70 percent to 80 percent.

To be effective, the spermicide must be inserted into the vagina as close to the time of intercourse as possible, but no more than an hour before. As it covers the cervix, the spermicide forms both a physical and chemical barrier to sperm. To avoid interfering with the contraceptive action, a woman should not douche for at least six hours after intercourse.

Because the spermicides can kill bacteria as well as sperm, they may help protect against venereal disease, although not as well as condoms. Sometimes a woman or her partner may develop an irritation or allergic reaction from use of a spermicide. Changing to another brand may solve the problem.

Sponge

A relative newcomer to the array of contraceptive products available without a prescription, the contraceptive sponge was first marketed in 1983. It is made of polyurethane and contains the spermicide nonoxynol-9. Preliminary data estimate its effectiveness to be 80 percent to 87 percent. Before intercourse, the sponge is inserted into the vagina to cover the cervix, forming both a physical and chemical barrier to sperm. It should be left in place for at least six hours after intercourse. The sponge may be left in place up to 24 hours and is still effective if intercourse is repeated during that time. It should be discarded after use.

As with spermicides, a small percentage of users may experience irritation or allergic reactions from use of contraceptive sponges. There have also been reports of difficulty in removing the sponge and its fragmenting in the vagina. A woman who experiences such problems should contact her physician.

There have been a few cases of the rare but potentially fatal illness called toxic shock syndrome (TSS) among women using contraceptive sponges. But the rate is very low—less than one TSS case per 3 million sponges used. And women can minimize this already low risk by carefully following the directions on the leaflet accompanying the product.

Diaphragm

The diaphragm is similar to the contraceptive sponge in that it is inserted into the vagina before intercourse to cover the cervix. But while the disposable OTC sponge comes in one-size-that-fits-all, the diaphragm is reusable, comes in several sizes, and must be fitted by a physician.

A round disk made of rubber with a flexible rim, the diaphragm must be coated with spermicidal jelly or cream before it is inserted. Although the diaphragm is a prescription device, the cream and jelly are available over-the-counter.

The diaphragm should be inserted within one hour of intercourse and should be left in place at least six hours after. If intercourse is repeated, the diaphragm is left in place while additional cream or jelly is inserted into the vagina. The diaphragm's effectiveness is estimated to be 80 percent to 98 percent.

As with all these methods, allergic reactions occur only rarely with diaphragm use, due to either the rubber or spermicide. Changing brands of spermicide may solve this problem. Other infrequently reported side effects include bladder infections, constipation, and, very rarely, TSS.

Cervical cap

The cervical cap has not been approved by FDA for contraceptive use. It is, however, available as an investigational device in a few clinics around the country. Like a diaphragm, the cap fits over the cervix, but it is more difficult to insert than a diaphragm. It is smaller than a diaphragm, fitting more snugly around the cervix, and requires less spermicidal cream or jelly than the diaphragm. Like the diaphragm, it comes in different sizes. Investigations are now under way to see if the cap can be left in place more than a day. While using the cap, intercourse may be repeated without adding more spermicide. Although this contraceptive seems to hold some promise, its safety and effectiveness are still under investigation.

Intrauterine device (IUD)

The intrauterine device (IUD) is inserted by a physician through the cervix into the uterus (womb). IUDs are made of plastic and come in a variety of shapes and sizes. In one type, the plastic is wound with copper, and another includes a hormone, progesterone, that is slowly released. These may be slightly more effective than the all-plastic types, but they must be replaced more frequently (every one to three years) because the copper or progesterone dissipates.

The effectiveness of IUDs is estimated at 95 percent to 96 percent.

After an IUD is inserted, the woman need do nothing more than check after each menstrual period to make sure she can feel the thread that is attached to the IUD and hangs down through the cervix. If she cannot feel the thread or if it feels longer or shorter than usual, this may mean the IUD is out of place or has been expelled and she should contact her doctor.

Some women experience some cramping or dizziness when an IUD is inserted. Some may also have bleeding, cramps and backache that may continue for a few days. During the first few menstrual cycles after insertion, there may be spotting between periods and menstruation itself may be longer and heavier than usual.

In addition to these relatively short-term side effects, there are some more serious adverse effects possible with IUDs. The incidence of pelvic inflammatory disease (PID) is estimated to be 1.5 to 4 times higher in IUD users than in nonusers. The rate is highest in women who have had PID before and in those with many sex partners. Symptoms of PID may include a vaginal discharge that is heavier or more uncomfortable than normal and lower abdominal pain, with or without fever. An IUD user with these symptoms should consult her doctor immediately. If left untreated, PID can cause sterility. (See accompanying article on the Dalkon Shield.)

A rare IUD adverse effect is perforation of the uterus, a serious medical problem. It usually occurs at the time of insertion or immediately thereafter.

If pregnancy should occur during IUD use, there are increased risks of septic abortion (a miscarriage with serious infection) and ectopic (tubal) pregnancy, both potentially life-threatening. An IUD user who suspects she may be pregnant should contact her doctor.

Birth control pills

Birth control pills, technically called oral contraceptives and known popularly as "the pill," are the most effective of all temporary methods of birth control. But because of their side effects they may not be the best method for some women. They are particularly risky for those who smoke, are over 35, or have high blood pressure, diabetes, or high cholesterol.

There are two types of birth control pills: combination pills, containing both estrogen and progestin (synthetic hormones similar to those produced naturally in a woman's body), and "mini-pills," containing only progestin. Although they both prevent sperm from uniting with an egg, they work in slightly different ways. The combination pill keeps a woman's ovaries from releasing an egg. The mini-pill is less reliable in suppressing egg release but creates changes in the cervix and uterus that are hostile to conception. The mini-pill is less effective than the combination pill, but does not have some of the risks attributed to estrogen, such as increased risk of blood clots and nausea. However, the mini-pill causes more problems with spotting and bleeding between periods. Therefore, its use is not widespread. It is claimed that biphasic and triphasic combination pills, which vary the levels of hormones to more closely approximate a woman's normal hormonal variations, may also have a lower risk of side effects. However, since these types of pills have been in use only a short time, definite conclusions about the reduction in risks cannot yet be drawn.

In addition to their effectiveness (about 99 percent for the combination pill and about 97 percent for the mini-pill), oral contraceptives offer other benefits. Menstrual periods are usually lighter, making iron deficiency anemia less likely, and there may be less cramping. Fibrocystic breast disease, ovarian cysts and pelvic inflammatory disease occur less frequently among pill users. There is also some evidence that oral contraceptives may offer some protection against ovarian cancer and cancer of the lining of the uterus, and that this protection may last up to 10 years after pill use is stopped. In addition, ectopic pregnancy, in which the embryo begins to develop outside the uterus, occurs less frequently among pill users in the rare instance when pregnancy occurs at all.

Women who use birth control pills should not smoke because cigarette smoking increases the risk of such serious adverse effects as heart attack and stroke. This risk increases with age, and dramatically increases in women older than 35 who smoke more than 15 cigarettes a day.

For most healthy women under 35 who do not smoke, the benefits of the pill appear to be greater than the risks. But there are some women who should not use oral contraceptives. Those who are pregnant or think they may be pregnant should not take the pill because it may increase the risk of birth defects. Other methods of contraception also should be considered by women who have, or have had, heart attacks or strokes, blood clots in the legs (thrombophlebitis) or lungs (pulmonary embolism), chest pain (angina pectoris) associated with heart disease, unexplained vaginal bleeding, cancer of the breast or of the lining of the uterus, liver tumors, or jaundice due to pregnancy or prior birth control pill use.

Blood clots are the most serious side effect of the combination birth control pill. They can cause stroke, heart attack, or pulmonary embolism. Any of these can result in death. Rarely, a clot may occur in the blood vessels of the eye, causing impaired or double vision or even blindness. Birth control pill use may also cause high blood pressure (which usually returns to normal when the woman stops taking the pills).

Other possible serious side effects include greater risk of gall bladder disease requiring surgery, and noncancerous (but nonetheless dangerous) liver tumors.

There is some evidence that oral contraceptive users may have an increased risk of cancer of the cervix; however, this finding may be related to factors other than pill use. One study has shown that birth control pills may increase the size of preexisting noncancerous fibroid tumors of the uterus. However, no other studies have confirmed this finding.

After reviewing recent studies, FDA has concluded that there appears to be no increased risk of breast cancer in oral contraceptive users or any subgroup of users, or with any particular type of oral contraceptive.

There are also several less serious side effects that may affect some combination pill users. The most frequent of these are nausea, vomiting, stomach cramps, bloating, weight change and water retention. Water retention may cause swelling of fingers or ankles.

Other side effects of oral contraceptives may include nervousness, depression, dizziness, change in appetite, loss of scalp hair, rash, vaginal infections, migraine headaches, missed menstrual periods and bleeding between periods. Contact lens wearers may notice a change in vision or more discomfort in wearing their lenses.

Some drugs interact with birth control pills, making the oral contraceptives less effective or causing bleeding between periods. Such drugs include barbiturates (for example, phenobarbital), phenytoin (Dilantin), phenylbutazone (Butazolidin) and some antibiotics, particularly isoniazid and rifampin. In addition, the need for some nutrients may be changed.

Pill users should have their blood pressure checked and should have physical examinations and PAP tests at least yearly. Because the risk of serious side effects in many cases decreases with a reduced hormone dose, patients should discuss with their physicians using the lowest effective dose.

Natural family planning (rhythm method)

Methods of contraception that rely on awareness of a woman's fertility pattern have none of the adverse side effects of artificial methods of contraception. But effectiveness is highly variable, with estimates generally ranging from 53 percent to 86 percent, and even lower for women who have irregular menstrual cycles.

The most common of these methods are the basal body temperature method, the vaginal mucus method, and the calendar method. They can be used together for increased effectiveness.

When using the basal body temperature method, a woman must take her temperature every morning before arising, preferably with a special oral thermometer, called a basal thermometer, precise enough to measure the very small changes in body temperature that occur normally during a woman's cycle. When the basal body temperature, or temperature of the body at rest, rises one-half to one degree and remains elevated for three days, this signals that ovulation is taking place. It is considered "safe" to have intercourse *after* temperature has been elevated three full days. "Unsafe" days are all those from the beginning of a woman's period to the beginning of the fourth day after temperature rises.

The vaginal mucus method relies on a woman observing the normal changes in the consistency of her vaginal mucus that occur during her cycle.

Intercourse should be avoided from the time when the consistency of the mucus indicates that ovulation is about to occur until at least three days afterward. It may be resumed on the fourth day and continued until menstruation begins. Days during menstruation are considered unsafe because mucus signs cannot be monitored.

The calendar method, which is effective only when used with one or both of the other methods, consists of keeping track of the number of days in the menstrual cycle in an attempt to pinpoint ovulation. If menstrual cycles are short, this method is highly unreliable.

Voluntary sterilization

Sterilization is a permanent form of birth control for couples who do not ever want more children. It involves cutting and closing off the tubes through which either the sperm (for men) or the egg (for women) travel.

Male sterilization, called vasectomy, is the less risky and less expensive of the two operations. Considered minor surgery, it is usually performed in the doctor's office under local anesthesia. Its effectiveness as a contraceptive is estimated to be at least 99 percent.

After a cut is made in each side of the scrotum, the vas deferens (the tubes through which the sperm travel) are closed off by cutting or clamping. The operation takes about 20 minutes. There may be some pain and swelling after the procedure, and very occasionally infection may occur.

Although there have been reports of adverse effects on the cardiovascular system in animal studies, human studies have shown no differences in cardiovascular problems between men who have had vasectomies and those who haven't. However, about 5 percent of vasectomized men report having psychological problems related to the procedure.

Female sterilization, called tubal ligation, is an operation usually performed under general anesthesia in a hospital. Depending on the type of procedure, it may be done on an outpatient basis or may require a hospital stay of one to four days.

According to the National Center for Health Statistics, among women over 30, female sterilization is the most common single type of contraception, with 41 percent of women who use birth control being sterilized by age 39.

There are several different methods of performing tubal ligation. The

A Guide to the Pros and Cons

Efficacy rates given in this chart are estimates based on a number of different studies. Methods which are more dependent on conscientious use and therefore are more subject to human error have wider ranges of efficacy than the others. For comparison, 60 to 80 percent of sexually active women using no contraception would be expected to become pregnant in a year. Because the contraceptive sponge has only been on the market a short time, effectiveness estimates for it are not based on as many studies as those for the other forms of contraception. This chart should not be used alone, but only as a summary of information in the accompanying article.

Type	Estimated Effectiveness	Risks	Non-Contraceptive Benefits	Convenience	Availability
Condom	64–97%	Rarely, irritation and allergic reactions	Good protection against sexually transmitted diseases, possibly including herpes and AIDS	Applied immediately before intercourse	OTC
Vaginal Spermicides (used alone)	70–80%	Rarely, irritation and allergic reactions	May give some protection against some sexually transmitted diseases	Applied no more than one hour before intercourse; can be "messy"	OTC
Sponge	80–87%	Rarely, irritation and allergic reactions; difficulty in removal; very rarely, toxic shock syndrome	May give some protection against some sexually transmitted diseases	Can be inserted hours before intercourse, left in place up to 24 hours; disposable	OTC

Method	Effectiveness	Side Effects/Risks	Benefits	Usage	Rx/OTC
Diaphragm with Spermicide	80–98%	Rarely, irritation and allergic reactions, bladder infection, constipation; very rarely, toxic shock syndrome	May give some protection against some sexually transmitted diseases	Inserted before intercourse; can be left in place 24 hours but additional spermicide must be inserted if intercourse is repeated	Rx
IUD	95–96%	Cramps, bleeding, pelvic inflammatory disease; rarely, perforation of the uterus	None	After insertion, stays in place until physician removes it	Rx
Birth Control Pills	97% (Mini) 99% (Comb.)	Not for smokers; blood clots, gall bladder disease, noncancerous liver tumors, water retention, hypertension, mood changes, dizziness and nausea	Less menstrual bleeding and cramping, lower risk of fibrocystic breast disease, ovarian cysts and pelvic inflammatory disease; may protect against cancer of the ovaries and of the lining of the uterus	Pill must be taken on daily schedule, regardless of the frequency of intercourse	Rx

Type	Estimated Effectiveness	Risks	Non-Contraceptive Benefits	Convenience	Availability
Natural Family Planning or Rhythm	Very variable, perhaps 53–86%	None	None	Requires frequent monitoring of body functions and periods of abstinence	Instructions from physician or clinic
Vasectomy (Male Sterilization)	Over 99%	Pain; infection rarely; possible psychological problems	None	No care after surgery	Minor surgery
Tubal Ligation (Female Sterilization)	Over 99%	Surgical complications; some pain or discomfort; possibly higher risk of hysterectomy later in life	None	No care after surgery	Surgery

oldest, laparotomy, involves a three- to five-inch abdominal incision. It is a 30-minute procedure requiring general anesthesia and a hospital stay of about four days. Recovery is about four weeks. Today, this procedure is rarely performed except in women who have already had some type of abdominal surgery or when tubal ligation is performed immediately after the woman has given birth.

The more frequently performed types of tubal ligation are minilaparotomy and laparoscopy. Their effectiveness rate is higher than 99 percent.

The minilaparotomy, as the name implies, requires an incision of only one inch. It is usually performed under general anesthesia and takes 20 to 30 minutes. The recuperative time is less than for a laparotomy but longer than for laparoscopy.

Laparoscopy has been nicknamed ''Band-aid'' and ''belly button'' surgery because of the small size of the incision near the navel. Inert gas is introduced by means of a needle into the abdominal cavity through the one-half-inch incision. The gas pushes the intestine away from the uterus and Fallopian tubes. A laparoscope (a kind of medical telescope in a thin flexible tube that also carries a fiberoptic light) is inserted through the same incision to allow the surgeon to see the internal area. Operating instruments can either be inserted through the laparoscope or through a second small incision at the pubic hairline. The Fallopian tubes are usually sealed off, most commonly by burning through electro-cauterization. However, because of the risks with this method (including burns of the intestine, bowel, and bladder and destruction of the blood supply to the ovary) many surgeons choose to use clips or rings to seal the tubes.

Laparoscopy is often done as an outpatient procedure, usually under general anesthesia. It takes about an hour, and recuperation is usually only one or two days. Postoperative discomfort from the gas is frequently reported.

Another procedure, vaginal tubal ligation, in which the surgeon makes an incision in the vagina, is currently done much less often than previously, primarily due to its higher risks of infection and bleeding and its higher failure rate.

There is a certain amount of discomfort and pain following all these operations. Although the complication rate may vary among surgeons and among procedures, the overall complication rate for tubal ligation has been reported to be between 0.1 percent and 15.3 percent. One recent report estimated the serious complication rate for laparoscopy to be 1.7 percent. Very rarely, there is a death during these procedures. This most often occurs as a complication of general anesthesia.

In addition to complications at the time of surgery, there have been reports of higher rates of hysterectomy later in life for women who have had tubal ligation with electrocautery, and of higher incidences of premenstrual syndrome (PMS), heavy menstrual bleeding, and irregular cycles. Other investigations, however, have not found these high risks.

Currently under investigation are procedures that may lessen the risks of tubal ligation and enable the operation to be more easily reversible. One of these methods now being studied involves the insertion of silicone plugs into the Fallopian tubes which could, at a later date, be removed if the woman wanted more children.

At present, although some attempts are made at rejoining the tubes in both men and women, these reversal operations have a low success rate; thus, both male and female sterilization must be considered permanent.

Judith Willis

Reprinted from May 1985, FDA Consumer, HHS Publication No. (FDA) 85–1123. Department of Health and Human Services, Public Health Service, Food and Drug Administration, 5600 Fishers Lane, Rockville, Md. 20857, Office of Public Affairs. U.S. Government Printing Office 1985—461-367/20069.

Dental Plaque
The Battle Is Endless But Worth It

When a horse trader looks into the horse's mouth, he's really inspecting the length of teeth to figure out the horse's age. The shorter the teeth, the older the horse, nature's mute testimony to the daily rations the animal has chomped on during a lifetime.

A dentist or periodontist looking at a human patient's teeth will see signs of aging too. In humans the exposed parts of the teeth appear to grow *longer* with age, unless the patient practices good mouth hygiene. Keeping the teeth and their anchorage—the gums—in good shape means regular toothbrushing, five minutes or so of daily dental flossing, and periodic visits to the dental hygienist to get plaque and tartar scaled or removed.

"Long in the tooth" has been a picturesque way to describe characters who are advancing in years. With aging, the teeth become both longer and looser, a condition that really has its beginning some time earlier when a colorless film of sticky, bacterially produced material called plaque forms on the tooth surfaces without the owner's knowledge and—in time—turns into deposits of tartar, or calculus.

As the stuff forms, it crowds, irritates, loosens and eventually pushes back the gumline. Inflammation and infection set in around the tooth's root, and the gum slowly recesses. As the infected area widens and deepens, the bone in which the tooth is set shrinks away. This makes the tooth's pocket deeper and gives the roots less anchorage. Sometimes it's years before the patient really knows what's happening.

This briefly describes the melancholy progress of periodontal disease, or periodontitis, also in its earlier stages referred to as gingivitis. Pyorrhea is another, older name no longer in fashion. Periodontal disease wipes out more teeth from our heads every year than any other major dental disease, including tooth decay (caries). The disease costs the American public an estimated $4 billion a year for repair of its ravages.

Cosmetically, the person with untreated periodontal disease is considered inelegant and will become only more so as the days, the weeks, the years go by. First comes bad breath, that bugaboo of romance and social acceptance. Foul breath is almost always caused by diseased or infected gums, not decayed teeth. All the mouthwash you can swill is not going to wash it away, but will temporarily trade one smell for another. The next consequence of periodontal disease is that uncertain smile, with its gappy look. And eventually false teeth, which just don't have the appeal of nature's own, no matter how white and even they may appear.

Nutritionally, advanced gum disease is a bummer. You find yourself swallowing food mostly unchewed, or giving up on it altogether. And some delights, such as corn on the cob, a hard roll, or an apple, are better avoided altogether.

The saddest part is that periodontal disease doesn't really have to happen. An 18-inch piece of dental floss used daily, proper brushing, and those trips to the hygienist's will keep that smile healthy, no matter what color settles on the top of your head.

That mouthwash ad of long ago was probably right in saying that even your best friends won't tell you about your bad breath. If they won't, who will? And where will you learn the significance of that halitosis? Unfortunately, many people find out the hard way.

Too many of us have been lulled by the sense of security we feel from simply brushing our teeth regularly. But brushing often misses those areas down at the gumline and between the teeth where the plaque gets a toehold. Too many of us do not take warning from the little tinge of red that shows up on our toothbrush, or from our sore or tender gums.

Then one day comes the discovery that a few teeth rock too freely, or stick out farther from the gum than they used to, or that our breath is fetid, even to ourselves. The extent of the problem comes to light when the dentist informs us that we may lose some teeth or that we face complicated gum surgery and maintenance because of a serious case of periodontitis. And now we know what our mouth has been trying to tell us: We're long in the tooth.

It's true that older persons are the ones who suffer most from periodontitis in its more advanced stages, though some people have severe cases in their twenties, thirties or forties. With one exception—a relatively rare disease called juvenile periodontitis, or periodontosis, whose cause has not been fully determined—neglect is the culprit in periodontal disease. Almost all periodontitis cases—98 percent—are the unpleasant consequence of earlier failure to practice good mouth hygiene, usually dating back to childhood, youth or early adulthood. Perhaps the victim didn't take the dentist seriously when told of the importance of dental flossing, of how to use a toothbrush regularly and properly, or how to use gum massaging devices, such as the rubber tip on the handle of some toothbrushes, Water Pik, and wood, plastic and brushing aids to massage the gums between the teeth.

To many people, unfortunately, the appearance of those parts of the teeth seen by friends or strangers is more important than the parts seen by the dentist's harder look. Meanwhile, that colorless, invisible bacterial plaque continues to develop and work its way insidiously into the gumline.

There are some factors that—although they are not causes of gum disease—contribute to or exacerbate the condition: tobacco smoking or chewing, badly aligned teeth, ill-fitting dentures, nail biting, clenching or grinding the teeth, poor nutrition, pregnancy, diabetes or certain blood diseases, and some medications, including oral contraceptives and some anti-epilepsy, steroid, and cancer drugs.

Granting that bacterial plaque is responsible for most of the trouble and that ordinary toothbrushing can't remove enough of it to provide the safety needed, isn't there some chemical, some cleaner capable of removing the plaque or loosening it so it will be easier to rinse or brush away?

Dr. Clarence Gilkes, of the division of surgical-dental drug products in FDA's Center for Drugs and Biologics, says that research for some substance to remove plaque has been going on for many years, but so far no New Drug Application for such a product has been approved by the agency.

One substance, chlorhexidine, used in a mouth or gums rinse, has been found effective to some extent, and in fact is in current use in some European countries, but there is no approved New Drug Application for a chlorhexidine product on file at FDA. The reported side effects are a bitter taste and a tendency to discolor natural teeth, as well as porcelain, plastic, and resinous composites used to fill and cap the teeth. Both the bitter taste and staining would be hindrances to market acceptance.

The methods and measures used to treat periodontitis vary in nature and extent and are based mainly on the progress the disease has made.

If the disease is still in its early stages, all that's needed may be scaling and root planing. Scaling and buffing of the teeth surfaces with scraping instruments, machine-rotated buffing pads, and sometimes ultrasonic vibration devices to remove plaque and calculus deposits are usually done by a dental hygienist in a dentist's or periodontist's office. Removal of calculus below the gumline and root planing are usually done by a dentist or periodontist. Root planing consists of removing plaque and calculus from the root to provide a smooth surface to which the gum may reattach.

Another practice in early stages of periodontitis is removing by curettage of (scraping away) the diseased gum tissue in the infected pocket to permit the infected area to heal.

When the pockets become deeper (five millimeters or more) it's difficult for patients to keep pockets clean and free from plaque. Infection can lead to bone resorption (shrinkage). Surgery is often called for. One procedure consists of cutting away the flap of outer tissue to remove the pocket and permit the gum to heal and reattach to the tooth. If the pocket is deep and bone has already resorbed, flap surgery may be necessary. This consists of cutting and lifting the gum away for access to the root of the tooth for removal of calculus, plaque and any diseased tissue. The gum is then sutured back into place. Sometimes the bone that forms the pocket around the tooth may be reshaped or partially removed to facilitate healing. There are several other surgical procedures, including bone grafting.

Periodontal treatment may also call for replacement of worn or defective fillings, removal of possibly infected pulp in the tooth and replacement with an inert substance, correction of chewing or biting problems by reshaping the teeth or orthodontic (shifting of teeth) treatment, use of splints, braces, plastic or other fixtures to stabilize loose teeth, and fitting of plastic mouthpieces to be worn over the teeth at night or at other times by patients who unconsciously clench or grind their teeth.

These and other periodontal techniques—even tooth implants are now coming into use—can give a person a serviceable set of teeth, but they're second best, at best. The best time to start practicing good oral hygiene was yesterday. The next best time is today.

Doing what has to be done to keep periodontitis away is a lifelong proposition. Because we can't see immediate results of the brushing, the flossing, and other hygienic practices, the job takes discipline and purpose.

The reward, assuming we're also attending to our less important dental problems, is a lifetime set of choppers that will always fit. Our own.

Harold Hopkins, reprinted from September 1984, *FDA Consumer*, HHS Publication No. (FDA) 85–3148. Department of Health and Human Services, Public Health Service, Food and Drug Administration, 5600 Fishers Lane, Rockville, Md. 20857. U.S. Government Printing Office 1985—461-367/185.

Depression

Using Drugs To Lift That Dark Veil of Depression

One day, Abraham Lincoln sat down and wrote to his law partner, John Stuart: "I am now the most miserable man living. If what I feel were equally distributed to the whole human family, there would not be one cheerful face on earth. Whether I shall ever be better, I cannot tell; I awfully forebode I shall not. To remain as I am is impossible. I must die or be better. . . ."

Lincoln suffered from a disorder that affects some 127 million people throughout the world and an estimated 9 to 11 million Americans at any given time. Depression—also known as clinical depression or depressive disorders—is the most prevalent mental illness in the United States.

As old as recorded civilization—ancient Egyptian manuscripts and the writings of Greek physicians refer to it as "melancholia" or madness—depression respects neither social class, race, sex, nor ethnic group. Children as young as age 5 have been treated, although the peak years for depression are ages 25 to 44. Outbreaks usually taper off after age 60.

But depression can be treated. A variety of therapies—electroconvulsive therapy (ECT), psychotherapy and antidepressant drugs—lessen the oppressive load.

Antidepressant drugs provide one of the most widely used therapies. These drugs have been credited with miraculous results and also blamed for false hopes and debilitating side effects. Patients who have spent years trying alternatives and finally discover the right antidepressant swear by the results. Those who can't be helped by the drugs—a sizable minority—lament the wasted time. But the fault lies not so much in the imperfections of the various therapies as in the disorder itself. We still don't know much about depression. The brain does not give up its secrets easily and any talk about "cures" for depression is premature.

The word "depression" evokes numerous—and often erroneous—interpretations. Many people think that depression is the feeling of sadness engendered by the vicissitudes of everyday living. Losing a loved one or a job, or suffering any setback, often makes the world seem like a dreary place.

"But those feelings fall into a class of normal emotional reactions and not clinical depression," says Dr. William Potter, a psychopharmacologist at the National Institute of Mental Health (NIMH).

Although one may cry, lose weight, or complain of sleeplessness these symptoms soon pass.

"What determines clinical depression is the severity and duration of symptoms," says Dr. Frederick Goodwin, chief of research at NIMH.

Instead of lasting only a few days, the symptoms of severe depression last for weeks or months, perhaps years. They fall into several categories: mood disturbances (enduring feelings of sadness, guilt or hopelessness); disturbance of biological functioning (sleep disturbance, appetite change, weight gain or loss, loss of sexual drive, fatigue); and disturbances of thought (morbid preoccupations, delusions, hallucinations). Clinical depression may be precipitated by the same losses and stresses that trigger "normal" depressed feelings. It also may occur spontaneously or in response to events that seem quite minor.

"At its extreme," says Dr. Potter, "individuals won't have a few good days or a few bad days. Depression's a long-lasting, bleak picture. Seriously depressed individuals lack the ability to take pleasure in anything—nothing cheers them up. They block, think slowly, and frequently can't answer questions directly."

Research shows that depression is a recurrent illness. Recent studies suggest that 70 to 90 percent of depressed individuals will experience more than one episode or have a chronic depression that is characterized by persistent symptoms and significant problems in social functioning.

Two serious complications frequently accompany depression: alcoholism and suicide. Dr. Kay Jamison, director of the Affective Disorders Clinic at the University of California at Los Angeles, reports that of those with a major depressive illness, 20 to 70 percent have drinking problems. And among those who are severely depressed, approximately one person out of every six will commit suicide. Although twice as many women as men attempt suicide, men more often succeed.

Since ancient times, healers have put their faith in medicines or drugs to cure mental illnesses. Potions, mineral baths, crushed herbs, vapors, and bromides all have been tried.

The successful breakthrough in treating mental disorders with drugs came in the early 1950s with the development of antidepressants and tranquilizers. The discovery of antidepressants was by accident. One of the antidepressant drugs had been used experimentally at first for treating TB. Another drug was intended as an antihistamine.

A second important breakthrough came when scientists discovered the existence of a variety of chemicals in the brain—the ramifications of which they are just beginning to appreciate. Called neurotransmitters or neurojuices, these chemicals perform an endless number of functions, including the regulation of pain, learning and memory, and the desire to eat, drink and sleep. Neurotransmitters also affect moods, feelings and behavior.

Approximately 40 have been identified, but according to Dr. Candace Pert of NIMH, co-discoverer of the endorphin neurotransmitters, ''there might be 100 to 200 different kinds of neurojuices that help regulate emotions and other body processes.''

Three neurotransmitters—dopamine, serotonin and norepinephrine—have been implicated as culprits in depressive illnesses. Too much of them, too little of them, or problems in regulating them as they journey through the brain may account for some types of depressive illnesses.

In fact, one clue as to why such a large number of depressed individuals commit suicide has been traced to lowered activity of the neurotransmitter serotonin. Significantly, low serotonin activity also has been linked to aggression and impulsiveness. Autopsies performed on the brains of suicide victims showed that those who committed violent suicide (gunshot and knife wounds) had lower levels of serotonin functioning than those who committed nonviolent suicide (such as an overdose of sleeping pills). Dr. Goodwin of NIMH hypothesizes that such suicides result from an interaction of depression with a biochemical predisposition to aggression and impulsiveness.

The biological basis for depression is demonstrated further by findings that the same neurotransmitter that influences moods also may regulate the appetite or sleeping habits. ''Obviously, the mind/body distinction is an artificial one because if the nervous system doesn't work, neither the mind nor the body functions very well,'' Dr. Potter says.

Since so many are seeking relief, prescribing of antidepressant drugs has become a multimillion-dollar business. According to survey data from the National Institute of Mental Health, 2 percent of adults took an antidepressant in one recent year. In 1981, 20 to 30 million prescriptions for such drugs were filled in U.S. drugstores.

"Depression is a very complicated disorder," says Dr. Jack Blaine, a clinical psychopharmacologist at NIMH. "There are clearly several kinds of depression with overlapping boundaries and symptoms ranging from moderate to severe."

Some depressions are chronic in nature; others are episodic, incorporating cycles of mania and depression (bipolar); still others consist of recurrent depressions alternating with normal or near-normal moods (unipolar).

Although the exact way an antidepressant works is not clearly understood, the drugs do alleviate many of the symptoms.

"Antidepressants also shorten the course of depression," says Potter. These drugs help many people to function day-to-day, keep them out of hospitals, and help them to keep their jobs and relationships intact.

Most antidepressants fall into three major classes: lithium, tricyclic drugs, and MAO inhibitors.

Lithium

Lithium is the recommended drug for patients suffering from manic depression or bipolar depression. This is a truly incapacitating form of depression and scientists suspect that genes play a large role in its incidence. During the manic phase, persons experience incredible highs, have frenetic and sustained bursts of energy (individuals have been known to stay up days at a time), have an unrealistic sense of well-being, exercise poor judgment, are aggressive, and experience delusions of grandeur. During the depressive phase, the individual plunges to such depths, and to despair so intense, that he or she may commit suicide. A young peoples' disease, this depression most often strikes those in their mid-20s.

Lithium, still a mysterious drug, brings down the euphoric highs of mania, but scientists do not understand why it also works against the depressive phase. The severity of the episodes, the potential impact of a future episode on an individual's functioning, the attitude of the patient toward taking medication for long periods, and many other factors will determine whether and how long a patient continues on treatment.

One of the major problems in prescribing lithium is getting patients to stay on the drug. Dr. Jamison found in a study on lithium compliance that 50 percent of the patients stopped taking the drug against medical advice. Their reason for stopping: They missed the euphoric feelings and sense of well-being experienced during mild manic states.

Side Effects According to the National Institute of Mental Health, "There is a narrow range between the therapeutic and toxic level." Periodic blood tests are needed to monitor the lithium level. Because lithium is excreted from the body almost entirely by the kidneys, any injury or weakening of the kidneys may allow lithium to accumulate to dangerous levels in the body. Since too little sodium also has been implicated in lithium build-up, the use of diuretics and low-sodium diets can be especially harmful to the patient taking lithium. Other side effects include nausea, lethargy, thirst, hand tremors, greatly increased urination, and possible weight gain.

Tricyclics

The most widely used class of the antidepressant drugs, tricyclics are usually prescribed for patients with depression characterized by "endogenous" symptoms. These include insomnia, loss of appetite and weight, psychomotor retardation, loss of energy, decreased capacity to feel pleasure, suicidal thoughts, and thought patterns dominated by hopelessness, helplessness and excessive guilt. Usually known as "classic depression," this depression most often strikes people in their late 30s or early 40s.

NIMH's Dr. Potter says 80 percent of those on the right dosage of tricyclic drugs eventually get better. For those who don't do well on a drug regimen, electroconvulsive treatment is sometimes recommended. There are even those who will spontaneously snap out of their depression after one or two episodes.

Side Effects   Tricyclics can be extremely toxic in excessive doses. Dr. Potter says coroners in metropolitan areas report that tricyclic drugs are a major culprit in deaths due to drug overdoses. Too high a dose also can produce irregularities in heartbeat. Other side effects include disturbed vision, sweating, dizziness, decreased or increased sexual desire, constipation, and edema.

MAO inhibitors

These antidepressants are usually prescribed for people who have not responded to tricyclics or else have "atypical" depression, a type of depression one psychiatrist described as "open to anyone's definition." Less common than classic depression, the condition includes high levels of anxiety and phobic and obsessive-compulsive symptoms. Some individuals also sleep and eat a lot—in contrast to the insomnia and loss of appetite associated with individuals who have classic depression.

MAO—monoamine oxidase—is an enzyme that breaks down neurotransmitter molecules into inactive substances. MAO inhibitors interfere with metabolic breakdown of amines. Therefore, amine levels increase in people taking these medications.

Side Effects The combination of certain foods with MAO inhibitors can trigger very high blood pressure, rapid pulse, headaches, problems with vision, and sometimes paralyzing or fatal strokes. Foods high in the amines tyramine or histamine should be avoided. These foods include beer, red wines, chocolate, pickled fish, cheese and yogurt. Stimulants, caffeine and allergy pills should also be avoided.

Keeping persons on antidepressants long enough for the antidepressive effects to be felt often proves difficult. During the first two to four weeks the patient feels the side effects of the drug but has little relief from the depression. "Physicians often make the mistake of taking their patients off the drug too soon for its antidepressive effects to be felt, or not raising the dose to an adequate level to be effective," says NIMH's Dr. Blaine. "It may take as long as six weeks for the drug to work."

Many physicians recommend that patients be kept on their drug regimen for six to eight months and even as long as a year. The relapse rate for patients taken off too early is 60 to 80 percent. A recent NIMH study showed that patients had to be almost completely symptom-free for approximately three months before the tricyclic drugs could be discontinued without excessive relapses.

Because antidepressant side effects can be dangerous to a few and nearly intolerable to a larger number, drug companies have tried to come up with variations on existing drugs which have fewer side effects.

Several new antidepressants await marketing approval from FDA, but long-term clinical trials will be needed to test both their effectiveness and the lack of or presence of deleterious side effects.

Dr. Mitchell Balter of NIMH, who has spent years conducting surveys of Americans' use of prescription drugs, says, "We're still looking for the perfect antidepressant."

The benefits of psychotherapy also should be emphasized. For mild depression, psychotherapy is usually the best treatment. But even for those who take drugs to control their depression, psychotherapy plays a necessary role in their treatment. As one patient so eloquently describes it:

"I cannot imagine leading a normal life without lithium. . . . Lithium keeps me in relationships, in my career, out of a hospital, and in psychotherapy. It keeps me alive, too. But psychotherapy heals, it makes some sense of the confusion, it reins in the terrifying thoughts and feelings; it brings back hope, and the possibility of learning from it all. No pill can help me deal with the problem of not wanting to take pills, but no amount of therapy alone can prevent my manias and depressions. I need both."

Antidepressant Drugs

Drug	Trade Name	Usual Dosage in Milligrams
Tricyclics		
Amitriptyline	Elavil	150 to 300
	Endep	
	SK-Amitriptyline	
	Amitid	
Amoxapine	Asendin	150 to 300
Desipramine	Norpramine	150 to 300
	Pertofrane	
Doxepin	Sinequan	150 to 300
	Adapin	
Imipramine	Tofranil	150 to 300
	SK-Pramine	
	Janimine	
	Imavate	
Nortriptyline	Aventyl	75 to 150
	Pamelor	
Protriptyline	Vivactil	10 to 60
Trimipramine	Surmontil	150 to 300
Antimanic		
Lithium Carbonate	Eskalith	300 to 2,400[*]
	Lithane	
	Lithonate	
MAO Inhibitors		
Phenelzine	Nardil	45 to 90
Tranylcypromine	Parnate	20 to 60
Isocarboxazid	Marplan	30 to 80
Triazolopyridines		
Trazodone	Desyrel	150 to 600
Tetracyclic		
Maprotiline	Ludiomil	150 to 300

[*] In some cases, large male manic patients may require 4,800 mg/day and do not experience toxic effects at this dose.

Judy Folkenberg, reprinted from October 1983, *FDA Consumer*, HHS Publication No. (FDA) 84–3140. Department of Health and Human Services, Public Health Service, Food and Drug Administration, 5600 Fishers Lane, Rockville, Md. 20857. U.S. Government Printing Office 1984—421–174/68.

Diabetes

An Overview

Diabetes, a disorder of carbohydrate, protein and fat metabolism, is one of the nation's leading health problems. Studies indicate that as many as 10 million Americans may be affected by this disease and that its incidence is rising in all age and socioeconomic groups.

Increased Federal support has markedly expanded the scope and depth of diabetes research and has resulted in several new and exciting advances in the understanding and management of diabetes. Scientists have identified several important factors related to the causes of diabetes. In recent studies, for example, they have found certain genetic factors that appear to be associated with both the insulin-dependent and noninsulin-dependent forms of diabetes, and have clarified differences in the patterns of inheritance between these two major types of the disease.

In related studies, researchers have demonstrated that beta cells grown in tissue culture can be infected and damaged by several common human viruses. A virus called "coxsackie B4" has been isolated from the pancreas of a youth who died from insulin-dependent diabetes. The virus was later shown to produce diabetes in animals. The association of genetic factors and virus infection in causing diabetes could eventually lead to methods of prevention in people who are genetically susceptible.

A number of promising new advances in diabetes treatment also have been made in recent years. For example, researchers have developed artificial devices that automatically deliver insulin to the body at programmed intervals. While NIH-supported studies suggest that these devices hold potential for significant improvement in the management of insulin-dependent diabetes, such artificial devices are still experimental. At present, use of these devices should be limited to patients of investigators with specialized experience in this research.

Another promising area of research is the transplantation of healthy insulin-producing islet cells into human diabetics. The major problem in transplantation is rejection by the human body. In recent research, NIH-supported investigators developed a procedure which has permitted transplantation of healthy pancreatic cells from rats into diabetic mice. These cells were not rejected by the mice, and were successful in reversing their diabetes. A number of problems must be resolved, however, before the procedure can be applied practically in man.

The clinical picture of diabetes is not complete without consideration of its long-term complications, which affect primarily the blood vessels, nervous system, kidneys, and eyes. Progress has been made in the management of some of these complications, most notably in the area of diabetic retinopathy—changes in the retina of the eye that can lead to blindness. This complication occurs in 90 percent of all persons who have had diabetes for 20 years or longer.

Recent research has shown that a procedure called photocoagulation reduces the risk of severe loss of sight by 50 percent in diabetics with advanced retinopathy. In this procedure, finely focused beams of light are used to seal off and destroy bleeding retinal vessels and diseased tissue. A new clinical trial is under way to determine whether earlier use of photocoagulation can halt the development of serious damage to the retina.

In related research, vitrectomy, the surgical removal of cloudy eye fluids that result from blood vessel bleeding, has been shown effective in providing vision to many diabetic patients with severe sight loss. In a new study, investigators are now seeking to determine the best time to remove the blood-clouded fluids (vitreous) from eyes with advanced retinopathy.

In other research, a blood test has been developed that may prove useful in screening for diabetes, in monitoring the effectiveness of treatment and in assessing patient compliance with prescribed treatment. The test involves measurement of a component of red blood cells (HbA_{1c} or hemoglobin A with glucose attached). Normally, this component forms less than 6 percent of total hemoglobin. When blood sugar is elevated, however, more glucose attaches to hemoglobin A. Because the sugar stays attached for the lifespan of the red blood cell—approximately four months—the HbA_{1c} level provides an accurate picture of diabetic control over that time period. The results of this blood test may signal the need for adjusting diet and/or drug therapy to achieve the best blood glucose control.

In response to increasing public and Congressional concern, the National Diabetes Mellitus Research and Education Act of 1974 proposed a "long-range plan to combat diabetes." Spurred by comprehensive legislation passed in October 1976, the plan's recommendations are being implemented through increased funding of research and research training, and the establishment of a specialized centers program for research, training, and education in diabetes.

The diabetes program of the National Institutes of Health crosses Institute lines in its research scope, drawing on the scientific expertise of all of the NIH components. In addition, community-based diabetes control demonstration projects have been developed in 10 states with the support of the Center for Disease Control.

The National Institute of Arthritis, Diabetes, Digestive and Kidney Diseases established the first Diabetes-Endocrinology Research Center (DERC) in 1973 to expand the scope of existing research efforts. Providing a nucleus of shared, comprehensive laboratory facilities, three DERC's now also furnish short-term support for new research initiatives and for studies to assess the feasibility of proposed research efforts.

Congress authorized the establishment of Diabetes Research and Training Centers (DRTC) in 1974 to intensify research and research training in diabetes and to accelerate the transfer of research information to physicians and allied health personnel. As in the DERC program, DRTC's provide core research facilities and short-term support for pilot and feasibility studies. Each of the eight DRTC's, however, also has special education or information activities, such as model care demonstration units that are used both for research and for training, education, and information programs. The type and scope of these information programs vary according to local needs and opportunities, and may relate to any component of the health care system.

Through the efforts of the National Diabetes Data Group, a component of the NIADDK, a new classification system for diabetes has been proposed as a uniform framework in which to conduct clinical and epidemiologic research. Its purpose is to ensure that more meaningful and comparative data will be obtained on the scope and impact of the various forms of diabetes and other classes of glucose intolerance. This classification system, recently endorsed by the international scientific community, will simplify the definition of diabetes and related conditions and make diagnosis easier.

The National Diabetes Information Clearinghouse functions within the NIADDK as the central point for the collection of diabetes educational information. The Clearinghouse has collected and classified hundreds of printed materials about diabetes and has compiled a number of topical annotated bibliographies. These listings provide a central reference source of valuable information and highlight important subject areas in professional and patient education.

The comprehensive plan developed by the National Commission on Diabetes represents the first important step in implementing the mandates of the National Diabetes Research and Education Act of 1974. The guidelines for research and administration provided by that plan and subsequent recommendations of the National Diabetes Advisory Board have aided greatly in the acceleration and coordination of the Federal attack on diabetes.

The combined efforts of the NIADDK, its sister Institutes and other involved Federal agencies are expected to lead to more effective methods of diabetes diagnosis and treatment and, eventually, to lessening of the impact of diabetes as a major public health problem.

National Institute of Arthritis, Diabetes, Digestive & Kidney Diseases, U.S. Department of Health and Human Services, Public Health Service, National Institutes of Health.

Diarrhea

Infectious Diarrhea and Other Causes

What is diarrhea?

Most people have frequent, watery bowel movements for one or two days each year. This change from the usual pattern of stools is recognized as diarrhea and called by many different names. Symptoms commonly disappear in a short time, and the only important effect is that water and salts are lost from the body. For most people, the episode is more an inconvenience than an illness. But sometimes diarrhea lasts for weeks or months, and then it can be an indication of major disease. This more serious form of diarrhea may be accompanied by blood, mucus, or undigested food in the stools. The disease causing diarrhea may also produce fever, abdominal cramps, weight loss, nausea, and/or vomiting. So, we should try to separate the mild and short-lived episodes of diarrhea from continuous and severe diarrhea with these other features.

What are the causes of diarrhea?

A hundred or more different diseases can cause diarrhea. Fortunately, most of the severe causes are rare and the most common form is the one that affects most of us for a few days each year. It is due to a simple infection usually caused by a virus. The more serious causes include ulcerative colitis (when blood is usually present in the stools), regional ileitis (Crohn's disease), some forms of intestinal cancer (when pain and weight loss might also be present), and some disorders of the intestine that lead to poor digestion of food. "Nervous diarrhea," which is part of the irritable bowel syndrome (IBS), is very common and often shows up briefly when we face the stress of a term paper or a job interview. However, some people suffer nervous stress fairly constantly and may have continuous diarrhea because of it. We shall not consider nervous diarrhea, ulcerative colitis, or cancer any further in this article.

What are the causes of infectious diarrhea?

The common illness, which may last several days, often called "intestinal flu," is often due to one of a number of viruses that infect the bowel, making it weep fluid. The excess of fluid in the bowel leads to liquid stools. The inflammation may also be associated with cramping abdominal pain, nausea, and vomiting.

Other common infectious diarrheas may be caused by bacteria. These bacteria irritate the bowel and make it pour out fluid. The inflammation may also be associated with cramping abdominal pain. "Travelers' diarrhea" is due to particular bacteria common in certain areas of the world. People living in these areas are usually well adjusted to the bacteria, but people who are new arrivals are susceptible to these bacterial infections. Although most infectious diarrheas are brief illnesses, some do not go away after a few days. More serious forms can be caused by microbes other than bacteria, such as amoebae and giardia, that can become established in the bowel and cause problems that persist for weeks or months. Contaminated food or water, public swimming pools, and communal hot tubs are possible sources of these infections.

How common is infectious diarrhea?

Mild forms are very common and insignificant, apart from minor discomforts and perhaps the loss of a few days from work. Nevertheless, mild gastrointestinal upsets are among the most common reasons for absences from work and are costly to society because of this. Between one-quarter and one-half of visitors to foreign countries develop travelers' diarrhea; most episodes are mild. However, infectious diarrhea can have serious consequences in certain persons. Young infants, very old people, or those who have major illnesses can be seriously weakened by even a minor infection. Simple infectious diarrhea is still a major killer in underdeveloped countries, where infections of the bowel are estimated to cause millions of deaths annually among infants.

Why is diarrhea dangerous to some people?

Watery stools also contain salt, and severe diarrhea causes the body to lose large amounts of water and salt. Since nausea or vomiting frequently accompanies the diarrhea, restricting the intake of food and liquids, the patient may suffer a loss of fluid and salt at the same time that the dietary intake is reduced. This can lead to dangerous dehydration, particularly in people poorly prepared to withstand losses of fluid and salt, such as the very young, the old, and the sick. Further, certain infections associated with diarrhea, such as typhoid fever, can involve other organs.

When should a doctor be consulted?

Anybody with diarrhea should be given fluids containing sugar and, preferably, salt. Regular (nondiet) soft drinks are a reasonable start;

commercial "quick energy" drinks, such as thirst quenchers containing sugar and salt, may be even better. (Additional salt should not be mixed with these fluids.) If the patient cannot take fluids by mouth and is still having symptoms of vomiting or diarrhea after 12 to 24 hours, medical advice should be sought, especially if the person is very young, old, or otherwise weak.

How is the diagnosis of an infection made?

In many instances, diagnosis of a particular infection may not be important, especially if the person is merely inconvenienced and is back to normal health in one to two days. No specific treatment will be needed for these infections. However, infections with salmonella (such as typhoid fever), shigella (dysentery), amoebae, and some other organisms might require specific treatment such as antibiotics. Examination of the stools and urine for the growth of the organisms by culture, or examination of the blood for antibodies, will then be required to establish the nature of the specific infection.

What is the treatment of infectious diarrhea?

The simple case needs no special treatment, only rest in bed, plenty of fluids by mouth, and perhaps an over-the-counter drug (such as paregoric) to reduce diarrhea and manage other digestive symptoms. More severe cases might require that the person be hospitalized and have intravenous fluids to replace lost water and salt. In infants it has been shown that when correct treatment is started at home, with commercially available liquids that contain proper concentrations of salt and sugar, there is less need for more intensive treatment in a hospital. In the past, many babies died from viral gastroenteritis before it was known how to keep them alive with fluids.

What should the traveler do?

Most forms of travelers' diarrhea are inconveniences rather than serious illnesses, so major treatment is usually not required. Travelers should be careful about nonprocessed water and ice, unwashed or uncooked foods (fruits and salads), and food bought from unlicensed sellers. If diarrhea is mild, bottled water, soft drinks, or clear soups will usually maintain hydration while the disease corrects itself. Antibiotics as a preventive measure may be useful but are not usually necessary.

Some drugs that have been used in the past to help prevent travelers' diarrhea (for instance, entero-vioform) are dangerous. Medical advice should be sought before any drugs are used. Some kinds of infectious diarrhea may be followed by temporary malabsorption, which means that the digestive system will not tolerate large amounts of milk and other dairy products and/or foods high in fat for one to three weeks after the infection subsides. Since temporary malabsorption causes symptoms similar to infectious diarrhea (cramping, nausea, vomiting, and diarrhea), it might be advisable to check with a doctor if your symptoms don't subside within 24 to 72 hours.

Sidney F. Phillips, M.D., Mayo Medical School. National Digestive Diseases, Information Clearinghouse, 1255 23rd Street, N.W., Suite 275, Washington, DC 20037, (202) 296-1138. NIH Publication No. 86–2749, December 1985. This publication is not copyrighted. The digestive diseases clearinghouse urges users of this fact sheet to duplicate and distribute as many copies as desired. Check with local printing firms for reproduction prices. Offset printing can be inexpensive. U.S. Department of Health and Human Services, Public Health Service, National Institutes of Health.

Diverticular Disease
New Hope

As the U.S. population grows older, experts have warned, Americans can expect to suffer from an increasing number of health problems. In recent years, however, attention has turned to the possibility that most Americans—by changing their lifestyles—may be able to avoid or control many of the diseases traditionally associated with aging, if they act in time.

One condition associated with aging for which new hope has emerged in recent years is diverticular disease—inflammation or infection of the large intestine, or colon. Diverticular disease rarely touches people under 40, but more than half of Americans have it by the time they reach 60.

Most people with a milder form of diverticular disease—a condition called diverticulosis—aren't aware they have it because they experience no symptoms. However, when it progresses to diverticulitis, they may suffer a variety of symptoms, including severe pain. Diverticulitis may lead to dangerous bowel complications requiring hospitalization and even major surgery. Though the disease itself is rarely fatal, complications from diverticulitis can cause death.

Diverticular disease consists of small sacs of grape-like protrusions formed when the lining of the intestine is forced out through the gut's muscular wall. The lesions may occur anywhere in the gut, but are found mostly in the colon. Doctors call them diverticula—or a diverticulum when there is only one. (It's from the Latin verb *divertere,* which means to turn aside.) These small, self-contained hernias of the colon wall vary in size from a fraction of an inch to slightly over an inch in diameter.

The small hernias in the gastrointestinal tract that give rise to diverticula usually occur in the last segment, called the sigmoid (for S-shaped), or descending, colon. So, to understand how diverticula develop, it's helpful to see how the large intestine functions.

The colon—five to seven feet long and three to four inches in diameter—is composed, in part, of two sets of muscles. One set runs lengthwise in three roughly parallel lines. The other encircles the colon in parallel rings, giving the organ a bumpy appearance like that of a long balloon ringed by strings that partially restrict its cross-section every inch or so.

The colon receives watery, undigested material from the small intestine. Acting in concert, the two sets of muscles push this residue from one end to the other in wave-like, squeezing motions. In the process, the colon wall may contract and expand up to 10 times a minute. As the undigested material moves through the colon, some vitamins, water and minerals are absorbed into the bloodstream. Finally, bacteria break down the residue before it is expelled through the rectum.

In diverticulosis, the colon contracts and its walls tend to thicken. This is particularly true of the sigmoid, the narrowest and most muscular section. The normally pillow-like external convolutions may take on a corrugated appearance instead. This process of constriction occurs as the sigmoid exerts more pressure on its contents. This added pressure is probably one of the causes of diverticula, although researchers are far from certain about how diverticulosis begins.

Weak spots often form in the intestinal wall—particularly along the corrugated ridges of the colon. At these weak spots, diverticula made up of mucous membrane and connective tissue may balloon through the muscle wall like bubblegum from the mouth of a child. They usually occur where arterioles—small arteries—enter the colon through small gaps in the muscle wall. Occasionally these arterioles balloon out with the diverticula.

According to one estimate, of the millions who harbor diverticula, only one in five will develop symptoms or become sick. Those with symptoms may complain of occasional nausea, constipation, gas, bloating and, sometimes, pain. (These same symptoms can arise from other diseases, such as irritable bowel syndrome, gastric ulcer, hiatal hernia, and liver disease.)

Physicians have two ways to diagnose diverticular disease: the diverticula can be seen on a barium enema X-ray of the lower digestive tract, and the tiny telltale hernias inside the colon wall often can be detected by examination with an endoscope—a flexible fiber device for seeing inside hollow organs of the body.

Physicians use such diagnostic procedures to follow up many gastrointestinal complaints. For example, sigmoidoscopy, an endoscopic examination of the sigmoid colon, is often part of routine physical checkups, particularly in middle-aged men, who tend to suffer a higher incidence of colon cancer. So diverticula may be discovered during routine physical examinations or as physicians diagnose other problems of the digestive tract.

When diverticula become inflamed, diverticulosis turns into diverticulitis. The likelihood of developing this inflammatory complication rises if diverticula are numerous or widely distributed in the colon, if they appear at an early age, or if they have been present 10 years or longer.

Inflamed diverticula may lead to several complications. The inflammation may give rise to an abscess when fecal matter, which occasionally lodges in diverticula, leaks out and contaminates the exterior surface of the colon; the inflamed tissue may adhere to nearby pelvic organs such as the bladder or vagina; a fistula, or hollowing, may develop between the colon and the organ stuck to the diverticula, allowing dangerous wastes to pass between them; a hole may open in a diverticulum and cause fecal matter or pus from an abscess to flow more freely into the pelvic or abdominal cavity, causing peritonitis, a dangerous inflammation of the abdominal cavity's lining; or tiny blood vessels that often form part of the diverticula may bleed.

Patients with diverticulitis may have pain, at times severe, and local tenderness near the groin in the lower left or, occasionally, the lower right abdominal quadrant. Some patients may complain of pain even when the disease is not inflammatory. Other symptoms may include pain when urinating; constipation, often interrupted by diarrhea or other changes in bowel movements; fever; and rectal bleeding.

Doctors advise patients with diverticular disease to stay away from harsh laxatives and avoid straining during bowel movements in order to lessen discomfort.

Diverticulitis often clears up spontaneously. When treatment is necessary, it depends on the nature and degree of inflammation. For severe and persistent cases, bed rest or hospitalization may be prescribed. In an acute phase of diverticular disease, the first objective may be to rest the colon. So a physician may prescribe a bland diet or even intravenous feeding until flare-ups subside. Antibiotics and pain-killing drugs may be indicated in some cases. However, physicians must be careful to differentiate cases of painful diverticulosis from diverticulitis because antibiotics are not prescribed for the former, which is not inflammatory or infected.

Although medical science lacks experimental evidence in humans to demonstrate exactly how diverticula arise, animal studies and epidemiological evidence support the view that dietary fiber plays a role. Before the turn of the century, diverticular disease was virtually unknown in the United States. But since then the number of cases has risen in Western countries, particularly the United States, England and Australia. Epidemiologists—doctors who study the causes and control of diseases in populations—note that the increased incidence of diverticular disease has paralleled the introduction of highly refined foods starting early in the 20th century. Some have associated the rise with the introduction, in the 19th century, of steel flour mills, which produce pulverized flour low in fiber.

Other epidemiologists have observed that diverticular disease is virtually unknown among rural Asian and African peoples who subsist largely on a high-fiber vegetable diet. Comparing the incidence of the disease in the developed countries and the Third World, some researchers, such as Dr. D. P. Burkitt—who spent many years studying nutrition and disease in Africa—have concluded that dietary fiber does play a key role in preventing diverticular disease.

After Dr. Burkitt and others published their epidemiological evidence in the *American Journal of Digestive Diseases* in 1971, physicians began to advise patients with diverticular disease to add fiber to their diets.

A study of 100 hospitalized patients with diverticular disease, published in the *British Journal of Surgery* in February 1980, showed that by adding fiber to their diets, over 90 percent of the patients remained symptom-free for five to seven years after release from the hospital. Older studies done before dietary fiber was used reported that only 38 percent to 64 percent of such discharged patients remained symptom free. So, although dietary fiber is not a cure, it appears that it can reduce or eliminate symptoms.

The precise role of fiber in preventing diverticular disease or controlling its symptoms is not yet known. However, dietary fiber increases the volume of the stool. The bulkier the stool, the faster it moves through the intestine. Stools high in fiber also retain moisture. This keeps them soft and bulky, thereby stimulating healthy colon function. Stools low in fiber, on the other hand, tend to lack water, leaving them compact and hard. The colon responds by exerting greater pressure to move the residue, giving rise to constipation and then diverticula.

How can you be sure that you are getting enough dietary fiber?

Foods rich in dietary fiber include breads, cereals and other products made from whole grains; brown rice; raw fruit (including edible skin and pulp) such as apples, peaches, berries, and citrus fruits; cabbage, broccoli, spinach and other leafy green vegetables, carrots, celery, most varieties of beans, squash, asparagus, and string beans.

One substance that has proven to be most effective in retaining the bulk and moisture of stool in the colon is wheat bran. Wheat bran is readily available either alone or as an ingredient in products such as breakfast cereals or muffins.

Egon Weck, *FDA Consumer,* July–August 1987.

Dizziness
Hope Through Research

Most of us can remember feeling dizzy—after a roller coaster ride, maybe, or when looking down from a tall building, or when, as children, we would step off a spinning merry-go-round. Even superbly conditioned astronauts have had temporary trouble with dizziness while in space. In these situations, dizziness arises naturally from unusual changes that disrupt our normal feeling of stability.

But dizziness can also be a sign that there is a disturbance or a disease in the system that helps people maintain balance. This system is coordinated by the brain, which reacts to nerve impulses from the ears, the eyes, the neck and limb muscles, and the joints of the arms and legs. If any of these areas fail to function normally or if the brain fails to coordinate the many nerve impulses it receives, a person may feel dizzy. The feeling of dizziness varies from person to person and, to some extent, according to its cause; it can include a feeling of unsteadiness, imbalance, or even spinning.

Disease-related dizziness, whether it takes the form of unsteadiness or spinning, is fairly common in the older population. Today, both older and younger people with serious dizziness problems can be helped by a variety of techniques—from medication to surgery to balancing exercises. Such techniques have been developed and improved by scientists studying dizziness.

Much of today's research on dizziness is supported by the National Institute of Neurological and Communicative Disorders and Stroke

(NINCDS). This Institute is a unit of the National Institutes of Health. It is the focal point within the Federal Government for research on the brain and central nervous system, including studies of the senses through which we interact with our surroundings.

With NINCDS support, scientists are searching for better ways to diagnose and treat dizziness, and are investigating the mechanisms that help us maintain our normal sense of balance. These studies, along with basic research on how the ear, the brain, and the nerves work, hold the best hope for relief for dizziness sufferers.

A delicate balancing act

To understand what goes wrong when we feel dizzy, we need to know about the vestibular system by which we keep a sense of balance amid all our daily twisting and turning, starting and stopping, jumping, falling, rolling, and bending.

The vestibular system is located in the inner ear and contains the following structures: vestibular labyrinth, semicircular canals, vestibule, utricle, and saccule. These structures work in tandem with the vestibular areas of the brain to help us maintain balance.

The vestibular labyrinth is located behind the eardrum. The labyrinth's most striking feature is a group of three semicircular canals or tubes that arise from a common base. At the base of the canals is a rounded chamber called the vestibule. The three canals and the vestibule are hollow and contain a fluid called endolymph which moves in response to head movement.

Within the vestibule and the semicircular canals are patches of special nerve cells called hair cells. Hair cells are also found in two fluid-filled sacs, the utricle and saccule, located within the vestibule. These cells are aptly named: rows of thin, flexible, hairlike fibers project from them into the endolymph.

Also located in the inner ear are tiny calcium stones called otoconia. When you move your head or stand up, the hair cells are bent by the weight of the otoconia or movement of the endolymph. The bending of the hair cells transmits an electrical signal about head movement to the brain. This signal travels from the inner ear to the brain along the eighth cranial nerve—the nerve involved in balance and hearing. The brain recognizes the signal as a particular movement of the head and is able to use this information to help maintain balance.

The senses are also important in determining balance. Sensory input from the eyes as well as from the muscles and joints is sent to the brain, alerting us that the path we are following bends to the right or that our head is tilted as we bend to pick up a dime. The brain interprets

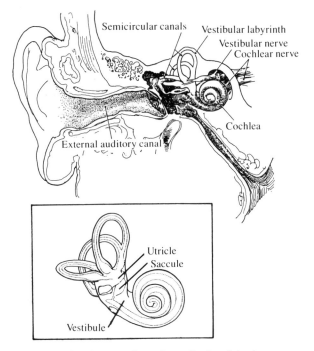

The semicircular canals and vestibule of the inner
ear contain a fluid called endolymph that moves in
response to head movement.

this information—along with cues from the vestibular system—and adjusts
the muscles so that balance is maintained.

Dizziness can occur when sensory information is distorted. Some people
feel dizzy at great heights, for instance, partly because they cannot focus
on nearby objects to stabilize themselves. When one is on the ground,
it is normal to sway slightly while standing. A person maintains balance
by adjusting the body's position to something close by. But when someone
is standing high up, objects are too far away to use to adjust balance.
The result can be confusion, insecurity, and dizziness, which is sometimes
resolved by sitting down.

Some scientists believe that motion sickness, a malady that affects
sea, car, and even space travelers, occurs when the brain receives conflict-
ing sensory information about the body's motion and position. For example, when someone reads while riding in a car, the inner ear senses the
movement of the vehicle, but the eyes gaze steadily on the book that is
not moving. The resulting sensory conflict may lead to the typical symptoms of motion sickness: dizziness, nausea, vomiting, and sweating.

Another form of dizziness occurs when we turn around in a circle
quickly several times and then stop suddenly. Turning moves the endo-

lymph. The moving endolymph tells us we are still rotating but our other senses say we've stopped. We feel dizzy.

Diagnosing the problem

The dizziness one feels after spinning around in a circle usually goes away quickly and does not require a medical evaluation. But when symptoms appear to be caused by an underlying physical problem, the prudent person will see a physician for diagnostic tests. According to a study supported by the National Institute of Neurological and Communicative Disorders and Stroke, a thorough examination can reveal the underlying cause of dizziness in about 90 percent of cases.

A person experiencing dizziness may first go to a general practitioner or family physician; between 5 and 10 percent of initial visits to these physicians involve a complaint of dizziness. The patient may then be referred either to an ear specialist (otologist) or a nervous system specialist (neurologist).

The patient will be asked to describe the exact nature of the dizziness, to give a complete history of its occurrence, and to list any other symptoms or medical problems. Patients give many descriptions of dizziness—depending to some extent on its cause. Common complaints are light-headedness, a feeling of impending faint, a hallucination of movement or motion, or a loss of balance without any strange feelings in the head. Some people also report they have vertigo—a form of dizziness in which one's surroundings appear to be spinning uncontrollably or one feels the sensation of spinning.

The physician will try to determine what components of a patient's nervous system are out of kilter, looking first for changes in blood pressure, heart rhythm, or vision—all of which may contribute to the complaints. Sometimes dizziness is associated with an ear disorder. The patient may have loss of hearing, discomfort from loud sounds, or constant noise in the ear, a disorder known as *tinnitus*. The physician will also look for other neurological symptoms: difficulty in swallowing or talking, for example, or double vision.

Tests and scans

After the initial history-taking and physical examination, the physician may deliberately try to make the patient feel dizzy. The patient may be asked to repeat actions or movements that generally cause dizziness: to walk in one direction and then turn quickly in the opposite direction, or to hyperventilate by breathing deeply for three minutes.

In another test, the patient sits upright on an examining table. The physician tilts the patient's head back and turns it part way to one side, then gently but quickly pushes the patient backward to a lying down position. The reaction to this procedure varies according to the cause of dizziness. Patients with benign positional vertigo may experience vertigo plus *nystagmus:* rapid, uncontrollable back-and-forth movements of the eyes.

One widely used procedure, called the caloric test, involves electronic monitoring of the patient's eye movements while one ear at a time is irrigated with warm water or warm air and then with cold water or cold air. This double stimulus causes the endolymph to move in a way similar to that produced by rotation of the head. If the labyrinth is working normally, nystagmus should result. A missing nystagmus reaction is a strong argument that the balance organs are not acting correctly.

NINCDS-supported scientists at The Johns Hopkins University in Baltimore observed that not all patients can tolerate the traditional caloric test. Some become sick when the ear is irrigated with the standard amount of water or air before physicians can measure their eye movements. So the scientists are designing a method of conducting the test more gradually by slowly adjusting the amount of water or air reaching the inner ear. Their goal is to reduce patient discomfort while allowing the test to proceed.

Some patients who cannot tolerate the caloric test are given a rotatory test. In this procedure, the patient sits in a rotating chair, head tilted slightly forward. The chair spins rapidly in one direction, then stops abruptly. Depending on the cause of dizziness, the patient may experience vertigo after this rotation.

In one variation of this test, the chair is placed in a tent of striped cloth. As the chair rotates, electrodes record movements of the patient's eyes in response to the stripes. The physician evaluates these eye movements, a form of nystagmus, to determine if the patient has a disorder of the balance system.

Because disorders of balance are often accompanied by hearing loss, the physician may order a hearing test.

Hearing loss and associated dizziness could also be due to damaged nerve cells in the brain stem, where the hearing and balance nerve relays signals to the brain. To detect a malfunction, the physician may order a kind of computerized brain wave study called a brain stem auditory evoked response test. In this procedure, electrodes are attached to several places on the surface of the patient's scalp and a sound is transmitted to the patient's ear. The electrodes measure the time it takes nerve signals generated by the sound to travel from the ear to the brain stem.

If there is reason to suspect that the dizziness could stem from a tumor or cyst, the patient may undergo a computed tomographic (CT) scan. In a CT scan, X-ray pictures are taken of the brain from several different angles. These images are then combined by a computer to give a detailed view that may reveal the damaging growth.

Sometimes anxiety and emotional upset cause a person to feel dizzy. Certain patients may be asked to take a psychological test, to try to find out whether the dizziness is caused or intensified by emotional stress.

The many tests administered by a physician will usually point to a cause for the patient's dizziness. Disorders responsible for dizziness can be categorized as:

- *peripheral vestibular,* or those involving a disturbance in the labyrinth.
- *central vestibular,* or those resulting from a problem in the brain or its connecting nerves.
- *systemic,* or those originating in nerves or organs outside the head.

Confused signals

When someone has vertigo but does not experience faintness or difficulty in walking, the cause is probably a peripheral vestibular disorder. In these conditions, nerve cells in the inner ear send to the brain confusing information about body movement.

Ménière's Disease A well-known cause of vertigo is the peripheral vestibular disorder known as Ménière's disease. First identified in 1861 by Prosper Ménière, a French physician, the disease is thought to be caused by too much endolymph in the semicircular canals and vestibule. Some scientists think that the excess endolymph may affect the hair cells so that they do not work correctly. This explanation, however, is still under study.

The vertigo of Ménière's disease comes and goes without an apparent cause; it may be made worse by a change in position and reduced by being still.

In addition to vertigo, patients have hearing loss and tinnitus. Hearing loss is usually restricted at first to one ear and is often severe. Patients sometimes feel "fullness" or discomfort in the ear, and diagnostic testing may show unusual sensitivity to increasingly loud sounds. In 10 to 20 percent of patients, hearing loss and tinnitus eventually occur in the second ear.

Ménière's disease patients may undergo electronystagmography, an electrical recording of the caloric test, to determine if their labyrinth is working normally.

Attacks of Ménière's disease may occur several times a month or year and can last from a few minutes to many hours. Some patients experience a spontaneous disappearance of symptoms while others may have attacks for years.

Treatment of Ménière's disease includes such drugs as meclizine hydrochloride and the tranquilizer diazepam to reduce the feeling of intense motion during vertigo. To control the buildup of endolymph, the patient may also take a diuretic, a drug that reduces fluid production. A low-salt diet—which reduces water retention—is claimed to be an effective treatment of Ménière's disease.

When these measures fail to help, surgery may be considered. In shunt surgery, part of the inner ear is drained to reestablish normal inner ear fluid or endolymph pressure. In another operation, called vestibular nerve section, surgeons expose and cut the vestibular part of the eighth nerve. Both vestibular nerve section and shunt surgery commonly relieve the dizziness of Ménière's disease without affecting hearing.

A more drastic operation, labyrinthectomy, involves total destruction of the inner ear. This procedure is usually successful in eliminating dizziness but causes total loss of hearing in the operated ear—an important consideration since the second ear may one day be affected.

Positional Vertigo　People with benign positional vertigo experience vertigo after a position change. Barbara noticed the first sign of this disorder one morning when she got up out of bed. She felt the room spinning. Frightened, she quickly returned to bed and lay down. After about 30 seconds the vertigo passed. Fearing a stroke, Barbara went to the emergency room of a hospital for a medical evaluation, which failed to show a problem. She had no symptoms for several days, then the problem returned. At this point, Barbara was referred to an otoneurologist, a physician who specializes in the ear and related parts of the nervous system.

Like Barbara, most patients with benign positional vertigo are extremely worried about their symptoms. But the patients usually feel less threatened once the disorder is diagnosed.

The cause of benign positional vertigo is not known, although some patients may recall an incident of head injury. The condition can strike at any adult age with attacks occurring periodically throughout a person's life.

In one type of treatment, the patient practices the position that provokes dizziness until the balance system eventually adapts. Rarely, a physician will prescribe medication to prevent attacks.

Vestibular Neuronitis　In this common vestibular disorder, the patient has severe vertigo. Jack experienced his first attack of this problem at 2 A.M. when he rolled over in bed and suddenly felt the room spinning violently. He started vomiting but couldn't stand up; finally, he managed to crawl to the bathroom. When he returned to bed, he lay very still—the only way to stop the vertigo. Three days later, he was able to walk without experiencing vertigo, but he still felt unsteady. Gradually, over the next several weeks, Jack's balance improved, but it was a year before he was entirely without symptoms.

Unlike Ménière's disease, vestibular neuronitis is not associated with hearing loss. Patients with vestibular neuronitis first experience an acute attack of severe vertigo lasting for hours or days, just as Jack did, with loss of balance sometimes lasting for weeks or months. About half of those who have a single attack have further episodes over a period of months to years.

The cause of vestibular neuronitis is uncertain. Since the first attack often occurs after a viral illness, some scientists believe the disorder is caused by a viral infection of the nerve.

Other Labyrinth Problems Inner ear problems with resulting dizziness can also be caused by certain antibiotics used to fight life-threatening bacterial infections. Probably the best-known agent of this group is streptomycin. Problems usually arise when high doses of these drugs are taken for a long time, but some patients experience symptoms after short treatment with low doses, especially if they have impaired kidneys.

The first symptoms of damage to the inner ear caused by medication are usually hearing loss, tinnitus, or unsteadiness while walking. Stopping the drug can usually halt further damage to the balance mechanism, but this is not always possible: the medicine may have to be continued to treat a life-threatening infection. Patients sometimes adapt to the inner ear damage that may occur after prolonged use of these antibiotics and recover their balance.

Balance can also be affected by a cholesteatoma, a clump of cells from the eardrum that grow into the middle ear and accumulate there. These growths are thought to result from repeated infections such as recurrent otitis media. If unchecked, a cholesteatoma can enlarge and threaten the inner ear. But if the growth is detected early, it can be surgically removed.

Brain and nerve damage

The vestibular nerve carries signals from the inner ear to the brain stem. If either the nerve or the brain stem is damaged, information about position and movement may be blocked or incorrectly processed, leading to dizziness. Conditions in which dizziness results from damage to the brain stem or its associated nerves are called central causes of dizziness.

Acoustic Neuroma One central cause of dizziness is a tumor called an acoustic neuroma. Although the most common sign of this growth is hearing loss followed by tinnitus, some patients also experience dizziness.

An acoustic neuroma usually occurs in the internal auditory canal, the bony channel through which the vestibular nerve passes as it leaves the inner ear. The growing tumor presses on the nerve, sending false messages about position and movement to the brain.

The hearing nerve running alongside the vestibular nerve can also be compressed by the acoustic neuroma, with resulting tinnitus and hearing loss. Or the tumor may press on other nearby nerves, producing numbness or weakness of the face. If the neuroma is allowed to grow, it will eventually reach the brain and may affect the function of other cranial nerves.

Computed tomography has revolutionized the detection of acoustic neuromas. If an early diagnosis is made, a surgeon can remove the tumor. The patient usually regains balance.

Stroke Dizziness may be a sign of a "small stroke" or transient ischemic attack (TIA) in the brain stem. TIA's, which result from a temporary lack of blood supply to the brain, may also cause transient numbness, tingling, or weakness in a limb or on one side of the face. Other signs include temporary blindness and difficulty with speech. These symptoms are warning signs: one should see a physician immediately for treatment. If a TIA is ignored, a major stroke may follow.

Systemic diseases: underlying illness

Dizziness can be a symptom of diseases affecting body parts other than the brain and central nervous system. Systemic conditions like anemia or high blood pressure decrease oxygen supplies to the brain; a physician eliminates the resulting dizziness by treating the underlying systemic illness.

Damaged Sensory Nerves We maintain balance by adjusting to information transmitted along sensory nerves from sensors in the eyes, muscles, and joints to the spinal cord or brain. When these sensory nerves are damaged by systemic disease, dizziness may result.

Multiple sensory deficits, a systemic disease, is believed by some physicians to be the chief cause of vaguely described dizziness in the aged population. In this disorder several senses or sensory nerves are damaged. The result: faulty balance.

People with diabetes, which can damage nerves affecting vision and touch, may develop multiple sensory deficits. So can patients with arthritis or cataracts, both of which distort how sensory information reaches the brain. The first step in treating multiple sensory deficits is to eliminate symptoms of specific disorders. Permanent contact lenses can improve vision in cataract patients, for example, and medication or surgery may ease pain and stiffness related to arthritis.

Symptoms of damaged sensory nerves may be relieved by a collar to eliminate extreme head motion, balancing exercises to help compensate for sensory losses, or a cane to aid balance. Some patients are helped by the drug methylphenidate, which can increase awareness of remaining sensations.

Systemic neurological disorders such as multiple sclerosis, Alzheimer's disease, Parkinson's disease, or Creutzfeldt-Jakob disease may also cause dizziness, primarily during walking. However, dizziness is rarely the sole symptom of these nervous system diseases.

Low Blood Pressure   One common systemic disease causing dizziness is postural or orthostatic hypotension. In this disease, the heart does not move the blood with enough force to supply the brain adequately. Symptoms include sudden feelings of faintness, light-headedness, or dizziness when standing up quickly.

Because the muscles in aging blood vessels are weak and the arteries inadequate in helping convey blood to the head, older people are particularly susceptible to this condition. Older persons who do not sit or lie down at the first sensation of dizziness may actually lose consciousness.

People who have undetected anemia or those who are taking diuretics to eliminate excess water from their body and reduce high blood pressure are also at risk of developing postural hypotension.

A physician can easily diagnose postural hypotension: the patient's blood pressure is measured before standing abruptly and immediately afterward. Treatment is designed to eliminate dizziness by reducing the patient's blood volume.

A Secondary Symptom   Dizziness may also be a secondary symptom in many other diseases. Faintness accompanied by occasional loss of consciousness can be due to low blood sugar, especially when the faint feeling persists after the patient lies down.

A common cause of mild dizziness—the kind described as light-headedness—is medicine. A number of major prescription drugs may produce light-headedness as a side effect. Two types of drugs that can cause this problem are sedatives, which are taken to induce sleep, and tranquilizers, which are used to calm anxiety.

When anxiety strikes

Tranquilizers may cause a type of dizziness referred to as light-headedness—but so may anxiety. Cynthia is a young woman who becomes light-headed under a variety of stressful circumstances. The light-headedness sometimes is accompanied by heart palpitations and panic. She can produce these symptoms at will by breathing rapidly and deeply for a few minutes.

Cynthia's light-headedness is due to hyperventilation: rapid, prolonged deep breathing or occasional deep sighing that upsets the oxygen and carbon dioxide balance in the blood. The episodes are typically brief and often associated with tingling and numbness in the fingers and around the mouth. Hyperventilation is triggered by anxiety or depression in about 60 percent of dizziness patients.

Once made aware of the source of the symptoms, a patient can avoid hyperventilation or abort attacks by breath-holding or breathing into a paper bag to restore a correct balance of oxygen and carbon dioxide. If hyperventilation is due to anxiety, psychological counseling may be recommended.

Some patients who report dizziness may be suffering from a psychiatric disorder. Generally these persons will say that they experience light-headedness or difficulty concentrating; they may also describe panic states when in crowded places. Tests of such patients reveal that the inner ear is working correctly. Treatment may include counseling.

Demystifying Dizziness through Research Scientists are working to understand dizziness and its sources among the complex interactions of the labyrinth, the other sense organs, and the brain. The research is offering new insights into the basis of balance, as well as improvements in diagnosis, treatment, and prevention of dizziness.

Innovative Surgery Delicate surgical instruments and operating microscopes have made possible new methods to help patients with dizziness. The symptoms of benign positional vertigo, for example, may be relieved by a microsurgical ear operation called a singular neurectomy in which a tiny portion of the vestibular nerve is divided and cut.

Patients with Ménière's disease may benefit from a microsurgical operation called the cochleosacculotomy. In this procedure, a small curette or wire loop is used to reach into the vestibule of the inner ear and remove the fluid-filled saccule. An investigator at the Massachusetts Eye and Ear Institute in Boston has found that this operation relieves symptoms of vertigo in about 80 percent of patients.

Space Biology Research also promises to help astronauts who suffer from dizziness or space sickness. In one study, a scientist aboard a space shuttle conducted experiments to find out why half the astronauts who have space sickness at the start of a flight overcome this problem before the end of the mission. The investigator, from the Massachusetts Institute of Technology, found that the space traveler's brain no longer relies on the gravity-sensitive inner ear structures for information about position and motion. Instead, the astronaut's brain realizes that the inner ear is sending false information and starts to depend more on the eyes to find out about the body's movements. This finding may enable space biologists to train astronauts before launch to avoid space sickness.

During that same space mission, a German scientist performed experiments that raised questions about the theory behind the caloric test. According to that theory, alternate heating and cooling of the endolymph causes the fluid to form wave-like swirling patterns called convection currents. These currents make the brain think the head is moving. The result is nystagmus.

In space, however, lack of gravity should prevent convection currents from forming, so the eyes were expected to remain still. Instead, they moved just as though the test was being done on Earth in normal gravity. These experiments indicate there is more than one explanation for why the caloric test works: when the endolymph is warmed, the fluid expands and moves the cupula, the top of the cochlear duct. The movement of the cupula cues the brain that the head is moving and the eyes respond.

This research helps scientists interpret methods used to test vestibular function. It also promises to increase our understanding of the balance system.

Currently, scientists at the Johnson Space Center in Houston and at the Good Samaritan Hospital in Portland are preparing to study space sickness and vestibular function in a microgravity (near zero gravity) laboratory. The astronauts' vestibular function will be analyzed in a series of experiments, including studies to test whether visual input becomes more important in maintaining balance as weightlessness increases. The scientists anticipate that this research will help all sufferers of motion sickness, not just astronauts.

Improved Diagnosis.   Back on Earth, improvements are being made in measuring precisely the eye movements of patients undergoing diagnostic tests for dizziness. Investigators at the NINCDS-funded research center at the University of California at Los Angeles have developed a computer-controlled chair in which a patient is shifted into a variety of body positions to stimulate the labyrinth. Eye responses are measured with newly designed computerized instruments. To further stimulate eye movements, a set of computer-generated visual patterns can be moved with the chair or independently of it.

These instruments will extract much information about a patient's ability to integrate information from the eyes and the inner ear, and will help distinguish patients with different disorders of the balance system.

Signaling the Brain.   To understand dizziness, scientists must find out how stimuli to the labyrinth are translated into information that the brain can use to maintain balance. How, for example, is information from the inner ear sent to the brain and interpreted? Among the scientists studying this question is an NINCDS grantee at the University of Chicago who is looking at the different ways hair cells react to the movement of inner ear fluid. He has identified a characteristic pattern of electrical response in hair cells. The next step is to discover how these messages are interpreted by the nerve cells carrying information to the brain.

Another NINCDS grantee at the University of Minnesota is studying the activity of the brain when it sends balance-preserving signals from the sense organs to the muscles. In one experiment, healthy persons are rotated in the dark at a constant rate. After a few minutes they no longer think they are moving. This is because the inner ear only senses changes in the rate of movement. If the lights are turned on and both the chair and the room rotate at the same constant speed, again the person doesn't sense movement. Both the inner ear and the eyes are fooled into thinking there is no motion.

But the investigator found that if the chair and the room are accelerated, the patient develops what is described as sensory conflict. The acceleration of the chair tells the inner ear that there is movement. But the eyes tell the brain that the body is stationary. How patients react in these conflict situations reveals how the brain puts together various types of sensory information to maintain balance. The results of this and related experiments will help scientists build a mathematical model of the balance system.

Hope for the future

For those who are healthy, equilibrium is a sense often taken for granted. People can't see their labyrinth, even though it is as much a sense organ as the ears or the eyes. But when it is injured, an ability vital to everyday living is lost.

Scientists already understand a great deal about the labyrinth's function and the way the brain maintains balance. Further research into this complex system should help those who are incapacitated by dizziness when the balance system goes awry.

Voluntary health organizations

The following organizations provide information on dizziness or on inner ear diseases that cause dizziness:

Acoustic Neuroma Association
P.O. Box 398
Carlisle, PA 17013
(717) 249-4783

American Academy of Otolaryngology-Head and Neck Surgery
Suite 302
1101 Vermont Avenue, N.W.
Washington, DC 20005
(202) 289-4607

Better Hearing Institute
P.O. Box 1840
Washington, DC 20013
(703) 642-0580
(800) 424-8576 (Toll free)

National Hearing Association
721 Enterprise
Oak Brook, IL 60521
(312) 323-7200

Human tissue banks

The study of ear tissue from patients with dizziness and deafness is invaluable in research. Temporal bones willed by people with balance or hearing problems and by people with normal hearing can be used to help research scientists and physicians training to be otolaryngologists. Physicians in training study the basic anatomy of the temporal bone and develop their surgical skills. Scientists use the bones for research on the inner ear and on congenital disorders that cause deafness. Middle ear bones (ossicles) and the eardrum are also used as grafts to surgically correct sound transmission problems of the middle ear.

NINCDS supports four temporal bone banks that supply scientists in every state with tissue from patients who have dizziness or deafness. The donated temporal bones includes the eardrum, the entire middle and inner ear, and the nerve tissues which combine into the brain stem. For information about tissue donation and collection, write to:

National Temporal Bone Bank
Eastern Center
Massachusetts Eye and Ear Infirmary
243 Charles Street
Boston, MA 02114
(617) 523-7900, ext. 2711

National Temporal Bone Bank
Midwestern Center
University of Minnesota
Box 396-Mayo
Minneapolis, MN 55455
(612) 624-5466

National Temporal Bone Bank
Southern Center
Baylor College of Medicine
Neurosensory Center—Room A523
Houston, TX 77030
(713) 790-5470

National Temporal Bone Bank
Western Center
UCLA School of Medicine
31-24 Rehabilitation Center
Los Angeles, CA 90024
(213) 825-4710

GLOSSARY

acoustic neuroma: tumor of the vestibular nerve that may press on the hearing nerve causing dizziness and hearing loss.

balance system: complex biological system that enables us to know where our body is in space and to keep the position we want. Proper balance depends on information from the labyrinth in the inner ear, from other senses such as sight and touch, and from muscle movement.

benign positional vertigo: condition in which moving the head to one side or to a certain position brings on vertigo.

brain stem auditory evoked response (BAER): diagnostic test in which electrodes are attached to the surface of the scalp to determine the time it takes inner ear electrical responses to sound to travel from the ear to the brain. The test helps locate the cause of some types of dizziness.

caloric test: diagnostic test in which warm or cold water or air is put into the ear. If a person experiences certain eye movements (nystagmus) after this procedure, the labyrinth is working correctly.

cholesteatoma: a tumorlike accumulation of dead cells in the middle ear. This growth is thought to result from repeated middle ear infections.

computed tomography (CT) scan: radiological examination useful for examining the inside of the ear and head.

diuretic: drug that promotes water loss from the body through the urine. Used to treat hypertension, diuretics may bring on dizziness due to postural hypotension.

dizziness: feeling of physical instability with regard to the outside world.

endolymph: fluid filling part of the labyrinth.

hair cells: specialized nerves found in the semicircular canals and vestibule. Fibers (hairs) sticking out of one end of the hair cells move when the head moves and send information to the brain that is used to maintain balance.

hyperventilation: repetitive deep breathing that reduces the carbon dioxide content of the blood and brings on dizziness. Anxiety may cause hyperventilation and dizziness.

inner ear: contains the organs of hearing and balance.

labyrinth: the organ of balance, which is located in the inner ear. The labyrinth consists of the three semicircular canals and the vestibule.

Ménière's disease: condition that causes vertigo. The disease is believed to be caused by too much endolymph in the labyrinth. Persons with this illness also experience hearing problems and tinnitus.

middle ear: the space immediately behind the eardrum. This part of the ear contains the three bones of hearing: the hammer (malleus), anvil (incus), and stirrup (stapes).

multiple sensory deficits: condition associated with dizziness in which damage to nerves of the eye and arms or legs reduces information about balance to the brain.

neurologist: physician who specializes in disorders of the nervous system.

nystagmus: rapid back-and-forth movements of the eyes. These reflex movements may occur during the caloric test and are used in the diagnosis of balance problems.

orthostatic hypotension: see **postural hypotension.**

otologist: physician who specializes in diseases of the ear.

peripheral vestibulopathy: vestibular disorder in which the vestibular nerve appears inflamed and paralyzed. Patients may have one or several attacks of vertigo.

postural hypotension (also called **orthostatic hypotension**):   sudden dramatic drop in blood pressure when a person rises from sitting, kneeling, or lying position. The prime symptoms of postural hypotension, which is sometimes due to low blood volume, is dizziness or faintness. The condition can be dangerous in older persons, who may faint and injure themselves.

semicircular canals: three curved hollow tubes in the inner ear that are part of the balance organ, the labyrinth. The canals are joined at their wide ends and are filled with endolymph.

stroke: death of nerve cells due to a loss of blood flow in the brain. A stroke often results in permanent loss of some sensation or muscle activity.

TIA: see **transient ischemic attack.**

tinnitus: noises or ringing in the ear.

transient ischemic attack (TIA):   temporary interruption of blood flow to a part of the brain. Because a TIA may signal the possibility of a stroke, it requires immediate medical attention. During a TIA, a person may feel dizzy, have double vision, or feel tingling in the hands.

vertigo: severe form of dizziness in which one's surroundings appear to be spinning uncontrollably. Extreme cases of vertigo may be accompanied by nausea.

vestibular disorders: diseases of the inner ear that cause dizziness.

vestibular nerve: nerve that carries messages about balance from the labyrinth in the inner ear to the brain.

vestibular neuronitis: another name for peripheral vestibulopathy.

vestibule: part of the labyrinth, located at the base of the semicircular canals. This structure contains the endolymph and patches of hair cells.

Prepared by the Office of Scientific and Health Reports, National Institute of Neurological and Communicative Disorders and Stroke. National Institutes of Health, Bethesda, Maryland 20892. NIH Publication No. 86–76, September 1986.

Dysmenorrhea

Dysmenorrhea and Premenstrual Syndrome

Many women experience some discomfort or distress associated with the menstrual cycle. For some women, the discomfort is mild and tolerable, but for others it is severe and disabling. The two most common problems of the menstrual cycle are dysmenorrhea and premenstrual syndrome.

Dysmenorrhea (painful menstruation) can disable a woman for a few hours before or at the onset of her menstrual period and last for several hours or as long as two days. Pain may be severe and daily activities may have to be modified.

Premenstrual syndrome (PMS) is the term given to the group of physical and behavioral changes that may affect some women in the week or so just before a menstrual period. For unexplained reasons, these women suffer moderate to severe distress and tension during that time. They may experience abdominal bloating, fatigue, irritability, or moodiness.

Often they may do and say things that alienate friends and family. Negative self-images may develop as these women attempt to cope with severe PMS symptoms.

In the past, women suffered menstrual discomfort in embarrassed, even guilty silence. Menstruating women were thought to be under a curse, unclean, or at the very least, unwell. The subject was not a topic for public discussion. Similar attitudes persist in certain cultures today. There is, however, an increasing awareness in most modern societies that menstruation is *not* an illness, but a normal and necessary function that is part of the process enabling women to bear children.

Dysmenorrhea and PMS have been the focus of recent public attention. Reports about both conditions in popular publications have suggested that effective treatment is readily available for menstrual cramps (the cause of pain during menstruation) and imminent for PMS. Scientific reports, however, are more conservative. They show that some medications for dysmenorrhea may help some women, but not all. Relief for PMS, however, is still largely a matter of treating symptoms in the absence of a known cause. Researchers first need to understand the precise workings of the menstrual cycle before they can know how and why hormonal imbalances occur.

The National Institute of Child Health and Human Development (NICHD) which supports research in the reproductive sciences, and the National Institute of Mental Health (NIMH) which studies hormone-related behavior changes, have primary responsibility within the federal government for research in menstrual disorders. This article reports what is known about dysmenorrhea and premenstrual syndrome, including new information from scientific research that may help women with either problem.

Hormones and the normal menstrual cycle

Hormones play an important role in the proper functioning of the menstrual cycle. In studying menstrual disorders, scientists have tried to determine how menstruation occurs normally.

The onset of menstruation (menarche) is the dramatic marker of the change from girl to woman. Usually occurring between ages of ten and sixteen, the beginning of menstruation means that a young girl is developing the ability to bear children. At first the cycle may be irregular. Usually, a regular menstrual cycle is established by the end of the first year after menarche. Interrupted only for pregnancies or specific health problems, it continues month after month until a woman is in her forties or fifties when menstruation ceases (menopause). A typical cycle is about 28 days, but cycles varying from 24 to 30 days are not uncommon. Generally, a woman keeps to the established pattern although stress, illness or the use of oral contraceptives may alter her cycle temporarily.

During each cycle, the inner wall or lining (endometrium) of the uterus thickens to provide a suitable environment for a pregnancy. A mature egg (ovum) is released from one of the two ovaries in midcycle (ovulation) and remains in the reproductive tract for about three days. For a pregnancy to occur, the ovum must be fertilized by a sperm. If there is no pregnancy, the lining of the uterus breaks down and is discharged as the menstrual flow (menses) over the course of three to eight days.

Although the reproductive organs are located in the body's pelvic area, the reproductive cycle is controlled by an area at the base of the brain containing the hypothalamus and the pituitary gland. The hypothalamus and the pituitary gland orchestrate menstrual cycle activities, sending "start" and "stop" signals each month to the ovaries and uterus.

On the first day of menstruation, hormone levels are low. But after one week and for most of the remaining cycle, *estrogens* are produced to promote ovulation and stimulate the development of the endometrium. During this time estrogens contribute to producing an appropriate environment in the reproductive organs for fertilization, implantation and nurturing of the early embryo. Estrogen production drops off a few days before the next cycle begins.

Progesterone, a hormone produced in large amounts during the latter half of the cycle, stimulates the development of the endometrium in preparation for a pregnancy. If there is no pregnancy, progesterone levels decrease and menstruation begins. If pregnancy occurs, production of progesterone continues throughout the nine months to help maintain the pregnancy.

Other hormone-like substances, *prostaglandins,* are also produced during the latter half of the cycle. Although the role of prostaglandins is not completely understood, they are believed to stimulate uterine contractions which are recognized as cramps during the menstrual period. The prostaglandins may be one of the possible factors that start labor.

Dysmenorrhea

Many women experience some discomfort when a menstrual period begins. Most can manage daily routines and responsibilities because the discomfort is mild and brief in duration. For others, the discomfort is severe, lasts for hours, and is disabling. In a recent health survey of adolescent women, more than half reported pain during menstruation.

Dysmenorrhea is the medical term for painful menstruation. It is primarily caused by moderate to severe cramping of the uterus. Headache, backache, diarrhea and nausea are associated symptoms.

Dysmenorrhea usually does not begin until six to twelve months following menarche, when a woman's system has developed fully and ovulation occurs regularly. The disorder appears to affect young women and women who have not borne children more so than older women who have had children.

In the past, the young woman's complaints of pain were dismissed with the advice, "It's just part of being a woman. You'll get over it after you have a baby." There is a measure of truth in that latter statement because dysmenorrhea diminishes in many women after a full-term pregnancy. This may occur because uterine muscles are stretched during pregnancy. Another possible explanation is that uterine blood supply and muscle activity may be improved by the process of having a child.

Research findings

Noting the similarity between menstrual cramps and mild labor pains, scientific investigation in the past had focused on the basic workings of uterine contractions. Prostaglandins were identified as one of the factors involved in causing contractions. These substances are secreted by the uterine lining and affect the smooth muscles of the uterus, thus assisting in the sloughing off of the lining during menstruation.

While attention was directed to this area of research, reports began to appear that oral contraceptive users seemed to have less menstrual problems than nonusers. One explanation given was that the decrease in menstrual flow associated with oral contraceptive use resulted in a reduction of prostaglandin concentration.

Other researchers, however, observed that oral contraceptives suppress ovulation, and in the absence of ovulation, uterine production of prostaglandins is diminished. This observation, combined with the knowledge that prostaglandins stimulate uterine contractions, led researchers to conclude that an oversupply of prostaglandins is a likely cause of painful contractions of the uterus.

Although oral contraceptives seem effective in relieving dysmenorrhea, their side effects have prevented many women from using them. As a result, other substances were sought to lessen or inhibit prostaglandin production. Now, through research and careful testing, such products are available. These agents, previously developed for the treatment of arthritis, are similar to aspirin, but many times more potent.

Treatment options

The first step in arriving at treatment for dysmenorrhea is a thorough pelvic examination. This can rule out certain medical conditions other than dysmenorrhea that can cause pelvic pain. At the time of the examination, other health factors and practices can also be discussed with the physician. For example, for some women reducing the amount of salt, caffeine and sugar in the diet, especially in the week before a period is due, often provides relief, as does moderate exercise and sufficient rest.

For a few women, menstrual disorders may stem from psychological problems and worries. Treating the psychological problems of these women often alleviates their menstrual problems. For most others who suffer dysmenorrhea, the source of their pain is the uterus, contracting too hard or too fast. Traditionally, analgesics and sedatives have been used to treat menstrual pain, although these drugs may affect a patient's normal activities, such as driving a car or taking an exam in school.

As a result of scientific research, new types of medication are available. For moderate to severe dysmenorrhea, drugs that prevent or lessen the production of prostaglandins in the first hours or day of the menstrual period have proved effective without serious side effects in about 75 percent of the patients. The drugs provide relief from pain by reducing the level of prostaglandins which in turn moderates the uterine contractions. Not all women can tolerate these drugs, however, especially those who have gastrointestinal problems.

Researchers continue to search for other possible causes of dysmenorrhea and to develop modes of treatment for women who are not helped by the present array of medications.

Premenstrual syndrome

While dysmenorrhea is a disorder more frequently reported by women in their teens and early twenties, premenstrual syndrome (PMS) is reported more often by women in their late twenties and thirties. Interestingly, PMS patients who have had hysterectomies (surgical removal of the uterus) may continue to have PMS symptoms. This observation has led researchers to conclude that the uterus appears not to be a significant factor in causing PMS.

Based on reviews of health surveys, it has been estimated that four out of five women surveyed experience varying degrees of premenstrual symptoms. Of these, one out of four suffer temporarily disabling symptoms. Behavioral symptoms range from depression, aggression, irritability and anxiety to mood swings, nervous tension, and food cravings. Physical symptoms include fluid retention, headache, acne, fatigue, and exhaustion.

Most women can cope with the mild form of PMS, but for others with moderate or severe PMS, the physical discomfort can be stressful. Because of fluid retention, a woman may feel bloated, with swelling in her ankles, abdomen and breasts. The enlargement of her breast can cause tenderness and discomfort. She may feel emotionally unstable and behave in seemingly odd and erratic ways.

As with dysmenorrhea, the traditional approach viewed premenstrual distress as "just part of being a woman." Until recently, the distress had been written off as something a woman could control if she would put her mind to it. The association of the various symptoms with menstruation was difficult to recognize because symptoms occur before a woman's period begins. The very nature of the syndrome often made objective reporting difficult. Only recently have the medical and scientific communities become sensitive to the possibility of physiological causes of the various symptoms.

When the symptoms were finally related to the *pre*-menstrual period, hormonal imbalance was suggested as a possible cause of the disorder. Other theories advanced included those linking PMS to nutritional or chemical deficiencies in a woman's body chemistry.

With the advent of oral contraceptives (usually a combination of estrogen and progestin, a synthetic progesterone), reports appeared that women on oral contraceptives experienced less premenstrual depression than nonusers. This observation led some investigators to theorize that progesterone deficiency in the last phase of the menstrual cycle might be involved in PMS.

Although hormone levels in a woman can be ascertained at a particular moment in time, these levels vary throughout the month and from woman to woman. Scientists do not fully understand what amount of progesterone is normal or adequate.

Nevertheless, for a number of years a few physicians in England have been prescribing progesterone to PMS sufferers, specifying only natural progesterone, a scarce, expensive drug that is difficult to administer. One has reported marked improvement in up to 95 percent of his PMS patients using progesterone therapy. Side effects of taking progesterone are rare, but headache, exhaustion, feelings of lightheadedness and uterine bleeding may be experienced.

Research findings

Although success with progesterone treatment has been reported, carefully controlled studies have failed to substantiate either the claim that progesterone deficiency is the cause of PMS or that progesterone therapy is beneficial. Currently, the U.S. Food and Drug Administration considers that progesterone treatment of PMS is not indicated.

A variety of other theories about the causes of PMS and methods of treatment for the disorder have been offered. Nutritional deficiencies, such as the lack of vitamin B_6, have been reported among women with PMS. As with progesterone therapy, replacement of the lacking nutrient has relieved PMS symptoms in some women although it is not certain that this is other than a placebo effect.

Most research projects are concerned with understanding the basic mechanisms of menstrual cycle activities. There are a few experimental treatment programs for PMS, usually associated with university medical schools or colleges. Limited success has been reported, such as in a research project using bromocriptine (a drug that suppresses lactation after childbirth) to treat PMS. In this study breast engorgement and tenderness were significantly reduced for some women, but other symptoms were not relieved.

The causes of premenstrual syndrome remain elusive. The subjective nature of the disorder contributes to the problem, as does the wide range of reactions to hormone activities that women can have. Some women react to the smallest shifts in body chemistry or functions, while others do not.

Researchers agree that this and other problems in studying PMS need clarification and further study. For example, one problem that both researchers and clinicians wish to clarify is the method of diagnosing PMS. Usually, when a patient tells a physician about symptoms of a medical problem, the physician can confirm the diagnosis with blood or urine analyses, X-rays, or with some other technology. But for PMS, no such tests are yet available. Scientists are looking for a way to assess the severity of occurrence of PMS. One recent project found lower levels of magnesium in the blood of women with PMS than in normal women. This observation may be useful in the future as a marker in diagnosing PMS. A federally funded study at the National Institutes of Health in Bethesda, Maryland, is attempting to document the relationship between the menstrual cycle and mood and behavior disorders.

A comprehensive study of the complex interrelationships of hypothalamic, pituitary, and ovarian function is currently supported by the NICHD. A new theory has emerged from this study indicating certain messenger chemicals from the pituitary (neuropeptides) as the possible source of mood and behavior symptoms reported in PMS. By blocking action of the neuropeptides with other chemicals, researchers hope to control the symptoms. To date, there has been wide variation in reaction to neuropeptide activity among the subjects in the study.

Scientists are just beginning to learn about neuropeptides and the effects the blocking agents may have. This research is expected to continue for the next several years as investigators search for a better understanding of hormones, neuropeptides, and the basic workings of the normal menstrual cycle. The nature of the research means, however, that studies often take months and sometimes years to collect data, perform analyses and reach conclusions.

Treatment options

Treatment for this disorder presents a challenge because of the many variables involved. To rule out any other medical or psychological problems that may be causing symptoms, a thorough physical examination by a gynecologist is the first step. Following this, a physician may treat the symptoms, recommending diuretics, special diets or medication. Some women may be referred to a university medical school department of gynecology or possibly to a PMS research program.

For help with the severe psychological aspects of PMS, physicians may recommend that women join behavior modification programs or support groups. Support groups can be valuable therapy for a PMS patient, particularly while attempting behavior modification such as changing diet or other health habits. Meeting other women who share the disorder and having access to current PMS information are important benefits of support groups.

Keeping informed

Professional, scientific and voluntary organizations interested in women's health can provide information on new developments in menstrual cycle research and in the diagnosis, treatment, and possible prevention of dysmenorrhea and premenstrual syndrome.

Another way to keep informed is by reading research reports published in scientific journals. Although generally very technical, the reports offer the reader an opportunity to learn first-hand what is new in scientific research. The journals can be found at medical school libraries or other medical libraries. The facilities of the National Library of Medicine are available for obtaining specific references and articles.

Some sources of information on dysmenorrhea and PMS are:

American College of Obstetricians and Gynecologists
600 Maryland Avenue, S.W.
Washington, D.C. 20024
Telephone: 202/638-5577

The Premenstrual Syndrome Program
40 Salem Street
Lynnfield, MA 01940
Telephone: 617/245-9585

Premenstrual Syndrome Action, Inc.
P.O. Box 19669
Irvine, CA 92713
Telephone: 714/752-6355

National Women's Health Network
224 Seventh Street, S.E.
Washington, D.C. 20003
Telephone: 202/543-9222

For more information about the studies reported in this pamphlet, contact Dr. David R. Rubinow, Chief, Unit of Peptide Studies, Biological Psychiatry Branch, National Institute of Mental Health, National Institutes of Health, Bldg. 10, 9000 Rockville Pike, Bethesda, MD 20205. "Facts About Dysmenorrhea and Premenstrual Syndrome" was written by Joan Z. Muller, Office of Research Reporting, National Institute of Child Health and Human Development (NICHD), and is reprinted from the August 1983 issue of *Ladycom* Magazine with permission of the publisher, Downey Communications, Inc., Washington, D.C. U.S. Government Printing Office 1985—461–338—814/25320.

Emphysema
Chronic Obstructive Pulmonary Disease

What are emphysema and chronic bronchitis?

Emphysema and chronic bronchitis make up the disease category called chronic obstructive pulmonary disease. At one time they were viewed as distinct clinical conditions, but it is now clear that in most patients these diseases coexist, although one or the other may predominate. These are chronic disorders and are characterized by progressive limitation of the flow of air into and out of the lungs. *Emphysema* is identified by its characteristic alteration of lung architecture. A person with emphysema has destruction of the walls of the smallest air passages, called *bronchioles*, and the walls of small air sacs, called *alveoli*, that function as the gas exchanging units of the lung. These alterations result in abnormally enlarged airspaces. *Chronic bronchitis* is characterized by excessive mucus secretion in the bronchial tree which leads to a persistent, productive cough. An individual is considered to have chronic bronchitis if cough

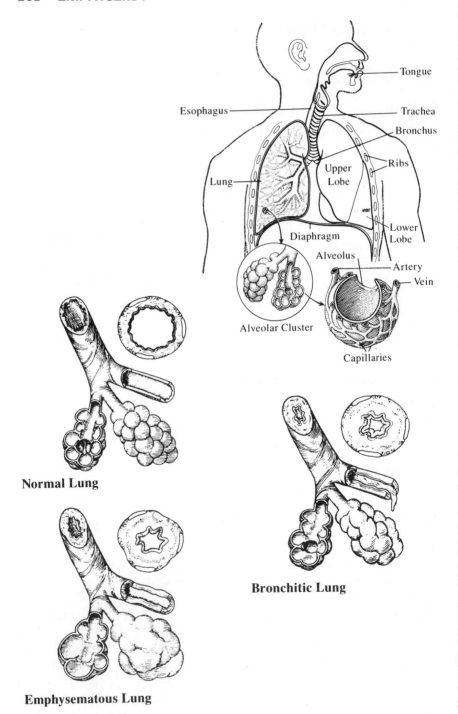

Tongue

Esophagus

Trachea

Bronchus

Ribs

Upper
Lobe

Lung

Lower
Lobe

Diaphragm

Alveolus

Artery

Vein

Alveolar Cluster

Capillaries

Normal Lung

Bronchitic Lung

Emphysematous Lung

and sputum are present on most days for a minimum of three months for at least two successive years, or for six months during one year.

In emphysema, the limitation of airflow is caused by abnormalities of lung *elastin,* an important structural material in the smallest air passages and the walls of the alveoli. The abnormalities in elastin result in collapse or narrowing of the small airways which in turn limits airflow out of the lung. Once this damage occurs, it is irreversible. In chronic bronchitis, on the other hand, airway obstruction is due to inflammatory changes in the walls of the bronchi which causes them to thicken. This thickening, together with excessive mucus production obliterates some of the smaller air passages and narrows larger ones. These changes are to some degree reversible.

How does chronic obstructive pulmonary disease affect the ability of the lungs to do their job?

The most important job that the lungs perform is to provide the body with oxygen and to remove carbon dioxide. This is called *gas exchange* and the normal anatomy of the lungs serves this purpose well. The lungs contain 300 million alveoli whose ultra-thin walls form the gas exchange surface. Enmeshed in the wall of each of these air sacs is a fine capillary network which brings blood to the gas exchange surface. When a person inhales, air flows from the nose and mouth through large and small airways and into the alveoli. Oxygen from this air then passes through the thin walls of the inflated alveoli and is taken up by the red blood cells for delivery to the rest of the body. Moving in the opposite direction, carbon dioxide leaves the blood and passes through the alveolar walls into the alveoli. During exhalation, the elastic properties of the lung push the used air out of the alveoli and through the air passages until it escapes from the nose or mouth.

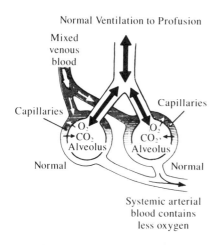

Normal Ventilation to Profusion

Mixed venous blood

Capillaries

Capillaries

O_2
CO_2
Alveolus

O_2
CO_2
Alveolus

Normal

Normal

Systemic arterial blood contains less oxygen

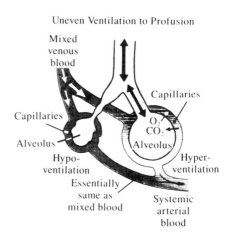

Uneven Ventilation to Profusion

Mixed venous blood

Capillaries

Capillaries

Alveolus

O_2
CO_2
Alveolus

Hypo-ventilation

Hyper-ventilation

Essentially same as mixed blood

Systemic arterial blood

With the development of COPD, the walls of the small airways and alveoli lose their elasticity. The walls of the small airways also become thickened and the passageways plugged with mucus. Air can get into unblocked alveoli, but may not be able to escape during exhalation because the air passages tend to collapse, trapping the "stale" air in the lungs. Overinflation of the already damaged alveoli may cause the walls to tear, leading to the formation of large air spaces called cavities or *bullae* which are filled with stagnant air. These abnormalities create two serious problems which affect gas exchange:

1) Blood flow and airflow to the alveolar walls where gas exchange takes place are uneven or mismatched. Some alveoli get plenty of blood but little air, while others get a good supply of fresh air but not enough blood. Under these conditions, fresh air cannot reach areas where there is good blood flow and oxygen cannot enter the bloodstream in normal quantities.

2) The work of pushing air through narrowed obstructed airways becomes more and more difficult. This tires the respiratory muscles and they may not be able to maintain an adequate airflow to the alveoli. The critical step for removal of carbon dioxide from the blood is adequate alveolar airflow. If airflow to the alveoli is insufficient, carbon dioxide builds up in the blood; blood oxygen also diminishes. An inadequate supply of fresh air to the alveoli is called *hypoventilation*. Breathing oxygen can often correct the blood oxygen levels but this does nothing to help in the removal of carbon dioxide. When carbon dioxide accumulation becomes a severe problem, mechanical breathing machines called respirators or ventilators must be used.

How does emphysema develop?

Twenty years of lung research has resulted in a much better understanding of the mechanisms of lung damage which cause emphysema. As mentioned previously, the symptoms of emphysema result primarily from destruction of elastin, a major structural protein of the lung. Essentially, the altered lung structure results from an imbalance between a lung protease called elastase, which breaks down elastin, and alpha-1-protease inhibitor (also called alpha-1-antitrypsin), the substance which inhibits elastase. Elastase is among the most important of the proteases produced by white blood cells, known as neutrophils.

In the normal individual, the relative amounts of protease and antiprotease are such that an abnormal amount of elastin destruction does not occur. The antiproteases can be thought of as forming a protective screen for the lung.

However, in some individuals there is a genetic defect which results in decreased levels of alpha-1-protease inhibitor. This upsets the balance between the protease and its inhibitor in favor of the protease. Most of the individuals with a severe deficiency of the inhibitor develop emphysema, sometimes quite early in life. It is important to understand that emphysema caused by a genetic deficiency of the antiprotease is very rare.

While emphysema is the result of a relative excess of protease, in the large majority of cases this imbalance is due to cigarette smoking. Research results indicate that the inhalation of the tobacco smoke stimulates excess release of protease from cells normally found in the lung. The inhaled smoke also stimulates more of these cells to migrate to the lung, which in turn causes the release of even more protease. To make matters worse, oxidants found in cigarette smoke inactivate a significant portion of the protease inhibitors that are present, thereby decreasing the amount of active antiprotease available.

While this process occurs to some degree in most smokers, it is still not known why only some of these smokers progress to the more serious and disabling forms of emphysema which eventually lead to death.

How serious a national health problem is chronic obstructive pulmonary disease?

More than 10 million Americans are thought to have chronic obstructive pulmonary disease. Since 1968, COPD has been the fastest rising major cause of death in the United States. In 1983, there were more than 62,900 deaths due to COPD, approximately 17.6 per 100,000 people. Although COPD is still much more common in men than women, the greatest increase in death rate was for white females, an increase which reflects the increased number of women who smoke cigarettes.

COPD attacks people at the height of their productive years, disabling them with unremitting shortness of breath. It destroys their ability to earn a living, causes frequent use of the health care system, and disrupts the lives of the victims' family members for one or two decades before death occurs.

In 1981, COPD was the cause of approximately 9.7 million office visits and 2.5 million hospital days. The economic costs of this disease are enormous, running into the billions of dollars annually.

What are the signs and symptoms of chronic obstructive pulmonary disease?

Early symptoms include mild shortness of breath and a slight morning cough. The sputum is usually clear. During acute respiratory tract infections such as "colds," shortness of breath and coughing may be much more noticeable and the sputum frequently turns a yellow or greenish color. Episodes of wheezing are likely to occur especially during or after colds or other respiratory tract infections.

Later, shortness of breath becomes more pronounced with severe episodes of breathlessness (dyspnea) occurring after only modest exertion. Minor respiratory tract infections may now become incapacitating and recovery may be protracted. Many patients sleep in a semisitting position because breathlessness prevents them from lying down. They often complain of awakening at night feeling "choked-up" and needing to sit up to cough.

Chronic obstructive pulmonary disease places a large burden on the heart, especially the chambers on the right side which are responsible for pumping blood into the lungs. As COPD progresses, the amount of oxygen in the blood decreases (see page 2) which causes important blood vessels in the lung to constrict. Also, many small blood vessels in the lung may be damaged or even destroyed as a result of the disease process. High pressures must now be produced by the right side of the heart to force blood through the remaining narrowed vessels. To perform this task, the right chambers of the heart enlarge and thicken. Under these circumstances the normal rhythm of the heart may be disturbed by abnormal beats. This condition, in which the heart is enlarged because of lung problems, is called *cor pulmonale.* Patients with cor pulmonale complain of easy fatigability, chest pains, and palpitations. If an additional strain is placed on the lungs and heart such as a "cold" the heart may fall behind in its pumping, resulting in swelling of the liver, legs, and ankles.

Another adjustment the body makes to inadequate blood oxygen is called *secondary polycythemia,* an increased production of oxygen-carrying red blood cells. The larger than normal number of red blood cells is helpful up to a point; however, a large overpopulation of red cells thickens the blood so much that it clogs small blood vessels causing a new set of problems. People who have polycythemia and a poor supply of oxygen usually have a bluish tinge to their skin, lips, and nailbeds, a condition called *cyanosis.*

Too little oxygen and too much carbon dioxide in the blood also affects the nervous system, especially the brain, and can cause a variety of unpleasant symptoms including headache, insomnia, impaired mental acuity, and irascibility.

How is chronic obstructive pulmonary disease detected?

Currently, there are a number of techniques for detecting chronic obstructive pulmonary disease. None of the tests detects the disease prior to the development of irreversible lung damage. While many measures of lung function have been developed, those most commonly used determine: 1) lung volumes, 2) the ability to move air into and out of the lung, 3) the rate at which gases diffuse between the lung and blood, and 4) blood levels of oxygen and carbon dioxide.

Lung volumes are measured by breathing into and out of a device called a spirometer. Some types of spirometers are very simple mechanical devices which record volume changes as air is added to or removed from them. Other kinds are more sophisticated and use various types of electronic equipment to determine and record the volume of air moved into and out of the lungs. There are many different volumes or capacities which are measured in the lung. The three volume measures most relevant to chronic obstructive pulmonary disease are vital capacity (VC), residual volume (RV), and total lung capacity (TLC). The *vital capacity* is the maximum volume of air which can be forcibly expelled after inhaling as deeply as possible. Not all of the air in the lungs can be removed when measuring the vital capacity. The amount remaining is called the *residual volume*. The *total lung capacity* is the combination of the vital capacity and residual volume. While most of the measured lung volumes or capacities change to some degree with chronic obstructive pulmonary disease, residual volume usually increases quite markedly. This increase is the result of the weakened airways collapsing before all the air normally expired can leave the lungs. The increased residual volume makes breathing even more difficult and labored.

Because chronic obstructive pulmonary disease results in narrowed air passages, a measure of the rate at which air can be expelled from the lungs can also be used to determine how severe the narrowing has become. In this test, the patient is asked to inhale maximally, and on signal, exhale as completely, and as rapidly as possible. This is called the *forced vital capacity* maneuver. The volume of gas exhaled within 1 second is then measured. This value is referred to as the *forced expiratory volume in 1 second* (FEV_1). This volume may also be expressed in terms of the percent of the vital capacity which can be expelled in 1 second. As chronic obstructive pulmonary disease progresses, less air can be expelled in 1 second.

Another measure of lung function is called *diffusing capacity*. This is a more complicated test which measures the amount of gas which can move in a given period of time from the alveolar side of the lung into the blood. There are a number of conditions which can cause the diffusing capacity to decrease. However, in chronic obstructive pulmonary disease, the decrease is the result of a destruction of alveolar walls, which leads to a significant decrease in surface area for diffusion of oxygen into the blood.

Because the primary function of the lung is to remove carbon dioxide from the blood and add oxygen, another indicator of pulmonary function is the measurement of blood levels of oxygen and carbon dioxide. As chronic obstructive pulmonary disease progresses, the amount of oxygen in the blood drops and carbon dioxide increases.

The above measures of pulmonary function are those most commonly used. No unanimous agreement exists, however, as to the single, best measure of lung function. In most cases, the results of several different tests are compared in order to make the best diagnosis. It is hoped that current research will result in more accurate and earlier measures of lung destruction and diminished function.

What is the course of chronic obstructive pulmonary disease?

A typical course of COPD might proceed as follows. For a period of about 10 years after cigarette smoking begins, symptoms are usually not prominent. After this, the patient generally starts developing a chronic cough with the production of a small amount of sputum. It is unusual to develop shortness of breath during exertion below the age of 40, after which it becomes more common and may be well developed by the age of 50. However, not all cigarette smokers develop a notable cough and sputum production, or shortness of breath. Researchers have been investigating the effectiveness of using a recently developed method, the Tecumseh Index of Risk, to provide an individualized assessment of a person's chances of developing airway obstruction.

Most patients with COPD have some degree of reversible airways obstruction, at least at the time they are first seen by a physician. It is therefore likely that initially, treatment will lead to some improvement or stability in lung function. Following this period, almost all signs and symptoms except cough and sputum production tend to show a gradual worsening. This trend can show fluctuations, but over the course of four or five years, a slow deterioration becomes evident. When FEV_1 is used as an indicator of lung function, the average rate of decline in patients with COPD is observed to be two to three times the normal rate of 20 to 30 milliliters per year.

Survival of patients with COPD is closely related to their initial level of lung function impairment and the rate at which it continues to decline. If the FEV_1 is approximately one-third that expected for an individual, then about two of every three patients under 65 years of age will probably survive 5 years or more. Approximately one-half of those surviving at 5 years will survive an additional 5 years.

How is chronic obstructive pulmonary disease treated?

There is no known cure for COPD, but in almost all cases the disease can be prevented. Numerous studies have shown that cigarette smoking is the most important risk factor; not smoking almost always prevents COPD from developing and cessation of smoking slows the disease process. Pulmonary function studies of large groups of people indicate that the ability to move air into and out of the lungs declines slowly with age in healthy nonsmokers, but in smokers, deterioration of lung function tends to be much more rapid. This is extremely important because the amount of air which a COPD patient can forcibly expel from his/her lungs in 1 second, the FEV_1, is a fairly good predictor of disability and early death. If a smoker without serious COPD stops smoking, the rate at which lung function deteriorates returns to normal. Unfortunately, pulmonary function is unlikely to return all the way to normal because some lung damage is irreversible.

However, if the patient and medical team develop and adhere to a program of complete respiratory care, disability can be minimized, acute episodes prevented, hospitalizations reduced, and some early deaths avoided. On the other hand, no treatment has been shown to slow the progression of the disease, and only oxygen therapy has been shown to increase the survival rate.

In most instances of chronic obstructive pulmonary disease, some irreversible damage has already occurred by the time it is diagnosed. At this point, every effort should be made by the physician and others providing medical care to educate the patient and the patient's family about the disease and how to live with it. The goals, limitations, and techniques of treatment must be understood by the patient so that symptoms can be kept under control and daily life proceed as normally as possible. Patients and family members can usually participate in an educational program through a local hospital or branch of the American Lung Association. Patients are generally advised to do the following:

- Stop smoking. Many programs are available to help smokers quit smoking and to stay off tobacco. Some programs are based on behavior modification techniques, others combine these methods with nicotine gum as an aid to help smokers gradually overcome their dependence on nicotine.
- Avoid occupational exposures to dusts and fumes.
- Avoid air pollution including smoke filled rooms, and curtail physical activities during air pollution alerts.
- Avoid respiratory infections:
  1. Refrain from intimate contact with people who have "colds," "flu," etc.
  2. Discuss with your physician the advisability of getting influenza and polyvalent pneumococcal vaccinations.
- Avoid excessive heat, cold, or very high altitude. (Note: Some commercial aircraft cruise at high altitude and maintain a cabin pressure equiva-

lent to that of an elevation of 5,000 to 8,000 feet (which can cause discomfort to some COPD patients).

- Stay well-hydrated by drinking a lot of water. This is a good way to keep phlegm (sputum) loose so that it can be brought up by coughing.
- Maintain good nutrition. Usually a high protein diet, taken as many small feedings, is recommended.
- Avoid gas producing foods. A dietitian may be helpful in planning an appropriate diet.
- If allergies or asthma complicate COPD, then "allergy shots" may be recommended.
- Medications frequently prescribed for COPD patients include:
  1. *Bronchodilators,* of which there are two main categories: *sympathomimetics* (isoproterenol, metaproterenol, terbutaline, albuterol, Proventil®, Ventolin®, etc.) which can be injected subcutaneously or intravenously, taken orally (tablets, capsules, and syrups), or inhaled as aerosol sprays; and *methylxanthines* (theophylline and its derivatives) which can be given intravenously, orally, or rectally.
  2. *Antibiotics* are frequently given at the first sign of a respiratory infection such as increased cough, sputum production, or change in color of sputum from clear to yellow or green. Tetracycline, ampicillin, erythromycin, and trimethoprim-sulfamethoxazol combinations, Bactrim®, and Septra®, are commonly used.
  3. *Corticosteroids* (steroids) are sometimes used in selected cases if wheezing cannot be kept under control with bronchodilators.
  4. *Expectorants* are sometimes used. Water is the best one, others (glycerylguaiacolate or a saturated solution of potassium iodide) are of questionable value.
  5. *Diuretics* are frequently given to prevent water retention. Patients should be followed carefully because a well-hydrated state is desirable, and the goal of this treatment is only to avoid excess water retention. Also, these drugs often cause potassium imbalances which may lead to abnormal heart rhythms.
  6. *Digitalis* (usually in the form of digoxin) is used to treat left-sided heart failure. It should be used very cautiously in patients who also have COPD, especially if their blood oxygen tensions are low, because they are extremely vulnerable to abnormal heart rhythms when taking this drug.
  7. *Other drugs* sometimes taken by patients with COPD are tranquilizers, pain killers (Demerol®, morphine, Darvon®, etc.), cough suppressants (codeine), and sleeping pills (barbiturates). All these drugs depress breathing to some extent; they should be avoided whenever possible and used only with great caution.

Approximately two dozen combination drugs containing various assortments of sympathomimetics, methylxanthines, expectorants, and sedatives are marketed and widely advertised. These drugs are undesirable for several reasons. It is difficult to adjust the dose of methylxanthines without getting interfering side effects from the other ingredients. The sympathomimetic drug used in these preparations is ephedrine, a drug with many side effects and less bronchodilating effect than other drugs now available. The combination drugs often contain sedatives to combat the unpleasant side effects of ephedrine. They also contain expectorants which have not been proven to be effective and may increase the side effects. The task of keeping air passages reasonably clear of secretions is a formidable one for patients with advanced COPD. Some commonly used methods for mobilizing and removing secretions are:

1. *Bland aerosols,* often made from solutions of salt or bicarbonate of soda are inhaled with or without the aid of a device called an *IPPB machine* (see page 273) that pushes air into the lungs. These aerosols are used to thin and loosen secretions. Treatments usually last 10 to 15 minutes and are taken three or four times a day. Bronchodilators (see page 270) are sometimes added to the aerosols.
2. *Chest percussion* or lightly clapping the chest and back is used to help dislodge secretions.
3. *Postural bronchial drainage* is another method for getting secretions out of airways. The patient lies in prescribed positions which allow gravity to drain different parts of the lung. This is usually done after inhaling an aerosol. The basic position is one in which the patient lies on a bed with his chest and head over the side and his forearms resting on the floor.
4. *Controlled coughing* techniques are taught to help bring up secretions.

Training programs fall into three main categories, general physical fitness exercises, breathing exercises, and breathing techniques, such as pursed lips breathing and relaxation. The goals are to improve overall physical endurance, strengthen and increase the endurance of the respiratory muscles, slow the respiratory rate, improve the coordination of the breathing effort, and decrease air trapping and the work of breathing.

Home oxygen therapy deserves special comment because it can improve survival in patients with advanced COPD who have *hypoxemia,* low blood oxygen levels. This treatment can improve a patient's exercise tolerance and ability to perform on psychological tests which reflect different aspects of brain function and muscle coordination. Oxygen can also lessen sleeplessness, irritability, headaches, and the overproduction of red blood cells. Continuous oxygen therapy is recommended for patients with severe hypoxemia. Many oxygen sources are available for home use; these include tanks of compressed gaseous oxygen or liquid oxygen and devices that concentrate oxygen from room air. However, oxygen is expensive with a cost per patient of approximately $200 to $350 per month, depending on the type of system and on the locale.

What research on chronic obstructive pulmonary disease is being supported by the National Heart, Lung, and Blood Institute?

The National Heart, Lung, and Blood Institute is supporting a number of research programs on COPD with the following objectives: 1) to understand the underlying causes; 2) to develop methods of early detection; and 3) to improve treatment. As was mentioned earlier, most scientists believe that emphysema is caused by an imbalance between proteases and antiproteases. This belief was initially based on research which had shown that when extra protease was placed in the lungs of experimental animals, they developed a "disease" which closely resembled emphysema. Recent work has demonstrated that many people with emphysema have more protease in their lungs than healthy people. Since cigarette smoking causes an increased number of neutrophils to enter the lung and release proteases, many scientists believe this is one reason why smoking increases the risk of developing emphysema. It has also been determined that chemicals called oxidants can cause a change in the antiprotease which prevents it from rendering the protease harmless. When cigarettes are smoked, oxidants present in the smoke are inhaled in large amounts into the lungs and produce this effect. Thus, not only does smoking tobacco increase the amount of protease in the lung, it also decreases the amount of useful antiprotease!

Currently, the only way to detect emphysema is to conduct different types of relatively expensive and time-consuming tests which measure lung function. Unfortunately, these tests are not very sensitive and cannot detect emphysema until irreversible damage has already occurred. However, recent advances from research on the basic changes produced by emphysema, may ultimately lead to a method to detect lung damage by measuring fragments of the lung protein, elastin, in the urine or blood. An increase in these fragments is believed to be one of the earliest signs of the onset of the disease. Although still in its most experimental stage, this may lead to a relatively simple, fast, and inexpensive method to detect early lung damage.

The Institute continues to support clinical studies to look at different ways of improving the patient's condition. A recently initiated study called the "Chronic Obstructive Pulmonary Disease Prevention Trial" is designed to enroll and follow approximately 6,500 smokers to find out more about the effects of quitting smoking and treatment with a bronchodilator drug (to keep air passages open) on pulmonary function. The results of this study should help to determine the extent to which identification and treatment of asymptomatic subjects with early obstructive lung disease would be useful as a preventive health measure.

A study completed several years ago examined the use of oxygen therapy for people who, because of chronic obstructive pulmonary disease, cannot get enough oxygen into their blood by breathing air. This study has determined that continuous oxygen therapy is more beneficial in extending life than giving oxygen for 12 hours at night.

Another clinical study compared inhalation therapy using a machine which administers medication to the lungs by intermittent positive pressure breathing (IPPB) with one that also delivers the medicine, but relies on the patient's own breathing. Although home use of IPPB machines was widespread, previous studies had not been able to show conclusively whether they were effective. In this study, 985 ambulatory patients with COPD were randomly assigned to a treatment group which received a bronchodilator aerosol solution by IPPB, or to a control group which received the medication via a compressor nebulizer. The only difference between the two groups was the positive pressure applied by the IPPB. There was no statistically significant difference between the two treatment groups in numbers of deaths, frequency and length of hospitalization, change in lung function tests, or in measurements of quality of life.

Methods to treat emphysema before it becomes disabling remain an important research objective. Since it is believed that either having excess protease, or too little useful antiprotease, can lead to development of disease, scientists have been using experimental animal models to see if natural or synthetic antiproteases can be used to prevent development of emphysema-like lesions in these animals. Preliminary results appear promising. Investigators are now attempting to develop a more sophisticated type of animal model which will mimic the human condition of inherited alpha-1-protease inhibitor deficiency. Further animal research needs to be done on the safety and effectiveness of these agents before they can be used to treat humans.

What are the risk factors for chronic obstructive pulmonary disease and how can I protect myself?

Scientists have identified several factors which increase the risk of developing COPD. If all of these factors are combined, it appears that a late middle-age male who is a heavy smoker, in a relatively low socio-economic setting, and has close relatives with COPD, is at high risk for developing emphysema. In addition, if this person has a history of wheezing, the chances of developing progressive airways disease are even greater.

People with a severe genetic deficiency of alpha-1-protease inhibitor run the greatest risk of developing emphysema. If these individuals smoke, they usually become symptomatic by the time they reach early middle age. Deficiency of alpha-1-protease inhibitor is a rare finding that can be detected by blood tests available through hospital laboratories. People from families in which other members have developed emphysema in their thirties and forties should be tested. If a deficiency is found, then it is of the utmost importance for these people not to smoke.

Of all the risk factors, smoking is by far the most significant. If you smoke, quit! It is the best way to decrease your risk of developing chronic obstructive pulmonary disease.

Prepared by Division of Lung Diseases, National Heart, Lung, and Blood Institute. U.S. Department of Health and Human Services, Public Health Service, National Institutes of Health. NIH Publication No. 86–2020, revised September 1986. U.S. Government Printing Office 1986—491-292:41186

Epilepsy
Removing the Dread

People suffering from epilepsy have been freed from much of the fear and stigma experienced by earlier victims, thanks to anti-convulsant drugs now available. There still is no cure for this nervous system disorder, which is characterized by a variety of symptoms including muscle spasms, mental confusion and loss of consciousness. However, an array of anti-convulsant drugs is available, and proper use of the appropriate medication can help make possible an active and fulfilling life for most with only a small chance of suffering an epileptic seizure.

Therapy for epilepsy is intended to prevent seizures in which brain cells, or neurons, create abnormal electrical discharges that cause temporary loss of certain body functions. These seizures can range from mild to severe and usually last only a short time. Epilepsy is not contagious, is not a mental illness, and is not indicative of a low intelligence level.

Anti-convulsant or anti-epileptic drugs are chemicals that may be prescribed singly or with other drugs. Some people who have epilepsy are subject to more than one kind of seizure, and treatment may require more than one anti-convulsant drug. When possible, physicians try to find a single drug that is effective and whose benefits can be balanced against possible side effects or other adverse reactions.

It is estimated that 2.1 million Americans suffer from epilepsy. The three main types of seizures are classified by the Epilepsy Foundation of America as generalized tonic-clonic (or grand mal), generalized non-convulsive (also known as petit mal or absence), and partial. Tonic-clonic is the most dramatic form of epilepsy. As nerve cells discharge throughout the brain the entire body stiffens and shakes, the arms and legs jerk violently, and the victim falls, loses consciousness, becomes rigid and begins breathing irregularly.

Tonic-clonic attacks last one to several minutes. A period of rigidity in the tonic phase is followed by the clonic aspect in which the major muscles alternately contract and relax. As the seizure subsides, a period of deep relaxation follows. Non-convulsive attacks last only a few seconds and consist of blank spells in which the victim loses awareness, twitches slightly, stares and blinks. Unlike tonic-clonic attacks, which are rarely continuous, generalized non-convulsive attacks may occur dozens or even hundreds of times a day and may even be mistaken for daydreaming or inattentiveness. Partial epilepsy results when nerve cells discharge in a part of the brain, causing a period of mental confusion followed by pointless movements such as pacing and hand rubbing, pain, dizziness and irritability. These seizures can last up to 20 minutes.

There are many less common types, including one in which abnormal electrical activity in a given area of the brain causes spasms in a specific part of the body while the ill person remains conscious. Another less common type causes infantile convulsions in which babies lose consciousness or muscle control for a short while.

Scientists still do not know why neurons build up and discharge in the brain, but epilepsy has been related to birth defects, prenatal damage or injury at birth to the central nervous system, head injuries, poisons, diseases such as measles, circulatory disorders, brain tumors, and poor nutrition. In some cases, it is impossible to identify the cause. Those that can be traced to a specific cause are classified as symptomatic; those that cannot are called idiopathic.

Researchers really don't know exactly how medication helps sufferers, but the drugs may work in one or more ways. Some may interrupt the spread of excess energy in the brain while others may increase the amount of a natural seizure inhibitor which turns brain cells on and off like a light bulb. Up to now, therapy has been largely based on experience, but researchers are trying to find better scientific answers that could lead to even more effective treatment.

The physician's skill is especially important in prescribing drugs for the treatment of epilepsy because patients react individually. The right dose needed to gain control of the disease may be determined quickly for some; in others, considerably more experience is necessary before a seizure-preventing level of the drug is reached in the patient's blood. In addition, individuals suffer different side effects from anti-convulsants.

With the development of a technique called anti-epileptic drug level testing, physicians can tell sooner what happens when medication enters a patient's body. This monitoring is carried out by analysis of a blood sample to find the amount of the medication present in the bloodstream, the route by which anti-convulsants reach the areas of the brain where the seizures begin. Levels too low can result in inadequate seizure protection. Levels too high can cause undesirable side effects, including drowsiness or confusion.

Generally, side effects are mild and usually occur at the beginning of therapy. Besides drowsiness or confusion, side effects can include irritability, nausea, rash, some thickening of facial features, increased growth of body hair, some physical clumsiness, overgrowth of gum tissue, and hyperactivity in children. Some individuals undergo emotional changes caused by the drug they are taking. Careful monitoring by the physician is required to customize the proper drug and dosage.

Interaction with other drugs, including non-prescription products, must be watched for and patients are urged to tell their physicians about the other medications they are taking.

Drugs used for treating epilepsy include quinacrine, methsuximide, clonazepam, valproic acid, methamphetamine, dextroamphetamine, acetazolamide, phenytoin, metharbital, chlordiazepoxide, mephobarbital, mephenytoin, primidone, paramethadione, ethotoin, phenobarbital, phenacemide, methylphenidate, carbamazepine, clorazepate, trimethadione, diazepam, and ethosuximide.

The Epilepsy Foundation says that anti-convulsant drugs are successful in preventing seizures in the majority of people who take them regularly and as prescribed. According to the foundation, at least 50 percent of all patients with epilepsy gain complete control of their seizures for substantial periods. For many of this group there may be no seizures for years, while for another 30 percent seizures may be as infrequent as once or twice a month or even once or twice a year, the foundation says.

A recent study published in *The New England Journal of Medicine* reported that certain epileptic children who remain free of seizures during four years of treatment probably can stop taking drugs without suffering relapses. These are children who do not fall into four high-risk categories: (1) those who had epilepsy for a long time before treatment was started,

(2) those with mental retardation or physical disability caused by neurological disturbances, (3) patients with certain types of unusual seizures, or (4) those with a combination of seizures.

The study, conducted at Washington University in St. Louis, involved 148 children whose treatment was stopped after four years without a seizure. For up to 23 years afterward, only 41, or 28 percent, suffered relapses, and these were in at least one of the four risk categories.

Any discontinuance of medication must be carefully monitored by the patient's physician, however, because of the danger of non-stop seizures, which could cause brain damage.

Some patients at all ages continue to experience seizures regularly, even when they take medication, because the right chemical combination has not been found to control their epilepsy. Because of this, researchers are still seeking to produce new drugs and find new ways to use them.

Women who have epilepsy and are also pregnant face a vexing choice between risk and benefit. Without medication there is a risk of having a seizure that could lead to a fall. This might damage the developing child more than a possible fetal defect caused by anti-convulsant medication.

There is not enough knowledge for an easy solution to this problem. However, sudden withdrawal of anti-convulsants could cause non-stop, severe seizures that might be injurious to the mother and to the unborn child. The Epilepsy Foundation says that 92 percent of mothers on anti-convulsant medication give birth to normal, healthy babies.

As in other regimens, the patient is a key member of the therapy team. To assist him or her, the Epilepsy Foundation has a publication, *Medication for Epilepsy,* which offers these suggestions for taking medications:

- Don't take less than prescribed. You may have a seizure.
- Don't ever stop your medication abruptly. If you do, you risk a medical emergency in the shape of non-stop seizures that can threaten your life.
- Don't try other people's pills. Even if a friend says he or she has better control with a different medication, check with your doctor instead.
- Don't mix large amounts of alcohol with your medication. This can be a deadly combination. Both anti-convulsants and alcohol act as depressants, and one may intensify the effect of the other.
- Don't drive when starting a new medication until you know how it affects you. You may be able to function perfectly, or it may make you drowsy at first. Find out before you get behind that wheel.
- Don't assume that if you've missed a few doses of your medication you can then make them up safely by taking them all at once. It

doesn't work that way. What you need is a certain amount of medication, taken at regular intervals.

- If you have trouble remembering to take your medication in sequence (this may be necessary if you are taking more than one type of anti-convulsant drug), give your memory some help by counting out each day's supply of pills and storing them in special containers, which you can buy at the drugstore.
- Don't let yourself run out of medication. Set up a schedule for reordering so that it becomes automatic.
- Keep all medication locked up and away from children.

John M. Couric, *FDA Consumer*, Vol. 16, No. 7, September 1982.

Fever

What to Do—and What Not to Do—When the Heat Is On

"Fever" can be a frightening word, particularly when it is part of the name of a disease, as in "yellow fever," "typhoid fever," "scarlet fever," "childbed fever," and so on. Literary descriptions of a heroine languishing with fevered brow or a hero dying of an unknown fever give the word an air of mystery, while "feverish activity" or similar phrases suggest frenzied excitement.

Unless it is very high, a fever is not to be feared. It is not a disease, simply a symptom, a warning sign that something is wrong with the body that needs investigation. A fever may even serve a useful purpose.

Fever usually occurs with a bacterial or viral infection or inflammation. Noninfectious conditions, such as thyroid and adrenal disease, dehydration in infants and the elderly, some skin conditions, stroke, cancer, and even some adverse drug reactions may also cause a fever.

The causes of some fevers, particularly in children, are not so easily pinned down. These "fevers of unknown origin," as they are called, are characterized by a rectal temperature of 101.3 degrees Fahrenheit or higher, measured on at least four occasions over a two-week period. They may often defy diagnosis for as long as a week. About half of these fevers in children are ultimately found to be caused by infections; 20 percent are caused by collagen inflammatory diseases, such as juvenile rheumatoid arthritis; and 10 percent are the result of cancer, primarily leukemia. The remainder are of miscellaneous or truly unknown origins.

That fever is associated with disease has been known and accepted for centuries. However, views on what should be done about it have not been as consistent. Ancient medical savants looked upon fever as something to be encouraged. It was considered the most important of the body's natural defenses against increases of phlegm, one of the four "humors" of ancient physiology. (An overabundance of phlegm was associated with apathy and indolence.) The 17th-century English physician Thomas Sydenham called fever "nature's engine," brought to the field to fight the enemy.

Medical attitudes toward fever changed in the 19th century when the French physiologist Claude Bernard reported that death in experimental animals quickly occurred when the body temperature rose to more than 107 degrees Fahrenheit. From then on, fever was deemed injurious to health and was treated vigorously with antipyretics—fever-reducing drugs—and "heroic measures" such as bleeding.

In modern medicine, the focus is on finding out what is causing the fever and treating that illness, rather than on treating the fever itself. Of course, if the fever results in severe weakness, causes major symptoms such as convulsions or dehydration, or is affecting the central nervous system, the doctor will take steps to reduce it, whether or not the cause has been discovered.

There are some very good reasons for not treating a fever. For one, there is some evidence that a fever may play a role in stimulating the body's natural defenses. The ups and downs of a fever also help in diagnosing an illness and following its course. And fever is often the only way to determine whether a particular treatment is working. If a patient is on an antibiotic, for instance, a persistent fever would indicate that the drug is probably not effective and that an alternative should be used.

A number of recent studies involving parents of young children have shown that the old fears about the dangers of fever still persist. Several researchers have dubbed this parental concern "fever phobia."

In general, the studies revealed that parents worry a lot about fever and its possible harmful effects. They do not understand what constitutes a "high fever," they fear that if the fever isn't treated it will continue to rise to dangerous levels, and they believe that even moderately high temperatures could cause permanent harm, such as "brain damage."

Many of the parents interviewed in these studies thought that temperatures as low as 100 degrees Fahrenheit were serious and said they would start giving their children medication as soon as the fever thermometer reached that point.

Some parents tend to check their children's temperatures frequently—

from five to eight times a day, sometimes even hourly. Quite a number of parents worry so much about fever that they wake the child to give additional medication to lower the temperature. Such aggressive treatment of childhood fevers isn't always necessary, according to pediatricians.

Fever is one of the most common reasons parents bring their children to see a doctor. About 90 percent of these fevers are minor and self-limiting, caused by some common infectious agent such as an influenza virus. Truly high fevers—105 F or higher—are rare and may be the result of a serious infection or other condition that has upset the body's temperature regulation.

Unless the fever is very high, the temperature of a feverish child who feels reasonably well otherwise (which is often the case) doesn't have to be reduced, experts say.

There are exceptions, of course. Persistent fevers over 103 F and fevers in infants and very young children and in those who have a history of convulsions require prompt medical attention.

Even though professional health care isn't needed for all feverish children, tender, loving care is still in order. There are a number of measures parents can take to make the young patient more comfortable.

- Help the body maintain its own temperature regulation. Many well-meaning parents bundle up a sick child, thus preventing natural heat loss. The sick room should be kept at a moderate temperature and the bed coverings kept to a minimum.
- Sponging with lukewarm water can also make the patient more comfortable. This increases heat loss by evaporation. Iced water, alcohol in water, or cold water enemas should *not* be used. Cooling mattresses are frequently used in hospitals to help reduce fever.
- Be sure that the child gets plenty of fluids.
- If treatment with antipyretic drugs is recommended, among the most effective are aspirin and acetaminophen (known by several trade names, such as Tylenol, Datril, and Panadol, and also sold generically).

Both drugs work equally well in reducing fever, but each has other advantages of its own. Acetaminophen is available in liquid form—a plus if a small child is being treated—but it is not effective in reducing inflammation. Aspirin does fight inflammation, but it can have serious side effects, including gastrointestinal bleeding and interference with blood clotting if given for prolonged periods or in excessive amounts. Both drugs can be toxic if taken in large amounts. Therefore, care should always be taken to keep the bottle out of the reach of the toddler or young child.

In addition, parents should be particularly aware that they should consult a physician before giving aspirin to children and teenagers with flu or chicken pox. Some studies have shown a possible association between such use of aspirin and the development of a rare but often fatal condition called Reye syndrome.

Symptoms of Reye syndrome include violent headache, persistent vomiting, lethargy, sleepiness, belligerence, disorientation and delirium. These symptoms are very serious and can develop quickly, sometimes within half a day after the child has apparently recovered from the original flu or chicken pox. Unless emergency medical treatment is initiated promptly in a hospital setting, Reye syndrome can cause brain damage and even death.

In most cases, a fever is not serious, but still, it can be a sign that something is seriously wrong. That is why it is important to follow the general rule that if the temperature goes above 103 F in an older child or adult, or the fever persists for more than three days (72 hours), or recurs, it's time to call the doctor. Fever in infants is potentially more serious, and if it persists or recurs, the doctor should be contacted within 24 hours.

Annabel Hecht

The body's thermostat

Physiologically speaking, a fever is an abnormal rise of the body's temperature. The normal temperature in most people is 98.6 F (37 Celsius), 99.6 F if measured rectally. However, even a normal temperature varies a bit depending on the time of day. The temperature is often higher in the afternoon than in the morning, for instance.

What keeps the body's temperature at a normal level is the hypothalamus, a tiny area in the center of the brain that serves as the command center for the most critical of the body's functions, including food intake, endocrine levels, water balance, sexual rhythms, and the autonomic nervous system.

Body heat, produced primarily by muscular activity, is carried via the bloodstream to the skin, where it dissipates into the surrounding air. If the body is hot, as it might be after a vigorous game of tennis, for example, the hypothalamus will send a message to dilate (widen) the blood vessels, thus increasing the loss of heat. Sweating also promotes heat loss through evaporation.

If the temperature of the blood drops, the hypothalamus will order the blood vessels in the skin to constrict (narrow), decreasing heat loss. The hypothalamus also signals the adrenal glands to increase their production of the hormones that cause further constriction of the blood vessels and increase cellular metabolism and, therefore, heat production. The muscle activity involved in shivering also helps produce more heat.

In the case of fever, the hypothalamic thermostat is reset at a higher level by the action of "endogenous pyrogens," proteins released by the cells when they are stimulated by infection or other trauma.

There's evidence that the pyrogens do not act directly on the hypothalamus, but are involved in the manufacture of certain compounds called prostaglandins, which are released from the tissues when the body is under stress. Supporting this theory is the fact that aspirin, the best-known fever-reducing drug, interferes with the production of prostaglandins.

Fever usually comes on gradually, but it can start suddenly with a chill. During a fever, the temperature-regulating mechanism continues to function at the higher "thermostat setting." The body attempts to conserve heat by constricting the blood vessels (hence the pale, cold skin) and by producing heat through shivering. When the heat conservation measures have been successful and the temperature is above the new set point, the blood vessels dilate and the patient begins to sweat, a sign that the fever is coming down—or, as they said in many a melodrama, "the fever is broken."

FDA Consumer, November 1985.

Flu

Flu/Cold—Never The Strain Shall Meet

According to ancient legend, the Greek goddess Thetis heard a prophecy that her son, Achilles, would die in battle. To protect him, she attempted what might be called the first inoculation by dipping him head first into the magical River Styx. This made him invulnerable—except for the part of his body that Thetis held onto, his heel. Thus, we get the colorful phrase "Achilles heel" for a weak point in an otherwise strong person. In terms of an invasion route for many bacteria and viruses, our Achilles heel is located at the other end of the anatomy, the respiratory tract: the nose, throat, windpipe, bronchial tubes and lungs.

Every day, as we inhale some 500 cubic feet of air, equivalent to a large walk-in closet, all kinds of unwanted visitors tag along: dust particles and the mites that often accompany them, pollen, a variety of airborne debris, and numerous bacteria and viruses. The body has various defenses protecting its respiratory tract. Strong, rough hairs in the nostrils stop the largest of these unwelcome guests. Smaller invaders then encounter the equivalent of flypaper, a sticky film of mucus that traps bacteria and particles. These are then pushed by the continual beating of legions of tiny whiplike hairs, the cilia, back to the gullet where they descend into the digestive tract and are consumed. Bacteria that make it past these obstacles encounter a variety of other defense mechanisms which together prevent the many organisms we inhale every day from causing disease.

Despite these formidable barriers, occasional harmful bacteria or viruses do manage to gain a foothold. Among these can be any of 200 viruses in eight groups or families that produce the common cold. There are also three types of influenza virus: type A, the most frequently encountered and often the most severe; B, which commonly causes localized outbreaks and occasionally severe epidemics; and C, which occurs rarely. Among the influenza A viruses, there are numerous subtypes that exist in the animal kingdom, three of which are known to be capable of infecting man.

The spread of influenza viruses from person to person depends on whether an infected individual comes in contact with someone who is susceptible. It is thought that infection with one influenza virus leaves a person resistant indefinitely to infection with the exact same virus. When a strain of influenza virus appears in a population for the first time, outbreaks that occur are likely to be limited in size. Outbreaks that affect large numbers of individuals over a wide geographic area are referred to as epidemics, and worldwide epidemics affecting all age groups are called pandemics.

The capacity of influenza viruses to produce significant outbreaks year after year is the result of their diversity. Pandemics occur when viruses of an influenza A subtype emerge that have not been present for many years. Such pandemics occurred with the emergence of "Spanish flu" in 1918, "Asian flu" in 1957, and "Hong Kong flu" in 1968. The viruses that caused these pandemics were each representatives of different subtypes of influenza A.

In addition to the differences in types of variation seen in influenza and cold viruses, there are important differences in the types of disease they cause. The common cold is well-known as a self-limited illness that is usually no more than a nuisance for two or three days. By comparison, influenza is a major killer worldwide. The Spanish flu pandemic of 1918 was the worst pestilence that ever afflicted mankind. It has been estimated that more than 30 million people died in the United

States, and perhaps billions died worldwide. In 1957, more than 50 thousand people died in the United States from Asian flu. Even in years between pandemics there are usually thousands of deaths in this country, mostly in elderly persons or those with chronic illnesses such as cystic fibrosis, asthma, or heart disease.

It is this capacity to produce sudden, widespread epidemics of varying severity that once made influenza appear to be a mysterious affliction. Many theories were proposed to account for the speed and intensity of a flu epidemic. In 1657, the English physician Thomas Willis, remarking on the sudden way so many were afflicted with chills, aches, and fever, attributed it to the malign influence of the stars—in Italian, *influentia coeli,* from which we get the word influenza. The word *grippe,* sometimes also *la grippe,* was once often used as a synonym for influenza. While this may seem like a precise French word for the harsh grip of the disease on the body, it actually comes from the Russian word *krip,* or hoarseness.

Those caught in influenza's grip are far from caring how the disease was christened but are more concerned with how to get rid of it.

During the 1918 pandemic, the question of whether the early signs of respiratory distress signaled only another common cold or the dreaded onset of Spanish flu and a brush with death was of sharp and immediate concern. *The Denver Post* of Oct. 11, 1918, seeking to conserve the energies of that city's physicians, who were exhausted from dealing with so many desperately ill persons, tried to tell its readers the difference between a cold and the flu. The beginning of a cold, the paper said, was not as sudden, its aches not as severe, its fever not as high. And, the *Post* added, a cold is distinguished by "chilliness rather than definite chills." In terms of diagnosis outside a laboratory, the truth is we haven't really progressed much past the vague advice in that 1918 newspaper. What is possible now that wasn't possible in 1918 is a sure way of knowing whether a person has flu by laboratory testing for presence of the specific antibody associated with the flu virus. It's also possible to provide a precise list of symptoms that distinguish flu from a cold. But the list deals with generalities and averages.

One reason it's so difficult to tell definitely from symptoms alone that a person has the flu or a cold is that humans differ widely in how they react to these respiratory infections. Some may become quite ill from a cold; others may exhibit only mild distress from the flu. In fact, there is no single symptom that distinguishes flu from the common cold—or even from the early stages of bronchitis or strep throat. From controlled experiments with volunteers, the best that can be said is the following:

- Regarding fever: colds rarely are accompanied by fever, except in children; flu usually begins with fever.

- Regarding onset: flu is swift and severe; colds tend to build more slowly.
- Regarding location: colds show localized symptoms such as sneezing, runny nose, etc.; flu has general symptoms such as weakness, muscular pain, chills, headache.
- Regarding other symptoms: 90 percent of flu victims have a dry, hacking cough; 60 percent have sore eyes; 50 percent have a flushed face and hot, moist skin. Such symptoms appear less often in cold sufferers.

The point to note is that there is no absolute way to tell by symptoms alone which infection a person is suffering from. The best that can be said is that if a patient is suddenly stricken with fever, chills, general weakness, headache and muscular pains, accompanied by a severe cough, sore eyes and flushed face, *and if there is a flu outbreak in the area,* then he or she *probably* has influenza. But since children and older persons differ in the severity of symptoms, and since symptoms are further clouded by differences between individuals—such as prior history of exposure to influenza, genetic endowment, stress or personal health— it is simply impossible to state on the basis of symptoms alone that a respiratory infection is or is not the flu.

Unfortunately, even if we could tell from symptoms whether a person has influenza, there is no medicine now known to cure it, although some drugs are being studied. Penicillin and other antibiotics have no effect on flu or other viruses, although they may help fight certain complicating infections, such as bronchitis and some types of pneumonia. A physician is the best judge of when to use antibiotics.

Nevertheless, while influenza cannot yet be cured, it can be prevented by vaccination. However, because flu virus often drifts or shifts into a form new to the body's immune defenses, inoculation against one flu strain does not necessarily protect against the next epidemic. Such protection requires inoculation with a vaccine specific for the strain or strains currently circulating.

If flu can only be prevented, not cured, how can it be treated, once caught? In the 1918 pandemic, nurses were in greater demand than physicians, since the main need for flu victims was tender loving care. That's still the best treatment. The patient should drink lots of water and fruit juice, keep warm and comfortable, and remain in bed until temperature returns to normal. To ease discomfort from muscle pains or headaches, aspirin or a substitute may be taken by an adult. An aspirin substitute (or aspirin, if directed by a physician) may be taken by children. It is important that the patient be closely observed to detect signs of complications. This includes just about every infectious respiratory tract disease, such as acute bronchitis, pharyngitis, tonsillitis, laryngitis, croup, sinusitis and pneumonia. Ordinarily such complications don't involve the digestive or intestinal system. Therefore, influenza virus is seldom if ever responsible for what is erroneously called "intestinal flu" or "stomach flu."

Finally, how serious is the flu? Obviously, as the Spanish flu pandemic of 1918 shows, flu can be a life-threatening disease. This is why, when a flu strain appeared in 1976 (the "swine flu") that seemed to resemble the 1918 flu virus, the government geared up for inoculation of every American. This proved to be a false alarm. But new flu strains that are far less virulent than that which caused the 1918 pandemic can still exact a huge toll in losses of life and in illness. For example, the Asian flu pandemic of 1957 caused 45 million cases of influenza in the United States alone.

In the absence of such potent influenza strains, the kinds of influenza we usually encounter tend to produce moderately severe illnesses, but are not serious health threats to most healthy individuals. Complete recovery can be expected within a week. For certain high-risk groups—old people, children, the chronically ill, and pregnant women—any form of flu can be a serious problem, since the disease or its complications may be life threatening. The mortality curve of influenza—the death rate for each age group—usually takes a U-shaped form on a graph, evidence of flu's special danger to the very young and the very old. (The single exception was the Spanish flu, which showed a W-shaped form, attesting that millions in the prime and healthiest years of life died either from the flu or its complications.) There is also some evidence that pregnant women may have more severe influenza than healthy, non-pregnant women. Any pregnant woman who catches influenza should report it promptly to her physician.

Special precautions are necessary with children who contract influenza. It can strike with far more severity than in an adult, and include fever above 104 degrees Fahrenheit, along with such complications as convulsions, croup, or pneumonia. With both types of flu (as well as with chickenpox) there is danger for children from infancy to the late teen years of a life-threatening illness called Reye syndrome (pronounced "rye"). Reye syndrome usually takes the following course: The child is recovering from a mild viral illness such as influenza. Suddenly, in rapid succession, the child has vomiting, violent headaches, listlessness, irritability (even combativeness), delirium, disturbed breathing, stiffness of arms and legs, and then coma. A parent should not wait until there is a full progression of these symptoms or enough of them to substantiate fear that the child has Reye syndrome. Immediate action is called for. The family physician should be called right away. If a physician cannot be reached, the child should be taken to a hospital emergency room. A Reye syndrome attack moves so fast, and the penalty for failure to respond with equal speed is so severe, that not a second should be lost.

The word "syndrome" is applied when medicine recognizes a fixed pattern of symptoms but doesn't fully understand their cause (or causes). Thus, no one yet knows what causes Reye syndrome. However, there are studies indicating that the appearance of Reye syndrome in children may be associated with (not the same as "caused by") aspirin and other drugs that contain salicylates (the chemical basis of aspirin). Therefore, the U.S. surgeon general has advised against giving aspirin and other salicylate-containing products to children with flu or chickenpox, unless directed by the child's physician. This is why the Food and Drug Administration announced that it is considering a regulation which would require the labels on aspirin and other salicylate-containing products to warn against giving such products to children under 16 with flu or chickenpox without consulting a physician.

Medicine has come a long way from the time when influenza was blamed on an evil star. The only certainty is that even the mildest illness must be treated with respect, and the patient not only cared for but observed carefully.

Tim Larkin, FDA Consumer Vol. 17, No. 7, September 1983

Food Poisons

Who, Why, When And Where Of Food Poisons (And What To Do About Them)

No one would intentionally put poison in his or her food. But sometimes food becomes toxic because of lack of care in processing or because people fail to take steps to prevent foodborne illness. This happens because people often are not aware of the variety of ways food can become contaminated.

The following chart identifies some of the more common organisms that cause food poisoning, the name of the illness each causes, conditions under which the organism thrives in food, symptoms of illness, and methods of preventing food contamination.

Much of the illness classified under the heading "food poisoning" involves the gastrointestinal tract (with one notable exception: botulism causes neurotoxic symptoms involving the respiratory tract). Gastrointestinal symptoms include nausea, vomiting and diarrhea, and are sometimes known as "gastroenteritis." Although the symptoms are all somewhat similar, the organisms or their byproducts that cause the illness are quite different. Those listed in the chart include bacteria, bacterial toxins, viruses, mycotoxins (from molds) and protozoa (one-celled microscopic parasites).

Similarly, the events that result in food poisoning are also different. For instance, some bacteria—such as the *Shigella*—cause illness when large numbers are eaten in food such as potato salad. Because the bacteria multiply rapidly in certain prepared foods left at room temperature, prompt and proper refrigeration of the susceptible foods is the way to prevent illness.

On the other hand, *Clostridium botulinum* bacteria are perfectly harmless to most people if eaten in foods that have not been preserved because they are in the spore, or inactive, stage that survives when there is oxygen in the environment (some infants, however, can become ill from eating botulinum spores). The spores remain inactive unless they are put into the anaerobic (oxygen-less), low-acid environment that they require for activation and growth—a can of green beans, for example. If spores have not been killed during the canning process by application of heat under high pressure, they will reactivate and resume their life cycle, or reproductive process. During this process, the botulinum toxin is manufactured. It is this substance that makes the food poisonous. Contamination of preserved foods may be prevented by following the recommended established canning or other preservation methods.

Viruses and protozoa have their source in the human intestinal tract and can get into food directly from handling by a person who fails to wash his or her hands after a visit to the bathroom. The more personal handling of a food, the greater the chance of contamination and resulting illness. The solution to the problem is to observe proper sanitary habits during food preparation—that is, wash both the hands and raw ingredients thoroughly.

Illness caused by foodborne poisons and poisonous organisms can vary in intensity. The malady can be so mild that it is barely noticed or is passed off as an upset stomach. Again, a lengthy hospitalization might result and, in some cases, the illnesses can kill. But regardless of intensity, food poisoning is unpleasant. It is also something that can be avoided.

Carol L. Ballentine and Michael L. Herndon, *FDA Consumer*, reprinted from July/August 1982. HHS Publication No. (FDA) 82–2167. U.S. Government Printing Office 1982—361-174/150.

Disease & Organism That Causes It	Source of Illness	Symptoms	Prevention Methods
salmonellosis *Salmonella* (bacteria; more than 1,700 kinds)	May be found in raw meats, poultry, eggs, fish, milk, and products made with them. Multiplies rapidly at room temperature.	Onset: 12–48 hours after eating. Nausea, fever, headache, abdominal cramps, diarrhea, and sometimes vomiting. Can be fatal in infants, the elderly, and the infirm	• Handling food in a sanitary manner • Thorough cooking of foods • Prompt and proper refrigeration of foods
staphylococcal food poisoning staphylococcal enterotoxin (produced by *Staphylococcus aureus* bacteria)	The toxin is produced when food contaminated with the bacteria is left too long at room temperature. Meats, poultry, egg products; tuna, potato and macaroni salads; and cream-filled pastries are good environments for these bacteria to produce toxin.	Onset: 1–8 hours after eating. Diarrhea, vomiting, nausea, abdominal cramps, and prostration. Mimics flu. Lasts 24–48 hours. Rarely fatal.	• Sanitary food handling practices • Prompt and proper refrigeration of foods
botulism botulinum toxin (produced by *Clostridium botulinum* bacteria)	Bacteria are widespread in the environment. However, bacteria produce toxin only in an anaerobic (oxygen-less) environment of little acidity. Types A, B and F may result from inadequate processing of low-acid canned foods, such as green beans, mushrooms, spinach, olives, and beef. Type E normally occurs in fish.	Onset: 8–36 hours after eating. Neurotoxic symptoms, including double vision, inability to swallow, speech difficulty and progressive paralysis of the respiratory system. OBTAIN MEDICAL HELP IMMEDIATELY. BOTULISM CAN BE FATAL.	• Using proper methods for canning low-acid foods • Avoidance of commercially canned low-acid foods with leaky seals or with bent, bulging, or broken cans • Toxin can be destroyed after a can is opened by boiling contents hard for 10 minutes—NOT RECOMMENDED

Disease & Organism That Causes It	Source of Illness	Symptoms	Prevention Methods
perfringens food poisoning *Clostridium perfringens* (rod-shaped bacteria)	Bacteria are widespread in environment. Generally found in meat and poultry and dishes made with them. Multiply rapidly when foods are left at room temperature too long. Destroyed by cooking.	Onset: 8–22 hours after eating (usually 12). Abdominal pain and diarrhea. Sometimes nausea and vomiting. Symptoms last a day or less and are usually mild. Can be more serious in older or debilitated people.	• Sanitary handling of foods, especially meat, meat dishes, and gravies • Thorough cooking of foods • Prompt and proper refrigeration
shigellosis (bacillary dysentery) *Shigella* (bacteria)	Food becomes contaminated when a human carrier with poor sanitary habits handles liquid or moist food that is then not cooked thoroughly. Organisms multiply in food stored above room temperature. Found in milk and dairy products, poultry, and potato salad.	Onset: 1–7 days after eating. Abdominal pain, cramps, diarrhea, fever, sometimes vomiting, and blood, pus or mucus in stools. Can be serious in infants, the elderly, or debilitated people.	• Handling food in a sanitary manner • Proper sewage disposal • Proper refrigeration of foods
campylobacterosis *Campylobacter jejuni* (rod-shaped bacteria)	Bacteria found on poultry, cattle and sheep and can contaminate the meat and milk of these animals. Chief food sources: raw poultry and meat and unpasteurized milk.	Onset: 2–5 after eating. Diarrhea, abdominal cramping, fever, and sometimes bloody stools. Lasts 2–7 days.	• Thorough cooking of foods • Handling food in a sanitary manner • Avoiding unpasteurized milk

gastroenteritis *Yersinia enterocolitica* (non-spore-forming bacteria)	Ubiquitous in nature; carried in food and water. Bacteria multiply rapidly at room temperature, *as well as* at refrigerator temperatures (4° to 9°C). Generally found in raw vegetables, meats, water and unpasteurized milk.	Onset: 2–5 days after eating. Fever, headache, nausea, diarrhea, and general malaise. Mimics flue. An important cause of gastroenteritis in children. Can also infect other age groups and, if not treated, can lead to other more serious diseases (such as lymphadenitis, arthritis, and Reiter's syndrome).	• Thorough cooking of foods • Sanitizing cutting instruments and cutting boards before preparing foods that are eaten raw • Avoidance of unpasteurized milk and unchlorinated water
cereus food poisoning *Bacillus cereus* (bacteria and possibly their toxin)	Illness may be caused by the bacteria, which are widespread in the environment, or by an enterotoxin created by the bacteria. Found in raw foods. Bacteria multiply rapidly in foods stored at room temperature.	Onset: 1–18 hours after eating. Two types of illness: (1) abdominal pain and diarrhea, and (2) nausea and vomiting. Lasts less than a day.	• Sanitary handling of foods • Thorough cooking of foods • Prompt and adequate refrigeration
cholera *Vibrio cholera* (bacteria)	Found in fish and shellfish harvested from waters contaminated by human sewage. (Bacteria may also occur naturally in Gulf Coast waters.) Chief food sources: seafood, especially types eaten raw (such as oysters).	Onset: 1–3 days. Can range from "subclinical" (a mild uncomplicated bout with diarrhea) to fatal (intense diarrhea with dehydration). Severe cases require hospitalization.	• Sanitary handling of foods • Thorough cooking of seafood

Disease & Organism That Causes It	Source of Illness	Symptoms	Prevention Methods
parahaemolyticus food poisoning *Vibrio parahaemolyticus* (bacteria)	Organism lives in salt water and can contaminate fish and shellfish. Thrives in warm weather.	Onset: 15–24 hours after eating. Abdominal pain, nausea, vomiting, and diarrhea. Sometimes fever, headache, chills, and mucus and blood in the stools. Lasts 1–2 days. Rarely fatal.	● Sanitary handling of foods ● Thorough cooking of seafood
gastrointestinal disease enteroviruses, rotaviruses, parvoviruses	Viruses exist in the intestinal tract of humans and are expelled in feces. Contamination of foods can occur in three ways: (1) when sewage is used to enrich garden/farm soil, (2) by direct hand-to-food contact during the preparation of meals, and (3) when shellfish-growing waters are contaminated by sewage.	Onset: After 24 hours. Severe diarrhea, nausea, and vomiting. Respiratory symptoms. Usually lasts 4–5 days, but may last for weeks.	● Sanitary handling of foods ● Use of pure drinking water ● Adequate sewage disposal ● Adequate cooking of foods
hepatitis hepatitis A virus	Chief food sources: shellfish harvested from contaminated areas, and foods that are handled a lot during preparation and then eaten raw (such as vegetables).	Jaundice, fatigue. May cause liver damage and death.	● Sanitary handling of foods ● Use of pure drinking water ● Adequate sewage disposal ● Adequate cooking of foods

mycotoxicosis mycotoxins (from molds)	Produced in foods that are relatively high in moisture. Chief food sources: beans and grains that have been stored in a moist place.	May cause liver and/or kidney disease	• Checking foods for visible mold and discarding those that are contaminated • Proper storage of susceptible foods
giardiasis *Giardia lamblia* (flagellated protozoa)	Protozoa exist in the intestinal tract of humans and are expelled in feces. Contamination of foods can occur in two ways: (1) when sewage is used to enrich garden/farm soil, and (2) by direct hand-to-food contact during the preparation of meals. Chief food sources: foods that are handled a lot during preparation.	Diarrhea, abdominal pain, flatulence, abdominal distention, nutritional disturbances, "nervous" symptoms, anorexia, nausea, and vomiting.	• Sanitary handling of foods • Avoidance of raw fruits and vegetables in areas where the protozoa is endemic • Proper sewage disposal
amebiasis *Entamoeba histolytica* (amoebic protozoa)		Tenderness over the colon or liver, loose morning stools, recurrent diarrhea, change in bowel habits, "nervous" symptoms, loss of weight, and fatigue. Anemia may be present.	• Sanitary handling of foods • Avoidance of raw fruits and vegetables in areas where the protozoa is endemic • Proper sewage disposal

Foot Problems

Caring For Corns, Bunions, And Other Agonies Of De-Feet

How often have you been offered a chair and invited, colloquially speaking, to "take the weight off your feet?" However inelegantly put, the invitation is usually welcome, for the feet bear a tremendous burden in the course of day-to-day living. Considering that an average day of walking subjects the feet to a force equal to several hundred tons, it is little wonder that they ache by nightfall.

Like other parts of the body, the feet are highly specialized structures. Each is made up of 26 bones, laced with ligaments, muscles, nerves and blood vessels. The principal functions of the feet are weight-bearing and locomotion. Their range of motion allows them to move with ease over practically any surface, whether it is rough, uneven or slippery. Their flexibility enables the ballet dancer to stand on one toe, the climber to gain a foothold on a rock face, the circus performer to walk the tight wire, or the small child to gain a few inches to reach the forbidden cookie jar.

But as versatile as they are, our feet are also prey to countless problems. Because of their location and the fact that they must support all our weight, the feet are subject to more pressure and injury than any other part of the body. They can also be affected by congenital or hereditary malformations, such as clubfoot. (Such problems can usually be corrected in infancy with special casts or braces.)

Other foot problems may be an indication of some other underlying health disorder. Circulatory problems, diabetes, anemia and even kidney disorders are often first detected in the feet. Foot joints are frequently the first to be involved when arthritis strikes.

Still other foot problems are brought on by personal habits, sometimes the result of following fashion rather than common sense in choosing shoes. Among the more common foot ailments are corns and calluses, warts, athlete's foot, ingrown nails, and bunions.

Corns and calluses are very much alike. Both have a marked thickening of the top layer of the skin, caused by long periods of pressure or friction against the skin. Calluses can develop anywhere on the weight-bearing areas, such as the sides and soles of the feet. They are usually raised, off-white in color, and have a normal pattern of skin ridges on the surface.

Corns come in two major varieties—hard and soft. Hard corns are the more common, usually occurring on the surfaces of the toes. They appear shiny and polished. Soft corns are whitish in color and are most often found on the web between the fourth and the little toe. Unlike calluses, corns have a central core, which consists of a base on the surface of the skin and an apex pointing inward. Pressure of the core on nerve endings in the skin causes the pain of corns.

Calluses and corns usually develop from wearing ill-fitting shoes, socks or stockings. They may also occur as a result of an underlying foot problem such as a bony growth on the toe.

Calluses and hard corns can be self-treated with over-the-counter (OTC) drug products, according to a panel of experts that assisted FDA in its review of ingredients in these products.

Salicylic acid is the only ingredient the panel found safe and effective for treating calluses and hard corns. The experts recommended it be used in concentrations of 12 to 40 percent in pads, plasters and disks and at concentrations of 12 to 17.6 percent in collodion (a solution of nitrocellulose), which leaves a transparent film when applied to the skin. The panel said there was insufficient data on which to recommend a concentration of salicylic acid that would be safe and effective for treating soft corns. They called for studies on soft corn treatment. (FDA's proposed rules on OTC drug ingredients for callus and corn treatment have not yet been published.)

Other types of treatment include removing some of the thickened skin—something that should be done only by a doctor—and using pads to relieve pressure over bony growths. Occasionally these growths are removed surgically.

Warts on the bottom of the feet, called plantar warts, are often mistaken for calluses, but they have nothing in common. Although the pressure of walking on plantar warts can cause pain, pressure does not cause them. Plantar warts, like warts on other parts of the body, are caused by a virus.

A plantar wart can grow only on the bottom of the foot and occurs in children as well as adults. It may appear singly or in clusters. The wart is flat and may be either hard or soft. Because they are caused by a virus, warts can be spread from one person to another either directly or indirectly in public areas such as swimming pools or showers. For this reason, many medical experts feel warts should be removed even though most of them will go away by themselves in time.

Salicylic acid is the only safe and effective OTC ingredient the panel found for removal of warts. This ingredient acts as a skin peeler, destroying the wart tissue. Because the drug can harm healthy skin, the panel recommended keeping the product away from surrounding skin, preferably by encircling the wart with a ring of petrolatum.

If there is any doubt about a wart, a doctor should be consulted.

Wart treatments that doctors use include freezing the wart with liquid nitrogen, removing it surgically, or using prescription drugs. Single-dose X-ray treatment is another option but is less common today than it once was.

Athlete's foot is a fungal infection that, despite its name, is not exclusive to the locker room. It usually occurs in men between the ages of 14 and 40, but women also may fall prey to the fungus.

Itching, burning, and redness are the common symptoms of athlete's foot (known medically as tinea pedis). White scale (flaking skin) develops in the toe-web, especially between the fourth and little toe. Blisters may also occur. On the sole of the foot, athlete's foot may appear as irregularly grouped blisters and superficial scale.

The fungi that most commonly cause athlete's foot—*Trichophyton mentagrophytes, T. rubrum* and *Epidermophyton floccosum*—are prevalent in homes, offices, and athletic facilities, but that doesn't mean everyone passing through will get the affliction. However, the chance of infection increases if there is broken skin or increased moisture from tight shoes, excessive sweating, humid summer weather, or a tropical climate.

To treat athlete's foot, FDA's expert advisory panel on OTC antimicrobial drugs recommended using OTC drugs that contain iodochlorhydroxyquin, tolnaftate, or undecylenic acid, and its calcium, copper, and zinc salts. Tolnaftate can also be used to prevent, as well as treat, this condition, the panel said.

The panel also recommended that haloprogin and miconazole nitrate be switched from prescription to OTC status for the treatment of athlete's foot. Nystatin, another prescription drug recommended for OTC use, should be used only in combination with other safe and effective OTC ingredients, the panel said. (Proposed rules covering these ingredients have not yet been published by FDA.)

An ingrown toenail almost always afflicts the big toe and occurs when a section of the nail curves into the flesh of the toe corners and becomes imbedded in the soft tissues, causing pain, swelling, inflammation and ulceration.

Incorrect trimming of the nails is usually the cause of ingrown toenails, although pointed-toe shoes and tight shoes and hosiery may also be to blame. People with nails that curl naturally are more likely to develop this condition.

To avoid ingrown toenails, the nails should be cut straight across without tapering the corners.

Unfortunately, FDA's expert advisory panel did not recommend any OTC ingredients as being safe and effective for self-treatment of the discomfort of ingrown nails. Medical treatment is aimed at relieving external pressure and includes prescription medications that will harden the nail groove or help shrink the soft tissue. Hot packs may be applied, as well as topical antiseptics and medications to control infection. In stubborn cases, surgery may be needed to remove part of the nail.

Few foot afflictions are more disfiguring and painful than bunions. Many experts blame ill-fitting shoes for this condition, while others consider this an over-simplification. Bunions have been known to occur in people who don't wear shoes and, conversely, don't always develop in people whose footwear is poorly fitted. Heredity, flat feet, and structural defects resulting from poliomyelitis or cerebral palsy also make some people more prone to bunions.

Bunions are actually misaligned big toe joints that become swollen and tender. The technical name is *hallux valgus*—*hallus* being the Latin name for the great toe and *valgus* another Latin word meaning bent outward. Normally the bones of the big toe lie more or less in a straight line with the large metatarsal bone of the foot. When a bunion develops, the large metatarsal bone angles outward, away from the other metatarsals, and the big toe bones are forced in the opposite direction (see illustration). Pressure over this joint causes inflammatory swelling of the bursa, a fluid-filled sac that prevents friction between two bones of a joint.

Bunions may not produce symptoms, but usually they become quite painful, swollen and tender. The skin over the bunion may become thick and rough. There are no topical medications that will make a bunion go away. Use of protective pads and shoes that do not constrict the front part of the foot may help in relieving symptoms. Often the only answer to this deformity is surgery, which ranges from removal of bony outgrowths on the toe to joint resection (cutting away parts of the bone itself), fusion, and toe realignment.

Corns, calluses, warts, athlete's foot, ingrown toenails and sometimes even bunions can, to a large extent, be prevented by proper foot care. This includes selecting shoes that fit correctly, keeping the feet clean and dry, and trimming nails properly.

Good foot care is particularly important in helping the elderly to live useful, satisfying lives. Foot ailments make it difficult for many older people to work or participate in social activities.

To keep older people mobile, the American Podiatric Medical Association (the professional organization of foot doctors) recommends walking as the best exercise for the feet. Shoes with a firm sole and soft upper are best for daily activities, the association says. Socks or stockings should be of the correct size and preferably seamless. Elderly people should not wear constricting garters. Feet should be bathed and inspected daily.

For diabetics of any age, these foot-care recommendations are not only important—they are essential. Any injury to the lower extremities can have serious consequences. Because diabetics tend to have poor circulation, they must avoid anything that will decrease blood flow to the feet, such as wearing tight shoes, constricting socks or garters, or even sitting cross-legged.

Diabetics are more prone to infection; thus any break in the skin is a danger sign. Because they often lose sensation in their feet, diabetics may cut themselves or develop an infection without knowing it. For this reason, it is important that the feet be bathed daily and inspected for cuts, swelling or sores. Bath water should be warm, never hot. And diabetics should never use hot water bottles or electric blankets on their feet.

Commercial corn, callus, and wart removers, which are caustic, are not for the diabetic, either. They can destroy tissue and pave the way for infections. Labels on such preparations usually warn against use by diabetics. Finally, diabetics should have a podiatrist remove corns, calluses, and warts and trim toenails, rather than doing this themselves. This not only provides an opportunity for a careful foot examination by a doctor but avoids the chance of infection from accidental cuts.

Annabel Hecht, *FDA Consumer*, Vol. 19, No. 5, June 1985.

Gallstone Disease

An estimated 25 million Americans—over 10 percent of the population—have gallstones. In the next year, 1 million more people will discover that they have them. Even though gallbladder disease is not usually fatal, approximately 6,000 people will die from complications this year.

Gallstones are lumps of solid material that form in the gallbladder. Though in many patients these stones remain "silent" and cause no problems, in many other patients they do. Indeed, each year 500,000 people have their gallbladders removed in order to treat or prevent serious or even life-threatening complications. This makes cholecystectomy (ko-lee-sis-TEK-toe-mee)*—the surgical removal of the gallbladder—the fifth most common operation performed in the United States.

Gallstone disease is a common and expensive illness that costs the

---

*Please refer to the end of this article for a glossary.

American public $1.5 billion annually. Who gets gallstones? Why do they form? What are the complications? Why is surgery often necessary?

How does the gallbladder normally function?

The gallbladder is a sac located beneath the liver on the right-hand side of the abdominal cavity. Its primary job is to store the bile secreted by the liver until it is needed in the small intestine for digestion. When digestion begins, the gallbladder contracts and sends the bile into the intestine through a series of ducts. When digestion is completed, the bile is routed to the gallbladder for storage.

Bile helps break up fat so that it can be further digested by pancreatic enzymes and absorbed by the intestines. Bile contains bile salts, cholesterol, bilirubin (bi-lee-ROO-bin), and lecithin. In one day, the liver may produce as much as 700 milliliters (almost three cups) of bile to aid in digestion.

What causes gallstones to form?

Gallstones form when there is a precipitation of chemicals in the bile. Two types of gallstones can occur: cholesterol gallstones, or pigment gallstones. Cholesterol gallstones are composed chiefly of cholesterol, and pigment gallstones are composed of bilirubin and other compounds. About 80 percent of the patients with gallbladder disease in the United States have cholesterol gallstones.

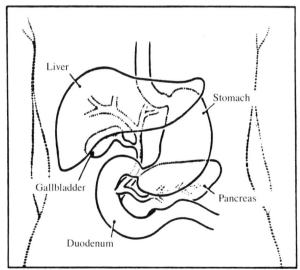

Figure 1 shows the location of the gallbladder in relation to other organs of digestion.

Cholesterol and other components of bile are collected in the gallbladder during periods of fasting—for instance, during sleep or between meals. For some reason that is not yet understood, in those patients who develop gallstones, the cholesterol comes out of solution and forms crystals. These crystals provide the cores around which the stones develop.

Researchers are uncertain about the relative importance of the liver and the gallbladder in the formation of gallstones. (But removing the gallbladder does prevent the formation of additional gallstones in the great majority of patients in the United States.) It is possible that the mixture of chemicals secreted by the liver of a patient with gallstones is not able to hold cholesterol in solution. On the other hand, some chemical may be present in the gallbladder of a patient with gallstones that disturbs the mixture and leads to the formation of crystals.

The cholesterol in bile and gallstones comes from the liver as a waste product of the body's metabolism. Even though researchers have determined that dietary cholesterol contributes to the pool of cholesterol, it has not been determined that the amount of cholesterol in the diet is directly related to the amount found in the gallbladder.

Who gets gallstones?

The people most likely to develop gallstones are women who have been pregnant, overweight people who eat a lot of dairy products and animal fats, and people over 60. In the 20 to 60 age group, women are three times more likely to develop gallstones than men. By the age of 60, however, almost 30 percent of all men and women have gallstones.

The incidence also varies by population and geographic location. For example, the occurrence in young Native American women can be as high as 75 percent, while the occurrence in Swedish women of all ages is 57 percent. The occurrence in Asian and African women is much lower.

Do hereditary and environmental factors play a role?

Both heredity and environment may play a significant role. In some tribes of Native Americans, for instance, 75 percent of the women have gallstones by the age of 25. Native American men have a similar incidence of gallstones by the time they reach 60. This incidence is far greater than that of the general population and suggests that heredity plays a role, though just how has not yet been determined. On the other hand, researchers have determined that people who are obese stand a greater chance of developing gallstones. This seems to indicate that environmental factors such as diet are involved in the formation of gallstones.

What are the symptoms of gallstone disease?

A great many people have gallstones but do not have symptoms. These people have silent gallstones and their stones may remain silent for the rest of their lives.

When symptoms are evident, a person with gallstones may have severe, steady pain in the upper abdomen. It lasts at least 20 minutes and usually up to two to four hours. There may be pain between the shoulder blades or in the right shoulder. There may be nausea or vomiting.

Gallstones cause more severe problems when they make their way out of the gallbladder. Gallstones can lodge in the channel that allows the bile to enter and leave the gallbladder. This channel is called the cystic duct. If gallstones block the channel for a prolonged period, the gallbladder may become inflamed. This condition is called cholecystitis (ko-lee-sis-TI-tis). Obstruction of the cystic duct is a relatively common complication of gallbladder disease.

Other complications are less common. For example, gallstones can enter and block the channel that drains the liver. This is called common

Figure 2 shows the sites of common complications of gallstone disease. Gallstones that escape from the gallbladder may lodge in the common bile duct, the cystic duct or the pancreatic duct and block vital organs.

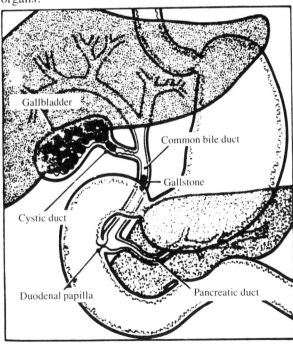

bile duct obstruction. Gallstones can lodge in the main channel that drains the pancreas, called the pancreatic duct, and cause pancreatitis.

The major symptom of all the complications of gallstone disease is abdominal pain. The pain is usually sudden, often severe, and located in the middle or right portions of the abdomen. The pain may spread out and it may be felt on both sides, in the back, or throughout the abdomen. It may shift from side to side or it may lodge in the right shoulder. This pain is often so intense that the sufferer may perspire heavily or vomit. The patient will have a chill with a high fever. An attack of this kind may be over in a few minutes, but usually lasts several hours. If this occurs, the patient should check with a physician as soon as possible.

How are gallstones diagnosed?

Many silent gallstones are identified when X-ray or ultrasound examinations are performed as part of a routine medical checkup or because some other illness is suspected. In patients who develop the typical symptoms of complications associated with gallbladder disease noted in the previous section, the physician will begin by taking a medical history and performing appropriate laboratory tests to help rule out other possible illnesses.

The diagnosis of patients with silent gallstones and those who have had complications that have subsided can be made with at least 95 percent accuracy. There are several methods available to do this. Oral cholecystography (ko-lee-sis-TOG-rah-fee) is a procedure in which X-rays of the gallbladder are taken after the patient has swallowed pills containing a dye that is absorbed and later appears in the bile outlining the gallbladder.

An ultrasound examination of the gallbladder is a test in which a picture of the organ and the duct network is produced by passing sound waves across the abdomen. These sound waves respond in a particular manner when stones are present. Based upon the same idea as sonar technology developed during World War II, ultrasonography is a valuable method of diagnosing gallstone disease.

Despite its relative expense and the fact that it requires a highly skilled person to administer and interpret the results, ultrasound provides many advantages. Ultrasound is a noninvasive technique (nothing is injected into or penetrates the body) that is painless, has no unpleasant side effects, and requires no exposure to radiation.

Ultrasonography is as sensitive as any method available to detect gallstones. It provides the physician with an immediate set of rules from which to make a diagnosis. Additionally, ultrasound pictures allow the physician to detect other disorders that may be present.

To get a picture of the extensive network of ducts and any stones that may be lodged in them, the doctor may perform a PTC—percutaneous transhepatic cholangiography (per-kyu-TAY-nee-us trans-heh-PA-tik ko-LAN-jee-OG-rah-fee). In this procedure, dye is injected into the small bile ducts in the liver. Once the dye has spread through the system into the common bile duct, an X-ray is taken.

Another method, ERCP (endoscopic retrograde cholangiopancreatography—ko-LAN-jee-oh-PAN-kree-ah-TOG-rah-fee), uses a flexible tube in the intestine to deliver the dye through another, smaller tube into the common bile duct. While both of these procedures provide a good look at the ducts, they carry a slight risk of complications. For this reason they are used only with certain patients.

What treatments are available and when should they be used?

The surgical removal of the gallbladder—cholecystectomy—is by far the most common course of treatment for patients who develop complications of gallbladder disease. This is because, until recently, removal of the gallbladder was the only way to get rid of gallstones. Even with the introduction of new drugs, many patients with gallstones will require surgery when life-threatening complications occur. Removal of the gallbladder does not seem to interfere with the normal digestive process. After the gallbladder is removed, the bile produced by the liver flows directly to the intestine.

Physicians will recommend surgery for most patients with cholecystitis and common bile duct obstruction and for nearly all patients with pancreatitis caused by gallstones. With both the common bile duct obstruction and pancreatitis caused by gallstones, the surgeon will have to remove the stones that are blocking the channels as well as removing the gallbladder. In patients who are in a seriously weakened condition, stones in the common bile duct can sometimes be removed through the opening in the intestine without abdominal surgery. This procedure is called endoscopic papillotomy (PAP-il-AH-toe-mee).

For patients with silent gallstones, research to determine the best course of treatment is needed. Physicians do not know, for instance, how to identify those patients with silent gallstones who will have complications in the future. Physicians are also unable to predict whether a patient who has had one or two episodes of cystic duct obstruction will have other episodes that could lead to more serious complications.

Preliminary information from several clinical studies provides some clues. Silent gallstones are common and chance favors that they will not cause problems in the future. Moreover, patients who have occasional symptoms of cystic duct obstruction do not appear to have other complications of gallstone disease with greater frequency than those with silent gallstones. This information has prompted many physicians to withhold surgical removal unless compelling reasons for surgery exist. Obviously, each patient's problem must be considered in light of all factors. For instance, a person with silent gallstones might be advised to have surgery before leaving the United States to spend five years in an underdeveloped country where optimal surgical treatment would not be available.

Also patients with silent gallstones who also have either diabetes or heart disease might be advised to have their gallbladders removed. This is because the risks of surgery increase the longer the patient lives with either of these diseases. The risk would also be increased if the surgery had to be performed as an emergency.

Until recently, no drugs have been available to treat gallstone disease. The report from the National Cooperative Gallstone Study (published in September 1981) offers some hope for the development of such treatment. Sponsored by the National Institute for Arthritis, Diabetes and Digestive and Kidney Disease (NIADDK), the two-year study tested the safety and effectiveness of chenodeoxycholic (KEE-no-dee-ox-ee-KOH-lik) acid in dissolving gallstones. Investigators concluded that this drug is most effective in dissolving stones in patients who are thin and have small cholesterol gallstones. The study recommended, however, that patients who take the drug be warned of its potential side effects (diarrhea and possible liver damage). The investigators also noted that once the drug is stopped, stones may again develop.

What are the promising areas of research?

Currently, researchers are addressing four major questions. Why do gallstones form in some people and not others? Why do some gallstones lead to complications while others remain ''silent''? How does a physician determine what the best course of treatment is? Can the available drugs be made both more potent and safer?

Investigators are studying the factors that determine whether cholesterol remains in the bile or whether it crystalizes and forms gallstones. The factors that influence the secretion of cholesterol and the other components of bile are also being studied.

Researchers are gathering information on the natural history of gallstone disease to determine the best course of treatment to follow. Patients with silent gallstones and those with cystic duct obstruction are being observed.

As previously mentioned, recent studies show that some gallstones can be dissolved by drugs taken by mouth. The drugs that have this effect are bile acids, the same bile acids that are made in the liver and that hold the cholesterol in solution in the bile. The drug that has been tested most extensively, chenodeoxycholic acid, will dissolve gallstones in a relatively small number of patients. Another drug under investigation is ursodeoxycholic (er-so-dee-ox-ee-KOH-lik) acid.

The potential side effects of these drugs and the relative benefits and risks are currently being evaluated. Investigations into how to make drugs more potent and at the time ensure their safety continue.

Finding an effective and safe drug to dissolve gallstones will offer patients who do not require surgery a safe and effective alternative.

GLOSSARY

Bile.   A complex fluid, produced by the liver, that aids in the digestion of fats and is used by the body to dispose of non-water-soluble wastes.

Bile Ducts.   The system of tubes that carries bile from the liver to the intestine.

Bilirubin (bil-ee-ROO-bin).   A brown or yellow bile pigment formed from hemoglobin when red blood cells are broken down. The condition called jaundice reflects increased blood levels of bilirubin.

Chenodeoxycholic (KEE-no-dee-ox-ee-KOH-lik) **Acid.**   A drug, identical to one of the natural bile acids, that can dissolve some types of gallstones.

Cholecystectomy (ko-lee-sis-TEK-toe-mee).   Surgical removal of the gallbladder.

Cholecystitis (ko-lee-sis-TI-tis).   Inflammation of the gallbladder.

Cholecystography (ko-lee-sis-TOG-rah-fee) (Oral Cholecystography).   A diagnostic test in which an X-ray is taken of the gallbladder after the patient has swallowed pills containing dye. The patient must take the dye the night before the test is performed and may not eat until after the X-ray is taken.

Cholesterol.   The most abundant steroid in animal tissue, especially in bile and gallstones.

Common Bile Duct Obstruction.   Blockage of the tube that allows the bile to flow from the liver to the small intestine.

Cystic Duct Obstruction.   Blockage of the tube that allows the bile to flow from the gallbladder into the common bile duct and on to the small intestine.

Endoscope.   A small, flexible tube-like instrument, consisting of thousands of tiny glass fibers, that allows a doctor to see into the esophagus, stomach, duodenum, and colon. It also allows a doctor to perform biopsies, take color photographs, and perform surgical and therapeutic procedures.

Endoscopic Retrograde Cholangiopancreatography (ERCP) (ko-LAN-jee-oh-PAN-kree-ah-TOG-rah-fee). A diagnostic examination performed by a physician through an endoscope. A catheter (tube) is placed through the endoscope into the opening of the bile ducts and pancreas, and dye is injected for visualization of the ductal systems. An X-ray is taken while the injection is being performed.

Endoscopic Papillotomy (PAP-il-AH-toe-mee). After ERCP has been performed, a catheter with a wire is placed into the bile duct draining into the duodenum. An electrical current is passed through the wire resulting in an opening being made into the common bile duct for common duct stone removal.

Gallbladder. A sac, located beneath the liver, that stores bile. The gallbladder can store about one-half pint of bile, which is squeezed out during digestion.

Gallstone Disease (Gallbladder Disease). The condition of having gallstones in the gallbladder or lodged in one of the ducts leading to or from the gallbladder.

Gallstones. Solid material that forms in the gallbladder or bile ducts. Though most stones are composed of cholesterol, some are made of bilirubin. In the United States, cholesterol gallstones contain 70 to 90 percent cholesterol. Pigment gallstones contain 50 to 70 percent bilirubin and less than 10 percent cholesterol. Pigment stones are common among people living in the Orient and among people with hemolytic disorders (abnormally short survival of red blood cells) such as sickle cell anemia.

Lecithin. A waxy substance, found in the bile, that is capable of dissolving fats.

Noninvasive. A term used to describe procedures that do not require any injection into or penetration of the body.

Obstruction. Blockage or clogging of an organ. The result is that liquids or solids can no longer flow through the area and there is a buildup of pressure near the obstruction.

Pancreas. A gland, located next to the duodenum, that produces juices that digest food.

Percutaneous (per-kyu-TAY-nee-us) **Transhepatic** (trans-heh-PA-tik) **Cholangiography** (ko-LAN-jee-OG-rah-fee). A diagnostic test in which an X-ray is taken of the gallbladder and bile ducts after a dye is inserted through the skin into the duct network of the liver.

Silent Gallstones. Gallstones that cause no symptoms and are discovered incidentally by X-ray or ultrasound, or during surgery.

Ultrasonography (Ultrasonic Imaging, Echoscanning, Ultrasound).

A diagnostic test in which sound pulses are sent into the body. The returning echoes from inside the body are collected and a picture is produced from them. It uses the same technology as sonar.

Ursodeoxycholic (er-so-dee-ox-ee-KOH-lik) **Acid.** A drug, similar to chenodeoxycholic acid, that is being tested for safety and effectiveness in dissolving gallstones.

Malcolm P. Tyor, M.D. *Chief, Division of Gastroenterology Duke University Medical Center, Durham, North Carolina.*

National Digestive Diseases, Education and Information Clearinghouse, 1255 23rd Street, N.W., Suite 275, Washington, DC 20037, (202) 296–1138. This publication is not copyrighted. The digestive diseases clearinghouse urges users of this fact sheet to duplicate and distribute as many copies as desired. Check with local printing firms for reproduction prices. Offset printing can be inexpensive. U.S. Department of Health and Human Services, Public Health Service, National Institutes of Health.

Gastrointestinal Tract
Happenings Along The GI Tract

The juice, eggs, toast, and coffee that a person eats for breakfast take about 24 hours to be digested and absorbed. During this time, the food and drink travel through about 30 feet of internal channels. The substances are churned and mixed with some powerful acids secreted along with enzymes. The route traveled is known as the alimentary canal, or the gastrointestinal (GI) tract, and goes from the mouth to the anus, the last segment of the rectum.

Digestion begins in the mouth where food is broken up by chewing and then mixed with saliva containing the enzyme amylase, which begins the breakdown of starch to sugar. Swallowing carries the food into the esophagus and sends it on its way to the stomach. Time down the 10-inch long esophagus varies by no more than a few seconds, depending on whether what is swallowed is a liquid or a solid.

The stomach is not located just below the belt line, as many people think, but is much higher up, on the left side of the abdomen just under the diaphragm. The stomach serves as a kind of holding tank where the food is further churned and mashed by its rhythmic contractions. Starch digestion continues and pepsin breaks protein down into simpler compounds. Pepsin needs the help of hydrochloric acid. The two substances are released from stomach cells by gastrin, a hormone that is stimulated by the presence of food in the stomach.

After it is thoroughly mashed and mixed, the food, now called chyme, moves into the small intestine through the pylorus, a muscular valve at the lower end of the stomach. Because the small intestine can handle only so much, the pylorus allows only a small amount of chyme through at a time. Carbohydrates, which require less work from the digestive system, move through the pylorus faster than high protein and fat foods. This may explain why Chinese meals, which tend to be more vegetable than meat, seem to leave the diner feeling hungry soon after the meal is over.

The small intestine, named for the size of its diameter rather than for its 20 to 22 foot length, consists of three sections: the duodenum, the jejunum, and the ileum. In the duodenum, chyme is subjected to pancreatic juices and bile from the liver. These juices neutralize the hydrochloric acid and cause a further breakdown of carbohydrates, proteins and fats. The final digestion of chyme and the absorption of nutrients takes place in the jejunum and ileum. Absorption takes place through the actions of tiny hair-like projections, called villi, that line the intestines. Fats and fat soluble components are carried partly to the liver and partly to the blood via the lymphatic system. Vitamins, minerals, amino acids, and sugars travel to the liver, the body's key unit in the processing of nutrients. By the time the chyme has completed its passage through the small intestine, 95 percent of the nutrients have been absorbed. What's left is sent on to the large intestine, or colon, which takes care of the absorption of water and electrolytes—i.e., sodium, potassium, chloride, and bicarbonate. What can't be absorbed is concentrated as fecal matter and periodically eliminated.

So much for breakfast.

Except for the conscious act of chewing and swallowing, most people don't give much thought to the digestive process. It is completely automatic. But ever so often they become acutely aware of the existence of the gastrointestinal tract. Fortunately, many digestive disorders are relatively minor—an upset stomach or a touch of gas. These conditions usually go away by themselves or, if they become too uncomfortable, can be treated with non-prescription, or over-the-counter, drugs. The ingredients in these products have been reviewed for safety and effectiveness by a number of panels of non-government experts assisting in FDA's massive review of OTC drugs.

There are, for instance, antacids that can be taken for an upset stomach associated with heartburn, sour stomach or acid indigestion. Simethicone can help relieve the symptoms of flatulence, or excess gas, according to FDA.

But another panel, in a recent report, has found no evidence that gas has anything to do with symptoms that occur in conditions called "immediate postprandial upper abdominal distress" (IPPUAD) and "intestinal distress" (ID). The group found no safe and effective ingredients in today's OTC products that will relieve IPPUAD symptoms of bloating, distention, fullness, or pressure. This uncomfortable feeling develops within 30 minutes after eating. Nor did the panel find any safe and effective ingredients to relieve ID, a similar uncomfortable feeling that occurs 30 minutes to several hours after eating.

There are 100 or more diseases that can cause diarrhea, including viral and bacterial infections, diseases of the gastrointestinal tract, or various hormone and metabolic disturbances. What is experienced most frequently, however, is a mild, two-day illness sometimes associated with loss of appetite, abdominal cramps, nausea and vomiting, usually caused by an intestinal virus. Rest in bed, plenty of fluids, and perhaps a drug such as paregoric to reduce diarrhea and abdominal cramps are what's needed to treat mild cases. Diarrhea lasting more than two days should be treated by a physician.

On the opposite side of the coin, of course, is constipation. Simple constipation results most often from improper diet, inadequate fluid intake, possibly lack of exercise, or a change in habits during travel. Laxatives can help get things moving again, but they should not be used too often. Overuse of laxatives can impair normal bowel function. Acute abdominal pain and vomiting could be symptoms of a serious condition such as appendicitis. Laxatives should never be used to treat such symptoms.

Much has been said about adding fiber to the diet to relieve constipation as well as a number of other bowel problems. Eating more whole grain breads, cereals, fruits, and fresh vegetables can add bulk to the diet, and that does help prevent constipation. However, too much fiber can have distressing side effects such as a feeling of being "stuffed" or "bloated." Large amounts of fiber also can impair the body's ability to absorb certain important minerals such as iron, copper, and calcium.

Lack of dietary fiber and overuse of laxatives are thought to lead to hemorrhoids, that universal and much maligned condition of the nether end of the GI tract. Whether increasing the fiber in the diet does any good for hemorrhoids is a matter of conjecture, but there are a number of OTC products that will relieve pain and itching, reduce swelling, and protect inflamed tissues.

Minor gastrointestinal upsets, such as those described above, are rarely serious, but there are some very serious, even life-threatening digestive diseases that are major health problems. According to the National Institute of Arthritis, Diabetes and Digestive and Kidney Diseases (NIADDK), some 20 million Americans are chronically ill due to digestive disease, and more people are hospitalized because of these conditions than for any other group of disorders. The economic cost is enormous: $17 billion yearly in medical care, $35 billion in lost wages. Approximately 200,000 deaths a year are attributed to digestive diseases.

Among the major digestive diseases are hiatal hernia, peptic ulcer, cirrhosis of the liver, gallstones, Crohn's disease, ulcerative colitis, and diverticulitis.

A hernia is the protrusion of an organ through a wall of the cavity in which it is enclosed. In the case of a hiatal hernia, it is the stomach that protrudes, and the hole through which it goes is a teardrop-shaped opening in the diaphragm where the esophagus and stomach join.

Hiatal hernia may develop in people of all ages and both sexes, although it is considered to be a condition of middle age. The most frequent cause is an increased pressure in the abdominal cavity produced by coughing, vomiting, straining at stool or sudden physical exertion. Pregnancy, obesity, or excess fluid in the abdomen also contribute to causing this condition. The hernia itself is painless. What brings the patient to the doctor is heartburn and indigestion caused by esophagitis, an irritation of the esophagus from stomach acid that is often, but not always, associated with hiatal hernia.

Most hiatal hernias do not need treatment. However, if the hernia is complicated by esophagitis, treatment is necessary because ulceration and scarring of the esophagus may eventually develop, making it impossible for the patient to swallow food. Most cases respond to antacids, bland diet, weight reduction and common sense about eating, drinking, and other living habits. If symptoms persist, surgery can restore the stomach to its proper position and strengthen the area around the opening.

A peptic ulcer is a crater-like sore in the lining of the esophagus, stomach, or duodenum, i.e., those areas bathed by the acid and pepsin in the digestive juices. The action of the acid on the sore place is what causes the pain. Duodenal ulcer occurs eight times more often than stomach or gastric ulcer. Why this is so is not fully understood. Anxiety, stress, alcohol, coffee, and aspirin can stimulate the flow of gastric acid even when there is no food in the stomach.

The most common symptom of duodenal ulcers is a steady gnawing or burning pain in a small area of the abdomen between the navel and lower end of the breast bone. This pain usually starts within 30 minutes to two hours after eating and can usually be relieved by eating more food or by taking antacids. Ulcer treatment is aimed at reducing the amount of acid or irritants in the stomach. Drugs such as antacids are used to neutralize the acid. Atropine or related drugs block nervous stimulation of stomach acid secretion. Cimetidine (Tagamet), in 1981 the No. 1 selling prescription drug in the nation, blocks the response to histamine, a chemical in the body that is a powerful stimulator of gastric acid. FDA recently approved a new drug, sucralfate (Carafate) that acts by forming a protective coating over the ulcer, preventing the digestive action of acid and pepsin.

Cirrhosis of the liver is a degenerative disease in which liver cells are damaged and replaced by scar tissue. When normal tissue is lost, the organ can't carry on some of its important work such as processing and disposal of nutrients, hormones, drugs, and toxins.

Chronic alcoholism is the most common cause of cirrhosis in the United States, but the disease may also result from hepatitis, other viruses, some chemicals and poisons, an excess of iron or copper in the system, or obstruction of the bile duct. The onset of the disease may be "silent," symptoms not appearing until the disease is far advanced. The patient may experience fatigue, weakness and exhaustion, loss of appetite and weight, jaundice, intense itching, abdominal distention, and copious hemorrhage from rupture of dilated veins in the esophagus.

Treatment depends on the type and stage of the cirrhosis and may include a strict diet, diuretics to decrease fluid retention, vitamins and, naturally, avoidance of alcohol. In some cases, surgery may be required to deal with the complications.

Gallstones are formed by aggregation of cholesterol, bile pigment, or calcium, or combinations of these, in the gallbladder. Their size can range from that of a pinhead to a golfball. When these stones get stuck in the bile ducts leading to the duodenum, the gallbladder and the duct try to dislodge them by muscular contractions, thereby causing severe abdominal pain. Blockage of the duct prevents flow of bile to the intestines and causes bile to back up in the bloodstream.

Gallstones are more common in people over 40, particularly in women and the obese. Surgery to remove the gallbladder is the traditional treatment for gallstones. Experimental drugs now being tested might prove effective in dissolving gallstones.

Crohn's disease and ulcerative colitis are two severe diseases of the intestines that have many things in common. The cause of neither is known, and each tends to occur most often in young people and to run in families. Neither is contagious. Both diseases can produce ailments outside the intestines such as skin changes, arthritis and eye inflammation.

Crohn's disease affects both the small and large intestines and is characterized by a thickening and inflammation of all layers of the intestinal wall. Since sections of diseased bowel often occur between normal sections, the disease is sometimes called regional enteritis. When the colon is the site of disease, it is called granulomatous colitis.

Symptoms of the disease may include anemia, abdominal pain, bloating, fever, diarrhea and malnutrition. Long hospitalization is common. Surgery may be required to remove diseased sections of the bowel, but the disease tends to recur in the remaining bowel. A long-term study sponsored by NIADDK has found sulfasalazine and prednisone to be effective in inducing remissions in some cases, but not in preventing exacerbation (increase in severity) of the disease.

Ulcerative colitis is an inflammation of all or part of the colon, or large bowel. The most common symptoms are abdominal cramps and bloody diarrhea. There also may be weight loss, anemia and loss of body fluids and minerals.

In general, treatment of ulcerative colitis is aimed at correcting malnutrition and halting the constant loss of blood, fluids, and mineral salts. This calls for administration of intravenous fluids, or certain steroid drugs and antibiotics. Sulfasalazine may be prescribed over a long period to control symptoms and prevent recurrent attacks. In some severe cases surgical removal of the colon may be necessary.

Some scientists believe the Western diet of refined foods leads to diverticulosis—sac-like pouchings in the colon. Although most people with diverticulosis notice no symptoms or complications, about 15 percent develop an inflammation called diverticulitis. This occurs more often in men than women and more often on the left side of the body than on the right.

The symptoms are like those of appendicitis or colon cancer—crampy or steady pain and local tenderness. Many attacks are mild and pass without treatment. In other cases there may be a rupture of the pouches into the abdominal cavity with a small amount of bleeding. Heavy bleeding from erosion of a large blood vessel may occur, but is uncommon. Inflammation can produce abscesses and fistulas, that is, abnormal pathways into other nearby organs, or can lead to a narrowing of the colon with partial or complete obstruction of the channel.

Medical treatment of acute diverticulitis involves putting the colon "at rest"—that is, the patient takes no food by mouth. Antibiotics are given to fight infection. Surgery may be required in chronic cases. At one time, it was thought that a bland diet was the way to treat diverticulosis, but now doctors tend to agree that more bulk is what is needed.

There are, of course, many other digestive disorders, some caused by infectious diseases, others by parasites. Inborn errors of metabolism can interfere with the proper absorption of certain foods. The condition of the teeth and the state of emotions also can have an effect on the digestive system. Cancer can develop almost anywhere along that 30-foot route.

Automatic as it may be, the digestive system is not something to be taken for granted.

Annabel Hecht, *FDA Consumer*, Vol. 16, No. 4, May 1982.

Glaucoma

Keeping An Eye On Glaucoma

Glaucoma is a relatively common eye disease which, if allowed to run its course, causes blindness. It is more prevalent in people over 40 and is often hereditary. However, as this article points out, the disease can be controlled with drugs or surgery.

Glaucoma is a well-hidden disease of the eye that bears watching. Glaucoma hides well because it works silently. For the most part, it provides no cosmetic signs of distress. But once discovered, it must be watched carefully and controlled with drugs or by surgery.

Glaucoma is simply pressure that builds up within the eye, threatening that complex mechanism's ability to function. The pressure that builds up is from an excess of aqueous humor—a liquid that circulates in the eye, providing nourishment to the tissues. For several reasons, that circulation system may become impaired, and the fluid has nowhere to go or drains too slowly. The increased pressure within the eye also puts a crimp on the blood supply to the optic nerve, which is the nerve of vision. Without the necessary supply of blood, the optic nerve becomes damaged, resulting in a loss in the field of vision for the victim. If the damage continues, the optic nerve, which sends impulses to the brain, dies and blindness results.

Glaucoma is one of the leading causes of blindness in this country. It need not be. The disease can be contained if diagnosed and treated soon enough. Early detection sometimes means looking back on the family genes (for some glaucoma is hereditary), observing the 40th birthday (glaucoma occurs most frequently—but not only—in individuals over that age), and of course having the eyes tested for aqueous humor pressure. Other signs of glaucoma may be loss of peripheral, or side, vision and delayed ability to adjust to semi-darkness or low light levels.

The most common form of the disease is called open angle or chronic simple glaucoma. Usually inherited, it results from the failure of the eye to drain the aqueous humor fast enough. It most often affects both eyes, and generally can be controlled by drugs.

Acute congestive or closed angle glaucoma almost invariably requires surgery for correction. That's because it is caused by physical blockage of the drainage area. Drugs may be used in closed angle glaucoma to alleviate the blockage. For example, a pupil-constricting drug may open up some of the drainage area that would be blocked by a normal-sized pupil. However, for the most part, surgeons need to get in and force openings. Congestive glaucoma also is often hereditary, with the individual's particular inherited pattern of growth tending to shut off the drainage canal.

Symptoms of acute congestive or closed angle glaucoma are usually less sneaky than those of simple glaucoma. Unless simple glaucoma goes undetected for a long time, there is no pain associated with it. However, with acute congestive glaucoma, the symptoms may begin with mild attacks that include blurred vision and some mild discomfort. They progress to severe attacks that may include pain extreme enough to induce vomiting, blurred vision with a red eye, and seeing halos around lights. The attacks will continue until medical treatment or surgery relieves them.

Other than being inherited, glaucoma can be caused by trauma (a blow to the head or eye), prolonged dilation of the pupil, and even emotional upset. Secondary glaucoma can also result from illness, infection, or cataracts. In addition, glaucoma can be a congenital defect, so it is not limited to 40-year-olds and beyond.

Chronic simple or open-angle glaucoma accounts for the vast majority of the cases of the disease—estimates range beyond 90 percent—with a fourth or more of the victims unaware of it. Just how many glaucoma patients there are in the United States and just how prevalent is the disease are two unknowns or at least two debatables. The National Society to Prevent Blindness estimates that 2 million Americans have the disease and that 60,000 have been blinded by it. But some researchers have come to the conclusion that true prevalence figures are elusive.

There is also debate over just how high the intraocular eye pressure has to be before the glaucoma diagnosis can be made. The conventional ophthalmologic wisdom has been that a pressure of 21 millimeters of mercury means that it's time to start thinking of treatment, a reading of 24 being considered in the glaucomatous level. However, many in the profession are quick to point out that different eyes can tolerate different levels of pressure.

A reading in the 10 to 20 mm range is considered normal. Readings can vary depending on a number of factors, including the time of day. Extremely low readings are also danger signs, as without the pressure the eye would collapse. The pressure is measured through tonometry, in which the force necessary to indent the eye is measured. This is done by devices pressed against or into the eye after it is anesthetized, or by measuring the force needed to penetrate the eye when a puff of air is blown into it.

High pressure isn't a sure sign of glaucoma. Indeed, only 5 to 10 percent of those with pressures above 21 may develop visual field loss and glaucoma. That's why a pressure reading must be followed by an eye specialist looking into the eye for signs of damage and by field of vision tests being given to discern signs of developing tunnel vision. Recently, an FDA advisory subcommittee on ophthalmology decried the medical practice of putting individuals on a new glaucoma treatment drug just because they had elevated pressures. The subcommittee recommended that Timoptic, the new and extremely popular pressure-controlling drug that is a beta blocker, be prescribed only for individuals "who are at a sufficient risk to require that intraocular pressure be lowered."

(The debate about intraocular eye pressure levels and glaucoma serves to illustrate just how insidious glaucoma can be. While the argument is basically about where in the low 20's glaucoma starts, it is significant to note that it usually takes a reading in the 40's for an individual to notice any pain from the pressure. In other words, a reading of, say, 35 would be intolerable medically but bearable to the individual. In fact, the individual wouldn't feel a thing, although a few hours at that pressure could leave permanent damage.)

Surgery to alleviate eye pressure usually consists merely of opening up drainage areas; however, two novel ideas have been offered recently. One involves implanting a tiny plastic valve into the eye to permit the aqueous humor to bypass blocked veins. It is used for a severe form of glaucoma in which blood vessels and other tissue grow over the drainage area.

The other surgical innovation is essentially nonsurgical; at least, it doesn't require a full-scale operation. Instead, a laser beam is used to drill a microscopic hole in the iris through which built-up fluid can drain. The laser technique is used mostly on closed angle glaucoma patients. It can be done on an outpatient basis, requiring only eye drops as anesthesia. In a few cases, the hole has filled up but it can be re-drilled.

However, for most glaucoma patients, no such exotic relief is in sight, even temporarily. The majority of the victims of the disease with the open-angle glaucoma find themselves on maintenance drugs—for the rest of their lives. The drugs cover a wide range. Most are in the form of eye drops, but some come in pill form to be taken orally. One drug may come in several strengths, and several drugs may be used together. They also do different jobs: Most are designed to cut down the output of fluid; others may increase the outflow.

Timoptic, which has the generic name of timolol maleate, is by far the most popular of the glaucoma maintenance drugs right now. Some 4 million prescriptions were written for it in 1979, according to the National Prescription Audit. Half of the glaucoma patients in the country who are being treated by drugs are on Timoptic, the National Disease and Therapeutic Index indicates.

Timoptic was first marketed in August 1978 and hailed as a breakthrough drug. Prescriptions were written rapidly because the drug produced no signs of the side effects associated with other glaucoma treatment agents. In 1979, new prescriptions totaled 1.1 million.

The manufacturer, Merck Sharp & Dohme, touted its new product for its effectiveness and lack of side effects. The firm offers the product in .25 percent and .5 percent solutions, packaged in plastic containers that are squeezed from the bottom. The 5 milliliter vial (about a teaspoon) sells at retail for $8 and $9; a 10 cc version is also available. The drops are taken once or twice a day, usually one drop at a time.

The manufacturer said the only adverse reactions from the drug are mild ocular irritation and a slight reduction of the resting heart rate. In the PHYSICIANS' DESK REFERENCE FOR OPHTHALMOLOGY, the firm said that actions of the drug are not completely known but that it reduces fluid formation and also seems to increase outflow.

According to the PDR, the firm's multi-clinic studies showed that Timoptic was 61 percent more effective in reducing pressure compared to 32 percent for pilocarpine (now the second most popular drug). Timoptic's reductions in pressure were 30.7 percent on an average, while pilocarpine averaged 21.7 percent reductions. Compared to epinephrine, the other most popular eye drop, Timoptic was better (69 percent compared to 42 percent) in reducing pressure, and better (33.2 percent to 28.1 percent) in the amount reduced.

However, adverse reaction reports collected by FDA's Division of Drug Experience and by the National Registry of Possible Drug Induced Ocular Side Effects show that the drug produces more side effects than the manufacturer had found in its pre-market testing. Those side effects included problems associated with nerves, digestion, vision, skin, respiration, and the heart. As a result, FDA has called upon the manufacturer to change the physician's labeling (essentially what is carried in the PDR cited above) to warn of some of these possible adverse reactions.

Pilocarpine, the No. 2 glaucoma treatment agent, was used by slightly better than one-fourth of the glaucoma patients, according to the National Disease and Therapeutic Index. Prescriptions in 1979 totaled 3.2 million for glaucoma. It has been in use for over 100 years and comes in strengths of ½, 1, 2.4, and 6 percent. The drops must be applied three or four times a day. Used for both open- and closed-angle cases, pilocarpine makes the pupil small, thereby increasing the fluid outflow.

Diamox is the trade name for acetazolamide and it is the No. 1 selling oral drug. It serves to cut the fluid production. Slightly more than a half million prescriptions for glaucoma patients were written for it last year. Older patients often prefer tablets for their medicine, finding the drops hard to administer. However, Diamox has some adverse effects, such as tingling of the toes and fingers, loss of appetite, drowsiness, and mental confusion in the short term, and in the long term a lowering of the alkali reserve in the blood.

Neptazane (generic: methazolamide) is another tablet form agent used for all types of glaucoma. It is often used when a postponement of surgery is desired. It, too, has a number of adverse reactions.

Epinephrine, which dilates the pupil, works to inhibit the flow of fluid. The National Disease and Therapeutic Index says that a half million patients used it in 1979. Local side effects include eye pain or ache, headache, and brief eye smarting. It may also be absorbed into the blood circulatory system, causing heart palpitations and nervousness. Epinephrine is prescribed frequently in tandem with pilocarpine.

Other, lesser-used drugs are stronger and are generally prescribed for special cases.

Much has been written and said in recent years about the effect that marijuana has on glaucoma patients. It does reduce intraocular pressure. Just how, is as yet uncertain. The National Eye Institute says that any possible advantages for marijuana over other glaucoma medications have not yet been established. The drug is now used legally to treat glaucoma only in clinical investigations that have been approved by FDA. Thus far, there are no indications that marijuana is the only drug that will do the pressure-lowering job for certain people.

Whatever the therapy, glaucoma will remain a public health concern. That's because of its furtive nature and because it affects so many people, particularly older individuals. However, with early detection and proper care, the disease can be thwarted before it runs its painless, sight-killing course.

Roger W. Miller, Reprinted from *FDA Consumer,* HHS Publication No. (FDA) 80–3105. U.S. Department of Health and Human Services, Public Health Service, Food and Drug Administration, 5600 Fishers Lane, Rockville, Md. 20857. U.S. Government Printing Office 1980—311-254/87.

Headache
Hope Through Research

For two years, Jim suffered the excruciating pain of cluster headaches. Night after night he paced the floor, the pain driving him to constant motion. He was only 48 years old when the clusters forced him to quit his job as a systems analyst. One year later, his headaches are controlled. The credit for Jim's recovery belongs to the medical staff of a headache clinic. Physicians there applied the latest research findings on headache, and prescribed for Jim a combination of new drugs.

- Joan was a victim of frequent migraine. Her headaches lasted two days. Nauseous and weak, she stayed in the dark until each attack was over. Today, although migraine still interferes with her life, she has fewer attacks and less severe headaches than before. A specialist prescribed an antimigraine program for Joan that included improved drug therapy, a new diet, and relaxation training.
- An avid reader, Peggy couldn't put down the new mystery thriller. After four hours of reading slumped in bed, she knew she had overdone it. Her tensed head and neck muscles felt as if they were being squeezed between two giant hands. But for Peggy, the muscle-contraction headache and neck pain were soon relieved by a hot shower and aspirin.

An estimated 40 million Americans experience chronic headaches. For at least half of these people, the problem is severe and sometimes disabling. It can also be costly: headache sufferers make over 8 million visits a year to doctor's offices. Migraine victims alone lose over 64 million workdays because of headache pain.

Understanding why headaches occur and improving headache treatment are among the research goals of the National Institute of Neurological and Communicative Disorders and Stroke (NINCDS). As the focal point for brain research in the Federal Government, the NINCDS also supports and conducts studies to improve the diagnosis of headaches and to find ways to prevent them.

Why does it hurt?

What hurts when you have a headache? Several areas of the head can hurt, including a network of nerves which extends over the scalp and certain nerves in the face, mouth, and throat. Also sensitive to pain, because they contain delicate nerve fibers, are the muscles of the head and blood vessels found along the surface and at the base of the brain.

The bones of the skull and tissues of the brain itself, however, never hurt, because they lack pain-sensitive nerve fibers.

The ends of these pain-sensitive nerves, called *nociceptors,* can be stimulated by stress, muscular tension, dilated blood vessels, and other triggers of headache. Once stimulated, a nociceptor sends a message up the length of the nerve fiber to the nerve cells in the brain, signaling that a part of the body hurts. The message is determined by the location of the nociceptor. A person who suddenly realizes "My toe hurts," is responding to nociceptors in the foot that have been stimulated by the stubbing of a toe.

A number of chemicals help transmit pain-related information to the brain. Some of these chemicals are natural painkilling proteins called endorphins, Greek for "the morphine within." One theory suggests that people who suffer from severe headache and other types of chronic pain have lower levels of endorphins than people who are generally pain free.

When you should see a physician

Not all headaches require medical attention. Some result from missed meals or occasional muscle tension and are easily remedied. But some types of headache are signals of more serious disorders such as head injury and call for prompt medical care. These include
- Sudden, severe headache
- Headache associated with convulsions
- Headache accompanied by confusion or loss of consciousness
- Headache following a blow on the head
- Headache associated with pain in the eye or ear
- Persistent headache in a person who was previously headache-free
- Recurring headache in children
- Headache associated with fever
- Headache which interferes with normal life

A headache sufferer usually seeks help from a family practitioner. If the problem is not relieved by standard treatments, the patient may then be referred to a specialist—perhaps an internist or neurologist. Additional referrals may be made to psychologists.

Diagnosis: what the physician looks for

Diagnosing a headache is like playing Twenty Questions. Experts agree that a detailed question-and-answer session with a patient can often produce enough information for a diagnosis. Many types of headaches have clear-cut symptoms which fall into an easily recognizable pattern.

Patients may be asked: How often do you have headaches? Where is the pain? How long do the headaches last? When did you first develop headaches?

The patient's sleep habits and family and work situations may also be probed.

Most physicians will also obtain a full medical history from the patient, inquiring about past head trauma or surgery and about the use of medications. A blood test may be ordered to screen for thyroid disease, anemia, or infections which might cause a headache. X-rays may be taken to rule out the possibility of a brain tumor or blood clot.

A test called an electroencephalogram (EEG) may be given to measure brain activity. EEG's can indicate a malfunction in the brain, but they cannot usually pinpoint a problem that might be causing a headache.

A physician may suggest that a patient with unusual headaches undergo a computed tomographic (CT) scan. The CT scan produces images of the brain that show variations in the density of different types of tissue. The scan enables the physician to distinguish, for example, between a bleeding blood vessel in the brain and a brain tumor. The CT scan is an important diagnostic tool in cases of headache associated with brain lesions or other serious disease. Experts generally agree, however, that this sophisticated and expensive technology is not required to diagnose simple or periodic headache.

An eye exam is usually performed to check for weakness in the eye muscle or unequal pupil size. Both of these symptoms are evidence of an aneurysm—an abnormal ballooning of a blood vessel. A physician who suspects that a headache patient has an aneurysm may also order an angiogram. In this test, a special fluid which can be seen on an X-ray is injected into the patient and carried in the bloodstream to the brain to reveal any abnormalities in the blood vessels there.

Thermography, an experimental technique for diagnosing headache, promises to become a useful clinical tool. In thermography, an infrared camera converts skin temperature into a color picture or thermogram with different degrees of heat appearing as different colors. Skin temperature is affected primarily by blood flow. Research scientists have found that thermograms of headache patients show strikingly different heat patterns from those of people who never or rarely get headaches.

A physician analyzes the results of all these diagnostic tests along with a patient's medical history in order to arrive at a diagnosis.

Headaches are diagnosed as

• Vascular
• Muscle contraction
• Traction
• Inflammatory

Vascular headaches—a group that includes the well-known migraine—are so named because they are thought to involve abnormal function of the brain's blood vessels or vascular system. Muscle contraction headaches appear to involve the tightening or tensing of facial and neck muscles. Traction and inflammatory headaches are symptoms of other disorders, ranging from stroke to sinus infection. Some people have more than one type of headache.

Migraine headaches: A painful malady

The most common type of vascular headache is *migraine*. Migraine headaches are usually characterized by severe pain on one or both sides of the head, an upset stomach, and at times disturbed vision.

Basketball star Kareem Abdul-Jabbar remembers experiencing his first migraine at age 14. The pain was unlike the discomfort of his previous mild headaches.

"When I got this one I thought, '*This* is a headache'," he says. "The pain was intense and I felt nausea and a great sensitivity to light. All I could think about was when it would stop. I sat in a dark room for an hour and it passed."

Symptoms of Migraine   Abdul-Jabbar's sensitivity to light is a standard symptom of the two most prevalent types of migraine-caused headache: *classic* and *common*.

The major difference between the two types is the appearance of neurological symptoms 10 to 30 minutes before a classic migraine attack. These symptoms are called an *aura*. The person may see flashing lights or zigzag lines, or may temporarily lose vision. Other classic symptoms include speech difficulty, weakness of an arm or leg, tingling of the face or hands, and confusion.

The pain of a classic migraine headache is described as intense, throbbing, or pounding and is felt in the forehead, temple, ear, jaw, or around the eye. Classic migraine starts on one side of the head but may eventually spread to the other side. An attack lasts one to two painwracked days.

The common migraine—a term that reflects the disorder's greater occurrence in the general population—is not preceded by an aura. But some people experience a variety of vague symptoms beforehand, including mental fuzziness, mood changes, fatigue, and unusual retention of fluids. During the headache phase of a common migraine, a person may have diarrhea and increased urination, as well as nausea and vomiting. Common migraine pain can last three or four days.

Both classic and common migraine can strike as often as several times a week, or as rarely as once every few years. Both types can occur at any time. Some people, however, experience migraines at predictable times—near the days of menstruation or every Saturday morning after a stressful week of work.

The Migraine Process   Research scientists are unclear about the precise cause of migraine headaches. There seems to be general agreement, however, that a key element is blood flow changes in the brain. People who get migraine headaches appear to have blood vessels that overreact to various triggers.

Scientists have devised one theory of migraine which explains these blood flow changes and also certain biochemical changes that may be involved in the headache process. According to this theory, the nervous system responds to a trigger such as stress by creating a spasm in the nerve-rich arteries at the base of the brain. The spasm closes down or constricts several arteries supplying blood to the brain, including the scalp artery and the carotid or neck arteries.

As these arteries constrict, the flow of blood to the brain is reduced. At the same time, blood-clotting particles called platelets clump together—a process which is believed to release a chemical called serotonin. Serotonin acts as a powerful constrictor of arteries, further reducing the blood supply to the brain.

Reduced blood flow decreases the brain's supply of oxygen. Symptoms signaling a headache, such as distorted vision or speech, may then result, similar to symptoms of stroke.

Reacting to the reduced oxygen supply, certain arteries within the brain open wider to meet the brain's energy needs. This widening or dilation spreads, finally affecting the neck and scalp arteries. The dilation of these arteries triggers the release of pain-producing substances called *prostaglandins* from various tissues and blood cells. Chemicals which cause inflammation and swelling, and substances which increase sensitivity to pain are also released. The circulation of these chemicals and the dilation of the scalp arteries stimulate the pain-sensitive nociceptors. The result, according to this theory: a throbbing pain in the head.

Women and Migraine Although boys and girls seem to be equally affected by migraine, the condition is more common in adult women than in men. Both sexes may develop migraine in infancy, but most often the disorder begins between the ages of 5 and 35.

The relationship between female hormones and migraine is still unclear. Women may have "menstrual migraine"—headaches around the time of their menstrual period—which may disappear during pregnancy. Other women develop migraine for the first time when they are pregnant. Some are first affected after menopause.

The effect of oral contraceptives on headaches is perplexing. Scientists report that some migrainous women who take birth control pills experience more frequent and severe attacks. However, a small percentage of women have fewer and less severe migraine headaches when they take birth control pills. And normal women who do not suffer from headaches may develop migraines as a side effect when they use oral contraceptives. Investigators around the world are studying hormonal changes in migrainous women in the hope of identifying the specific ways these naturally occurring chemicals cause headaches.

Triggers of Headache The existence of a migraine personality is a controversial theory which suggests that migraine patients are compulsive, rigid, and perfectionistic. Most scientists believe, however, that not all migraine patients have these traits and that not all individuals with these personality characteristics have migraine.

Rather than focusing on character traits, says one headache specialist, it would be better to view people who get migraines as having an inherited abnormality in the regulation of blood vessels. Many sufferers have a family history of migraine, but the exact hereditary nature of this condition is still unknown.

"It's like a cocked gun with a hair trigger," explains the specialist. "A person is born with a potential for migraine and the headache is triggered by things that are really not so terrible."

These triggers include stress and other normal emotions, as well as biological and environmental conditions. Fatigue, glaring or flickering lights, the weather, and even certain foods can set off migraine. It may seem hard to believe that eating such seemingly harmless foods as yogurt, nuts, and lima beans can result in a painful migraine headache. However, some scientists believe that these foods and several others contain chemical substances such as tyramine which constrict arteries—the first step of the migraine process. Other scientists believe that foods cause headaches by setting off an allergic reaction in susceptible people.

While a food-triggered migraine usually occurs soon after eating, other triggers may not cause immediate pain. Scientists report that people can develop migraine not only during a period of stress but also afterwards when their vascular systems are still reacting. The "Preacher Monday-Morning Headache" is named for those clergymen who get migraines a day after the stress of delivering a Sunday sermon. Migraines that wake people up in the middle of the night are also believed to result from a delayed reaction to stress.

Other Forms of Migraine In addition to classic and common, migraine headache can take several other forms:

Patients with *hemiplegic migraine* have temporary paralysis on one side of the body, a condition known as hemiplegia. Some people may experience vision problems and vertigo—a feeling that the world is spinning. These symptoms begin 10 to 90 minutes before the onset of headache pain.

In *ophthalmoplegic migraine,* the pain is around the eye and is associated with a droopy eyelid, double vision, and other sight problems.

Basilar artery migraine involves a disturbance of a major brain artery. Preheadache symptoms include vertigo, double vision, and poor muscular coordination. This type of migraine occurs primarily in adolescent and young adult women and is often associated with the menstrual cycle.

Benign exertional headache is brought on by running, lifting, coughing, sneezing, or bending. The headache begins at the onset of activity, and pain rarely lasts more than several minutes.

Status migrainosus is a rare and severe type of migraine that can last 72 hours or longer. The pain and nausea are so intense that people who have this type of headache must be hospitalized. The use of certain drugs can trigger status migrainosus. Neurologists report that many of their status migrainosus patients were depressed and anxious before they experienced headache attacks.

Headache-free migraine is characterized by such migraine symptoms as visual problems, nausea, vomiting, constipation, or diarrhea. Patients, however, do not experience head pain. Headache specialists have suggested that unexplained pain in a particular part of the body, fever, and dizziness could also be possible types of headache-free migraine.

Treating migraine headache

During the Stone Age, pieces of a headache sufferer's skull were cut away with flint instruments to relieve pain. Another unpleasant remedy used in the British Isles around the ninth century involved drinking "the juice of elderseed, cow's brain, and goat's dung dissolved in vinegar." Fortunately, today's headache patients are spared such drastic measures.

Drug therapy, biofeedback training, stress reduction, and elimination of certain foods from the diet are the most common methods of preventing and controlling migraine and other vascular headaches. Joan, the migraine sufferer, was helped by treatment with a combination of an antimigraine drug and diet control.

Regular exercise, such as swimming or vigorous walking, can also reduce the frequency and severity of migraine headaches. Joan found that yoga and whirlpool baths helped her relax.

During a migraine headache, temporary relief can sometimes be obtained by using cold packs or by pressing on the bulging artery found in front of the ear on the painful side of the head.

Drug Therapy There are two ways to approach the treatment of migraine headache with drugs: prevent the attacks, or relieve symptoms after the headache occurs.

For infrequent migraine, drugs can be taken at the first sign of a headache in order to stop it or to at least ease the pain. People who get occasional mild migraine may benefit by taking aspirin or acetaminophen at the start of an attack. Aspirin raises a person's tolerance to pain and also discourages clumping of blood platelets. Small amounts of caffeine may be useful if taken in the early stages of migraine. But for most migraine sufferers who get moderate to severe headaches, and for all cluster patients, stronger drugs may be necessary to control the pain.

One of the most commonly used drugs for the relief of classic and common migraine symptoms is ergotamine tartrate, a vasoconstrictor which helps counteract the painful dilation stage of the headache. For optimal benefit, the drug is taken during the early stages of an attack. If a migraine has been in progress for about an hour and has passed into the final throbbing stage, ergotamine tartrate will probably not help.

Because ergotamine tartrate can cause nausea and vomiting, it may be combined with antinausea drugs. Research scientists caution that ergotamine tartrate should not be taken in excess or by people who have angina pectoris, severe hypertension, or vascular, liver, or kidney disease.

Patients who are unable to take ergotamine tartrate may benefit from other drugs that constrict dilated blood vessels or help reduce blood vessel inflammation.

For headaches that occur three or more times a month, preventive treatment is usually recommended. Drugs used to prevent classic and common migraine include methysergide maleate, which counteracts blood vessel constriction, propranolol, which stops blood vessel dilation, and amitriptyline, an antidepressant.

In a study of propranolol, amitriptyline, and biofeedback conducted by the Houston Headache Clinic, scientists found that migraine patients improved most on a combination of propranolol and biofeedback. Patients who had mixed migraine and muscle-contraction headaches received the greatest benefit from a combination of propranolol, amitriptyline, and biofeedback.

Another recent study showed that propranolol may continue to prevent migraine headaches even after patients have stopped taking the drug. The scientists who conducted the study speculate that long-term therapy with propranolol may have a lasting effect on blood vessels, training them to react less than usual to the triggers of migraine.

Antidepressants called MAO inhibitors also prevent migraine. These drugs block an enzyme called mono-amine oxidase, which normally helps nerve cells absorb the artery-constricting chemical, serotonin.

MAO inhibitors can have potentially serious side effects—particularly if taken while ingesting foods or beverages that contain tyramine, a substance that closes down arteries.

Several new drugs for the prevention of migraine have been developed in recent years, including papaverine hydrochloride, which produces blood vessel dilation, and cyproheptadine, which counteracts serotonin.

All these antimigraine drugs can have adverse side effects. But they are relatively safe when used carefully. To avoid long-term side effects of preventive medications, headache specialists advise patients to reduce the dosage of these drugs and then to stop taking them as soon as possible.

Biofeedback and Relaxation Training Drug therapy for migraine is often combined with biofeedback and relaxation training. Biofeedback is a space-age word for a technique that can give people better control over such body function indicators as blood pressure, heart rate, temperature, muscle tension, and brain waves. *Thermal biofeedback* allows a patient to consciously raise hand temperature. Some patients who are able to increase hand temperature can reduce the number and intensity of migraines. The mechanism of this hand-warming effect is being studies by research scientists.

"To succeed in biofeedback," says a headache specialist, "you must be able to concentrate and you must be motivated to get well."

A patient learning thermal biofeedback wears a device which transmits the temperature of an index finger or hand to a monitor. While the patient tries to warm his hands, the monitor provides feedback either on a gauge that shows the temperature reading or by emitting a sound or beep that increases in intensity as the temperature increases. The patient is not told how to raise hand temperature, but is given suggestions such as "Imagine that your hands feel very warm and heavy."

"I have a good imagination," says one headache sufferer who traded in her medication for thermal biofeedback. The technique decreased the number and severity of headaches she experienced.

In another type of biofeedback called *electromyographic or EMG training,* the patient learns to control muscle tension in the face, neck, and shoulders.

Either kind of biofeedback may be combined with relaxation training, during which patients learn to relax the mind and body.

Biofeedback can be practiced at home with a portable monitor. But the ultimate goal of treatment is to wean the patient from the machine. The patient can then use biofeedback anywhere at the first sign of a headache.

The Antimigraine Diet   Scientists estimate that a small percentage of migraine sufferers will benefit from a treatment program focused solely on eliminating headache-provoking foods and beverages.

Other migraine patients may be helped by a diet to prevent low blood sugar. Low blood sugar, or hypoglycemia, can cause dilation of the blood vessels in the head. This condition can occur after a period without food: overnight, for example, or when a meal is skipped. People who wake up in the morning with a headache may be reacting to the low blood sugar caused by the lack of food overnight.

Treatment for headaches caused by low blood sugar consists of scheduling smaller, more frequent meals for the patient. A special diet designed to stabilize the body's sugar-regulating system is sometimes recommended.

For the same reason, many specialists also recommend that migraine patients avoid oversleeping on weekends. Sleeping late can change the body's normal blood sugar level and lead to a headache.

Beyond migraine: Other vascular headaches

After migraine, the most common type of vascular headache is the toxic headache produced by fever. Pneumonia, measles, mumps, and tonsillitis are among the diseases that can cause severe toxic vascular headaches. Toxic headaches can also result from the presence of foreign chemicals in the body. Other kinds of vascular headaches include "clusters," which cause repeated episodes of intense pain, and headaches resulting from a rise in blood pressure.

Chemical Culprits   Repeated exposure to nitrite compounds can result in a dull, pounding headache that may be accompanied by a flushed face. Nitrite, which dilates blood vessels, is found in such products as heart medicine and dynamite. Hot dogs and other meats containing sodium nitrite can also cause headaches.

"Chinese restaurant headache" can occur when a susceptible individual eats foods prepared with monosodium glutamate (MSG)—a staple in many Oriental kitchens. Soy sauce, meat tenderizer, and a variety of packaged foods contain this chemical which is touted as a flavor enhancer.

Vascular headache can also result from exposure to poisons, even common household varieties like insecticides, carbon tetrachloride, and lead. Children who eat flakes of lead paint may develop headaches. So may anyone who has contact with lead batteries or lead-glazed pottery.

Painters, printmakers, and other artists may experience headaches after exposure to art materials that contain chemicals called solvents. Solvents, like benzene, are found in turpentine, spray adhesives, rubber cement, and inks.

Drugs such as amphetamines can cause headaches as a side effect. Another type of drug-related headache occurs during withdrawal from long-term therapy with the anti-migraine drug ergotamine tartrate.

Jokes are often made about alcohol hangovers, but the headache associated with "the morning after" is no laughing matter. Fortunately, there are several suggested remedies for the pain, including ergotamine tartrate. The hangover headache may also be reduced by taking honey, which speeds alcohol metabolism, or caffeine, a constrictor of dilated arteries. Caffeine, however, can cause headaches as well as cure them. Heavy coffee drinkers often get headaches when they try to break the caffeine habit.

Cluster Headaches   Cluster headaches, named for their repeated occurrence in groups or clusters, begin as a minor pain around one eye, eventually spreading to that side of the face. The pain quickly intensifies, compelling the victim to pace the floor or rock in a chair. "You can't lie down, you're fidgety," explains a cluster patient. "The pain is unbearable." Other symptoms include a stuffed and runny nose and a droopy eyelid over a red and tearing eye.

Cluster headaches last between 30 and 45 minutes. But the relief people feel at the end of an attack is usually mixed with dread as they await a recurrence. Clusters can strike several times a day or night for several weeks or months. Then, mysteriously, they may disappear for months or years. Many people have cluster bouts during the spring and fall. At their worst, chronic cluster headaches can last continuously for years.

Cluster attacks can strike at any age but usually start between the ages of 20 and 40. Unlike migraine, cluster headaches are more common in men and do not run in families. Research scientists have observed certain physical similarities among people who experience cluster headache. The typical cluster patient is a tall, muscular man with a rugged facial appearance and a square, jutting or dimpled chin. The texture of his coarse skin resembles an orange peel. Women who get clusters may also have this type of skin.

Studies of cluster patients show that they are likely to have hazel eyes and that they tend to be heavy smokers and drinkers. Paradoxically, both nicotine, which constricts arteries, and alcohol, which dilates them, trigger cluster headaches. The exact connection between these substances and cluster attacks is not known.

Despite a cluster headache's distinguishing characteristics, its relative infrequency and similarity to such disorders as sinusitis can lead to misdiagnosis. Some cluster patients have had tooth extractions, sinus surgery, or psychiatric treatment in a futile effort to cure their pain.

Research studies have turned up several clues as to the cause of cluster headache, but no answers. One clue is found in the thermograms of untreated cluster patients, which show a "cold spot" of reduced blood flow above the eye.

The sudden start and brief duration of cluster headaches can make them difficult to treat. By the time medicine is absorbed into the body, the attack is often over. However, research scientists have identified several effective drugs for these headaches. The antimigraine drug ergotamine tartrate can subdue a cluster, if taken at the first sign of an attack. Injections of dihydroergotamine, a form of ergotamine tartrate, are sometimes used to treat clusters.

Some cluster patients can prevent attacks by taking propranolol or methysergide. Investigators have also discovered that mild solutions of cocaine hydrochloride applied inside the nose can quickly stop cluster headaches in most patients. This treatment may work because it both blocks pain impulses and it constricts blood vessels.

Another option that works for some cluster patients is rapid inhalation of pure oxygen through a mask for 5 to 15 minutes. The oxygen seems to ease the pain of cluster headache by reducing blood flow to the brain.

In chronic cases of cluster headache, certain facial nerves may be surgically cut or destroyed to provide relief. These procedures have had limited success. Some cluster patients have had facial nerves cut only to have them regenerate years later.

Painful Pressure   Chronic high blood pressure can cause headache, as can rapid rises in blood pressure like those experienced during anger, vigorous exercise, or sexual excitement.

The severe "orgasmic headache" occurs right before orgasm and is believed to be a vascular type. Since sudden rupture of a cerebral blood vessel can also occur during orgasm, this type of headache should be promptly evaluated by a doctor.

Muscle-contraction headaches: The everyday menace

It's 5:00 P.M. and your boss has just asked you to prepare a 20-page briefing paper. Due date: tomorrow. You're angry and tired and the more you think about the assignment, the tenser you become. Your teeth clinch, your brow wrinkles, and soon you have a splitting *tension headache*.

Tension headache is named not only for the role of stress in triggering the pain, but also for the contraction of neck, face, and scalp muscles brought on by stressful events. Tension headache is a severe but temporary form of muscle-contraction headache. The pain is mild to moderate and feels like pressure is being applied to the head or neck. The headache usually disappears after the period of stress is over.

By contrast, chronic muscle-contraction headaches can last for weeks, months, and sometimes years. The pain of these headaches is often described as a tight band around the head or a feeling that the head and neck are in a cast. "It feels like somebody is tightening a giant vise around my head," says one patient. The pain is steady, and is usually felt on both sides of the head. Chronic muscle-contraction headaches can cause sore scalps—even combing one's hair can be painful.

Many scientists believe that the primary cause of the pain of muscle-contraction headache is sustained muscle tension. Other studies suggest that restricted blood flow may cause or contribute to the pain.

Occasionally, muscle-contraction headaches will be accompanied by nausea, vomiting, and blurred vision, but there is no preheadache syndrome as with migraine. Muscle-contraction headaches have not been linked to hormones or foods, as has migraine, nor is there a strong hereditary connection.

Research has shown that for many people, chronic muscle-contraction headaches are caused by depression and anxiety. These people tend to get their headaches in the early morning or evening when conflicts in the office or home are anticipated.

Emotional factors are not the only triggers of muscle-contraction headaches. Certain physical postures—such as holding one's chin down while reading—can lead to head and neck pain. Tensing head and neck muscles during sexual excitement can also cause headache. So can prolonged writing under poor light, or holding a phone between the shoulder and ear, or even gum-chewing.

More serious problems that can cause muscle-contraction headaches include degenerative arthritis of the neck and temporomandibular joint dysfunction, or TMJ. TMJ is a disorder of the joint between the temporal bone (above the ear) and the mandible or lower jaw bone. The disorder results from poor bite and jaw clenching.

Treatment for muscle-contraction headache varies. The first consideration is to treat any specific disorder or disease that may be causing the headache. For example, arthritis of the neck is treated with anti-inflammatory medication, and temporomandibular joint dysfunction may be helped by corrective devices for the mouth and jaw.

Acute tension headaches not associated with a disease are treated with muscle relaxants and analgesics like aspirin and acetaminophen. Stronger analgesics, such as propoxyphene and codeine, are sometimes prescribed. As prolonged use of these drugs can lead to dependence, patients taking them should have periodic medical checkups and follow their physicians' instructions carefully.

Nondrug therapy for chronic muscle-contraction headaches includes biofeedback, relaxation training, and counseling. A technique called *cognitive restructuring* teaches people to change their attitudes and responses to stress. Patients might be encouraged, for example, to imagine that they are coping successfully with a stressful situation. In *progressive relaxation therapy,* patients are taught to first tense and then relax individual muscle groups. Finally, the patient tries to relax his or her whole body. Many people imagine a peaceful scene—such as lying on the beach or by a beautiful lake. *Passive relaxation* does not involve tensing of muscles. Instead, patients are encouraged to focus on different muscles, suggesting that they relax. Some people might think to themselves, *Relax* or *My muscles feel warm.*

People with chronic muscle-contraction headaches may also be helped by taking antidepressants or MAO inhibitors. Mixed muscle-contraction and migraine headaches are sometimes treated with barbiturate compounds, which slow down nerve function in the brain and spinal cord.

People who suffer infrequent muscle-contraction headaches may benefit from a hot shower or moist heat applied to the back of the neck. Cervical collars are sometimes recommended as an aid to good posture. Physical therapy, massage, and gentle exercise of the neck may also be helpful.

When headache is a warning

Like other types of pain, headaches can serve as warning signals of more serious disorders. This is particularly true for headaches caused by traction or inflammation.

Traction headaches can occur if the pain-sensitive parts of the head are pulled, stretched, or displaced, as, for example, when eye muscles are tensed to compensate for eyestrain. Headaches caused by inflammation include those related to meningitis as well as those resulting from diseases of the sinuses, spine, neck, ears, and teeth. Ear and tooth infections and glaucoma can cause headaches. In oral and dental disorders, headache is experienced as pain in the entire head, including the face.

Traction and inflammatory headaches are treated by curing the underlying problem. This may involve surgery, antibiotics or other drugs.

Characteristics of the various types of traction and inflammatory headaches vary by disorder:

- *Brain tumor.* Brain tumors are diagnosed in about 11,000 people every year. As they grow, these tumors sometimes cause headache by pushing on the outer layer of nerve tissue that covers the brain or by pressing against pain-sensitive blood vessel walls. Headache resulting from a brain tumor may be periodic or continuous. Typically, it feels like a strong pressure is being applied to the head. The pain is relieved when the tumor is destroyed by surgery, radiation, or chemotherapy.
- *Stroke.* Headache may accompany several conditions that can lead to stroke, including hypertension or high blood pressure, arteriosclerosis, and heart disease. Headaches are also associated with completed stroke; the latter occurs when brain cells die from lack of sufficient oxygen.

  Many stroke-related headaches can be prevented by careful management of the patient's condition through diet, exercise, and medication.

  Mild to moderate headaches are associated with so-called ''little strokes,'' or transient ischemic attacks (TIA's), which result from a temporary lack of blood supply to the brain. The head pain occurs near the clot or lesion that blocks blood flow.

  The similarity between migraine and symptoms of TIA can cause problems in diagnosis. The rare person under age 40 who suffers a TIA may be misdiagnosed as having migraine; similarly, TIA-prone older patients who suffer migraine may be misdiagnosed as having stroke-related headaches.
- *Spinal tap.* About one-fourth of the people who undergo a lumbar puncture or spinal tap develop a headache. Many scientists believe

these headaches result from leakage of the cerebrospinal fluid that flows through pain-sensitive membranes around the brain and down to the spinal cord. The fluid, they suggest, drains through the tiny hole created by the spinal tap needle, causing the membranes to rub painfully against the bony skull. Since headache pain occurs only when the patient stands up, the "cure" is to remain lying down until the headache runs its course—anywhere from a few hours to several days.

- *Head trauma.* Headaches may develop after a blow to the head, either immediately or months later. There is little relationship between the severity of the trauma and the intensity of headache pain. One cause of trauma headache is scar formation in the scalp. Another is ruptured blood vessels which result in an accumulation of blood called a *hematoma.* This mass of blood can displace brain tissue and cause headaches as well as weakness, confusion, memory loss, and seizures. Hematomas can be drained to produce rapid relief of symptoms.
- *Arteritis and meningitis.* Arteritis, an inflammation of certain arteries in the head, primarily affects people over age 50. Symptoms include throbbing headache, fever, and loss of appetite. Some patients experience blurring or loss of vision. Prompt treatment with corticosteroid drugs helps to relieve symptoms.

  Headaches are also caused by infections of meninges, the brain's outer covering, and phlebitis, a vein inflammation.
- *Tic douloureux.* Tic douloureux, or trigeminal neuralgia, results from a disorder of the trigeminal nerve. This nerve supplies the face, teeth, mouth, and nasal cavity with feeling and also enables the mouth muscles to chew. Symptoms are headache and intense facial pain that comes in short, excruciating jabs set off by the slightest touch to, or movement of trigger points in the face or mouth. People with tic douloureux often fear brushing their teeth or chewing on the side of the mouth that is affected. Many tic douloureux patients are controlled with drugs, including carbamazepine. Patients who do not respond to drugs may be helped by surgery on the trigeminal nerve.
- *Sinus infection.* In a condition called acute sinusitis, a viral or bacterial infection of the upper respiratory tract spreads to the membrane which lines the sinus cavities. When one or all four of these cavities are filled with bacterial or viral fluid, they become inflamed, causing pain and sometimes headache. Treatment of acute sinusitis includes antibiotics, analgesics, and decongestants.

  Chronic sinusitis may be caused by an allergy to such irritants as dust, ragweed, animal hair, and smoke. Research scientists disagree about whether chronic sinusitis triggers headache.

A childhood problem

Like adults, children experience the infections, trauma, and stresses that can lead to headaches. In fact, research shows that as young people enter adolescence and encounter the stresses of puberty and secondary school, the frequency of headache increases.

Migraine headaches often begin in childhood or adolescence. According to a recent health interview survey, over a million children age 16 and under experience migraine and other vascular headaches.

Children with migraine often have nausea and excessive vomiting. Some children have periodic vomiting, but no headache—the so-called "abdominal migraine." Research scientists have found that these children usually develop headaches when they are older.

Phenobarbital, cyproheptadine, and certain anticonvulsant drugs are used to treat migraines in children. A diet may be prescribed to protect the child from foods that trigger headache. Sometimes psychological counseling or even psychiatric treatment for the child and the parents is recommended. NINCDS-supported scientists at the State University of New York in Albany find that thermal biofeedback can help children with migraines control their headaches.

Childhood headache can be a sign of depression. Parents should alert the family pediatrician if a child develops headaches along with other symptoms such as a change in mood or sleep habits. Antidepressant medication and psychotherapy are effective treatments for childhood depression and related headache.

Research intervenes

Modern methods of diagnosis and treatment enable physicians and psychologists today to help about 90 percent of chronic headache patients, according to the director of a major U.S. headache clinic. These methods are based on years of scientific research. New research should lead to even more advanced techniques of headache management.

Some scientists explore the role that certain foods play in causing this disorder. Others are more concerned with the function of the autonomic nervous systems of headache-prone people. The autonomic nervous system automatically controls a variety of essential body functions, including the flow of blood throughout the body and the working of the pupils of the eyes.

At the Philadelphia College of Osteopathic Medicine, scientists supported by the National Institute of Neurological and Communicative Disorders and Stroke are gauging the autonomic nervous system activity of normal controls and headache patients with a technique called "pupillometry." This technique measures the response of the iris, or eye muscle, to light and darkness. Migraine, cluster, and muscle-contraction headache patients are included in the study. Each patient sits in a chair with his or her head in a chin rest. The eye is stimulated with light and then with darkness. A television camera in front of the patient picks up the reaction of the iris and translates it into a graph which provides clues about the functioning of the patient's autonomic nervous system.

Another experiment with the pupillometer involves measuring eye muscle reaction to light and darkness after stress. In this study, stress is simulated by dipping the patient's arm in very cold water for up to 20 seconds.

Preliminary findings from these studies suggest that, under stress-free conditions, the autonomic nervous systems of both people with common migraine and of people without headaches react normally. Paradoxically, migraine patients during stress show reduced autonomic nervous system activity, a condition that should prevent the decreased blood flow thought to cause headaches.

However, NINCDS-supported scientists at Southern Illinois University in Carbondale report a different connection between blood flow and migraine headache.

Using an infrared light sensor that measures the diameter of blood vessels, the investigators have found that, after stress, blood flow returns to normal more quickly in headache-free people than in patients with migraine and muscle-contraction headache. This finding supports the theory that restricted or decreased blood flow may cause or contribute to headache.

The scientists also found that different types of headaches are characterized by different blood flow patterns. After stress, the temporal arteries in the foreheads of migraine patients expand to a greater degree than the arteries of muscle-contraction headache patients. People with the same type of headache also show differences in blood flow patterns— offering evidence that there are a variety of causes for each headache type.

Testing New Treatments   Scientists are also developing new therapies and analyzing the effectiveness of current treatment methods for headache. The research team at Southern Illinois University is comparing a biofeedback method that monitors blood flow with a method that monitors muscular tension in the head. This research should lead to improved understanding of individual differences in treatment response.

Several scientists are studying the value of biofeedback and other forms of treatment carried out in the patient's home. Home-based programs may be a boon to patients in rural areas who have limited access to medical care and cannot afford frequent visits to headache specialists.

In NINCDS-supported research at the State University of New York in Albany, scientists are comparing the effectiveness of a standard office-based relaxation training program for muscle-contraction, migraine, and mixed-headache patients with a similar program conducted by patients at home. Patients in the home-based program are seen in the office once a month but rely heavily on manuals, cassettes, and portable biofeedback devices.

Preliminary results suggest that home-based and office-based programs are equally effective. "If these relaxation techniques are learned at home," speculates the investigator, "they may transfer more readily to the home situation—where they will be used to cope with daily stresses."

Furthermore, at the University of Washington in Seattle, an NINCDS-supported investigator is finding that home-based treatment involving only dietary changes is as effective in treating migraine patients as a home-based program of biofeedback and stress management.

Thermal biofeedback training, which involves the conscious warming of parts of the body through thought control, is believed to work because it gives people a feeling of control over their headaches. An NINCDS-supported study at Midwest Research Institute in Kansas City, Missouri, raises the possibility that this feeling of control is a more important factor in decreasing headaches than is the actual warming of the hands.

Patients who had frequent migraines were told that they would be given one of two types of biofeedback: "real temperature biofeedback," where a sound indicated their real hand temperature, or "bogus biofeedback," where a prerecorded sound emitted from the monitor would be unrelated to the patient's effort to warm the hands. Neither the patients nor the technicians training them knew whose feedback was real or bogus. Throughout the six weeks of training, the scientists emphasized to the patients that biofeedback should become an integral part of their lives because it was giving them control over their headaches.

Patients in the bogus biofeedback group had a success rate that rivaled the one in the real biofeedback group. More than 80 percent of patients in both groups reduced the frequency and intensity of their headaches, as well as the quantity of medication they had been taking to control pain.

"It isn't so much the physical mechanism of migraine that matters," explains the principal investigator, "but a person's ability to cope with the syndrome and to take charge of his or her body. The emphasis on self-control is what made these people improve."

Another important area of research is the study of beta-blocking drugs like propranolol, which are used to prevent migraine.

Beta-blockers stop the activities of beta receptors—cells in the brain and heart which control the dilation of blood vessels. The ability of beta-blockers to halt the dilation of blood vessels in the brain is believed to be a major reason for their antimigraine action. But because the drugs also affect heart receptors—slowing the heart rate—they cannot be used by people who have certain heart conditions.

This problem may be resolved by NINCDS-supported research at Massachusetts General Hospital in Boston. A research team there is using biochemical techniques to find out if there is a certain type of beta receptor that exists in the blood vessels of the brain but not in the heart. The discovery of this receptor could lead to the development of beta-blocking agents that would affect brain receptors only.

Another NINCDS-funded study at the University of Kansas Medical Center is comparing the effectiveness of propranolol with that of the antidepressant amitriptyline in the prevention of migraine. Physical and psychological characteristics of migraine patients are being correlated with their responses to the two drugs.

Investigators supported by the National Institutes of Health General Clinical Research Center at the University of Colorado in Denver are studying the antimigraine properties of a class of drugs called calcium-channel blockers. Research on these drugs is also under way at the U.S. Air Force Medical Center, Wright-Patterson AFB in Ohio. Calcium-channel blockers interfere with the constriction of arteries, an effect that appears to be responsible for reducing the frequency of headaches in patients studied so far.

High Technology in Diagnosis Physicians of the future may diagnose their patients' headaches with the aid of a computer. A computer might take a patient's medical history, store information on headache characteristics, and keep data on patients and their treatments. Programs might even be devised to explain to patients the way to take prescribed medications and the side effects of those drugs.

Scientists at Beth Israel Hospital in Boston are taking the first steps toward computer-assisted headache practice in a study funded by the National Library of Medicine. They are creating a working model for a headache interview program in which a computer will collect patient histories and symptoms. The scientists envision that an ''automated physician's assistant'' will eventually free health care providers from collecting routine medical information, allowing them to devote more time to physical examination and treatment.

A final word of hope

If you suffer from headaches and none of the standard treatments help, do not despair. Some people find that their headaches disappear once they deal with a troubled marriage, pass their law board exams, or resolve some other stressful problem. Others find that if they control their psychological reaction to stress, the headaches disappear.

"I had migraines for several years," says one woman, "and then they went away. I think it was because I lowered my personal goals in life. Today, even though I have 100 things to do at night, I don't worry about it. I learned to say no."

For those who cannot say no, or who get headaches anyway, today's headache research offers hope. The work of NINCDS-supported scientists around the world promises to improve our understanding of this complex disorder and how to treat it.

Where to get help

Finding a clinic or physician who specializes in headache is a task made easier by the National Migraine Foundation. The foundation provides a list of clinics in the U.S. as well as the names of physicians in a specific geographic area who are members of the American Association for the Study of Headache. The foundation also supports research and education in migraine headache.

National Migraine Foundation
5252 North Western Avenue
Chicago, Illinois 60625
(312) 878-7715

Inquiries about NINCDS research on headache may be directed to:

Office of Scientific and Health Reports
National Institute of Neurological and
Communicative Disorders and Stroke
Building 31, Room 8A-06
National Institutes of Health
Bethesda, Maryland 20205
(301) 496-5751

Diane Striar, Office of Scientific and Health Reports, NINCDS, NIH; U.S. Department of Health and Human Services, Public Health Service, National Institutes of Health. Prepared by the Office of Scientific and Health Reports, National Institute of Neurological and Communicative Disorders and Stroke. National Institutes of Health, Bethesda, Maryland 20205. NIH Publication No. 84–158, September 1984.

Hearing Loss
Hope Through Research

Some years ago pollsters asked a sample of adults, "If you had to choose between becoming blind or becoming deaf, which would you choose?" A surprisingly large number chose blindness. As terrifying as a world of darkness may have seemed, a world of silence seemed even worse.

When you think about it, the reasons are not hard to fathom. Human beings are talkers, social creatures who seek out their fellow beings for conversation and contact. From birth on we cry and coo, look and listen, in our first attempts to communicate. But for over 200,000 newborns and young infants who are born deaf or suffer severe hearing loss in the first years of life, that vital communications link never gets forged. Not only are deaf children denied the wealth of experience that comes from listening to the sounds of nature, of music, and of the human voice, but they must also struggle hard to master speech and language.

For those who become profoundly hard of hearing later in life, the impact is hardly less tragic. At present nearly 2 million Americans are either totally deaf or suffer such significant hearing loss in both ears that they cannot hear conversation, a phone ringing, traffic noises, or a fire alarm. Another 14 to 15 million are moderately to severely impaired.

All these people know the loneliness, isolation, and frustration that comes from hearing loss. They know what it's like to sit in company and miss the joke or the gist of conversation. Worse, they soon realize that society can be cruel. People are impatient. They don't like repeating their words or raising their voices. They show by facial expression and gesture how annoyed they are when talking to someone "who doesn't understand what I'm saying." It is only a short step from that attitude to the assumption that people who are hard of hearing are soft in intelligence. Ages ago that assumption led to the vulgar use of the word *dumb* to mean stupid. *Dumb* derives from Old English roots that mean mute, unable to speak; once the common fate of those born deaf.

Fortunately, many elements in society—including the hearing impaired themselves—have rallied to fight ignorance and prejudice. Such well-known figures as Henry Fonda, Nanette Fabray, Lou Ferrigno (TV's Incredible Hulk), and *New Yorker* cartoonist and children's book author William Steig have publicly acknowledged their hearing problems. Their example, along with individuals as celebrated as Beethoven, Thomas Edison, Helen Keller, and Winston Churchill, has helped dispel the embarrassment that many hearing-impaired people feel, an embarrassment that often makes them deny they have a problem and avoid seeking treatment or wearing a hearing aid.

Pediatricians, family physicians, ear specialists and parents are increasingly aware of the need to diagnose hearing impairments early in life, so that remedial measures and language and speech training can begin. Many lay and professional organizations have formed to aid those with hearing impairments.

In 1975, one of the 11 research Institutes of the National Institutes of Health in Bethesda, Md., added *communicative disorders* to its name to emphasize its increasing attention to research on hearing, speech, and language problems. The National Institute of Neurological and Communicative Disorders and Stroke (NINCDS) is the principal Federal agency supporting research on the many causes of hearing loss, as well as on prevention, treatment, and rehabilitation. Support includes the development of better hearing aids and other ways to augment hearing: research on hearing *gains,* one might say, to counter hearing *losses.*

Through basic studies of normal hearing and studies targeted on specific impairments, the primary goal of the NINCDS research program is to develop improved methods of *prevention.* But until this goal of prevention is achieved, research attention will continue to be directed toward better therapies for the hearing impaired.

Sound and hearing

Human hearing depends on a series of mechanical and electrical events that enable sound waves in air to be converted to electrical impulses carried by nerves to the brain.

Sound itself is a form of energy. Suppose you snap your fingers. The snap generates a force that presses against the molecules of air surrounding your fingertips. The molecules are pushed out a short distance in all directions, crowding into space occupied by other air molecules so that a densely packed shell of air molecules forms. That shell—sound experts call it a ''shell of compression''—in turn presses against other air molecules nearby so that they, too, are pushed out to form a second, slightly larger shell of compression, which nudges a third layer of air, and so on.

Meanwhile, the air around your fingertips has become less dense as a result of those first molecules being pushed out. A partial vacuum is created by this ''rarefied'' air, and the molecules that moved out now rush back to fill that vacuum. Their return creates a second partial vacuum in their wake, which the molecules of the second shell rush back and fill. And so it goes. Thus, the original sound energy generated by your fingersnap moves through the air on a "wave" which is really a succession of shells of compression and rarefaction created by molecules moving back and forth—vibrating.

The number of shells of compression that pass a given point every second determines the frequency of the sound, measured in cycles per second (cps) or Hertz (Hz). Human beings interpret frequency as pitch: the greater the frequency, the higher the pitch. How far the molecules move back and forth as they vibrate is a measure of the energy or intensity of sound. Human beings interpret sound intensity as loudness.

Our ears are sensitive to only certain ranges of frequency and intensity. Healthy young adults can hear notes as low as 20 Hz—lower than the lowest notes of a bass fiddle—as well as sounds at 20,000 Hz, beyond the upper reaches of a flute. The intensity range to which our ears respond is enormous. When sound is just audible—the threshold level of hearing— the force of sound waves acting on the ear is about 140 million times smaller than the force needed to lift a 1-ounce weight. At the other extreme, human ears can respond—painfully—to sonic booms, explosions, or the noise of jackhammers breaking up city streets.

Because the ear can respond to such enormous ranges of sound energy, intensity is measured in ratios. That is the basis of the decibel (dB) scale. A sound 10 times more intense than another at the same frequency differs from it by 10 dB; a sound 100 times more intense differs by 20 dB. The decibel scale is usually set at an arbitrary zero level (0 dB), which does not mean the absence of sound, but the average threshold level of hearing of healthy young adults. On that basis, a whisper is about 20 dB, and normal conversation about 60 dB. The noise of a jet taking off is on the order of 160 dB—10 quadrillion times the zero level!

Tuning in

Understanding these fundamentals of sound explains a lot of what goes on—and what can go wrong—with the hearing process. Initially the job of the ears is to pick up sound waves and conduct them accurately to the inner ear. That the ears can manage this task with great skill and efficiency is due in part to the design of the outer and middle ear.

When sound waves enter the ear they travel for an inch or so down a narrow tube, the external auditory canal, before striking the delicate, skin-covered tympanic membrane, or eardrum. The drum is shaped like a broad flat cone about ½-inch across and less than ⅟₅₀-inch thick. The drum vibrates in tune with the sound waves striking it and transmits the vibrations accurately to three tiny bones in the middle ear, the ossicles. These bones—the malleus, the incus, and the stapes—amplify the vibrations so that the waves can pass on to the inner ear.

It's not hard to understand why specialists find the ear a stunning example of design as well as a challenge for study. For the ear's high-fidelity equipment is miniaturized. The ossicles are the smallest bones in the human body; they fit into a stringbean-seed sized cavity that has been carved out of the temporal bone of the human skull.

Two other features of the middle ear are important: One is that the compartment connects to the throat by a narrow canal with collapsible walls, the eustachian tube. When you swallow, the eustachian tube opens so that air pressure in the middle ear and throat is equalized. That mechanism protects your middle ear from harmful pressure differences that can occur in a fast-rising elevator, for example, or on takeoff and landing in an airplane. The second important middle ear feature is also protective. Muscles attached to the ossicles automatically contract in response to loud noises. These automatic reflexes may prevent strong sound pressures from damaging the delicate structures of the inner ear.

To summarize, when the eardrum and middle ear bones are working properly, sound waves striking the drum are faithfully conducted across the middle ear and boosted in energy. The energy boost helps prepare sound waves that have been traveling in air for the more resistant watery medium of their next stop: a fluid-filled bony shell in the inner ear called the cochlea.

Conductive problems

A variety of problems can affect hearing before sound reaches the cochlea. Because these early stages in the hearing process are concerned with picking up and conducting sound signals, specialists refer to the hearing impairments involved as *conductive* problems. Among the most common problems are:

- *External blockage.* Sometimes there is a buildup of wax in the ears. Sometimes children put things in their ears. Sometimes a bug crawls in. These are obvious plugs that partially block sound. The removal of impacted wax and foreign objects is best left to experts to avoid the possibility of damaging the eardrum.
- *Perforated eardrum.* A hole or a tear in the eardrum can occur as a result of injury, sudden pressure change, or infection. Ear specialists can repair or completely rebuild the eardrum using the latest techniques of microsurgery.
- *Genetic and congenital abnormalities.* Malformations of the outer and middle ear sometimes occur in connection with hereditary disease or as a result of injuries and illnesses that affect a baby before or around the time of birth. Surgery can sometimes correct these problems.
- *Otitis media.* By far the most prevalent cause of conductive impairments is a common middle ear disease, otitis media. The problem can occur

at any age but is particularly prevalent in children. An estimated two-thirds of preschoolers have at least one episode. The reason that children are so vulnerable may be that their eustachian tubes are shorter and positioned more horizontally than in adults. Infectious agents causing colds or other upper respiratory disease can easily spread to the middle ear. At the same time, mucus, pus, or other fluids accumulating in the middle ear tend not to drain off. Thus the middle ear can become inflamed, swollen, fluid-filled, and painful—the classic symptoms of otitis media that can result in temporary and sometimes permanent hearing impairment. Thanks to today's medications, most middle ear infections can be cleared up with no lasting damage.

Some children are particularly prone to middle ear disease, however, suffering five or six bouts a year. When the condition recurs that often and is accompanied by fluid in the ear, it is called chronic otitis media with effusion (also serous otitis media). NINCDS-supported scientists at the University of Minnesota are currently studying chronic otitis media to determine if changes in the body's immune system are involved. One possibility is that the body's immune defenses successfully fight off the initial infection, but that some residue of the virus or infectious agent remains to stimulate an immune reaction, leading to the accumulation of fluid. NINCDS is also supporting a major Otitis Media Research Center in Pittsburgh, Pa., in association with Children's Hospital of the University Health Center. The center will study all aspects of otitis media in animals and in human patients.

Patients with chronic middle ear disease with effusion need careful supervision and treatment by ear specialists (otologists) or ear, nose, and throat specialists (otolaryngologists). Not only is there danger of permanent hearing impairment, but frequent bouts of temporary hearing loss may in themselves be serious. The auditory system, especially in the developing years, needs the regular stimulation of sound for healthy growth. Periodic episodes of hearing loss may starve the auditory cells in the brain and contribute to impairments in speech and language skills. Studies of such "auditory deprivation" are under way by NINCDS grantees at Louisiana State University in New Orleans.

Physicians treating otitis media with effusion can drain the fluid by making a small incision in the eardrum. The incision will heal and the problem may disappear. If fluids continue to build up, however, the physician may insert a small drainage tube in the eardrum in an operation called a tympanostomy. Tympanostomy tubes are sometimes dislodged accidentally and may be rejected by the body, but often they may stay in place for as long as a year and effectively control the problem. Because there is a small risk that the tubes can give rise to scarring or thickening of the drum after removal, some doctors prefer not to use them, and choose instead to wait and see if the ear problem will improve in time.

- *Otosclerosis.* An example of a hereditary hearing problem that develops in adults is otosclerosis, a condition in which there is an overgrowth of bone in the middle ear. Usually the tiny stirrup-shaped stapes bone is the most affected and becomes fixed in place, impeding sound conduction. Otosclerosis can often be remedied by surgery to remove the excess bone and replace all or part of the stapes with an artificial part. Those who have undergone successful surgery describe the results as miraculous. "I was completely deaf before the operation," one woman said. "As soon as I woke up I could hear again!"

- *Presbycusis.* Specialists have coined the word *presbycusis*—literally, old hearing—to describe hearing impairments that occur in aging. While presbycusis is primarily associated with changes in the inner ear and brain (discussed later), conductive impairments may also occur. The bones of the middle ear may become stiff, for example, or the eardrum thicker and less flexible. Both those changes may reflect a less rich blood supply to the ear as a result of heart disease, high blood pressure, or other circulatory problems in older people.

Conductive impairments can be detected in the course of an ear examination that includes a variety of diagnostic tests. Before we describe the tests, let us pick up the story of what happens to sound when it reaches the cochlea.

From ear to brain

When sound vibrates the three middle ear bones, the last in line, the stapes, presses against a membrane called the oval window. This membrane is fitted into a thin shell of bone that encloses all the inner ear structures. About an inch down from the oval window, the bone spirals to form the snail-shaped cochlea, another ministructure less than ½-inch across at its base, rising a mere ¼-inch to its tip.

The cochlea is composed of three fluid-filled compartments. The center and smallest compartment is a duct of soft tissue that contains the organ of hearing, called the organ of Corti, after the Italian scientist who first described it. Like the retina of the eye, the organ of Corti contains special cells called sensory receptors that take incoming energy—light in case of the eye, sound for the ear—and transform that energy into electrical signals. The ear cells that do the transforming are called hair cells because the cell tops are fringed with fine hairs that stick up into the fluid filling the duct. The hair cells are sandwiched between two membranes: one membrane rests lightly on the hair tips; the other forms the floor or base of the duct, and so is called the basilar membrane.

Research had led to greater understanding of how the organ of Corti works and to a Nobel prize for the investigator who contributed significantly to that understanding, Georg von Békésy. Put very simply, when the stapes kicks in the oval window, the fluid in the cochlea is stirred and sets the basilar membrane moving in a very special way: Sounds of high frequency cause the greatest movements of the membrane under hair cells at the base of the cochlea, agitating the tips of the cells' protruding hairs. Sounds of middle frequency cause maximum movements of the membrane further toward the center of the cochlea, while sounds of lowest frequencies cause peak membrane movements near the top of the cochlea.

The movements of the hairs cause changes inside the cells that lead to the production of electrical signals. These signals excite nearby nerve cells whose long fibers—some 30,000 in each ear—spiral out from the cochlea to form the eighth, or auditory nerve, which goes from the ear to the brain.

Soon after entering the brain, eighth nerve fibers contact nerve cells in the first of many nerve centers concerned with hearing. Ultimately the auditory signals reach the cortex, the outermost covering of the brain. The cortex contains centers associated with interpreting speech and music, with thinking, memory, learning, and other higher mental faculties.

There are a great many details and subtleties about human hearing that scientists are continuing to work out. How do we manage to block out unwanted sounds, for example, enjoying an intimate conversation in the midst of a noisy party? How do we detect subtle differences in loudness as well as pitch? What enables some of us to hear a tune for the first time and repeat it perfectly? How do we locate the source of sound and judge how near or far it is?

Much of this research requires a detailed analysis of what happens at the cochlea and at auditory centers in the brain. In recent years NINCDS-supported scientists have been able to remove embryonic cochlear tissue and grow it in the laboratory. Small animals like guinea pigs or chinchillas are often used in these studies because their cochleas are relatively large and their brains not very complex.

Work with human volunteers is also essential. Persons with normal hearing are often studied in experiments in which different messages are piped into each ear or where computers are used to generate garbled or synthetic speech. These studies are aimed at analyzing how people recognize speech and how they detect a meaningful message amidst noise.

Also of great interest are studies of how the two ears and the two halves of the brain work individually and together in the perception of speech, music, and other complex sounds. Experiments with hearing-impaired individuals are equally important, leading to a better understanding of the cues hearing-impaired people use to recognize speech—and how noise affects them.

Hearing problems higher up

Hearing impairments that result from damage to the sensory apparatus (the hair cells and other parts of the inner ear) or to the eighth nerve and auditory centers higher up in the brain (the neural apparatus) are often lumped together as "sensorineural" problems. These include:

- *Hearing loss at birth.* Some 4,000 infants are born deaf every year in the United States. Close to half those cases are due to hereditary disorders.

  A larger group of babies is born deaf or with major hearing impairments as a result of congenital disorders or difficult labor and delivery. Mothers who contract certain infections during pregnancy or who take certain drugs may give birth to hearing-impaired infants. Sometimes the hearing loss accompanies other prenatal or birth-related problems that result in cerebral palsy, seizures (epilepsy), or mental retardation.

  Before the advent of a vaccine for German measles (rubella), this viral disease in pregnant women was a notorious cause of hearing impairment at birth. Common measles (rubeola) in pregnant women also imposed a threat to the unborn child. Fortunately, there are now vaccines for both these viral diseases so that women can (and should) be immunized well before becoming pregnant.

  There are other virus infections for which no effective treatments or vaccines exist as yet. Of these, cytomegalovirus and herpes simplex type 2 virus (which causes a genital infection) can seriously affect the nervous system of infected newborns. Cytomegalovirus infection is estimated to affect one out of every 100 children born in the U.S. Between 5 percent and 10 percent of those children develop hearing impairments, especially for high frequencies, and have IQ scores less than 80 later on in school.

- *Hereditary hearing loss.* It is important to realize that hereditary conditions not only can result in deafness at birth, but also account for a variety of hearing impairments occurring later. Hereditary disorders can affect the outer and middle ear, as in otosclerosis, but generally involve damage to the cochlea or higher nerve centers. Because there are so many kinds of hereditary disorders, with different risks of inheritance, couples with a history of deafness on either side of the family should consult genetic counselors for information.

- *Trauma-induced problems.* A severe blow to the head, an accident, stroke, brain hemorrhage, or other trauma that affects the ear or any of the auditory pathways and brain centers will obviously take its toll on hearing ability.
- *Tumors.* Patients with eighth nerve tumors—called acoustic neuromas—may complain of hearing loss in one or both ears, headaches, dizziness, ringing in the ear (called tinnitus), or numbness over the face. Such symptoms deserve prompt attention. If an eighth nerve tumor is detected early, surgery to remove the tumor can be completely successful, leaving no hearing or other impairment. Tumors diagnosed at later stages may have grown large enough to be life-threatening, or their surgical removal may result in hearing loss, disturbances in the sense of balance (also located in the inner ear), loss of sensation in the face, or facial paralysis.

  Acoustic neuromas can occur for no known reason, but can also arise as a result of a hereditary disease called neurofibromatosis.

- *Noise damage.* Brief exposures to high intensity sound can cause a temporary but reversible hearing loss. But continued exposure to loud noise means trouble: Eventually the hair cells sustain permanent damage, resulting in gradual hearing loss.

  During the early days of industrialization nobody doubted that the din surrounding boilermakers, hydraulic press operators, or steel mill workers rendered their hearing less than perfect. Nowadays specialists are concerned that the everyday sounds of our highly technological society are also wilting our hair cells. Think of the power mowers and chain saws, the disposals, stereo sets, dishwashers, and food processors we live with . . . and the sounds of airplanes, motorcycles, city and highway traffic, fire and emergency trucks. Think, too, of joggers wearing earphones or young people at rock concerts or disco clubs, and you have the reason so many hearing specialists are worried.

  Concern about noise has inspired research at several major hearing laboratories supported by NINCDS. Scientists at Washington University Medical School in St. Louis, Mo., for example, are systematically changing the frequency, intensity, and duration of noise to see how each of these factors affects the structures of the inner ear. Investigators at the Central Institute for the Deaf, also in St. Louis, are analyzing the effects of noise on the inner ears of animals and also observing how such stress affects the animals' behavior. Other NINCDS-supported investigators are studying how noise damage may lead to degeneration of eighth nerve fibers, why some people are more affected by noise than others, and why the ear, once impaired by noise, often becomes hypersensitive—even more vulnerable to noise damage.

- *Drug-induced hearing loss.* Drugs as common as aspirin, the antibiotics streptomycin or neomycin, and certain of the water pills (diuretics) used to treat high blood pressure can damage the hair cells or other vital parts of the inner ear. Anyone who, while under medication, has a sudden change in hearing, or experiences dizziness or ringing in the ears (tinnitus), or has other problems with hearing or balance should report the symptoms to a physician at once. Often changes in the prescription can eliminate the symptoms and prevent permanent damage to the ear.

  Certain powerful anticancer drugs may also damage hearing. NINCDS is currently conducting research studies of patients undergoing cancer chemotherapy at the Clinical Center, the research hospital of the National Institutes of Health. Audiologists measure the patient's hearing before treatment and then at periodic intervals thereafter to determine if the drugs have affected hearing.

- *Tinnitus.* Many people have experienced one or more occasions when they felt a ringing or buzzing in the ears or inside the head. But a surprising number of people, especially in middle age or later years, complain of a constant ringing in the head for no known reason. In some cases the symptoms may be unnoticed if a person is busy at work, talking, or otherwise distracted. For other people, however, the unpleasant sounds are present during every waking hour, interfering with all activities. In the most severe cases, tinnitus even interrupts sleep. The hapless victim is tormented by an incessant internal siren sounding off. The psychological effects on a person can be devastating.

  Tinnitus is considered a sensorineural disorder, but what causes it and where in the ear or brain the trouble lies are unknown. Because excessive amounts of aspirin and related drugs produce temporary tinnitus in human beings, NINCDS-supported investigators are studying the effects of these drugs in animals. The scientists can detect whether the animal is experiencing tinnitus by first training the animal to behave in specific ways in response to typical tinnitus sounds. They then observe whether the animal behaves the same way after drug treatment. Other NINCDS grantees are studying sounds that may be generated within the cochlea itself. Still a third NINCDS-supported group at the University of Oregon is developing an ear device designed to mask the tinnitus sounds, a method of treatment that appears to help some tinnitus sufferers. A variety of tinnitus maskers can now be obtained commercially.

- *Presbycusis.* Changes associated with aging are responsible for the majority of hearing impairments in adults. Many people in their forties and fifties experience a decline in sensitivity to high frequencies. The decline is gradual and progressive so that by their sixties and seventies as many as 25 percent of the elderly are noticeably impaired. However, investigators are beginning to question whether "aging factors" *per se* are at fault. There are cultures in the world—the Mabaan people of the African Sudan, for example—where presbycusis doesn't exist. Both men and women have excellent hearing in old age. The environment of the Mabaans is exceptionally quiet by Western standards. Further, the Mabaans do not suffer from heart disease, high blood pressure, ulcers or asthma. They lead relatively stress-free lives. No conclusions can yet be drawn, except that presbycusis is clearly not an inevitable result of aging.

Many experts now think that lifelong exposure to noise, as well as the high prevalence of heart disease, high blood pressure, and other blood vessel disorders increase the odds of hearing loss in later years.

In addition, some hereditary predisposition may be involved: As one investigator puts it, "Some of us may simply be programmed to suffer a decline and fall of our hair cells or our auditory neurons starting at a particular age—as young as the twenties and thirties in some people." Further, the decline may be selective: The hair cells and inner ear structures may be healthy in some older individuals so that they can pass a hearing test for pure tones with flying colors. Yet those same people may have trouble understanding speech, especially under trying conditions. Experts suspect that the listener's confusion is associated with tissue damage or loss of nerve cells in the brain where centers for speech perception and discrimination are located.

With the realization that people are living longer, the problem of presbycusis has become an area of growing concern to the National Institute on Aging (NIA) as well as NINCDS. At present, 6 million Americans 65 or over have moderate to severe hearing losses. By the year 2000 an estimated 32 million Americans will be 65 or older. If 25 percent continue to be affected by presbycusis that means that 8 million Americans may know only too well the limitations on activities, the lack of enjoyment, the isolation and boredom that severe hearing impairments can impose. To deal with this problem, cooperative research ventures are being initiated by the NINCDS with its sister organization, the NIA.

Currently NINCDS-supported research on presbycusis includes programs at the University of Michigan, focusing on the causes of presbycusis and microscopic changes in the inner ear, and a program at the University of California at Los Angeles concerned with how age affects the transmission of nerve signals along the auditory pathways in the brain.

Detecting hearing loss

In the case of a simple infection or impacted wax, the diagnosis and treatment of a hearing problem may begin and end in the family doctor's office. More complicated cases call for the expertise of the otologist. He or she will conduct a thorough ear examination, note the patient's medical history, and inquire about hearing problems affecting other members of the family. Certain blood tests or other laboratory analyses may be necessary, as well as standard hearing tests. The specialist may also want X-rays of the head or the computerized X-ray images of the brain called CT scans.

Hearing tests are usually conducted by audiologists, professionals educated in the science of hearing and in the battery of tests used to assess and analyze hearing impairment. Audiologists also provide counseling and nonmedical rehabilitation for the hearing impaired, such as lipreading and hearing aid evaluation.

Persons undergoing audiological testing sit in a small soundproof room. The examination usually includes tests to determine how well the eardrum and middle ear bones conduct sound. These tests depend on inserting a snug-fitting probe with wires attached into the external canal of the ear. Then air pressure between the probe tip and the eardrum is varied at the same time that a tone is sounded through the probe tip. A machine analyzes the movements of the drum and middle ear bones, printing out the results on a graph—the "tympanogram."

The probe can also be used to check the acoustic reflex to loud noise. The tympanogram and acoustic reflex tests take only a few minutes. Since the tests depend on automatic responses of the auditory system, they can be used to test hearing in infants and others who cannot respond voluntarily.

The audiologist then measures the patient's thresholds for two-syllable words and for pure tones in a range from 250 Hz to 8000 Hz. The patient wears headphones and indicates when he or she can just barely detect sounds as the decibel level is varied. The graph that plots sound frequency against decibel level is the audiogram. The audiologist also measures the ability to discriminate speech by having the individual repeat one-syllable words. The audiologist may conduct further tests to determine the nature of the hearing loss. These tests may involve manipulations of pure tones and noises or the use of tape recordings that introduce distortions into voice or sound signals.

An EEG for hearing

In the past decade, investigators have developed ways of recording the electrical activity of brain centers associated with hearing. Electrodes are attached to the top of the head and at each side, near the ear. The individual wears earphones and sits quietly in a soundproof room listening to clicks at different intensities. A computer analyzes the nerve cell activity in response to the clicks and displays the brain wave pattern on a video screen. Audiologists know the normal shape of the waves and the time it takes for nerve signals to move from center to center along the auditory pathways. Delays in the appearance of certain waves or changes in their pattern help localize the problem. Because the brain cells recorded lie in the brainstem—a core of brain tissue located below the cortex—the brain wave recording is called the auditory brainstem response. Like tympanometry, the auditory brainstem response test is automatic and so can be used to study hearing in infants. However, the test takes up to an hour and the subject must remain stationary and quiet, so testing in young children usually requires mild sedation.

Many people think that you can't measure children's hearing in the first months or years of life. Even without the newer automatic tests, however, there have always been ways of measuring infants' hearing. Parents can approach a baby from behind and sound a bell or rattle. The child who hears will be startled, and, depending on the stage of brain development, may turn toward the direction of the sound. Audiologists can also test an infant's hearing with standard pure tone tests. The infant wears earphones and sits on its mother's lap in the test room. The audiologist trains the child to associate a certain sound with the appearance of a toy or other interesting object displayed on a screen. By observing the child's behavior in response to speech or noises at various intensities, the audiologist can measure how well the child can hear.

The results of medical and audiological examinations may indicate a problem that can be helped by surgery, medication, or a hearing aid. Sometimes preventive measures are urged: Adults with middle ear infections are cautioned to avoid flying; workers who are beginning to show noise-induced hearing losses are advised to transfer to less noisy departments or at least wear ear protection. Often, however, the hearing loss is longstanding and irreparable. In those instances there is no instant remedy or miraculous cure. But there *are* important things that can be done.

What hearing aids do

A hearing aid amplifies sound. The aid provides the extra power to boost sound so that it can stimulate the cochlear cells. Hearing aids can benefit anyone, as long as some hearing remains. How well hearing aids work is another matter. Their effectiveness depends not only on the design of the aid (is it a quiet, high-quality, easy-to-maintain instrument?), but also on how well the aid matches the individual's needs. Present-day aids are a far cry from the ear trumpets used generations ago. A modern aid is lightweight, battery-operated, and miniaturized. It can be molded to fit inside the ear, worn behind the ear, or fitted into eyeglasses.

Many individuals with hearing impairments become sensitive to amplified sound. This does not mean they cannot wear a hearing aid; it does mean that the aid must accommodate their sensitivities. Some investigators now suspect that hard-of-hearing people occasionally retain "islands of hearing"—frequency ranges where sound is still perceived at near normal levels. Such individuals might find the amplification provided by hearing aids uncomfortable. Scientists at Louisiana State University in New Orleans are currently investigating islands of hearing in hearing-impaired people to see how common the phenomenon is, and whether special aids making use of these frequencies could be designed to enable individuals to understand speech.

But no matter how well designed and appropriate to the wearer's hearing impairment, the chances of the aid benefiting the user largely depend on attitude and motivation. It is important to realize that adjustments in the aid have to be made and all wearers go through a period of learning and adaptation. In short, the recommendation and fitting of a hearing aid is not the end of an audiological examination, but the beginning of a new way of life. Followup in the first few weeks, proper maintenance, and periodic checkups to see how the human ear and aid are both doing are a necessary part of the process.

At the same time, a person can learn simple skills to enhance the usefulness of an aid. Speechreading (lipreading) is one. Most people already possess this skill to a remarkable degree. If you think you are not a speech reader, consider the times you have watched a TV movie where sound was not quite synchronized with lip movement.

Hearing handicaps before age 3

The problems of communication are vastly more complicated for the child who has never heard speech than for those whose hearing problems develop later.

Normally we learn to speak by imitating others and listening to the sounds we make. That instant replay—auditory feedback—allows us to correct our speech and continuously adjust the tone, rhythm, and loudness of our voices. Children who suffer a hearing loss in infancy must overcome a double hurdle: They are cut off from a major source of learning about the people, places, and things of this world. And they cannot benefit from the natural feedback system that makes speaking one's native tongue the inevitable event in development that it is for most of us.

Children who become moderately to severely impaired before age 3 (the prelingual years) can be helped by hearing aids, but as one specialist put it, "Rehabilitation begins with parent education . . . the audiologist and hearing therapist must use considerable skill in helping parents (and children) adjust to the benefits and the limitations of a hearing aid." How much progress can be made also depends on what other handicaps a child may have. Visual problems, movement disorders or mental retardation compound the basic communication and learning problems.

It is testimony to human resourcefulness and to progress in hearing research that people no longer despair of overcoming the problems of hearing loss in infancy. In times past those afflicted often remained mute or chose not to make vocal sounds. They communicated with the speaking world through notes, gestures, and signs—not unlike the tourist struggling in a foreign land. Society tended to enforce the communications barrier by ignoring the problem or else relegating deaf people to special schools or institutions. One result has been that deaf people have tended to form a separate culture among themselves, employing their own means of communication and seeking each other's company. Even today 95 percent of deaf people marry other deaf people. Many have the native intelligence and creativity to succeed at professional careers, but communication and social barriers continue to work against their achieving their full potential.

At the end of the 19th century, authorities urged reforms in education aimed at solving the problem of the isolation of the deaf: Enforce a strictly oral mode of speech training, they declared. Forbid children to use any form of sign language, finger spelling, or other manual communication. Instead, teach speechreading and vocal training exercises so that the deaf will have to master the sounds of speech and the principles of spoken language. This strictly oral approach has been effective in many cases and remains the guiding philosophy of many training centers and schools for the deaf throughout the world.

In the United States, however, opposition to the oral-only tradition remained active, in part due to the efforts of such teachers as Thomas Gallaudet, for whom Gallaudet College for the Deaf in Washington, D.C., is named. Gallaudet believed that the all-important goal for the deaf individual was to be able to communicate with *anyone*. He strongly advocated sign language. Others agreed, urging that whatever means aided communication—speechreading, vocal training, gestures, or sign language—should be encouraged. Today this "total communication" approach, as it has come to be called, coexists with the oral-only school, each with strong adherents and notable successes.

Important in the development of the total communication approach has been the growing use of American Sign Language, *Ameslan*. Ameslan uses subtle combinations of hand, face, and body movements to comprise a vocabulary and grammar that are distinct from English. Ameslan "signers" now make it possible for profoundly hearing-impaired people who have learned the language to watch the television news or attend some public meetings. In the hands of the creative actors and writers of the National Theater of the Deaf, Ameslan has also developed as a vehicle for imaginative expression in poetry and drama.

Hearing horizons today . . .

The hearing-impaired individual has more learning opportunities and communications aids available now than at any other time in history. Legislation enacted in 1973 prohibits discrimination against the handicapped in employment or education by any organization receiving any amount of Federal funds. This has meant new opportunities for the profoundly hard of hearing in the job market and at all levels of education.

In addition, variants on the training methods followed by either oralist or total communication practitioners have been developed. "Cued speech" is an outgrowth of the desire to make speechreading more effective. Speakers learn to augment their lip movements by finger signs to indicate particular consonantal or vowel sounds. The signs clarify whether the lips are saying "bad" or "pad," "road" or "load." (Only about a third of spoken English can be understood by interpreting lip movements alone.)

There has also been renewed interest in teaching the deaf to understand speech by having the deaf person feel the muscles of the throat and neck as the speaker pronounces words. This was the method Helen Keller's teacher used, and NINCDS-supported investigators at Massachusetts Institute of Technology (Cambridge, Mass.) are currently exploring its effectiveness.

An increasing variety of amplifying devices and signals are now available for the hearing impaired. Telephones can be equipped with lights to signal when the phone is ringing and amplifiers can be built into the receiver. Other communication equipment includes teleprinters which enable a sender to type a message that is then coded electronically for transmission over the phone. A decoder at the other end reconverts the signals to a printed message.

. . . and tomorrow

Meanwhile scientists are exploring how to use the body's other sense systems as a means of communication when hearing fails. The skin is sensitive to vibrations over a range of frequencies. By attaching a set of vibrators around the waist or chest, the wearer can learn to interpret a sequence of vibrations as words and sentences. Such "vibrotactile aids" are currently being investigated by NINCDS-supported scientists at the University of Washington in Seattle and the Callier Center for Communication, Dallas, Texas.

Perhaps the most ambitious scientific program on the design boards today is the cochlear implant, a device to aid individuals with sensorineural deafness. The implant uses tiny electrodes to apply electrical stimulation directly to auditory nerve fibers. NINCDS currently supports implant research at Stanford University, Palo Alto, Calif., the University of California at San Francisco, and the University of Washington in Seattle. In some designs, the electrodes are implanted in the cochlea itself, positioned to stimulate selected nerve fibers as they spiral around the shell. In other designs, the electrodes are applied to nerve fibers after they have been bundled together in the eighth nerve. Either way, the trick is to stimulate fibers associated with a selection of different frequencies so that the brain can distinguish different tones. So far, the implants use only a few electrodes, too crude to enable even the rudiments of speech to be encoded and deciphered. But in the few instances where profoundly deaf individuals have volunteered to have the devices surgically implanted, the hardware seems to be well tolerated and the wearers generally report pleasure in being able to hear any sound at all.

The state of the art of cochlear implants is in its infancy. A dozen or so microelectrodes cannot be expected to replace the 30,000 nerve fibers we are born with in each ear. But advances in electronics, in computers, in audio engineering, and in hearing science have been great and continue to develop at an impressive rate. Tomorrow's cochlear implants may be even more miniaturized, allowing greater numbers of fibers to be stimulated with less risk that the implant itself may damage tissue. And if, in the end, the cochlear implant is not the ideal device, the same kind of thinking that led imaginative men and women to try it in the first place will stimulate other research directions, ultimately more successful solutions for the problems of the hearing impaired. That is the hope through research.

Voluntary health organizations

There are many organizations concerned with the problems of the hearing impaired. One of the largest groups is the American Speech-Language-Hearing Association, which is both a professional and lay organization. Another important professional organization is the American Academy of Otolaryngology/Head and Neck Surgery, which provides information to the general public.

Some groups espouse particular philosophies in speech education and training. The Alexander Graham Bell Association for the Deaf, for example, adopts the oralist approach. All the groups listed provide literature and advice, and can generally indicate schools and other resources available in local communities. Some organizations, like the National Easter Seal Society, have local chapters providing information and rehabilitation for a variety of handicapping conditions. One organization, the Better Hearing Institute, provides information on a toll-free Hearing HelpLine: (800) 424-8576. In addition, some organizations also support research. Most can supply practical information for individuals interested in donating temporal bone tissue to Temporal Bone Banks for research study. The temporal bone of the skull, collected at autopsy, contains the organs of hearing and balance and is valuable source material for scientists studying the tissue changes that occur in communicative disorders.

Organizations:

Alexander Graham Bell Association for the Deaf, Inc.
3417 Volta Place N.W.
Washington, D.C. 20007
(202) 337-5220

American Academy of Otolaryngology/Head and Neck Surgery
1101 Vermont Avenue, N.W., Suite 302
Washington, D.C. 20005
(202) 289-4607

American Speech-Language-Hearing Association
10801 Rockville Pike
Rockville, Md. 20852
(301) 897-5700

American Tinnitus Association
P. O. Box #5
Portland, Ore. 97207
(503) 248-9985

Better Hearing Institute
1430 K St., N.W.
Washington, D.C. 20005
Toll-free Hearing HelpLine: (800) 424-8576

The Deafness Research Foundation
9 East 38th Street
New York, New York 10016
(212) 684-6556

National Association for Hearing and Speech Action
10801 Rockville Pike
Rockville, Md. 20852
(301) 897-8682 (Call Collect)

National Association of the Deaf
Suite 301
814 Thayer Avenue
Silver Spring, Md. 20910
(301) 587-1788

National Black Association for Speech, Language, and Hearing
P. O. Box 50214
Washington, D.C. 20004

National Easter Seal Society, Inc.
2023 West Ogden Avenue
Chicago, Ill. 60612
(312) 243-8400

National Hearing Association
P. O. Box 8897
Metairie, Louisiana 70011
(504) 888-HEAR(4327)
Dr. Wallace Rubin, President

Self-Help for Hard of Hearing People, Inc.
7800 Wisconsin Avenue
Bethesda, Maryland 20814
(301) 657-2248

Publications

The following publications are published for people with hearing impairment and others concerned with the problem. (Subscription prices are not given since they are subject to change.)

Silent News
193 Main Street
Lincoln Park, N.J. 07035

Deaf American
(Published by the National Association of the Deaf, listed above)

NINCDS Information

Additional information concerning hearing research supported by the Communicative Disorders Program of the National Institute of Neurological and Communicative Disorders and Stroke can be obtained from:

Office of Scientific and Health Reports
National Institute of Neurological and Communicative Disorders and Stroke
Building 31, Room 8A-06
National Institutes of Health
Bethesda, Md. 20205
(301) 496-5751

U.S. Department of Health and Human Services, Public Health Service, National Institutes of Health. Prepared by the Office of Scientific and Health Reports, National Institute of Neurological and Communicative Disorders and Stroke. National Institutes of Health, Bethesda, Maryland 20205. NIH Publication No. 82–157, January 1982.

Heart Attacks
The magnitude of the problem

Cardiovascular disease is a major health problem, with 60 million Americans having high blood pressure or one or more forms of heart or blood vessel disease. Heart disease has been the number one cause of death since 1910. Since 1949 it has caused about one-half the deaths in the United States, accounting for 987,000 deaths in 1983. Two forms of cardiovascular disease, heart disease and stroke, rank as the first and third causes of death respectively.

In economic terms, data available for 1982 give an idea of the huge cost of cardiovascular diseases to the Nation. That year, the cost to the U.S. for cardiovascular diseases was an estimated $94 billion. Of this total, $41 billion was for direct health care costs; and an additional $53 billion was the estimated loss of productivity resulting from illness and premature deaths from cardiovascular diseases.

How the heart works

To understand what happens in a heart attack, think of the heart as a four-chambered pump. Blood from the body enters the upper chamber, atrium, on the right side of the heart and flows from there into the lower chamber, the ventricle. The blood is then pumped under relatively low pressure into the lungs where it releases excess carbon dioxide and picks up oxygen. The oxygenated blood flows from the lungs to the atrium on the left side of the heart and then into the lower chamber, left ventricle. The left ventricle, the main pumping chamber, then pumps the blood under relatively higher pressure to the rest of the body to supply oxygen and nutrients to the tissues.

So, the heart is like a pump, squeezing and forcing blood throughout the body. The most important part of the heart is the heart muscle, or myocardium. Like all muscles in the body, the myocardium must have oxygen and nutrients in order to do its work. The myocardium cannot use oxygen and nutrients directly from the blood within the chambers of the heart. Instead, nutrients and oxygen are furnished by three main blood vessels outside the heart. These are the left anterior descending and circumflex arteries (which start out together as the left coronary artery) and the right coronary artery. They in turn have further branches.

What causes heart attacks?

Arteriosclerosis, which involves both hardening and blocking of the blood vessels, is the major cause of cardiovascular disease. Arteriosclerosis of the coronary arteries, also known as coronary artery disease, continues to be the most important medical problem, in spite of a number of advances in medical and surgical treatment. It causes the most death, severely limits activity, and is the leading cause of social security disability. It also ranks first in number of hospital bed days utilized.

Arteriosclerosis is a general medical term for a number of diseases of the arteries. Atherosclerosis is the most common form of arteriosclerosis and it affects primarily the larger arteries of the body. In this condition the lining of the artery becomes thickened and irregular with deposits of fatty substances.

Atherosclerosis develops by a process that is totally silent. At birth the vessels are perfectly smooth and open, but all through one's life fatty deposits, or atheromata, develop in the blood vessels. Fortunately, in most people they develop at a very slow rate and only in certain areas.

Moreover, medical evidence shows that more than two-thirds of a coronary artery may be filled with fatty deposits without causing symptoms. Symptoms may show themselves as chest pain, called angina pectoris; heart attack, or sudden death. Arteriosclerosis is responsible for 77 percent of all cardiovascular disease, or using 1981 statistics, for more than 760,000 deaths a year. Twenty percent of deaths due to arteriosclerosis, about 150,000 a year, occur in people younger than 65.

Heart attacks account for nearly 56 percent of all cardiovascular deaths. In 1983 more than 550,000 deaths were due to arteriosclerosis of the coronary arteries resulting in heart attack. Another 160,000 deaths were due to strokes caused by arteriosclerosis of the vessels of the brain.

When a heart attack occurs

A heart attack happens when any of the coronary vessels become blocked and blood reaches the more distant heart muscle. Recent studies have shown that most heart attacks are caused by the formation of a clot, thrombus, in a coronary vessel at the site of narrowing and hardening. If an area of the myocardium is supplied by more than one vessel, the heart muscle may live for a period of time even if one vessel becomes blocked. However, the extent of heart muscle damage occurring with a heart attack depends on which vessel is blocked, on whether it is a big or small one, and on the remaining blood supply to that area of the myocardium. When heart muscle does not get adequate oxygen and nutrients, it dies. This process is called a myocardial infarction. A further area of heart muscle may be deprived of blood flow and oxygen to a lesser degree causing a temporary injury called myocardial ischemia. This dead and injured heart muscle causes the heart to lose some of its effectiveness as a pump, since reduced muscle contraction means reduced blood flow.

Symptoms

Many different symptoms may indicate a heart attack. Certainly the one most people have is chest pain, but this pain differs among individuals. Most often the pain is under the breastbone, or sternum. Sometimes it radiates to the neck, jaw or left shoulder or goes down the left arm. Some describe the pain as viselike, or constricting, as if a rope were being pulled tightly around the chest. Heart attack patients often experience weakness, shortness of breath, and nausea. A patient acutely ill with a heart attack often appears pale, cold, and sweaty.

Unfortunately, the first sign of disease in the heart and its vessels in about one-quarter of the patients who suffer heart attacks is sudden death. Also, approximately 60 percent of the deaths due to heart attacks occur outside of the hospital.

Risk of death is greatest within the first two hours of the heart attack. What does this mean? It means that anyone who has a new onset of chest pain or anyone with coronary disease who has continuing chest pain should seek medical help as quickly as possible.

What to do, where to go for help

If you have any sign of a heart attack, have someone get you to a hospital and obtain medical help as quickly as possible. But what if you or someone in a crowd suddenly collapses? A lifesaving technique has been developed to help someone who suffers heart arrest before an ambulance comes. This procedure is called cardiopulmonary resuscitation.

Cardiopulmonary Resuscitation (CPR)
If someone has had a heart attack so severe that the heart and breathing have stopped, CPR can keep the person alive until an ambulance and medical treatment is available. CPR is an emergency procedure that can be started immediately when the heart stops.

CPR involves using a combination of mouth-to-mouth resuscitation to maintain the patient's breathing and compression of the chest to maintain circulation. It has been used successfully for some time by doctors and nurses and an increasing fraction of the general public. It is recommended that the public be trained to use CPR. If you are interested in learning CPR, consult the white pages of your telephone book and call your local chapter of the American Heart Association or the American Red Cross.

Medical Aid
What happens when an ambulance does come, when a paramedic or doctor arrives on the scene? The first effort is to relax the patient and relieve pain. Doctors handle this primarily by giving an injection of pain-relieving drugs which will relieve chest pain and relax the patient. In addition, oxygen often may be given to try to make up for a deficient blood supply and to keep the heart muscle working.

Electrocardiograms are used to find out whether a heart attack really is happening. By placing electrodes on the chest and arms, the area of heart damage can be located. An electrocardiogram can also characterize rhythm disturbances.

Defibrillators
Should the heart develop ventricular fibrillation, a quivering of the heart with no effective beat, what happens then? Most ambulances now carry special equipment called defibrillators. Using a defibrillator, a paramedic or physician shocks the heart with an electrical impulse that can correct a chaotic, ineffective rhythm or start the heart beating again. Defibrillation is very effective and has saved many lives that otherwise would have been lost.

Coronary Care Units
When the ambulance reaches the hospital, the patient is admitted immediately to a coronary care unit where vital signs—blood pressure, heart rate, temperature, respiration—can be monitored.

Blood pressure is measured in order to determine the adequacy of blood circulation and blood is drawn for tests that can help diagnose a heart attack.

In the coronary care unit, medicines will be given that can relax the patient, relieve pain, or control the blood pressure. Also there are medicines that can help the heart to beat regularly.

Electrical Heart Problems
The heart is normally paced by electrical impulses from specific areas of the heart. If part of the heart's electrical system is injured by disease or heart attack, it may slow dramatically or it may stop beating. A much more common electrical problem is early or extra beats, which may progress to the chaotic, fatal ventricular fibrillation if not treated with drugs.

Twenty-five years ago, over half the heart attack deaths were from electrical problems in the heart. Today, in-hospital deaths due to electrical rhythm disturbances of the heart have become relatively uncommon because of the ability to monitor electrical impulses, to control heart rhythm with drugs or pacemakers, and to restart the heart with defibrillators. As a result, the death rate in hospitalized heart attack patients has been reduced from 30 to 40 percent to 15 percent or even less. Most of these remaining deaths result from weakening of the heart. The heart muscle may have been so extensively damaged that the heart cannot beat effectively. The result is not enough blood pumped out to serve the rest of the body.

Problems of Heart Function
Doctors are also making inroads in problems of maintaining adequate heart function. Techniques are now available that allow estimating the

amount of heart muscle that has been damaged when a patient has a heart attack. Blood tests measure the amount of specific enzymes released by dying and dead heart muscle and help diagnose how severe the heart attack is. Using a still experimental procedure, doctors can find and measure specific areas of heart damage and follow the extent of a heart attack by mapping the heart. This is done by placing a special vest with many small electrodes on the patient's chest.

In addition, new tests allow visualization of the area of heart damage. When certain radioisotopes are injected into a patient's vein, they accumulate in heart tissue. Some radioisotopes have an affinity for dead tissue, which allows the doctor to determine the extent of the damaged area. Others collect in healthy heart muscle, and thus indicate areas of inadequate perfusion or injury. Still others remain in the blood, allowing measurement of the dimensions and movements of the heart chambers.

The amount of muscle damaged during a heart attack is not fixed when a patient enters a coronary care unit. There are now treatments that may decrease the amount of heart muscle damage. These include giving oxygen or altering the blood pressure in some circumstances. Clinical studies are being conducted to identify other treatments to decrease the amount of heart muscle damage. Some studies are testing thrombolytic agents which are infused by catheter into the coronary circulation or injected into a vein to enter the general circulation. A thrombolytic agent is one that dissolves (lyses) a blood clot (thrombus) that may be obstructing a vein or coronary artery. Also being tested are special catheters that may dilate partially obstructed vessels. These agents and techniques may reduce heart muscle damage and mechanical failure, which are the major causes of death in patients hospitalized with heart disease.

After a heart attack

Rehabilitation for the patient with a heart attack begins at the time of hospitalization, as the patient enters the coronary care unit. Doctors now know that many symptoms experienced by patients after heart attacks are not due to heart muscle damage but to physical inactivity. Today, patients begin to exercise arm and leg muscles while in the coronary care unit. Shortly after hospital discharge, they can go on to full activity under medical supervision. Often, an exercise test is done before leaving the hospital to test endurance and to look for abnormal heart rhythm associated with exercise.

Coronary bypass surgery

Chest pain, angina, may continue in some people after they have a heart attack. Activity may provoke pain in the chest or left arm. Bypassing the area of obstruction with a procedure called coronary artery bypass surgery has been shown to relieve angina in many patients. In this procedure, as most commonly performed, a large vein called the saphenous vein is removed from the leg. One end of the vein is implanted into the aorta and the other end is connected to a coronary vessel beyond its obstruction. The coronary bypass operation supplies blood to an area of the heart with deficient blood supply, thereby relieving chest pain. Patients who were once incapacitated and limited to low-level activity can generally be relieved of pain with this procedure. There is also evidence that coronary bypass surgery in properly selected patients improves the function of the left ventricle or makes the heart pump better.

A recently reported study sponsored by the National Heart, Lung, and Blood Institute has demonstrated that the great majority of patients with stable and mild or moderate symptoms can defer having a bypass operation without fear of premature death. The Coronary Artery Surgery Study included 780 men and women who were randomly assigned to either a surgical group, which received a bypass operation, or a medical group, which was maintained on drug therapy.

Patients were followed for more than five years after entering the study to determine the number of heart attacks and deaths in both groups. Those in the medical group whose chest pain became a problem despite medical treatment had bypass surgery as needed for management of their symptoms.

At the end of the study, investigators found no significant difference in survival between the two major groups. In one subgroup—patients with both a limited pumping ability of the heart and substantial narrowing of all three major coronary arteries—those who received surgery initially had a better survival rate than those in whom surgery was deferred. The investigators concluded that for patients who fit the criteria of the study—patients with stable and only mild or moderate symptoms—bypass surgery could be postponed safely by medical management with appropriate heart medications unless the patients had both poor pumping function of the heart and involvement of all three major coronary arteries.

PTCA

A small percentage of patients who are candidates for bypass surgery may qualify for a simpler procedure, performed under local anesthetic, called PTCA (percutaneous transluminal coronary angioplasty) or the balloon catheter. For this procedure, the doctor inserts a balloon-tipped catheter into an artery through a small incision in the groin. The tip of the catheter is fed through the arterial system and positioned in the coronary artery at the site of the blockage. The small sausage-shaped balloon on the tip of the catheter is then inflated briefly to press the blockage against the walls of the artery and open up the narrowed artery. The balloon may have to be inflated and deflated several times to accomplish this. The doctors follow the progress of the procedure on an image intensifier so they can see when the channel of the artery has been opened. Once the opening has been enlarged, the balloon catheter is removed.

This procedure seems to offer a number of advantages over bypass surgery, but a rigorous comparison has not yet been made. It does not involve opening the chest, general anesthesia, or the use of the heart lung machine; and hospitalization and recovery are quicker. However, an occasional patient needs emergency bypass surgery. For a substantial fraction of patients, coronary narrowing recurs, requiring PTCA again or bypass surgery. Furthermore, the procedure is appropriate for only a fraction of patients who would otherwise need bypass surgery, and patient selection must be very carefully carried out.

Some new techniques

By monitoring the heart during exercise, doctors can spot possible problems. As exercise causes the heart to work harder, electrocardiography can measure one aspect of the heart's response to the increased exercise.

Also by injecting a small amount of radioactive dye into an arm vein, cardiologists can use imaging procedures to check the condition of the heart. The radioactive thalium will go into normal heart muscle but not into any area of ischemia. This method is being applied more often together with exercise tests. Within the next few years new techniques such as digital subtraction angiography, positron emission tomography, and magnetic resonance imaging may become important in letting cardiologists get a better view of the heart and its coronary arteries. These improved imaging techniques may result in even better diagnosis and treatment for selected patients.

Prevention

Cardiovascular epidemiologists have provided clues for preventing heart disease. They have defined traits and habits, called risk factors, that identify a person with an increased chance of having a heart attack long before the heart attack occurs. Risk factors can be divided into those that cannot be changed and those that can be modified to reduce the chances of having a heart attack.

Certain risk factors are built-in such as age, sex, and family history. The older you get, the more likely it is you will have a heart attack. Also a male is at higher risk than a female. A family history of your father, mother, brother, or sister having had a heart attack increases your chances of having one.

There are three important, or primary risk factors that can be changed. These are cigarette smoking, high blood pressure, and high blood cholesterol. The presence of any of these risk factors increases your chances of having a heart attack, and two or three of them together may make you as much as eight times more likely to have a heart attack. In addition, there are some less powerful, or secondary, risk factors including obesity, diabetes, and lack of exercise.

Cigarette Smoking
The Surgeon General of the United States has said that cigarette smoking "should be considered the most important of the known modifiable risk factors for coronary heart disease in the United States." Also, cigarette smoking is a graded risk factor, so the more you smoke the greater your risk of heart attack. Someone who smokes two packs of cigarettes a day is more at risk than the person who smokes one pack a day, and both are at greater risk than the nonsmoker.

Of course, cigarette smoking is associated with other diseases such as emphysema, lung cancer and other forms of cancer. Giving up cigarettes or never smoking in the first place is a major step to disease prevention.

High Blood Pressure
High blood pressure, or hypertension, is another of the major risk factors for heart disease. Probably up to 58 million Americans have high blood pressure. High blood pressure may eventually lead to a heart attack, stroke or kidney disease, so taking steps to control it will pay off. Scientific studies over the years have proven the benefits of controlling elevated blood pressure.

Blood pressure is measured using the familiar inflatable cuff and the stethoscope. The reading is reported in two numbers such as 120/80. The top number is the systolic blood pressure, which is the pressure exerted against the artery walls when the heart contracts. The bottom number is the diastolic blood pressure, which is the lowest pressure remaining in the arteries between heartbeats when the heart is at rest. A systolic reading of 140 or more, or a diastolic reading of 90 or more, or both, on repeated occasions indicates high blood pressure.

High blood pressure also is a graded risk. That is, if an individual's blood pressure rises from a normal of 120/80 to 150/95, that person's risk for a heart attack doubles. If other risk factors such as smoking are present, the risk may increase even more. High blood pressure has no symptoms, so a person is not able to tell whether he or she has it unless it is measured.

It is very important to lower elevated blood pressure to normal levels. Often this can be accomplished by changes in lifestyle. Weight reduction for the overweight individual is often very effective in lowering blood pressure. Other means such as avoiding salt and starting a regular exercise program are steps that can be taken to lower blood pressure. However, if these lifestyle alterations are not successful in lowering blood pressure, the doctor will prescribe medication for the condition. Even though no symptoms are noted, it is important to remain on the medication to keep the blood pressure under control.

High Blood Cholesterol

Cholesterol is a blood fat that is essential for certain body functions, but too much blood cholesterol can result in buildup of deposits in the arteries which may lead to a heart attack. Keeping cholesterol to a low level is an effective way to help prevent a heart attack. High blood cholesterol is another graded risk; that is, the person who has total cholesterol of 260 mg/dl is at greater risk of heart attack than is the person whose cholesterol is 220 mg/dl (mg/dl means milligrams of cholesterol per deciliter of blood; a deciliter is $\frac{1}{10}$ of a liter or about $\frac{1}{10}$ of a quart).

Although the relationship of high blood cholesterol to the increased risk of heart attack has been well known for some time, it was not proven until recently that reducing blood cholesterol will also reduce the risk of heart attack. The results of a recent clinical study, involving patients with substantial elevations of blood cholesterol, showed conclusively that lowering elevated blood cholesterol effectively lowers the risk of heart attack. For every 1 percent that the cholesterol level was reduced, the risk of heart attack was reduced by 2 percent. The person who reduced blood cholesterol by 25 percent potentially cut the risk of having a heart attack in half.

If blood cholesterol is elevated, steps should be taken to bring it down. The first method is to modify diet. Limit intake of saturated (animal) fat found in foods such as butter, whole milk, cheese and fatty red meats. Limit your intake of cholesterol-rich foods like egg yolks and organ meats. Eat more poultry (with skin removed) and fish. If you eat beef, pork, or lamb, trim off the fat and bake or broil it so the fat drains away from the meat. Read food labels so that polyunsaturated fats can be substituted for saturated fats, where possible.

Polyunsaturated fats come from vegetable sources such as sunflower, corn, or safflower oils. A registered dietitian can help you achieve changes in food choices and preparation to best reduce your blood cholesterol level.

Some people with high blood cholesterol may not be able to lower it enough through diet and exercise and may need to be placed on cholesterol-lowering drugs.

Other Risk Factors

Diabetes, or high blood sugar, is a significant problem that usually can be controlled. More than 80 percent of people who have diabetes die of some form of premature cardiovascular disease, usually heart attack. Control of the diabetes is thought to be important in decreasing cardiovascular risk. Elimination or reduction of other risk factors like hypertension, smoking, high blood cholesterol, and obesity is especially important for the diabetic.

A sedentary, or inactive, lifestyle is another factor that contributes to heart disease. People who are sedentary also may be adding another risk factor in the form of obesity. Excess weight in the form of fat, especially to the point that one is considered obese, adds to the work of the heart and increases the blood pressure. Also, it may be associated with elevated blood cholesterol. Overweight individuals are also more likely to develop diabetes.

A program of regular exercise is important in helping to guard against heart attacks. If you do not exercise regularly now, do not begin a rigorous program immediately. Start with a moderate exercise such as extra walking and gradually increase the exercise level until the heart and the other muscles in the body are in relatively good condition. If your health is not good to start with or if you experience symptoms such as chest pain while exercising, consult your doctor. All of the coronary risk factors significantly increase a person's chance of having a heart attack. However, many risk factors can be controlled, and taking steps to do so will lower the risk of heart disease.

You are changing

Although making these changes is extremely difficult, the American public seems to be changing. In 1964, the Surgeon General's report stated that smoking was hazardous to health and that smoking cigarettes would produce lung cancer, chronic bronchitis, emphysema, and early heart attack. In the years since then, the number of male smokers has decreased by 27 percent and the number of female smokers has decreased by 14 percent (however, young girls ages 12 to 20 are smoking more). Doctors have also decreased their smoking by over 45 percent during this time.

In 1971 the National High Blood Pressure Education Program was started because more than half of all Americans who had high blood pressure did not know it, and only about one-eighth were on adequate therapy. Since that program began, the number of Americans who do not know they have high blood pressure has fallen precipitously. Persons with high blood pressure have increased their visits to physicians by 50 percent. The number of patients on effective treatment for high blood pressure has increased from about 4 million to more than 11 million.

We have evidence of change. Americans are exercising more and have changed their dietary habits; per capita food consumption has changed. Since 1963, per capita consumption of whole milk is down 16 percent, use of butter and eggs is down 38 percent and 17 percent respectively, and the eating of animal fats and oils is down 39 percent. During this same time period, intake of vegetable fats and oils is up 63 percent.

Americans are changing their habits and their lifestyles, and they are reaping rewards for these behavior changes. Cardiovascular death rates are going down. Heart attack death rates, which began to decline about the time of the Surgeon General's report on smoking in 1964, have continued to decline at a greater rate since 1972.

In addition, a decline is seen in the absolute number of deaths due to heart disease. Beginning in the mid-1960's, more than 1 million Americans have died each year of cardiovascular disease, primarily heart attack. However, despite a growing and aging population, each year from 1975 through 1984, fewer than 1 million people died from this cause.

This decrease emphasizes the fact that prevention of heart attacks and improved medical care are resulting in great progress against heart disease. Everyone, however, must take the responsibility for maintaining his or her own health. So far, many Americans have acted on available evidence. Heart attack rates are decreasing. By controlling risk factors—cigarette smoking, high blood pressure, high blood cholesterol—the number of heart attacks will continue to decrease.

This publication is a revision of *Medicine for the Layman: Heart Attacks* (NIH Publication No. 79–1803) produced by the Information Office of the National Institutes of Health Clinical Center. The original publication was adapted from a lecture delivered by Robert I. Levy, M.D. while he served as Director of the National Heart, Lung, and Blood Institute. U.S. Department of Health and Human Services, Public Health Service National Institutes of Health. NIH Publication No. 86–2700, September 1986.

HEART CHARTS

Keeping track of cholesterol, blood pressure, and pulse rate is useful in keeping the heart healthy. Below are some charts that offer guidance on desirable ranges. Cholesterol counts are obtained by health professionals from blood samples. Blood pressure readings and pulse rates can be done at home or by a health professional. These readings are usually included in routine physical examinations, results of which are generally available to individuals.

Blood Pressure Classifications
Diastolic Blood Pressure
(The Lower of the Two Numbers)

Reading	Category
Less than 85	Normal blood pressure
85 to 89	High normal blood pressure
90 to 104	Mild hypertension
105 to 114	Moderate hypertension
115 or more	Severe hypertension

Systolic Blood Pressure
(The Higher of the Two Numbers and Coupled with a Diastolic Reading of Less than 90)

Reading	Category
Less than 140	Normal blood pressure
140 to 159	Borderline isolated systolic hypertension
160 or more	Isolated systolic hypertension

These categories are for persons 18 and older.

Source: The 1984 "Report of the Joint National Committee on Detection, Evaluation and Treatment of High Blood Pressure."

Cholesterol
(in Milligrams Per Deciliter)

Age	Moderate Risk	High Risk
2–19	Over 170	Over 195
20–29	Over 200	Over 220
30–39	Over 220	Over 240
40 and up	Over 240	Over 260

Source: National Institutes of Health consensus conference statement, *Lowering Blood Cholesterol*, 1984.

Exercise Pulse Rates

Age	Target Zone
20	120–150
25	117–146
30	114–142
35	111–138
40	108–135
45	105–131
50	102–127
55	99–123
60	96–120
65	93–116
70	90–113

"Target zone" is the pulse or heart rate in beats per minute. Exercise that sustains that target zone level for 30 minutes should be undertaken at least three times a week. Persons over 40 who have not been exercising regularly should consult a doctor before embarking on such a program.

Source: *Exercise and Your Heart,* National Heart, Lung and Blood Institute. FDA Consumer, February 1986, HHS Pub. No. (FDA) 86–1126.

Planning a Diet for a Healthy Heart

Coronary heart disease accounts for more U.S. deaths annually—in excess of 550,000—than any other disease, including all forms of cancer. (The term coronary is derived from the Latin word corona, meaning crown, and refers to the two arteries that originate in the aorta and supply blood directly to the heart, surrounding it much like a crown.)

Coronary heart disease is the most common cause of disability in this country. It is costly in other terms, too—imposing a financial burden in excess of $60 billion a year in direct and indirect costs.

The National Institutes of Health estimates that there are more than

5.4 million Americans "with symptomatic coronary heart disease and a large number of others with undiagnosed coronary disease, many of them young and highly productive."

One major contributor to coronary heart disease is atherosclerosis, or "hardening of the arteries." A high blood cholesterol level contributes to this condition, although it is not the only risk factor: Individuals are also at greater risk if they have high blood pressure or diabetes, smoke cigarettes, or are overweight.

Atherosclerosis results from a buildup of solid material called plaque in and on the walls of blood vessels. The buildup of plaque, which contains cholesterol and other substances, can restrict blood flow. Why plaque deposits are formed, what role cholesterol levels play in plaque formation, and to what extent the consumption of fat—especially saturated fat—and cholesterol influences blood cholesterol levels are questions that continue to plague scientists and medical authorities.

Despite the uncertainties, FDA, in the regulation it proposed recently for cholesterol labeling of foods, noted that most experts believe there is "a correlation between the severity of the plaque deposits and the levels of cholesterol in the blood."

The number of health experts who accept the cholesterol-heart disease connection has been growing steadily. In 1979, the U.S. Surgeon General issued a report that said Americans would be healthier if they consumed less saturated fat and cholesterol. In 1980, and again in 1985, the Department of Health and Human Services and the Department of Agriculture jointly published their "Dietary Guidelines for Americans," which called for similar dietary changes.

At a December 1984 conference held by the National Institutes of Health, a panel of experts reported that "elevated blood cholesterol level is a major cause of coronary artery disease" and proper dietary changes could reduce blood cholesterol levels. The panel cited data from more than a dozen clinical studies to support its conclusion.

One of the more important of these was a 7- to 10-year clinical study reported in January 1984 by the National Heart, Lung, and Blood Institute (NHLBI). A total of 3,806 men who were considered at high risk of developing coronary heart disease were in the study. The principal aim was to determine how well blood cholesterol levels could be treated by drug therapy, but findings about dietary changes also made the study noteworthy.

The participants in this study were put on a diet that contained about 400 milligrams of cholesterol a day and was designed to lower cholesterol levels by 3 to 5 percent. The diet included a high ratio of polyunsaturated fats to saturated fats. After three months, the dietary changes resulted in a 3.5 percent reduction in total cholesterol in the blood and a 4 percent drop in low-density lipoprotein (LDL) cholesterol. (High levels of LDL cholesterol have been associated with an increased risk of heart disease.)

The study also showed that an 8 percent reduction in blood cholesterol could reduce the risk of coronary heart disease by 19 percent. And the risk was reduced by 50 percent for those participants who had reduced their total blood cholesterol by 25 percent. In effect, NHLBI said, the study showed that "for every 1 percent drop in plasma cholesterol, there was a 2 percent reduction in coronary heart disease risk."

Because of such findings, the NIH panel recommended that Americans change their diets to reduce the level of blood cholesterol. The panel urged everyone except children under 2 to reduce fat intake from the current level of about 40 percent of total calories to no more than 30 percent. Particularly, Americans should reduce their intake of saturated fat from the current 16 to 18 percent of total calories to less than 10 percent. Consumption of polyunsaturated fats should be *increased* from the current 5 percent to 8 percent, but to no more than 10 percent of total calories. And, finally, these experts said, cholesterol intake should amount to no more than 250 to 300 milligrams a day.

Similar recommendations have been made by the American Heart Association, the American Medical Association, the federally created Inter-Society Commission for Heart Disease Resources, the World Health Organization, and other public and private health authorities.

Chris W. Lecos

Cutting Back on Fat and Cholesterol

	Maximum Percent of Total Calories
Total Fat*	Reduce to no more than 30%
Saturated Fat	Reduce to no more than 10%
Polyunsaturated Fat	Increase, up to 10%
Cholesterol	No more than 250–300 milligrams a day

The National Heart, Lung, and Blood Institute has recommended that all Americans over 2 years old moderate their intake of fat, especially saturated, fat, and cholesterol. The chart above is based on a 1984 Consensus Development Conference Statement issued by the institute.

* Total fat includes not only saturated and polyunsaturated fat, but also mono-unsaturated fat, which would make up the remaining 10 percent of total fat.

How Much Fat Should You Eat?

Total Daily Calories	Maximum Amount of Fat (in Grams)
1,500	50
2,000	67
2,500	83
3,000	100

Americans are being urged to reduce their consumption of fat from the current average of 40 percent of total calories to no more than 30 percent. Above is a rough guide to help show the amount of fat that will provide 30 percent of total daily calories. For example, if you eat an average of 2,500 calories a day, 83 grams represents 30 percent of your total calories.

If you're not sure of your typical calorie intake, here's a rough guide: 2,000 calories is the average suggested for women 23 to 50, and 2,700 calories is the average for men. Whether these levels are right for you depends on your age, body size, and level of activity.

The problem that confronts many people is how to translate recommendations for a reduced-cholesterol, reduced-fat diet into a shopping list and menu for themselves and their families.

In general, this means eating more fruits, vegetables, cereal grains, and starches, which have less fat (particularly saturated fat) and no cholesterol, and choosing vegetable oils such as safflower, sunflower, corn, and soybean oils, which have higher levels of polyunsaturated fatty acids and low levels of saturated fatty acids.

Here are some tips to help consumers pick and prepare foods lower in saturated fat and cholesterol:

- Switch from butter or a hydrogenated margarine high in saturated fatty acids to one higher in polyunsaturates. Soft tub margarines made from corn, safflower, or sunflower oils are the best choices.
- Use skim or low-fat (1 percent) milk.
- Buy lean grades of meat and trim visible fat. Prepare mixed dishes that combine meat with other foods (vegetable stews or pasta, for example). Eat organ meat, such as liver, brain and kidney, only occasionally.
- Broil, bake, or roast meat, fish, and poultry instead of pan-frying or deep-fat frying. Basting with wine, broth, lemon or tomato juice will prevent drying and give good flavor.
- Eat more fish, poultry (without skin), and dried peas and beans.
- Substitute low-fat sandwich meats for higher fat cold cuts, and use low-fat hot dogs instead of regular varieties. Serve sliced turkey breast,

Dairy Products

When selecting dairy products in a healthy-heart diet, try the low-fat options. Low-fat milk, for example, contains the vitamins, minerals and protein found in whole milk, but with less fat and cholesterol and fewer calories.

	Calories (Approximate)	Total Fat (Grams)	Saturated Fat (Grams)	Cholesterol (Milligrams)
MILK, YOGURT AND CHEESE:				
Milk, whole, 1 cup	150	8.1	5.1	33
Milk, 2 percent fat, with nonfat milk solids, 1 cup	125	4.7	2.9	18
Milk, 1 percent fat, with nonfat milk solids, 1 cup	105	2.4	1.5	10
Skim milk with nonfat milk solids, 1 cup	90	.6	.4	5
Yogurt, plain, low-fat, 8-ounce carton	145	3.5	2.3	14
Yogurt, fruit-flavored, low-fat, 8-ounce carton	230	2.4	1.6	10
Cottage cheese, creamed, ½ cup	120	5.2	3.3	17
Cottage cheese, 1 percent fat, ½ cup	80	1.1	.7	5
Cottage cheese, dry, ½ cup	60	.3	.2	5
Natural Cheddar cheese, 1 ounce	115	9.4	6.0	30
Mozzarella cheese, part skim milk, 1 ounce	70	4.5	2.9	16
Pasteurized process low-fat cheese product, 1 ounce	55	3.0	2.0	5
Pasteurized process filled cheese food (low cholesterol), 1 ounce	90	6.5	.8	1

CREAM AND COFFEE CREAMERS:

Sour cream, 1 tablespoon	25	2.5	1.6	5
Cream, table or light, 1 tablespoon	30	2.9	2.8	10
Cream, half-and-half, 1 tablespoon	20	1.7	1.1	6
Coffee creamer with coconut or palm oil, frozen liquid, 1 tablespoon	20	1.5	1.4	0
Coffee creamer with coconut or palm oil, dry powder, 1 teaspoon	10	.7	.6	0

DESSERTS:

Vanilla ice cream, ½ cup	135	7.2	4.4	30
Vanilla ice milk, ½ cup	90	2.8	1.8	9
Frozen yogurt, ½ cup	95	1.5	1.0	6
Orange sherbet, ½ cup	135	1.9	1.2	7

Source: *Food 3*, published by the American Dietetic Association based on material originally developed by the U.S. Department of Agriculture, 1982. One ounce = approximately 28 grams.

low-fat ham, and tuna or chicken salad instead of bologna and other processed sandwich meats.

- Use salad dressings made from oils other than coconut or palm (olive oil, for instance). Use yogurt as a substitute for sour cream.
- Substitute sherbet, ice milk, or nonfat frozen yogurt or tofu desserts for ice cream.
- When baking, cut back on cholesterol-laden egg yolks by using only the whites or by discarding every other yolk and substituting a teaspoon of polyunsaturated oil for each discarded yolk.
- Reduce the amount of fat in recipes by a third to a half. If you use commercial cake mixes, for example, buy those to which you add the fat or oil. Use a polyunsaturated oil and reduce the amount by a third, while increasing the water. For example, if the recipe calls for three tablespoons of oil, use only two, but add an extra tablespoon of water.
- Cut down on baked goods made with lard, coconut oil, palm oil, or shortening, and those deep fried in fat, such as doughnuts.
- Instead of two-crust pies, serve single-crust (open-face) pies.
- Use low-fat dried milk instead of non-dairy creamers for coffee. These creamers are generally high in coconut oil, which contains saturated fats.
- Use herbs or herb-flavored croutons instead of bacon bits or cheese to flavor salads or soups.
- Instead of whipped cream or commercial toppings (which are high in fat, especially saturated fats), make your own with nonfat dried milk, or use a yogurt, tofu or fruit topping.
- Substitute low-fat cheese such as part-skim mozzarella and ricotta in place of regular varieties. Some products are promoted as substitutes for cheese; read the label to see if they contain saturated fat.
- Use low-fat cottage cheese blended with yogurt instead of cream cheese. Adding cornstarch will help prevent curdling when using this combination in cooking.
- Avoid already breaded chicken, fish, and meat, as well as packaged breading mixes. Instead, make breading with plain bread crumbs. Coat food with crumbs after dipping in skim milk mixed with an egg white.
- Instead of buttered popcorn, spray popcorn lightly with a non-stick vegetable coating and then sprinkle with chili powder, onion powder, or cinnamon.
- Use a non-stick pan and vegetable-oil pan-coating instead of butter, margarine or oil when sautéing or frying foods.
- Read labels for terms that reveal the presence of cholesterol or saturated fats—for example, egg and egg-yolk solids; whole-milk solids; palm, palm kernel, or coconut oils; imitation or milk chocolate; shortening; hydrogenated or hardened oils; lard; butter; and suet and animal byproducts. Substitute other products for foods that have these ingredients.

Meat, Poultry, Fish, Beans and Eggs

The trimmable fat contributes much of the total fat and saturated fat to meat, while both the lean and the fat contain cholesterol. In comparison to meat, a greater percentage of the fat in fish is polyunsaturated.

	Total Fat[1] (Grams)	Saturated Fat (Grams)	Poly-unsaturated Fat (Grams)	Cholesterol (Milligrams)
Beef rib roast, Choice grade, roasted, 2 ounces				
Lean and fat	22.5	10.8	0.4	54
Lean only	7.6	3.7	.2	52
Beef rump, Choice grade, roasted, 2 ounces				
Lean and fat	15.6	7.5	.3	54
Lean only	5.3	2.5	.1	52
Beef rump, Good grade, roasted, 2 ounces				
Lean and fat	13.3	6.4	.3	54
Lean only	4.0	1.9	.1	52
Ground beef patty, cooked, 2 ounces				
Regular	11.5	5.5	.2	53
Lean	6.4	3.1	.1	53
Extra lean	3.5	1.7	.1	52
Pork loin, lean, roasted, 2 ounces				
Lean and fat	16.2	5.8	1.5	50
Lean only	8.0	2.9	.7	50
Liver, beef, cooked with fat added, 2 ounces	6.0	1.7	.6	248
Liver, chicken, simmered, 2 ounces	2.5	.6	0	423
Chicken, roasted, 2 ounces				
Light meat with skin	6.2	1.7	1.3	48
Light meat without skin	2.6	.7	.6	48
Dark meat with skin	9.0	2.5	2.0	52
Dark meat without skin	5.6	1.5	1.3	53
Turkey, roasted, without skin, 2 ounces				
Light meat	1.8	.6	.5	39
Dark meat	4.1	1.4	1.2	48

Meat, Poultry, Fish, Beans and Eggs (Continued)

	Total Fat[1] (Grams)	Saturated Fat (Grams)	Poly-unsaturated Fat (Grams)	Cholesterol (Milligrams)
Halibut fillets, broiled, 2 ounces	.8	.1	.3	35
Cod fillets, broiled, 2 ounces	.5	.1	.2	35
Tuna, canned, oil packed, drained, 2 ounces	4.6	1.2	1.0	37
Shrimp, steamed, shelled, 2 ounces	.9	.1	.4	117
Crab, cooked meat, 2 ounces	.9	.1	.3	57
Oysters, shucked, cooked, 2 ounces	1.5	.4	.4	36
Great northern or navy beans, cooked, ½ cup	.5	.1	.3	0
Canned beans with pork, ½ cup	.6	.1	.3	0
Canned pork and beans in tomato sauce, ½ cup	3.3	1.2	.3	5
Egg, large, 1				
Whole	5.6	1.7	.7	274
Yolk	5.6	1.7	.7	274
White	Trace	0	0	0

[1] Total fat includes mono-unsaturated fat as well as the amounts of saturated and polyunsaturated fats shown in the two columns.

Source: *Food 3*, published by the American Dietetic Association from material originally published by the U.S. Department of Agriculture, 1982.

Fats and Oils

Animal fats tend to be higher in saturated fat than vegetable oils, which are generally higher in polyunsaturated fats. Vegetable shortenings and margarines that have been hardened by hydrogenation contain varying amounts of saturated fat, depending on the brand. Only animal fats contain cholesterol. Amounts given are for one tablespoon.

	Total Fat[1] (Grams)	Saturated Fat (Grams)	Poly-unsaturated Fat (Grams)	Cholesterol (Milligrams)
ANIMAL FATS:				
Beef fat	12.8	6.4	0.5	14
Chicken fat	12.8	3.8	1.7	11
Lard	12.8	5.0	1.4	12
Butter	11.5	7.2	.4	31
VEGETABLE OILS:				
Corn	13.6	1.7	8.0	0
Cottonseed	13.6	3.5	7.1	0
Peanut	13.5	2.3	4.3	0
Safflower	13.6	1.2	10.1	0
Soybean[2]	13.6	2.0	7.9	0
Mixed (*mostly soybean and some cottonseed*)[2]	13.6	2.4	6.5	0
Sunflower	13.6	1.4	8.9	0
Olive	13.5	1.8	1.1	0
Coconut[3]	13.6	11.8	.2	0
Palm[3]	13.6	6.7	1.3	0
MARGARINE:				
Hard (*stick*)	11.4	2.1	3.6	0
Soft (*tub*)	11.4	1.8	4.8	0
Vegetable shortening, hydrogenated	12.8	3.9	1.8	0
SALAD DRESSINGS:				
Mayonnaise	11.0	1.6	5.7	8
Mayonnaise-type	4.9	.7	2.6	4
Italian	7.1	1.0	4.1	0

Fats and Oils (Continued)

	Total Fat[1] (Grams)	Saturated Fat (Grams)	Poly-unsaturated Fat (Grams)	Cholesterol (Milligrams)
Blue cheese	8.0	1.5	4.3	3
French	6.4	1.5	3.4	0
Thousand Island	5.6	.9	3.1	4

[1] Total fat includes mono-unsaturated fat as well as the amounts of saturated and polyunsaturated fats shown in the two columns.
[2] Soybean oils and soybean oil mixtures are the vegetable oils most commonly available to consumers.
[3] Used in commercially prepared foods.
Source: *Food 3,* published by the American Dietetic Association form material originally developed by the U.S. Department of Agriculture, 1982.

Selected Snacks

Choose snacks with care. Be careful of trading off high fat and cholesterol for high sodium content. (Dietary sodium has been linked to high blood pressure in some people; high blood pressure, like high blood cholesterol levels, is a risk factor for heart disease.)

	Total Fat (Grams)	Saturated Fat (Grams)	Cholesterol (Milligrams)	Sodium (Milligrams)
CRACKER AND CHIP-TYPES:				
Potato chips, 10	8.0	2.0	0	200
French fries, salted, 10 long strips	10.3	2.6	0	189
Corn chips, ½ cup	6.1	1.3	0	188
Popcorn, plain, 1 cup	.3	Trace	0	1
Popcorn, salted and buttered, 1 cup	2.0	.9	4	175
Butter crackers, 1	2.3	.8	0	142
Saltine crackers, 4	1.4	.3	0	140
Whole-wheat crackers, 4	2.2	.5	0	120
Pretzels, salted, 10 thin sticks	.1	Trace	0	51

Selected Snacks (*Continued*)

	Total Fat (Grams)	Saturated Fat (Grams)	Cholesterol (Milligrams)	Sodium (Milligrams)
NUTS AND SEEDS:				
Peanuts, roasted, salted, ¼ cup	17.9	3.9	0	200
Peanuts, dry-roasted, salted, ¼ cup	17.6	3.1	0	200
Peanut butter, 2 tablespoons	15.3	2.8	0	162
Sunflower seeds, roasted, salted, ¼ cup	16.8	3.2	0	196
DESSERT-TYPE:				
Chocolate chip cookies, 2	4.4	1.3	8	69
Frosted brownie, 1	6.6	2.2	12	69
Gingersnaps, 2	1.2	.3	5	80
Sandwich-type cookies, chocolate or vanilla, 2	4.5	1.2	8	96
Chocolate-frosted cupcake, 1	4.5	1.8	17	121
Frosted cream-filled cupcake, 1	5.2	1.7	26	194
Doughnut, cake-type, 1	6.0	1.5	19	160
Doughnut, raised, 1	11.2	2.8	10	99

Source: *Food 3*, published by the American Dietetic Association from material originally developed by the U.S. Department of Agriculture, 1982.

GLOSSARY

Cholesterol A fat-like substance found in all foods of animal origin (meat and dairy products), but not in food from plants. Some cholesterol is needed by the body, but too much can build up in arteries, leading to heart disease, heart attack, or stroke.

Fat A component of most foods of plant or animal origin. Fat is an essential part of the diet. Not only is it a major source of energy, but it also plays a key role as a carrier of the fat-soluble vitamins, A, D, E, and K. Dietary fat also supplies the body with essential fatty acids, particularly linoleic acid, necessary for proper growth and healthy skin.

Fatty acids   The basic chemical units of fat. They can be either saturated, mono-unsaturated, or polyunsaturated, depending on how many hydrogen atoms they hold. All dietary fats are a mixture of the three types of fatty acids, but vary in the amount of each that they contain.

Mono-unsaturated fatty acids   Found in varying amounts in both plant and animal fat. Olive oil, peanut oil, some margarines, and vegetable shortening tend to be high in mono-unsaturated fatty acids.

Polyunsaturated fatty acids   Tend to lower blood cholesterol levels. They are found mainly in the fat of foods from plants. Safflower, sunflower, corn, soybean, and cottonseed oils contain large amounts of polyunsaturated fatty acids.

Saturated fatty acids   Tend to raise blood cholesterol levels. They are found in largest amounts in meat and dairy products, but also in some vegetable oils, including coconut and palm kernel oils.

FDA Consumer, March 1987

Herpes
Drug Eases Symptoms, But Still No Cure

When genital herpes began to grab the attention of the American public in the early 1980s, the fear and loathing this venereal disease evoked were mainly due to its incurable, and even untreatable, nature. Now, after being discussed on virtually every talk show and written about in thousands of magazines and newspapers across the country, the uproar over this "epidemic of the '80s" has diminished somewhat. But the fear and loathing remain, as does the search for a cure.

Progress has been made, however, in finding effective treatments for this disease, which afflicts millions of Americans, with some 300,000 new cases every year. In January 1985, the Food and Drug Administration approved an oral form of the anti-virus drug acyclovir, which had previously been available as an intravenous solution for hospital use and as an ointment. The oral medication is approved not only for the treatment of initial genital herpes infections, as are the intravenous and ointment forms, but also for treating and suppressing recurrent genital infections.

Genital herpes is the third most common form of venereal disease in the United States today, behind chlamydial infections and gonorrhea. Unlike chlamydial infections, gonorrhea, or syphilis, genital herpes cannot be cured by antibiotics, because it is caused not by bacteria but by a virus. In most cases, the culprit is herpes simplex virus Type II, although about 15 percent of the cases are caused by herpes simplex virus Type I, which more commonly is the cause of oral herpes—not a venereal disease. Herpes simplex Type I is extremely prevalent throughout the population. Blood tests to detect the presence of herpes-fighting antibodies show that most people have been infected with the Type I virus by age 50, with some 30 million Americans suffering from the resulting cold sores, fever blisters, eye infections, or other symptoms.

Both types of herpes simplex viruses are members of a larger family of herpesviruses that cause several diseases in men and women, young and old, even children. To date, five human herpesviruses have been identified. Besides the two herpes simplex viruses, they are: varicella zoster virus, which causes chicken pox in children and shingles in adults; Epstein-Barr virus, which causes infectious mononucleosis and some other less common syndromes; and cytomegalovirus, which can cause birth defects and potentially life-threatening problems in organ and bone marrow transplant patients.

Genital herpes is a lifelong, sexually transmitted disease that has a tendency to recur again and again. It is characterized by blistery, fluid-filled sores around the genital organs. Once the virus enters the body, an active infection may develop. These first cases of herpes are generally the most severe. After the initial episode, the virus becomes latent, retreating to nerve cells near the spine. The virus may emerge at any time and cause renewed outbreaks, usually at the original site of the infection.

During the initial infection the symptoms usually appear a few days to three weeks after sexual contact. However, some infections can occur without symptoms, or the symptoms may be so mild that they are not noticed. Typically, the first signs include itching or numbness in the genital area, a burning sensation during urination, and a discharge from the vagina or penis. These are followed by headache, fever, muscle ache, and swollen glands in the groin. About 10 days later the painful blisters appear, and it may take two to six weeks for them to crust over, scab and heal.

In recurrent cases, warning signs, such as itching, burning, tingling and numbness, may precede the development of blisters by only a few hours or a few days. Recurrent attacks are generally less severe and last about 10 days. They can, however, be severe enough to mimic the original outbreak in some people. What causes the herpesvirus to move back down the nerve pathway and instigate a new episode of the disease is unknown. But many factors are considered possible triggers, including emotional stress, lack of sleep, poor diet, upper respiratory infection, sexual intercourse, or menstruation. In addition, wearing tight clothing, such as jeans, may provoke a recurrence. In many cases, recurrences appear without any obvious "trigger." Most people who have genital herpes experience one to six of these outbreaks a year, although some may get them at least once a month. A small percentage of people never have recurrences.

Herpes sufferers are most contagious when symptoms are present. Contagion results from "shedding" of viruses, and this typically occurs when the virus is reproducing itself in sufficient quantities to produce sores. Live viruses present in the blisters can be transferred from person to person through direct contact, almost always sexual contact. (Oral sex also can transmit the virus from one location to another.) However, a person can sometimes shed viruses without having sores. This may explain why some people can acquire the disease from those with no evidence of infection.

There is no consensus on whether the use of condoms helps reduce the risk of transmitting or catching herpes.

The virus can also be transmitted when a person touches herpes sores on his or her own body and then touches another site, such as the mouth, eyes or a break in the skin. Therefore, it is important to avoid touching the sores whenever possible, and to wash one's hands immediately afterward if sores are touched.

In fact, good personal hygiene, good nutrition, and plenty of rest are essential in helping patients recover from active outbreaks of herpes, so that the body's natural defenses can fight the virus. The affected area should be kept clean and dry. Bathing with soap and water and using a drying agent such as epsom salts may help relieve the pain and itching and hasten healing.

An active genital herpes infection during pregnancy is a cause for special concern. Some studies have shown that women with such infections run a greater risk of spontaneous abortion. Also, about 90 percent of cases of herpes in newborns can be traced to infection from the mother, usually during the baby's passage through an infected birth canal. An infant delivered vaginally during an active case of genital herpes in the mother has a 40 to 50 percent chance of being infected.

The chances for a baby so infected aren't good. Some 50 to 60 percent of newborns with herpes simplex infections die, and half to two-thirds of the survivors suffer permanent visual or neurological damage.

Until recently, it was generally recommended that a woman with a history of herpes infections deliver by cesarean section to reduce the chance of the baby being infected. However, the Committee on Infectious Diseases of the American Academy of Pediatrics has determined that if weekly testing during the pregnancy shows no sign of active infection during the two weeks before delivery, and if the membranes have been ruptured for less than four to six hours, the mother can deliver vaginally with a high degree of safety. Recently, scientists at the National Institutes of Health have developed a test that can provide more rapid detection—one day compared to a week for other methods—of an active herpes infection, allowing closer monitoring of pregnant women as they near the time of delivery.

Women with genital herpes also appear to have an increased risk of developing cervical cancer. Since this form of cancer can be cured if detected early, women with genital herpes should have routine cervical cancer checks (Pap smears), preferably twice a year.

Until the approval of oral acyclovir in January 1985, the intravenous and ointment forms of the medication were the only drugs approved by FDA as safe and effective for treating outbreaks of genital herpes. The ointment was approved in March 1982 for treating initial episodes of the disease. In studies of the ointment, female patients with initial infections had faster healing of sores and reduced viral growth. There was, however, no significant decrease in the pain associated with the disease in women. In men using the ointment for initial infections, studies showed a significant decrease in the healing time of sores and in the pain. In both men and women with recurrences of the disease, acyclovir ointment showed no important benefits.

The ointment is also used in patients with either oral or genital herpes whose immune systems are impaired (as a result of cancer chemotherapy, for example), making such infections potentially life-threatening. The ointment reduces the growth of the viruses and the duration of pain in these patients.

Later in 1982, the intravenous form of acyclovir was approved for treating herpes infections in hospitalized patients with impaired immune systems. It is also being used in patients with initial genital herpes infections severe enough to warrant hospitalization.

The newly approved oral form of acyclovir is useful in treating not only initial infections but also in treating and suppressing recurrences of genital herpes. The drug can be prescribed for extended periods (daily therapy for up to six months) to help prevent further attacks, or can be given on a short-term basis for five days to treat less severe recurring episodes and for 10 days to treat first infections.

In initial cases, oral acyclovir can reduce the duration of the infection and speed healing of the sores. It also reduces the development of new blisters and may shorten the time patients experience pain.

When used daily to suppress recurrences, the oral acyclovir capsules can greatly reduce the number of attacks and, in many cases, completely prevent them while the drug is being taken. However, because acyclovir does not rid the body of latent herpesviruses, patients are likely to experience renewed recurrences when they stop taking the drug, and the first such recurrence following long-term therapy may occur sooner or more severely than usual, or both.

In two studies, supported by the National Institutes of Health, of patients with frequent recurrences of genital herpes, oral acyclovir taken regularly for up to four months reduced the number of recurrences or their severity or both in more than 95 percent of the cases. Recurrences were prevented entirely in 40 percent to 75 percent of these patients.

For patients whose recurrences are not frequent or severe enough to warrant long-term therapy, oral acyclovir can be used just during the time of recurrent outbreaks. In such cases, the patient should begin to take the capsules as soon as early symptoms begin to appear in order to achieve the best results. By halting viral activity in the herpes sores, the drug can reduce the formation of new blisters and lead to faster healing—within five days for most people. The effect on the duration of pain in these patients is less clear.

Patients with very mild cases of genital herpes may choose not to use the drug at all.

Burroughs Wellcome Co., Research Triangle Park, N.C., the manufacturer of all three forms of acyclovir (under the brand name Zovirax), is providing written information for physicians and pharmacists to give to patients when acyclovir capsules are prescribed. The leaflet cautions users that acyclovir can treat the symptoms of genital herpes. But the drug does not cure the disease, and patients can still spread it, so sexual contact should be avoided during outbreaks. This is particularly important because of concern that use of acyclovir may increase the virus's resistance to the drug; thus, the viruses transmitted to another person could be harder to treat.

The patient information booklet also advises users to consult with their physician if they do not get sufficient relief, if they experience severe or troublesome adverse reactions, or if they become pregnant or wish to do so or to breastfeed while taking the drug.

Adverse reactions noted with use of acyclovir capsules have included nausea, vomiting, and headache in a very small number of patients using the drug for short periods; and headache, diarrhea, nausea, vomiting, vertigo, and joint pain in a small number of long-term-therapy patients. The effects were generally mild and did not require stopping the medication. Studies of the drug's long-term use will continue. The studies submitted for its approval support its use for no more than six months.

Acyclovir should not be taken during pregnancy unless the potential benefit justifies the potential risk to the fetus. Although animal tests did not show a risk of birth defects, the labeling states that "there are no adequate and well-controlled studies in pregnant women."

The drug should also be used with caution in nursing mothers because it is not known whether acyclovir is excreted in the milk. The safety and effectiveness of the drug in children have not been established.

While the three forms of acyclovir are the only drugs approved by FDA for treating genital herpes, others are being studied by researchers across the country. Studies will have to show them to be safe and effective before they can be marketed.

Studies are also being conducted to see if a vaccine can be developed to immunize people against genital herpes infections. But here, again, much work remains to be done before FDA can license a vaccine as proven safe and effective.

The fact remains that no drug, diet, vaccine, or other product has been shown to be effective in preventing or curing genital herpes, and only acyclovir has been found effective in treating outbreaks of the disease. Nevertheless, many sufferers have been lured into trying any of a number of quack remedies that have appeared on the market in the last few years. FDA has taken regulatory action against several of these products, among them LSO-1 (lithium succinate), marketed by Health From The Sun Products, Needham Heights, Mass.; Herpitex (butylated hydroxytoluene, or BHT, a food preservative), marketed by Advanced Nucleics, Atlanta, Ga.; and Herpetrol, from Standard Pharmacal, Elgin, Ill.

For many herpes victims the psychological suffering can be as difficult to handle as the physical symptoms. Some have found help through the Herpes Resource Center of the American Social Health Association, P.O. Box 100, Palo Alto, Calif. 94302. Individuals with questions about the disease can also contact the National VD Hotline at (800) 227–8922.

Bill Rados, Reprinted from April 1985, *FDA Consumer*, HHS Publication No. (FDA) 85–3151. Department of Health and Human Services, Public Health Service, Food and Drug Administration, 5600 Fishers Lane, Rockville, Md. 20857, Office of Public Affairs. U.S. Government Printing Office 1985—461-367/20030.

Hodgkin's Disease
What You Need To Know

Introduction

This article is written for you, the *cancer** patient. It also may be useful for members of your family.

We believe it is important for you and your family to understand your illness so you can face it together, with courage and hope.

Much has been learned about the nature of cancer in recent years. As a result, strides have been made in diagnosing the disease and treating it effectively. These modern methods are described in this pamphlet. You also will find information on sources of assistance, areas of research, and definitions of medical terms.

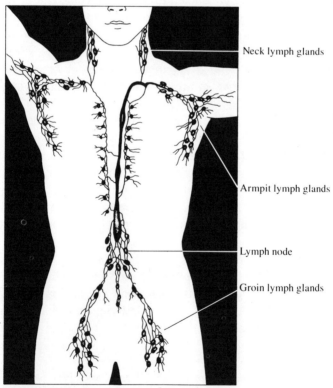

Neck lymph glands

Armpit lymph glands

Lymph node

Groin lymph glands

Location of some of the lymph nodes in the human body.

Words in italics are explained at the end of the article.

Hodgkin's disease is a form of cancer affecting the *lymphatic system.* The lymphatic system is part of the circulatory system that plays a major role in your ability to fight infection.

The disease usually begins by a painless swelling of *lymph glands* (*nodes*) in the neck, the armpits, or the groin. Normally, these glands are no larger than beans. The lymph glands manufacture *lymphocytes,* a type of white blood cell that fights the spread of infection. In Hodgkin's disease, these cells grow rapidly in a variety of abnormal forms. This leaves the body fewer normal lymphocytes with which to fight infection.

Some doctors believe that Hodgkin's disease begins in one area of the lymphatic system and, if left untreated, spreads throughout the system and even to other tissues and organs. As the disease progresses, changes in blood composition may take place and *anemia* (a reduction in the number of red blood cells) may develop. The body becomes less able to combat infections, and damage to vital organs occurs.

Symptoms

You may find the first symptom of this disease to be a painless enlargement of one or more of your lymph glands. The swelling will probably first appear in your neck, armpits, or groin. This does not definitely indicate that you have the disease because other conditions can cause enlargement of the *lymph nodes,* such as rheumatoid arthritis or infectious mononucleosis. However, if you have a lymph node that remains swollen for more than three weeks, you should see your doctor.

Other symptoms of Hodgkin's disease that can occur, usually in later stages of the disease, include fever, persistent fatigue, weight loss, itching and night sweats.

Because these symptoms also can occur in many other and often minor diseases, you should consult your physician.

Diagnosis

Your doctor can make a definite diagnosis by making a thorough clinical examination, special *X-rays,* laboratory tests, and a minor surgical procedure called a *biopsy.*

When your doctor finds a tumor or other evidence of an unusual growth, he will arrange for a *biopsy* to determine for certain whether the growth is *malignant* or *benign.* A small sample of tissue from the suspected area will be removed for close examination under a microscope. The doctor who examines the tissue is a pathologist, a physician who interprets and diagnoses the changes caused by disease in body tissues. The biopsy is used to confirm or rule out a diagnosis of cancer.

If your doctor suspects that you have Hodgkin's disease, he may need to take samples from your spleen, liver, and other organs. This can be done with a major operation known as a *laparotomy* in which an incision is made in your abdomen. This can also be done with a simpler procedure called a *peritoneoscopy*. This requires a much smaller incision in the abdomen through which a slender fiberoptic instrument, called a peritoneoscope, can be inserted to examine the internal organs and take tissue samples of suspicious areas.

These procedures and other laboratory tests and diagnostic X-rays help your physician to determine if the disease is confined to one lymph node region—such as the neck, armpit, groin, midchest, or abdominal cavity—or if it has spread to other areas. All of these tests to determine the extent of the disease are called *"staging."*

"Staging" may include a diagnostic X-ray examination called *lymphangiography*. In this procedure, a radio-opaque dye is injected into the lymph system. Under X-ray examination the dye outlines the lymph system and abnormalities in it.

Other X-rays also are used to determine the extent of the disease. Cancer specialists believe that appropriate diagnosis and "staging" are crucial to selecting the most effective treatment for a particular patient.

Hodgkin's disease is classified into one of four stages depending on the extent of the disease. When localized (confined to one lymph area), it is classified as Stage I. If it has spread to adjacent lymph regions but is confined either above or below the diaphragm, it is called Stage II. When the disease is present in lymph regions both above and below the diaphragm, it is classified as Stage III disease. Hodgkin's disease that has spread to lung, liver, bone, kidneys, or other tissues outside the lymph node system is called Stage IV. Each of the various stages is subdivided into groups A and B according to whether or not the patient experiences such symptoms as weight loss, fever, or night sweats.

After a diagnosis of cancer is confirmed, it is best for you to begin treatment in a hospital that has an expert staff and resources to apply all forms of effective treatment right from the beginning. Before treatment, you may, if you wish, request a second opinion from another physician to confirm the diagnosis and recommendations for therapy.

Treatment

Your doctor will consider a number of factors in determining the best treatment for you. Among these are your medical history, your general health, and the type and location of the cancer or cancers you have. Your treatment must be tailored to your individual needs.

X-ray (radiation therapy) is usually the most effective treatment for early stages of Hodgkin's disease. Each lymph node region involved and the adjacent region may be subjected to intensive X-ray therapy over a period of several weeks.

In some cases radiation therapy may be more extensive, involving high doses to all cancer patients, their families, and health professionals. Cancer Information Service offices are based in major cancer programs around the country.

For additional information on this subject, write to the Office of Cancer Communications, National Cancer Institute, Bethesda, MD 20892, or call the toll-free telephone number of the Cancer Information Service at

1-800-4-CANCER[*]

[*]In Alaska, call 1-800-638-6070; in Hawaii, on Oahu call 524-1234 (neighbor islands call collect). Spanish-speaking staff members are available to callers from the following areas (daytime hours only): California, Florida, Georgia, Illinois, northern New Jersey, New York, and Texas.

Emotional aspects

You may feel many different emotional reactions from the time cancer is diagnosed. "Why me?" every patient asks. This is a normal reaction to the diagnosis of cancer. You also may have periods of anxiety or depression. You may need to go through these feelings before you can accept the diagnosis and learn to live with it.

Talking with your doctor, other health professionals, your family, and even other cancer patients can give you emotional support during and after treatment. Because your doctor knows your condition, he is in the best position to answer questions about your individual case. Making a list of questions before you see the doctor can help you remember to ask him everything you want to know. You may be assured that your doctor and other health professionals will continue to offer you the best care that medicine has available.

You and your family may be able to handle the emotional strain of cancer better by discussing your problems openly with each other and with your doctor. But you may need help. You should feel free to ask for counseling if your problems become too difficult to handle.

Questions you may want to ask your doctor

You or your family may find it difficult to know how to ask your doctor some of the questions you may have about cancer. This is understandable. Cancer and its treatment are complex. Even your doctor may not always be able to give definite answers. But he or she will be happy to discuss your questions with you. Some typical questions might include these:

What kind of cancer do I have?

Is the tumor benign or malignant?

If it is benign, has it been cured?

If it is cancer, has it spread?

Can you predict how successful an operation or radiation treatment would be?

What are the risks?

Should I get an opinion from another doctor?

If an operation is done, will I need other treatment?

How helpful will this be in resuming normal activities afterward?

If I take anticancer drugs, what will the side-effects be?

How often will I need medical checkups?

What should I tell my relatives and friends?

Research

The National Cancer Institute, a bureau in the U.S. Department of Health and Human Services, is the Federal Government's principal agency for cancer research. The Institute supports research in many of the nation's universities, medical centers and laboratories, and conducts research in its own laboratories and clinics.

The National Cancer Institute has developed PDQ (Physician Data Query), a computerized database designed to give doctors quick and easy access to the latest treatment information for most types of cancer; descriptions of clinical trials that are open for patient entry; and names of organizations and physicians involved in cancer care. To access PDQ, a doctor may use an office computer with a telephone hookup and a PDQ access code or the services of a medical library with online searching capability. Most Cancer Information Service offices provide a physician with one free PDQ search and can tell doctors how to get regular access. Patients may ask their doctor to use PDQ or may call 1-800-4-CANCER themselves.

In addition to laboratory and clinical research, the National Cancer Institute studies patterns of cancer occurrence in the population. These studies show that Hodgkin's disease, like all forms of cancer, is not contagious. No one can catch cancer from another person. Cancer is not transmitted by coughing or sneezing, nor by sexual intercourse or any other kind of physical contact.

Hodgkin's disease often responds well to treatment. Even though its causes have not yet been determined, with proper treatment it can be controlled for long periods of time. Recent developments in the treatment of this type of cancer indicate that most patients treated in the early stages of disease may be cured. Encouraging results from new methods of treating patients with advanced Hodgkin's disease suggest that these patients may lead normal, productive lives for many years.

Although the causes of Hodgkin's disease, like those of most cancers, remain unknown, new research findings may suggest ways of preventing the disease. At the same time, the trend toward improved diagnosis and treatment provides hope that more patients with this disease will be treated effectively.

GLOSSARY

Anemia   A reduction in the number of red blood cells.

Biopsy   The removal and microscopic examination of tissue from the living body for purposes of diagnosis.

Cancer   A general term for about 100 diseases characterized by uncontrolled, abnormal growth of cells. The resulting mass, or tumor, can invade and destroy surrounding normal tissues. Cancer cells from the tumor can spread through the blood or lymph (the clear fluid that bathes body cells) to start new cancers in other parts of the body.

Chemotherapy   The use of anticancer drugs for treatment.

Hodgkin's Disease   A form of cancer affecting the lymphatic system.

Laparotomy   An incision or opening of the abdominal wall to permit examination of internal organs; obtaining samples of tissue or removal of diseased tissue.

Lymphangiography   An X-ray procedure using a radio-opaque dye to examine the lymph system.

Lymphatic System   Circulatory network of vessels carrying lymph, the almost colorless fluid that bathes body cells, and the lymphoid organs such as the lymph nodes, spleen, and thymus, that produce and store infection-fighting cells.

Lymph Nodes   Bean-shaped structures scattered along vessels of the lymphatic system. The nodes act as filters, collecting bacteria or cancer cells that may travel through the lymph system.

Lymphocytes   A type of white blood cell that fights infection.

Malignant   Cancerous. A growth of cancer cells (See definition of CANCER).

Pathologist   A physician who interprets and diagnoses the changes caused by disease in body tissue.

Peritoneoscope   A slender, flexible instrument used to examine internal organs and take samples of suspicious tissue.

Peritoneoscopy   A small incision of the abdomen to examine internal organs with a peritoneoscope.

Radiation Therapy   Treatment using high-energy radiation from X-ray machines, cobalt, radium, or other sources.

Remission   Temporary disappearance of all evidence of disease.

Staging   Tests to determine the extent of the disease.

X-ray   High-energy radiation used in high doses to treat cancer or in low doses to diagnose the disease.

U.S. Department of Health and Human Services, Public Health Service, National Institutes of Health, National Cancer Institute. NIH Publication No. 88–1555, reprinted December 1987.

Hypertension

Protect Your Lifeline! Fight High Blood Pressure

What is blood pressure?

Everyone has blood pressure. It is the amount of force required to circulate the blood through the body. As your heart pumps the blood through the arteries (vessels) the push of this blood on the walls of these vessels determines the amount of pressure.

The arterial walls are elastic and muscular. They stretch and contract to take the ups and downs of blood pressure. Each time the heart contracts, or beats—some 70 to 90 times a minute—the blood pressure in the arteries increases; each time the heart relaxes between beats the blood pressure goes down. Thus there is an "upper" and a "lower" blood pressure. Both pressures are measured when you are examined.

These two pressures are known as *SYSTOLIC* and *DIASTOLIC*. The systolic—the first and highest reading is the pressure in the arteries when the heart contracts (empties) in order to pump blood through the body. The diastolic—the second and lower reading—is the pressure in the arteries when the heart relaxes and rests between beats in order to fill again with blood. When your pressure is recorded, the highest number is written first (systolic) and then the lowest number (diastolic). An example would be 120/80. The 120 is the high or systolic pressure and the 80 is the low or diastolic pressure.

How is blood pressure measured (read)?

Your blood pressure is measured by using a gauge or machine which consists of several parts: A cuff, a rubber bulb, and a glass mercury tube or dial. The cuff is like a wide band. It is placed snugly around your arm just above your elbow. It has two rubber hoses attached. One of these has a bulb connected at the end and the other is attached to the mercury pressure indicator.

The cuff is inflated with air when the bulb is squeezed. As the cuff gets tighter, it compresses or closes a large artery in your arm. This temporarily shuts off the flow of blood through the artery because the squeeze from the air pressure in the cuff is greater than the push of the blood in the artery. At this point the mercury is high in the glass tube and the numbers alongside the column of mercury show the height of air pressure in the cuff.

A stethoscope is applied to your arm over the compressed artery just below the cuff. The air is then slowly let out. When the air pressure in the cuff is slightly lower than the blood pressure in the artery, blood begins to flow through the artery with each heart beat. This escape of blood in the artery produces a distinct sound or beat which can be heard through the stethoscope. As soon as this sound appears, the height of the mercury is noted. The air continues to be let out of the cuff until this distinct beat disappears as the blood is flowing steadily through the artery. At this point, the height of the mercury shows the least amount of pressure in the artery. By matching the sounds with the numbers indicated on the dial your blood pressure is read. The beginning sound is recorded as the systolic pressure and the last beat as the diastolic pressure.

What is high blood pressure?

There is no blood pressure reading that is normal for everyone. Your age, sex, and overall health determine what is "normal" for you. Blood pressure not only varies among people but it varies in the same person at different times. It decreases during sleep and increases during exertion or excitement. There is a normal pressure range from a systolic reading of 90 over a diastolic reading of 60 (90/60) to systolic of 139 over a diastolic of 89 (139/89). When pressure goes above that and remains elevated (up) it becomes the disease called high blood pressure (hypertension).

Over a period of time, the constant impact of hypertension, even when slight, takes its toll in several ways. Complications resulting from untreated hypertension affect vital areas of the body, particularly the heart, brain, and kidneys. Here's what happens.

High blood pressure can make your heart pump harder than normal and the arteries become less elastic. After a while the heart may get larger, then weaken and stop pumping effectively. This alone kills about 50,000 Americans each year. Or hypertension can speed up the progression of atherosclerosis, a kind of hardening of the arteries in which the inner layer of artery walls thickens and deposits of a fatty substance are formed. Atherosclerosis is involved in coronary heart attacks which every year kills some 400,000 in the United States.

In the eyes, wear and tear on the retina's blood vessels may bring on swelling, tiny hemorrhages, and eventually blindness. Vessels of the kidneys are often hardest hit, and eventually the kidneys are no longer able to perform their task of clearing wastes from the blood stream.

While a stroke (hemorrhage of a brain blood vessel) is not inevitable if you are hypertensive, it is another possible complication and the risk of stroke is much higher than among persons with normal blood pressure. As deposits build up in the arteries they narrow. Thus their capacity to carry blood is reduced or sometimes completely blocked. When this happens to an artery feeding the brain, a stroke is suffered. Some 200,000 persons die of stroke each year in this country.

What causes high blood pressure?

The main artery leaving the heart is the aorta. It is the largest of the body's arteries. It can be thought of as a tree trunk, with smaller and smaller arteries branching out from it. The smallest twigs of this arterial tree, the arteriolies, regulates your blood pressure. They control blood pressure by making it hard—or easy—for the blood to get through to the capillaries—those blood vessels which actually deliver the blood and its nutrients to all body tissue.

If the arterioles clamp or close down, the blood cannot easily pass through them to the capillaries. When this happens, the heart must pump harder to push the blood through. This increases the blood pressure in the arteries. The way arterioles control blood pressure is sometimes compared to the way a nozzle regulates water pressure in a hose. If you turn the hose nozzle to make its opening narrower, the pressure of the hose increases. With a larger opening, less pressure is needed to force the water through the hose.

It is known that if for some reason the arterioles clamp down all over the body, blood pressure will rise and stay up, the result is high blood pressure. Why does this happen?

In a small percentage of individuals high blood pressure can be traced to a specific disease or condition which is called *Secondary Hypertension*. More than 50 conditions that can cause "secondary" hypertension have been described and have been roughly placed in seven groups. Many of these can be specifically cured by surgery or treated by a special medicine. The seven groups are as follows:

1. *Kidney Defects:* The most common cause for correctable secondary hypertension is obstruction of blood flow to the kidney.

2. *Adrenal Cortex Defects:* Such defects may cause secretion of excessive quantities of a hormone, usually aldosterone, which causes the body to hang on to too much sodium. This excessive amount of hormone can come from a small non-cancerous tumor or from an inherited defect in hormone formation.

3. *Defects of Adrenaline Hormones:* Adrenaline chemicals come from nerve endings and from the inner part of the adrenal gland. Some people develop a tumor, called a pheochromocytoma, that produces excessive amounts of the adrenaline compounds. Others have an inherited lack of an enzyme that inactivates adrenaline, or they may be taking a monoamine oxidase inhibitor medicine that may prevent the working of that enzyme. These persons may develop severe high blood pressure from dexedrine sulfate ("bennies") used for weight reduction or from "cold" tablets, or after eating fermented foods such as yellow cheese, or after drinking wine.

4. *Other Hormone and Regulation Defects:* Certain diseases of the pituitary, thyroid, or parathyroid glands may also cause hypertension.

5. *Defects of Blood and Blood Vessels:*

6. *Nervous System Disorders:*

7. *Chemicals and Drugs:* There are several specific chemicals that can cause high blood pressure. Eating too much salt over a period of years is one example. Heavy metals, such as lead, mercury, or cadmium are also known to elevate blood pressure, but these usually cause other symptoms that tip off the doctor that they may be the cause.

The most common (approximately 80 to 85 percent) kind of high blood pressure is *Primary Hypertension* (also known as *Essential* Hypertension). This condition does not seem to be related to any other disease. At present its cause is unknown. Researchers are working hard to find its cause, or causes. Although they do not have the final answer yet, they do have a few good leads:

1. *Heredity:* Experts who studied high blood pressure report that a tendency towards this condition is often inherited. Therefore,

individuals whose parents had high blood pressure are more likely to develop it than those whose parents did not. Consequently, if there is someone in your family who has high blood pressure, all members of the family should be checked periodically to see whether their blood pressure is elevated.

2. *Body Chemistry:* In high blood pressure as in any other disorder, something may have gone wrong with the way some body part or organ works. The kidneys, or the adrenal glands, located just above the kidneys, may send substances into the blood stream which start a chain of chemical events. These events raise blood pressure. Moreover, the kidneys' handling of water, sodium, and other electrolytes may often be abnormal in people with primary hypertension. However, current evidence favors the view that abnormalities in the kidneys are probably a result of high blood pressure rather than a cause.

3. *Emotions:* When you're angry or fearful, your blood pressure goes up, that's natural. But, as the American Heart Association points out, some people who are "hyper-reactors" or "pre-hypertensive" tend to develop hypertension in time. Their bodies simply get accustomed to responding to events in daily life as if they were a series of emergencies. As we all know, with the complexity of today's living, it is almost impossible to avoid stress. For this reason, individuals with high blood pressure should consistently be on the alert, and those on medicine must take it regularly so that the increases in pressure due to emotional tension may be minimized.

4. *Smoking:* Heavy cigarette smoking is implicated. Nicotine is known to raise blood pressure.

5. *Diet:* High-fat and high-salt foods may contribute to hypertension. Chemically, fats and salts help accelerate the development of atherosclerosis (narrowing of the large and medium size arteries due to deposits forming on the inside walls). This in turn can lead to heart attacks and strokes.

6. The above leads are some of the ones advanced by medical researchers. However, probably the most widely accepted theory is the *Mosaic Hypotheses.* This is the view which holds that any of a number of factors may be involved in hypertension and its various phases. The factors that launch the hypertension state may not necessarily be responsible for maintaining it, and those of greatest importance at one stage of the disease may not be the main ones during other stages.

It is important to note that *Primary Hypertension* cannot be cured, but it can be controlled.

A third type of hypertension is *Severe and Malignant Hypertension.* In a "severe" case of hypertension, readings may jump to 200/115. In the grave, accelerating type (240/140–150), which physicians term "malignant," the course of the disease is steadily downhill as patients get progressively worse.

"Malignant," in this sense, has no relation to cancer. This worst type of hypertension is often fatal unless vigorous treatment has been provided.

What are the symptoms of high blood pressure?

In most cases, individuals with high blood pressure have no unusual symptoms and only find they have it when it is checked. When a sign does crop up, it may be bothersome headaches now and then, characteristically in the back of the head and upper part of the neck; they seem to strike most acutely when blood pressure is relatively low in the early morning. Other symptoms might be fatigue or insomnia, tension or excessive flushing of the face. It must be noted however, that these symptoms are also common in our general population and may result from other disorders.

It is thus unwise to try to rely on symptoms, or to try to diagnose and treat them yourself. Usually, high blood pressure creates symptoms only after it has produced disease in some organ, such as the kidney or heart, and that can take years.

So it is up to you to see your physician or go to a clinic to have your blood pressure checked. If you have some symptoms, tell the doctor who will do the detective work for a diagnosis.

Are some groups of people more affected by high blood pressure?

One out of every 10 Americans has high blood pressure. Or 23 million people in this country have high blood pressure that if untreated can take 15 years off their lives. To put these numbers into perspective, the number of deaths directly or indirectly linked to high blood pressure exceeds the combined total of all deaths due to accidents in the entire U.S., including highway deaths.

In the above statistics, there are groups of individuals who are more affected by high blood pressure; they are as follows:

1. Blacks are more affected by high blood pressure than whites. One in four has the disease. It is the single biggest cause of deaths among blacks. Generally, the hypertensive death rates among blacks

in young adulthood and in middle age are from three to 12 times greater than those among whites.

High blood pressure seems to be different among black people. Developing earlier in their life, it is frequently more severe and results in a greater number of deaths at a younger age—more commonly from stroke than from coronary artery disease.

No one knows why blacks get high blood pressure more often than whites. Some researchers noted that many blacks live in cities and that the stress of city living may lead to high blood pressure, although blacks in the Bahamas and West Indies have a high incidence of high blood pressure. Others link high blood pressure to the amount of salt a person eats and point out the high salt content in a normal black diet.

2. High blood pressure can present special problems for women in the following ways:

Statistics have shown that women who have never had high blood pressure may develop it rapidly during pregnancy. Sometimes it disappears after delivery. If it does not, it is important for the woman to follow her doctor's advice and treatment. It has also been noted that as a woman grows older her chances of having high blood pressure increase. Doctors don't know the reason yet, but they think that if a woman is overweight, her chances of developing high blood pressure as she grows older increases further.

There is also a link between contraceptives and high blood pressure. Estrogen causes an increase in blood pressure in perhaps one out of five women. It is thus a good idea for a woman to ask her doctor to take her blood pressure before prescribing the pill and then have it checked every six months or so. Special caution should be observed in prescribing oral contraceptives for a woman with a history of high blood pressure and excessive weight gain and edema during menstruation.

3. If high blood pressure runs in your family, you are probably in a higher risk group of developing hypertension.
4. Age is also a factor, in that most cases of primary hypertension have their onset before the age of 40. When a high level of blood pressure is detected in the 15 to 30 age group, the prognosis is poor unless it's treated as early as possible.

Blood pressure levels increase as we grow older, and systolic hypertension is one of the most familiar findings in the elderly. As blood vessels get less elastic, the systolic hypertension is one of the most familiar findings in the elderly. As blood vessels get less elastic, the systolic pressure may increase, while the diastolic remains relatively normal. But after 65 the rise is not as consistant as it was before that age.

What should you do if you have high blood pressure?

Your physician can do much to help control your high blood pressure. When it is definitely diagnosed, whether mild or very severe, it's wise to start treatment as soon as it is prescribed.

Whatever the treatment, the dual purpose is not only to keep your blood pressure down but also to avoid possible complications. The following are some of the ways high blood pressure can be treated and/or reduced:

Sometimes hypertension can be controlled without medication. In people who are overweight, losing excess weight may be enough to lower blood pressure. As you are probably aware, obesity imposes an added circulatory burden on your heart, blood volume increases with body weight, and the body's fat reserves must be supplied with blood. Thus the heart of an overweight person is forced to pump more blood through a much larger system of blood vessels. The diet prescribed would limit the amount and type of fat in your food, as well as your total calorie intake. The diet would also reduce the amount of salt. Your doctor may tell you to avoid salty foods and not to add salt at the table or you may have your salt intake limited more severely. The reduction in salt helps the body curb retention of fluids.

Many physicians believe that drug therapy treatment of mild hypertension is warranted; medical opinion is not unanimous on this point. Some specialists recommend that drug therapy for mild cases be reserved for individuals with additional risk factors such as high cholesterol levels, heart or kidney involvement, or a family history of vascular disease. Severe primary hypertension invariably does call for medication and only rarely does it prove impossible to bring a rampaging blood pressure under some control.

Your physician knows how to choose medicines best suited to your needs. However, since people respond to medicine in different ways, you may find your doctor trying out a variety of drugs, or a combination of them, in order to see what's going to work best for you.

It is good to remember once a program of treatment has been decided upon for you, it is usually easier and less complicated than you thought it would be. Even more important is to know that effective control of your blood pressure may be expected to prolong your life and reduce the threat of the dreaded complications: stroke, heart attack, kidney failure, and heart failure.

A last comment on this area of therapy is that even though most patients can achieve effective blood pressure control through the now available anti-hypertensive drugs as well as other measures, the goal of developing a uniformly effective, completely non-toxic, inexpensive single drug has of yet not been reached. The research in this area continues.

There are some general health habits which when practiced can help you in your battle with high blood pressure.

Rest and Recreation

Having high blood pressure doesn't mean you should make an invalid or even simi-invalid out of yourself. Many individuals whose condition has been adequately controlled carry on their usual activities. Recreation should be a part of your regular schedule. Your physician can recommend the amount and kind of exercise best suited for you.

Getting plenty of sleep is important because blood pressure is lowest during sleep and rises during waking hours. If feasible, make a habit of taking a short nap during the day. Whatever else relaxes you, whether it's watching a movie or TV, reading a book, or taking a warm bath, is good therapy.

If you have been overly tense or perhaps worrying too much, you can do much to ease this nervous tension by reviewing the way you've been living. Then apply moderation whenever and wherever possible.

Tobacco

Research reports on cigarette smoking have been widely published. Thus the dangers to one's health is well known. Its relation to high blood pressure is serious because if you smoke, there is a constriction of the blood vessels which boosts your blood pressure.

Alcohol

Alcohol consumption does not raise blood pressure, but some people react poorly to it. Therefore, it is wise to discuss with your physician the advisability of drinking alcoholic beverages. This is especially true if you are taking any kind of medications, because alcohol is a drug (depressant) and the mixing of drugs can be dangerous.

The question is always raised as to why some people don't get, or keep taking treatment for their high blood pressure. First of all, treatment is not a cure in primary hypertension. Persons who have high blood pressure must treat it for the rest of their life. Second, treatment sometimes involves drugs that cause drowsiness and other side effects that may impair daily activities. Unfortunately, this is the treatment people hear about. In eight out of ten cases, changes in diet, moderate exercise, a simple pill, or perhaps abstinence from smoking is enough to control the disease.

Nevertheless, it is often hard for a person who looks and feels fine to adhere to even the simple treatment. Such individuals need constant reminding. Oftentimes they do not see a doctor regularly, or when they do, the doctor may not have the time and initiative to deal with people whose blood pressure is "a few points above normal"—the "few points" that over the years may eventually kill or cripple.

The regimen and expense of daily pills and regular blood pressure tests often does not seem worth it to an individual who patronizes a clinic and finds himself faced with long waiting periods and possibly unfamiliar doctors just to get another prescription for a disease he or she doesn't see or feel. Thus they become one of the "dropout" hypertensives who are no longer receiving the treatment they so desperately need.

In summary, taking your medicine and carefully adhering to a prescribed diet may become a lifelong routine. Such a routine will involve seeing your physician regularly to check your blood pressure and the effects of your treatment program. Remember, however, your doctor cannot lower your blood pressure without your full cooperation. So it's really up to you whether or not you want to feel better and possibly live longer.

Diet and Your Hypertension
Much can be done with diet to assist in the treatment of high blood pressure and its complications. It's best to eat foods with a minimal amount of salt, sugar, and grease (saturated fats) for the following reasons:

1. Saturated fats play a very significant role in the development of cholesterol deposits in the arteries. The formation of these deposits proceeds at a more rapid pace in people who have hypertension than in those with normal blood pressure. A diet low in saturated fats will decrease the rate at which the cholesterol is deposited in the arteries and help avoid the strokes and heart attacks that may result.

A person with hypertension should avoid greases, such as animal fats, shortening, hydrogenated (partially hardened) oils. Oils which are liquid at room temperature (polyunsaturated oils) should be substituted in their place, but even these should be used in moderation. Since the body can convert table sugar into saturated fats, intake of this should also be limited.

2. One of the medications prescribed by your physician may be a diuretic which is a drug that lowers blood pressure in some people with high blood pressure. The diuretic helps the body remove excess salt and water. However, it also removes another mineral, potassium, but usually severe potassium loss can be prevented by eating the right foods. Sometimes too much potassium is lost, most often in older people, those with kidney disease or who are taking another medication, Digitalis. For these people, potassium may be given in a pill or liquid form.

The diuretic will do the best possible job for your hypertension if you eat foods that are low in salt and high in potassium. The foods (see list below) are not exotic—you are probably eating them now. Foods very high in salt are also listed. Try to eat less of them. Remember, an important source of salt in anyone's diet is the salt they sprinkle on their food at the table. Taste your food first, before you salt it, and maybe you'll decide not to add any at all.

Foods for you to watch for

These foods are good for you. (They have the perfect combination: high in potassium and low in salt.)

Fruits
apples
apricots
avocados
bananas**
cantaloupes
dates
grapefruits
nectarines
melons (casaba or honeydew)
prunes
raisins**
watermelon
peaches
(Dried fruit is usually good, but make sure to read the label on the package.)

Fruit Juices
apple
grapefruit
prune
orange**

Vegetables
asparagus
beans (white, green, snap, etc.)
Brussels sprouts
cabbage
cauliflower
corn on the cob
lima beans (not frozen)
mushrooms
green peppers
potatoes (sweet, white, raw, baked,** boiled without skin)
radishes
squash
tomatoes

Unsalted nuts
peanuts
pecan halves

**especially good

Try to avoid these foods. (They all have a great deal of salt or sodium).
buttermilk
cheese (except unsalted cottage or pot)
dried, salted, smoked or canned meats (bacon, ham, bologna, etc.)
canned tuna, or salmon (unless unsalted)
mayonnaise

relishes
sauces (soy, Worcestershire, ketchup, chili, bar-b-q)
bottled dressings
crackers (soda and graham)
pretzels
potato chips
packaged snack foods
instant potatoes
commercially prepared desserts
frozen dinners
foods made with baking powder or baking soda
soups (except homemade)

Foods that might fool you
(These have a great deal of potassium but also have a high salt content.)
canned tomato juice
clams, raw
pickles
olives
frozen peas
frozen lima beans
celery
sauerkraut
most canned vegetables (read the labels)

Summary

There are an estimated 23 million Americans with hypertension. Less than 15 per cent of these are receiving adequate anti-hypertensive treatment.

Because this condition can be so readily detected and because certain types can be cured and others controlled, it is of utmost importance that persons with high blood pressure learn of their condition and secure proper treatment.

Your doctor is the only one who can decide if you have hypertension that needs to be treated. It is important to know that blood pressure changes in every person—when you are sleeping it is lower, when you are smoking it rises, it is different if you are sitting or standing. People with hypertension have too much blood pressure most of the time—it is almost always elevated.

Your doctor will work with you to find a treatment that is best for your hypertension. During the first few months this may require changes in the treatment. Remember—you have an important part in this treatment. Call your doctor with any questions or problems.

In order to assist you in using less or no salt the following chart of "Where To Use Herbs" is offered as a cooking guide:

Where to Use Herbs

	Basil	Bay Leaf	Cay-enne	Celery Seed	Ginger	Marjoram
Appetizers	tomato juice	tomato juice				
Soup	tomato spinach	stock			cold tomato	spinach onion
Meat	lamb	roast stew fricassee	beef veal lamb			pot roast lamb veal
Fish	all			all		broiled baked creamed
Game Fowl	duck					
Eggs Dairy	scramb. eggs		all eggs			cottage cheese omelet scramb.
Sauces Gravies	tomato					cream
Vegetables	tomato peas squash beans	boiled potato carrots tomato		tomato potato	squash	carrots zucchini peas spinach
Salads	tomato greens					greens

The following items *should NOT* be used for seasoning on a 1000 mg. Sodium Diet: Salt, Seasoned Salts, Ketchup, Chili Sauce, Worcestershire Sauce and other steak sauces, Pickles, Relish, Olives, Salt Pork, Ham Hocks, Soy Sauce, Accent (monosodium glutamate), Bouillon Cubes or Granules, Cheeses.

Sage	Thyme	Oregano	Rosemary	Tarragon	Savory
	tomato juice	guacamole	fruit cup		
cream	borscht vegetable	tomato	pea spinach chicken	consomme chicken mushroom tomato	
	meatloaf veal	meatloaf pork lamb	lamb stews	veal	veal
	all		salmon	broiled	broiled baked
poultry game stuffing	poultry	stuffing	stuffing	poultry	chicken
scramb. eggs cottage cheese	cottage cheese	boiled or poached eggs		all eggs	scramb. eggs
chicken gravy	tomato	spaghetti sauce spanish		vinegar	
eggplant tomato	onions carrots beets	tomato	peas spinach	baked potato	rice
	tomato			greens	greens green beans

The following items *may be used* for seasoning on a 1000 mg. Sodium Diet: Tabasco Sauce, Garlic Powder, Vinegar, Pepper and all other dry spices such as curry, paprika, cinnamon, etc., All herbs listed on this page, Special dietetic Low Sodium Ketchup and Chili Sauce, Low Sodium Mustard, Special dietetic Low Sodium Bouillon Cubes, Salt Substitutes, Dry Mustard.

More Potassium-Rich Foods

Foods	Average Portion	Potassium (in mg.)	Calories
Fruits			
Orange	1 medium	360 mg.	95
Grapefruit	1 cup	380 mg.	75
Banana	1 medium	630 mg.	130
Strawberries	1 cup	270 mg.	55
Avocado	one half	380 mg.	275
Apricots	3 medium	500 mg.	55
Dates	1 cup	1390 mg.	500
Watermelon	one half slice	380 mg.	95
Cantaloupe	one half melon	880 mg.	75
Raisins	1 cup	1150 mg.	425
Prunes	4 large	240 mg.	90
Juices			
Orange	8 oz. glass	440 mg.	105
Grapefruit	8 oz. glass	370 mg.	130
Prune	8 oz. glass	620 mg.	170
Pineapple	8 oz. glass	340 mg.	120
Meats			
Hamburger	3 ounces	290 mg.	310
Beef Chuck	3 ounces	310 mg.	260
Beef Round	3 ounces	340 mg.	200
Rib Roast	3 ounces	290 mg.	270
Turkey	4 ounces	350 mg.	300
Vegetables			
Tomato	1 medium	340 mg.	30
Artichoke	1 medium	210 mg.	30
Brussels sprouts	1 cup	300 mg.	35

The information contained in this article has been compiled by the Veterans Administration Wadsworth Hospital Center, Employees Hypertension Clinic, from material published by The American Heart Association. National High Blood Pressure Education Program, "Hypertension," and "Life and Health" magazines.

The purpose for putting this all together is to help you find out what high blood pressure is, what it can do to you and your body, and how you can help control it. U.S. GOVERNMENT PRINTING OFFICE: 1986 0–157–040

Incontinence

Incontinence Comes Out of the Closet

>   *Unless 9-year-old Linda is wakened for a trip to the bath-*
> *room several times a night, she wets the bed. She's afraid*
> *to go on "sleep-overs" with friends, and time after time she*
> *comes home with her sweater tied around her hips to hide*
> *the fact that she's wet her clothes.*
>   *Greg, a successful young businessman, quit his job right*
> *after being promoted. The new position involved travel and,*
> *on the road, he was required to share hotel rooms. But he*
> *couldn't face his co-workers' finding out about his inconti-*
> *nence. Greg settled for a lower-paying job elsewhere.*
>   *Marion, age 72, dreads returning to her dentist. She wet*
> *the dental chair during her last visit because her appointment*
> *took longer than she had anticipated.*

For Linda, Greg, Marion, and others who suffer from urinary incontinence, or the involuntary passing of urine, here's good news: Incontinence can be treated and often cured, even in the elderly.

The National Institute on Aging estimates that over 12 million Americans are incontinent. In nursing homes, more than 50 percent of patients over 65 are so affected; in fact, incontinence is the second most common reason for institutionalizing older people. (Dementia, or mental deterioration, is the first.) Outside nursing homes, incontinence afflicts about 17 percent of elderly men and 37 percent of elderly women. It's particularly troubling for older women because they generally live longer than men.

Incontinence is costly, in dollars and in psychological trauma. U.S. Surgeon General C. Everett Koop has estimated that, in nursing homes alone, the annual cost of caring for incontinent people is nearly $8 billion. And though incontinence isn't life-threatening, the stigma attached to clothes-wetting, bed-wetting, and the resultant odor can inflict profound consequences: humiliation, depression and social withdrawal. Even in the lives of people with only mild leakage, incontinence can be a ruling force.

Sad to say, only one in 12 people with incontinence seeks medical help—a fact perhaps due to embarrassment, isolation, or the mistaken notion that incontinence is normal with aging.

"Incontinence is no more a normal part of aging than is chest pain or diabetes,'' said Dr. Neil Resnick, of the Harvard Medical School, at a national conference sponsored in 1986 by the Food and Drug Administration and the Public Health Service Coordinating Committee on Women's Health Issues.

Normally, the urinary system removes waste products from the body in a well-coordinated fashion. Through nerve pathways, the brain synchronizes the individual housecleaning tasks that nature has assigned to different body parts: The two kidneys move wastes from the blood into the urine, tubes called ureters (one per kidney) channel the urine to the sac-like muscle called the bladder for storage, and then, as needed, two sphincter muscles open and close the bladder outlet to control urine flow to the outside via a tube known as the urethra.

But sometimes the system doesn't work the way it's supposed to. As Harvard's Resnick put it: ''Either the bladder contracts when it should not, leading to the patient's being wet, or it fails to contract when it should, so that urine builds up and spills over. . . . Either the outlet is open when it ought to be closed or it is closed when it ought to be open.'' Resnick added that factors generally associated with aging, such as illness, medicines, and the weakening of the urinary system, can increase a person's risk of incontinence.

Incontinence occurs when one of those working parts is adversely affected—by an obstruction in the urethral tube, for instance, or by an abnormality in the sphincter muscle, bladder muscle, or both. It may result from a condition as common as chronic constipation, particularly if stool is impacted, or from the lack of nearby toilets, as may be the case for some patients in institutions. It may develop after a hysterectomy or prostate, rectal, or lower intestinal surgery. Obesity and childbirth also can contribute to incontinence. Other causes include drug side effects, multiple sclerosis, cancer, spinal cord injury, diabetes mellitus, stroke, Parkinson's or Alzheimer's disease, and birth defects—80 to 90 percent of children born with spina bifida are incontinent.

When acute (relatively severe, but of short duration) incontinence occurs, it's generally the result of another acute medical problem. For instance, a heart attack or some type of infection may cause a mental state called delirium, in which consciousness can become so clouded that the patient has difficulty controlling the bladder. Persistent incontinence, on the other hand, is not associated with an acute medical problem; it often worsens over time and can occur in different ways:

- **Stress incontinence.** Minor physical stress such as coughing, sneezing, laughing or lifting results in small amounts of urine leakage. This is common in older women, but is usually not seen in men unless there has been sphincter damage during surgery.
- **Overflow incontinence.** The person doesn't feel the urge to void or

isn't able to urinate normal amounts ("normal" generally being 8 to 20 ounces), so the bladder overfills and spills small amounts of urine.

- **Urge incontinence.** The person feels a strong desire to urinate, but can't get to a toilet before the bladder empties.
- **Primary enuresis (EN-you-REE-sis).** This is the term most commonly used for bed-wetting in children beyond the age (5 years) when they should be capable of bladder control and in adults who never gained nighttime control.
- **Reflex incontinence.** The bladder fills and empties without the person's having any mental control over it at all.

The key weapon in the psychological and physical battle to stay dry is: Tell your physician about the incontinence, so that a correct diagnosis can be made and treatment options can be discussed. Ask whether you should consult a specialist in treating incontinence (for children, for example, a urologist who specializes in pediatric problems; for adults, a geriatrician, gynecologist, or urologist). Early diagnosis and treatment are important for many reasons, but they can be life-saving when the incontinence is the first sign of a serious medical condition, such as a tumor. If help isn't forthcoming, see another doctor.

To begin the medical investigation, the physician usually takes a patient's history and performs an examination. Urine and blood specimens are collected, and tests are performed—how many and what type depend on the patient's symptoms and history.

Patients may be asked to undergo procedures called "urodynamic" tests to help the physician pinpoint whether the problem lies in the urinary system and, if so, where. They're done on an outpatient basis. One such test measures the speed of urine flow from the bladder as the person urinates into a special toilet connected to a machine. An obstruction would cause the flow to be slower than normal. Other procedures test the sphincter and bladder muscles, as follows: One end of a catheter (a small plastic tube) is passed up the urethra to the bladder, and an electrode carried by the catheter is attached to the sphincter. Then, electrical impulses coming from the sphincter muscles and pressure changes within the bladder are recorded. The physician evaluates the readings to see whether the muscles are functioning normally.

Other types of tests may be ordered as well.

Physicians treat incontinence by treating its underlying cause. Treatments include:

- **Battery-operated alarm.** Used for bed-wetting, the alarm is triggered by the wetting. Initially, for children, it may be necessary for someone in the household to respond to the alarm and waken the patient. Once patients become conscious of the alarm, they should waken on their own when it rings. Eventually, the patients are supposed to become so used to waking when wetting occurs that they start waking *before-hand*.

- *Scheduled voiding regimens.* For urge incontinence, patients may be asked to wait longer before urinating, gradually increasing the "waiting period," or to urinate only at assigned intervals. Mentally impaired patients may be prompted to stay dry by simply being asked if they need to urinate and, if so, helped to the toilet. What works for one incontinence problem may not work for another, so it's best to get medical advice before beginning a regimen. And, generally, women shouldn't put off urinating, as that can promote bladder infections.

- *"Kegel" exercises.* In 1948 Arnold Kegel, M.D., who was practicing in Los Angeles at that time, introduced exercises to strengthen the pelvic floor muscles in women with stress incontinence, so as to preserve or regain bladder control. It's possible to feel where these muscles are, at one end of the pelvic floor, by interrupting the flow several times during urination and, at the other end, by drawing in the muscle around the anus as if to stop a bowel movement. The patient is supposed to repeat the exercises—interrupting each urination and tightening the pelvic floor muscles from back to front—many times throughout the day.

  Harvard's Resnick advises that all women who aren't pregnant practice Kegel exercises to strengthen the pelvic floor muscles, which, in turn, may help ward off incontinence later in life. But, he says, people usually need professional instruction to do them correctly.

- *Drugs.* Estrogen therapy is prescribed for women with estrogen deficiency. The condition can cause the tissue lining of the urethra to become inflamed, and the irritated tissue can cause or worsen urge incontinence. The antispasmodic drug flavoxate is prescribed to treat incontinence associated with such conditions as cystitis (inflammation of the bladder). Flavoxate decreases muscle spasms in the bladder. However, the large dosages that are often required can be hazardous to other tissue, and the patient may have to contend with undesirable side effects, such as dry mouth, constipation, and blurred vision.

- *Reevaluation of drug therapy.* Incontinence may be due to drugs the person is taking for some other condition: Sedatives or tranquilizers may dull the senses so much that the urge to urinate isn't felt; anticholinergics prescribed for bowel spasm can decrease the bladder's ability to contract; diuretics, often given to lower blood pressure, increase urine production; and cold medicines may increase the bladder outlet's resistance so that the bladder doesn't completely empty. Upon reevaluation, the physician may find that a different drug will work without causing incontinence.

- *Surgical procedures.* Even frail, elderly patients can easily tolerate a number of newer corrective procedures, says Resnick. Deep abdominal surgery is usually not required; rather, the surgeon works through the vagina or a tiny abdominal incision and uses an endoscope (a narrow tube-like instrument inserted via the urethra or the incision) to see inside the bladder. This way, the surgeon can relieve an obstruction, tie up pelvic floor tissues to return a sagging urethra or bladder to a normal position, or repair a constantly opening bladder outlet so that it closes properly. The hospital stay is usually only a day or two; a younger person may be in and out of the hospital the same day. Other surgical options may be to implant an artificial sphincter or to reconstruct the bladder. (See illustration.)

Sometimes the underlying cause of the incontinence can't be cured, but the situation is still far from hopeless. There are many measures to help a person stay dry: more frequent trips to the toilet, a portable commode for invalids, and self-catheterization (after proper instructions) to empty the bladder several times a day. There are urine collection devices and disposable pads and pants available from medical supply stores, certain drugstores, and home health-care catalogs. One product may work better than another, so a person may want to try several. Also, oral deodorant tablets can be taken as an aid to reduce urinary odor. The active ingredient, chlorophyllin copper complex, helps to mask the odor.

Incontinence will probably never lead the list of tea-time topics of conversation. But health professionals, public health officials, women's groups, the media, makers of incontinence-related products, and others personally acquainted with the difficult problem are erasing the incontinence stigma. Actress June Allyson, appearing in ads that promote disposable absorbent pants, unashamedly acknowledges that her mother became incontinent after a stroke and that they're dealing with it. By being so frank, Allyson also promotes the idea that it's all right to talk about incontinence. Two support groups for incontinent patients were incorporated in 1983: HIP, or Help for Incontinent People, and The Simon Foundation, whose founder-director is herself incontinent. The groups offer information about such topics as recovery after prostate surgery, cleaning urine stains from clothing, incontinence-treatment products, and treatment options. To receive an information packet (there may be a charge), send the request and a stamped, self-addressed, business-size envelope to:

HIP, P.O. Box 544, Union, S.C. 29379 (phone 803-585-8789), or

The Simon Foundation, P.O. Box 835, Wilmette, Ill. 60091 (phone 1-800-23SIMON).

Dixie Farley

FDA Consumer, March 1987

Some patients with urinary incontinence — due to cancer, for instance — may be candidates for a surgical procedure in which a portion of the small intestine is used to make a substitute bladder. The resultant "Kock pouch," pictured here, is named for the procedure's developer, Nils Kock, M.D., of Sweden. The surgeon first removes the bladder and detaches a segment of the small intestine to make the pouch and two valves, one for each end of the pouch. Collars of synthetic material are used to hold the valves in place. One end of the pouch is connected to the ureters; the valve there allows urine to flow freely from the kidneys into the pouch, but prevents backward flow. The other end opens to the outside through the abdomen; that valve prevents leakage and allows the patient to insert a catheter for drainage, as needed. No external collecting device is required.

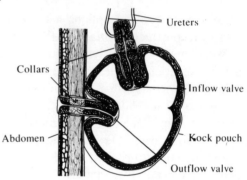

(Based on a drawing by Patricia Kynes, R.N., in the November-December 1986 Journal of Enterostomal Therapy.)

Urinary System

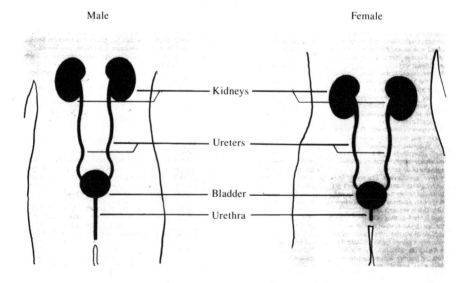

Infertility

Infertility, And How It's Treated

We are led to believe that couples aren't into children much anymore. That if a man and a woman want to have a really meaningful relationship, they'll continue childless. At the most, we are told, a couple might agree to sharing their lives with a single child. That's where they're coming from today.

That may sound very trendy, but the fact is that having children remains very popular. In the United States, live births still top 3 million a year. Raising a family may seem to some to be old-fashioned but to many it is a fond desire.

And to thousands it is, unfortunately, unrealized. The burden of being barren has weighted down women throughout history. At the same time, it has often crushed the male ego. That the problem hasn't gone away is best exemplified by figures from the National Disease and Therapeutic Index compiled by IMS America, a pharmaceutical marketing research firm. Those figures indicate that women visited doctors about fertility problems some 1.5 million times in the year ending Sept. 30, 1982. About 19 percent, or 285,000, of those visits were first visits. One study concluded that 15 percent of U.S. marriages are infertile.

While the problem hasn't gone away, we do know a little more about it today. We know that 30 to 40 percent of the cases may be traced to male infertility, and that although there are many causes of female infertility, a few of the major problems can very often be cured with drugs.

For men, infertility is generally associated with insufficient or weak sperm. A normal male provides 400 million sperm in an emission. When the sperm count gets below 100 million, the odds on one of them fertilizing an egg are extremely thin. Weak or defective sperm may be unable to make that tremendously difficult 9- or 10-inch upstream swim to the Fallopian tubes where the ready-to-be-fertilized egg waits.

Male sterility problems may be caused by diseases or may result from physical or metabolic disorders. Elevated scrotum temperatures can limit the production of sperm. A hot bath can cause it, as well as an infection. Today's fashionably tight clothing is also believed to contribute to higher testicular temperatures.

Often the problem is a physical condition called varicocele, which is actually varicose veins in the testes area. The enlarged veins block the return flow of blood from the testes, causing the blood to pool in the testes and elevating temperatures there. The condition has been treated for years by surgery, usually involving an overnight hospital stay. Nearly 40,000 such operations are believed to be performed annually. Recently, FDA gave approval for an investigational new device designed to solve the problem. Inserted into a vein, the tiny reed-like device has a balloon on one end that is inflated to stop the blood flow. Thus, the pooling of blood is stopped, and the area is cooled normally. A major advantage of the procedure using the device is that it can be done on an outpatient basis.

While the causes of infertility in women are many, they are often traced to blocked Fallopian tubes, or failure to produce eggs or to retain fertilized eggs. Blocked Fallopian tubes prevent the egg, which is traveling down from the ovaries, from meeting up with the upcoming sperm. The reason for the blockage may be physical or may be due to scars left from diseases. In such cases, surgery may alleviate the problem. However, many Fallopian tubes are blocked by a condition called endometriosis.

Endometriosis is a painful condition in which tissue from the lining of the uterus is found in other parts of the abdominal cavity. The strayed tissue grows, causing much pain and any number of other problems, including blocked tubes. An accidental discovery involving a long-time endometriosis sufferer who had a Caesarean section performed led to the treatment of the disease with a hormone-suppressing drug. In addition to creating a pseudomenopause condition, the drug causes the endometrial tissue to atrophy and die. Treatment usually lasts six to nine months. Pregnancy, if desired, follows in about 50 percent of the cases.

The drug Danocrine (chemical name: danazol) is prescribed mainly for treatment of endometriosis and not for infertility. However, according to IMS America, 10 percent of the 327,000 prescriptions written for it in 1982 were for treating infertility.

Drugs are often used successfully for inducing ovulation. However, they may have a major side effect—multiple births.

Lack of ovulation or infrequent and irregular ovulations may be a cause of up to half of female infertility problems. Drug therapy can result in pregnancy in about 25 percent of those cases.

The drugs used in such cases work by stimulating the pituitary gland to produce needed hormones. The hormones, known as FSH and LH, are believed to act on the ovaries in the following ways: FSH helps the follicle or egg sac to grow in the early stages of a woman's menstrual cycle. The follicle also releases an estrogen hormone at mid-cycle that will prompt the pituitary to release enough LH to cause the follicle to rupture and release its egg.

Clomid (clomiphene citrate) is a drug quite widely used in infertility cases. Taken orally, it is usually prescribed for days five through nine after menstrual bleeding has ended. The National Prescription Audit put the number of Clomid prescriptions at 658,000 in 1982.

Women who take Clomid and become pregnant deliver more than one child in 7 to 10 percent of the births. Three-fourths of the multiple births are twins. By comparison, in the population as a whole, multiple births represent but 1 percent, with twins accounting for slightly better than 98 percent of those.

The multiple births result because the ovaries are overstimulated by the drug. Thus, more than one egg may be ripe and ready for fertilization at the mid-cycle time of conception.

If Clomid doesn't result in pregnancy and if tests show that not too many ovary sacs are ripening, a more powerful drug, Pergonal (menotropins), may be prescribed. Injected into the muscle, Pergonal provides both FSH and LH and is given for nine to twelve days. Pergonal is known technically as human menopausal gonadotropin. It is extracted and purified from the urine of postmenopausal women. Human chorionic gonadotropin (HCG) (trade names: Antuitrin-S, A.P.L., Pregnyl and Follutein) is injected one day after the last dose of Pergonal.

HCG is extracted from the urine of pregnant women and is used in pregnancy tests. HCG acts to sustain the action of progesterone, a hormone important to the early growth and nesting of the fertilized egg.

Because Pergonal and HCG are injected in a doctor's office, it is difficult to track their usage records through prescription audits. Use of the combination is effective, bringing on pregnancy in 25 percent of the patients, if the women are properly selected. Multiple births result in 20 percent of the pregnancies. That's 20 times the national average. As with Clomid, a fourth of those multiple births are triplets or more.

After use in women for some years, Pergonal with HCG has been approved by FDA for males with pituitary gland problems. The combination may stimulate sperm production.

Infertility cases are not always so difficult as to need the more powerful drugs. Sometimes for women, doses of the single hormones estrogen or progesterone will do the job. And sometimes a douche with baking soda is all that is needed. Such a pre-intercourse douche can neutralize overly acidic cervical secretions that might be killing off sperm.

A hormone has also been used on men to suppress sperm count so that advantage can be taken of the rebound effect that follows when the hormone is withdrawn.

In addition, a study reported recently (March 3, 1983) in the *New England Journal of Medicine* noted success in achieving pregnancies for previously infertile couples by treating the husbands for a relatively minor but prevalent social disease caused by the microorganism *T mycoplasma* or *Ureaplasma urealyticum*. This infection of the genital tract was treated with a tetracycline type antibiotic. Researchers believe that the mycoplasma infection may be a major cause of infertility.

Roger W. Miller, reprinted from June 1983, *FDA Consumer*, HHS Publication No. (FDA) 83–3136. Department of Health and Human Services, Public Health Service, Food and Drug Administration, 5600 Fishers Lane, Rockville, Md. 20857. U.S. Government Printing Office 1983—381–174/43.

Kidney Stones
Prevention and Treatment

Stones that form in the kidneys and urinary tract are one of the most painful disorders to afflict human beings. This ancient health problem is known to have tormented numerous famous historical figures such as Benjamin Franklin, Frances Bacon, Isaac Newton, Peter the Great, and Louis XIV. In fact, scientists have found evidence in an Egyptian mummy of the occurrence of stones, dating from about 4,800 B.C. Although considerable progress has been made in treatment and in prevention of stones over the past two decades, the problem continues to plague mankind today.

More than a million Americans are hospitalized each year for the treatment of kidney and urinary tract stones. Surgery is still often necessary, but recent medical advances have improved understanding and increased the possibility that many cases of stone disease can be cured or controlled with nonsurgical therapies.

What is a kidney stone?

A kidney stone is usually a hard mass that builds up gradually when various salt or mineral crystals deposit on the inner surfaces of the kidney. As stones grow on the lining of the drainage system of the kidneys or urinary tract, bleeding may occur in the tissues there. This bleeding often leads the patient to visit a physician, who may detect the stone if it is opaque on X-ray examination. Sometimes a stone will break off from its location in the kidney pelvis, resulting in severe pain as it moves down the urinary tract.

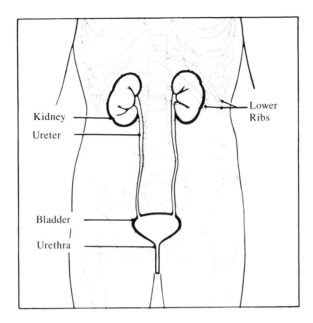

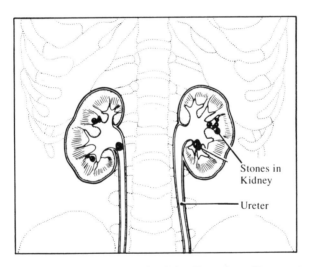

What are "urinary" and "bladder" stones?

The urinary system consists of two kidneys, located below the ribs toward the middle of the back; two drainage tubes called ureters, which connect the kidneys to the bladder in the lower abdomen; and the urethra, the tube through which urine flows from the bladder to outside of the body. Kidney stones that remain in the kidney or that break loose from the lining of the kidney and move to other parts of the urinary system are sometimes referred to as "urinary stones." Sometimes smaller stones pass through the ureters and lodge in the bladder where they enlarge, or stones may originate in the bladder. In either case, these are referred to as "bladder stones."

When stones grow so large that they cannot be passed out of the body easily, they obstruct the normal flow of urine, causing pain and possibly infection or kidney damage. Many stones are too large to pass out of the kidney pelvis. Other stones may become lodged in the ureter or at the outlet of the bladder.

Causes and types of stones

Stones produced within the urinary system are not the disease, of course, but the end product of the disease process. Scientists suggest many different causes or factors in stone formation such as age, genetic disorders, occupation, climate, metabolic disturbances, presence of infection, dietary patterns, and the amount of water consumed. Heredity may play an important role in the tendency to form stones. Black people tend to have far fewer stones than white people do. About three males are afflicted for every female. Stones occur in more than 70 percent of patients with the hereditary disease known as *renal tubular acidosis. Cystinuria* is a prime example of a genetic defect that often results in formation of urinary stones. In this disorder, the body excretes excessive amounts of the amino acid *cystine,* which is insoluble in urine and may accumulate in the urinary system to form stones. Another genetic defect that causes stone formation is *hyperoxaluria.* This metabolic disorder leads to overproduction of the chemical oxalate by the body, and increased excretion of this salt into the urinary tract.

Stones are composed of substances such as *calcium oxalate, calcium phosphate,* and *uric acid.* Calcium stones are the most common. In fact, about 90 percent of all urinary stones contain calcium, which dissolves poorly in urine. Calcium oxalate is the most common crystal found in stones. This organic acid is produced within the body, and it is also taken in through foods such as broccoli, spinach, asparagus, rhubarb, oranges, various berries, apples, grapes, pineapples, cranberries, beer, coffee, tea, cocoa, cola drinks, pepper, and others.

Both calcium and phosphorus, of course, are basic parts of the normal diet needed for bone and cell metabolism. Oxalate, which cannot be broken down by the cells of the body, must be flushed out in the urine. When too much calcium oxalate accumulates in the urine, crystals form and a kidney stone develops. This imbalance can result from ingestion of certain diuretics or antacids, or from eating foods high in oxalate. Formation of calcium oxalate stones also occurs frequently in patients who have suffered from chronic inflammation of the bowel, or who have had an intestinal bypass operation.

A urinary stone may consist entirely of one compound, but most stones are a combination of salts. Determining exactly what type of stone a patient has passed and the mechanism by which it was formed can be very important. The physician must have this information in order to provide rational preventive treatment.

Medical scientists are not always sure just why kidney stones form, or why one person forms them and another person does not. Sometimes anatomical abnormalities predispose a person to stone formation. There is evidence that drinking too little fluid, which can result in dehydration, decreases the amount of urine and increases the concentration of the elements that accumulate to form stones. Stones may accompany metabolic disturbances that result in excessive levels of calcium in the blood and urine. Sometimes stones occur in conjunction with chronic urinary tract infections or with the misuse of certain medications. The immobilization, for several weeks or longer, of a patient who is subject to stones can be the initiating event in stone formation.

While certain foods may promote formation of stones in susceptible people, scientists do not believe that eating any specific food causes stones to form in healthy individuals. *Absorptive hypercalciuria* is a condition in which a person's body absorbs calcium from food at an abnormally high rate, and empties the excess calcium through the bloodstream and kidneys into the urine. This high level of urinary calcium sometimes may cause crystals of calcium oxalate or calcium phosphate to form and grow in the kidneys or urinary tract. In some cases, a person may habitually eat too much food that is high in calcium, resulting in excessive calcium being passed through the kidneys. Normally, urine contains chemical substances that inhibit the formation of crystals. These inhibitors do not seem to work for everyone, however, and some people form stones even though their urine does not show abnormally high levels of calcium. Other causes of stone formation are hyperuricosuria (a disorder of uric acid metabolism), gout, overactivity of the parathyroid glands, excessive consumption of vitamin D, urinary tract infection, and blockage of the urinary tract.

Symptoms

Excruciating pain is usually the first symptom of a kidney stone. The pain often begins suddenly when a stone moves from the kidney into the ureter, causing irritation or obstruction. Typically, the patient experiences pain in the back and side in the vicinity of the kidney or in the lower abdomen. Later, the pain may radiate to the groin.

If the stone is too large to pass easily, the severe, constant pain continues as the muscles in the walls of the tiny ureter try to squeeze the stone along into the bladder. Sometimes the patient will find blood in the urine, and may experience a burning sensation during urination, or frequency of urination. Other symptoms may include the presence of urinary infection accompanied by fever, vomiting, nausea, loss of appetite, and chills. The patient may find that his kidney and abdomen in the region of the stone are very tender to the touch.

Diagnosis and treatment

Sometimes "silent" kidney stones are diagnosed as a result of X-rays taken in the course of a general health examination. More often, it is the sudden pain that signals the stone's presence. X-ray examination can be used to verify the presence of a stone. The exam often provides the physician with valuable information about the composition, location, and the factors that caused the stone. The physician will also perform analyses of the blood and urine to help determine the cause of the episode, and to enable him to plan the proper course of treatment. In some cases, the doctor may use specialized X-ray techniques or ultrasound to scan the kidney and urinary system in order to assess the degree of stone formation and plan necessary therapy.

"Silent" stones—those that are not causing any problem for the patient—normally do not require treatment. Acute attacks, on the other hand, usually require hospitalization, because the pain is so severe. In most cases, the stone is small and the patient needs only pain relief and instructions concerning recovery of the stone after it is passed. About 90 percent of stones pass spontaneously through the urinary system. Sometimes the stone becomes stuck in the ureter or bladder. In this event, the physician often decides that the best thing to do is just to wait and see if the stone will pass if it is given a little time.

In some cases, the doctor must attempt removal by passing a cystoscope (a hollow tubular instrument) up into the bladder, trying to grasp and withdraw the stone with a basket-like device. Sometimes stones that are stuck in the bladder can be crushed using a tiny instrument inserted with a catheter. Some stones (those composed of uric acid) may be dissolved by medical treatment. In other cases, surgery may be necessary to extract stones stuck in the urinary system.

In recent years, clinicians have developed still other means of extracting stones from the kidney and upper ureter. In some instances, a needle and probe can be inserted through the skin creating a channel straight to the area of the stone. Through this channel, the stone can be viewed using a fiberoptic nephroscope. In some cases, the doctor can insert an ultrasonic probe through the channel, placing it against the stone and gradually disintegrating it. Then the stone fragments are removed using special forceps, loops or baskets that grasp and draw out the pieces. Sometimes an alternative technique employing an electrohydraulic instrument is used to shatter the stone. As the stone breaks up, the area is continuously irrigated and the pieces of stone are sucked up by a vacuum apparatus.

Another procedure known as *coagulum pyelolithotomy* can sometimes offer a simple, rapid means of removal of multiple stones in the kidney. In this treatment, a liquid containing calcium chloride, cryoprecipitate, thrombin, and indigo carmine is injected into the kidney and allowed to form a jelly-like clot. Within minutes the stones are trapped inside the clot, which the surgeon then extracts with forceps. He sutures the incision, and the patient is free of the painful stones.

Shock wave therapy

Researchers are hopeful that the need for surgery may be reduced by a new therapy that uses high energy shock waves to pulverize kidney stones. In this procedure, developed in West Germany, high energy acoustic shock waves are produced by an underwater high voltage condensor spark discharge that causes an explosive evaporation of water surrounding the condensor. This action in turn leads to generation of shock waves through the surrounding fluid. In the first year of clinical use in West Germany, this treatment was used for over 750 patients.

Before treatment, the patient is anesthetized and positioned in a water bath so that the kidney stone is precisely localized and targeted to receive the highest energy of the shock wave. The blast, which does not harm any other area of the patient, penetrates the kidney stone and shatters it as the waves bounce back from the surrounding soft tissue of the body and collide with oncoming waves.

Preliminary studies of shock wave therapy are under way in the United States. American urologic investigators are collaborating with physicists and other basic scientists in these studies, and, in fact, several urology departments in the U.S. have made arrangements to secure the high energy shock wave equipment.

Prevention

"With a surprising lack of fanfare," wrote a noted scientist recently, "recurrent renal stones have become a preventable disease." In the past, it is true, little could be done for most patients with stones. There were treatments for some of the rarer forms, but patients with the most common kinds of kidney stones faced the prospect of drinking a lot of liquids and the likelihood of surgery. Today, however, scientific progress has brought greater understanding of the causes and mechanisms of stone formation and far more effective clinical management of stone disease.

Stones tend to be multiple and tend to recur even after spontaneous passage or surgical removal. Therefore, effective prevention depends on determining the specific cause of stone formation.

After a patient has passed a kidney stone, the physician usually orders a careful metabolic workup, and has the stone analyzed to identify its exact composition. The workup may include several blood tests, and the patient may be asked to collect 24-hour urine samples. The urine tests enable the doctor to determine if hypercalciuria (an abnormal level of calcium in the urine) or hyperuricosuria (excessive uric acid in the urine) are present. Patients with these conditions account for about two-thirds of those with calcium stone disease. In some cases, diuretics such as hydrochlorothiazide may be prescribed to decrease the excretion of calcium. Such "water pills" often are very effective in preventing the recurrence of calcium stones. Patients with hypercalciuria who also have hyperuricosuria may be treated with a drug called allopurinol.

Patients with hypercalciuria often can control stone formation simply by drinking a lot of fluids and following a moderately low calcium diet. Some patients with absorptive hypercalciuria may be placed on a low-oxalate diet and receive the drug sodium cellulose phosphate, which has been found to inhibit formation of these stones.

Physicians sometimes find that by using chemical agents to manipulate the acidity or alkalinity of the urine, crystal formation can be inhibited and stone formation prevented. Patients with calcium oxalate stones are usually advised to avoid foods with high oxalate content, and in some cases are advised to avoid foods fortified with vitamin D, and antacids that have a calcium base. An age-old treatment, increasing the patient's daily consumption of liquids (primarily water) is a worthwhile preventive measure regardless of the type of stones involved.

Uric acid stones

Hyperuricosuria can result from eating an excessive amount of meat, fish, or poultry, and almost always can be controlled if the patient changes his diet. For those who find it difficult to change their dietary habits, stone formation can be prevented through use of a drug called allopurinol, which reduces production of uric acid. Uric acid stones can also be prevented in many cases through use of an alkaline agent that regulates the acidity of the patient's urine, a key factor controlling crystallization of uric acid. Gout, a disorder of purine metabolism associated with arthritis, may also cause hyperuricemia, hyperuricosuria, and uric acid stones. This disorder requires specific drug treatment.

Struvite stones

Struvite stones are composed of magnesium, phosphate, and ammonium. They can be very difficult stones to treat, because they result from infection of the urinary tract that can recur even after the stones have been removed. This type of stone can fill the entire inside of the kidney, spreading into the smallest passages, blocking drainage of urine, and resulting in severe kidney damage.

Struvite stones occur mainly due to infection with a certain type of bacteria that tends to flourish and invade the kidney following a course of antibiotic therapy. For this reason, the best preventive measure against this type of kidney stone is to be aware of the need to be careful in the use of antibiotics. One should take them only when the doctor determines that it is absolutely necessary. In recent research, scientists also have found that an agent called *acetohydroxamic acid* (AHA), an inhibitor of the chemical action caused by the invading bacteria, can be used to effectively retard struvite stone formation.

Hyperparathyroidism

Overactivity of the parathyroid glands (hyperparathyroidism) is also a frequent cause of calcium stone disease. The parathyroids are tiny glands in the neck that produce a hormone that regulates the level of calcium in the blood. When these glands are overactive, too much parathyroid hormone in the system causes bone cells to release calcium that is retained in the blood. At the same time, abnormally high amounts of calcium also build up in the blood, and eventually the calcium level increases so much that it spills over into the urine where it promotes formation of kidney stones.

Once the physician makes the diagnosis of hyperparathyroidism, future stones from this cause can be prevented through surgical removal of all or part of the abnormal parathyroid gland. In most cases, only one of the glands is enlarged and its removal ends the patient's problem with kidney stones.

Cystine stones

Another type of stone occurs in patients with the relatively rare inherited defect of kidney function causing cystinuria. In this disorder, the amino acid cystine overloads the urine where it crystallizes and forms stones. Prevention of cystine stones is difficult, because there is no definitive treatment. The main therapy is for the patient to drink enough water to dissolve the cystine that escapes into the urine each day. This therapy can be difficult, because cystine is eliminated continuously, and so the patient may be required to drink over a gallon of water every 24 hours.

At night, about a third of a gallon of water may be consumed on this regimen, filling the bladder repeatedly and interfering with sleep. Sometimes when stones cannot be controlled through increased fluid consumption, the drug penicillamine is administered to make the cystine more soluble. This approach is always used cautiously, however, because patients often have severe allergic reactions to this drug.

The Division of Kidney, Urologic and Hematologic Diseases

The Division of Kidney, Urologic and Hematologic Diseases of the National Institute of Arthritis, Diabetes, and Digestive and Kidney Diseases supports most of the research on kidney and urinary tract stones and a significant portion of the kidney research of the National Institutes of Health. Through NIADDK support, many fundamental and clinical studies are conducted to expand the knowledge of kidney function. The emphasis of much research is on further understanding of the causes and mechanisms of stone formation. Other studies are aimed at preventing, controlling, and curing, not only kidney stones and related infections of the urinary tract and kidney, but many other disorders that take a great toll in disability and mortality.

U.S. Department of Health and Human Services, Public Health Service, National Institutes of Health. National Institute of Arthritis, Diabetes, & Digestive & Kidney Diseases, NIH Publication No. 83–2495, August 1983.

Leukemia
What You Need to Know

Introduction

This article is written for you, the cancer[*] *patient. It also may be useful for members of your family.*

We believe it is important for you and your family to understand your illness so you can face it together, with courage and hope.

Much has been learned about the nature of cancer in recent years. Modern methods of diagnosing and treating leukemia

---

[*]Words in italics are explained at the end of the article.

*are described herein. You also will find information on sources
of assistance, areas of research, and definitions of medical
terms.*

Leukemia is a generalized disorder of blood cell production in which
abnormal white blood cells accumulate in the blood and *bone marrow.*
In lymphocytic leukemia, these white cells are *lymphocytes,* produced
in the lymph nodes. Myelocytic leukemia (also known as granulocytic
or myelogenous leukemia) affects the *granulocytes,* white blood cells
produced in the bone marrow. Both lymphocytic and myelocytic leukemia
occur as acute (fast-growing) or chronic (slow-growing) diseases.

Leukemia, like other cancers, is a disease of the body's cells. Cells
of different shapes and functions make up various parts of the body:
the skin, heart, lungs, bones, and so forth. All cells reproduce themselves
by dividing. Normal growth and repair of body tissues take place in
this orderly manner.

When cell division is not orderly, abnormal growth takes place. In
leukemia, among the tiny cells which make up the blood are *blast cells,*
or immature cells, instead of normal cells.

To understand the nature of leukemia, it is necessary to know about
function and composition of the blood. It supplies food, oxygen, hormones, and other chemicals the body's cells must have to function properly. The blood transports these substances to and from storage centers,
helps in the removal of waste products, and is also one of the body's
most effective defenses against infection.

To carry out these and other important functions, the blood contains
many components, each with a specific task. Those that are involved
in leukemia are *red cells, platelets,* and *white cells.*

The red blood cells, along with the platelets and certain of the white
blood cells, are formed primarily in the bone marrow and are then released
into the bloodstream as they become mature. The bone marrow, a spongy
meshwork of tissue which fills up the cavities of the bones, is important
in leukemia because this is where the disease seems to begin.

The red cells, or *erythrocytes,* carry the oxygen necessary for life to
all the various organs and tissues of the body. Each of these cells contains
a small amount of a compound called hemoglobin, which is capable of
taking up oxygen as the blood passes through the lungs, and releasing
it in the tissues.

The bone marrow contains certain tiny disc-shaped cells, called platelets, that break off and circulate in the blood. Platelets are necessary
for the prevention of abnormal bleeding.

The third group of elements in the blood consists of the white blood
cells, or *leukocytes.* The two types of white cells are the granulocytes

(sometimes referred to as *neutrophils*), and the lymphocytes. These cells play a major role in the body's defense against disease-producing bacteria, viruses, and fungi.

The neutrophils are able to rid the body of harmful bacteria and other foreign particles by engulfing and destroying them. The number of these white cells in the blood varies greatly and can increase quite rapidly when needed to combat infection. Once an infection is overcome, the number of neutrophils in the blood usually returns to normal.

The lymphocytes act in a different way to maintain good health. When the body is invaded by viruses or bacteria, the lymphocytes and other specialized cells respond by producing antibodies. These are substances which react with the infectious agent so that it is ultimately destroyed and removed from the body. Because each antibody is generally effective against only one type of bacterium or virus, different ones must be produced to combat each infectious agent.

Leukemia may occur at any age. Since the disease affects children and adults in a different way, "What You Need to Know About Childhood Leukemia" is the subject of a separate pamphlet in this series.

Symptoms

Symptoms of acute lymphocytic leukemia and acute myelocytic leukemia are varied and can progress rapidly. The *lymph nodes, spleen* and *liver* become infiltrated with white blood cells and may be enlarged. Other common symptoms are bone pain, paleness, tendency to bleed or bruise easily, and frequent infections.

Chronic myelocytic leukemia is also known as chronic granulocytic leukemia, chronic myeloid leukemia, chronic myelogenous leukemia, or chronic myelosis.

The patient most often seeks medical treatment because of increasing fatigue, or weight loss. There may be a sense of fullness or heaviness under the left ribs, and the doctor may discover a mass in the abdomen. Less frequently, the complaints result from anemia, abnormal perspiration, fever, bleeding, pain in the spleen, or an attack of gout. Sometimes the discovery of the disease may be accidental, in the course of routine clinical or laboratory examinations.

Chronic lymphocytic leukemia usually occurs in older people and develops slowly. In fact, symptoms are entirely absent in some cases, and the disease discovered accidentally when a patient is examined for another complaint. When symptoms do occur, they may be a general feeling of ill health, fatigue, lack of energy, fever, loss of appetite and weight, or night sweats. Enlarged lymph nodes in the neck or groin may be noticed in some patients. Some may show signs of anemia or infections.

Diagnosis

Leukemia can be diagnosed only by microscopic examination of the blood and the bone marrow. If leukemia cells are present in these tissues, they can be identified and the diagnosis made.

The blood test may show low hemoglobin, low white cell levels and a low platelet level. Blast cells (immature cells) also may be present in the blood.

Because these findings suggest the diagnosis of leukemia, a bone marrow *biopsy* may be done. A sample of bone marrow is obtained by inserting a needle into the bone and withdrawing a tiny amount of tissue. The bone marrow is examined under the microscope by a pathologist. A pathologist is a physician who interprets and diagnoses the changes caused by disease in body tissues. The bone marrow biopsy establishes the specific type of leukemia, which is essential in determining the best form of treatment. It also is used as a way of checking on the progress of therapy.

When a diagnosis of leukemia is confirmed, it is best for you to begin treatment in a hospital that has an expert staff and resources to apply all forms of effective treatment right from the beginning. Before treatment you may, if you wish, request a second opinion from another physician to confirm the diagnosis and recommendations for therapy.

Treatment

Your doctor will consider a number of factors in determining the best treatment for you. Among these are your medical history, your general health, the type of leukemia you have, and the extent of your disease. Your treatment must be tailored to your individual needs.

Acute myelocytic leukemia and acute lymphocytic leukemia are treated with various combinations of drugs, or *chemotherapy*. Chemotherapy (treatment with anticancer drugs) kills cancer cells. Your physician must maintain a delicate balance of enough drugs to kill cancer cells without destroying too many healthy ones.

Some anticancer drugs may make you feel sick for a while, but your doctor tries to work out a treatment schedule that disrupts your daily routine as little as possible. The length and frequency of drug treatments depend on a number of factors. These include your type of leukemia, the kind of anticancer drugs prescribed, how long it takes you to respond to the treatment, and how well you tolerate any side-effects.

Therapy to the *central nervous system,* discussed below, may also be added to your regular treatment program. Combinations of drugs are then used in maintenance of *remission.*

A remission is a temporary—and potentially permanent—arrest of leukemia. When a complete remission occurs, there is a complete return to a state of normal good health: the symptoms disappear, the physical findings become normal, and abnormal cells are no longer found in the bone marrow and blood. Sometimes the remission is only partial and one or more of the signs of leukemia may not completely disappear. Examination of the blood at frequent intervals and of the bone marrow from time to time enables your doctor to follow the course of your disease and to select the proper dosage of the appropriate drugs.

Sometimes leukemic cells accumulate in the brain. Here, due to unique properties of the blood vessel walls that prevent certain substances from passing from the blood to the central nervous system, the leukemic cells may be relatively safe from attack by anticancer drugs.

Patients are now being treated before central nervous system symptoms appear with drugs administered directly into the spinal fluid, and in some cases with *radiation therapy* to the brain as well.

Chronic myelocytic leukemia often can be controlled at the beginning by a variety of treatments. One or more anticancer drugs often are administered. Irradiation with *X-rays* or radioactive phosphorus may benefit some patients. After a few weeks the patient often goes into remission and can resume his normal activities.

When a patient relapses, the abnormalities reappear and are similar to those seen in acute leukemias. Infections and hemorrhaging are frequent and may be severe. The methods for treatment are the same as for the acute leukemias during this stage of the disease.

Chronic lymphocytic leukemia may be left untreated when there are no symptoms and few or no abnormal physical signs. Patients may live normal lives with the disease for a number of years. However, the patient should be examined at regular intervals.

When the disease becomes active, one or more anticancer drugs may be of value. Radiation therapy also may be given in some cases.

Supportive care

Other problems in treating leukemia are the result of drug side-effects as well as leukemia itself. Both drugs and leukemia damage the bone marrow and impair the patient's ability to produce two important blood elements. These elements are platelets that prevent bleeding, and white blood cells that help control bacterial and fungal infections.

Transfusions of blood platelets have proved effective in preventing or stopping hemorrhage. A supply of platelets from a donor can be obtained by a technique known as *plateletpheresis,* in which platelets are removed from normal whole blood by centrifugation. Because the red cells are returned promptly, the donor may be able to give platelets as frequently as twice a week for periods up to three months. (In contrast, donors can give whole blood only once every six to eight weeks). Platelet-pheresis enables a single adult donor—often another family member—to provide the major portion of the platelets required by the patient.

The use of platelet transfusions has reduced the occurrence of hemor-rhage during the last decade, making it possible to use effective anticancer drugs even though they depress platelet production.

However, patients may become resistant to platelets obtained from persons of different platelet types. When this occurs, the donated platelets are rapidly destroyed, and the patient is again in danger from hemorrhage. Fortunately, platelets can be typed according to a *histocompatibility sys-tem. (HL-A).* HL-A matched platelets often survive normally in patients who have become resistant to nonmatched platelets. HL-A typing can thus frequently identify a suitable donor. Platelets obtained from the patient himself (while he is in remission) can be frozen and reinfused into the patient during relapse. Such platelets are often effective when the patient is resistant to platelets from available donors.

The success achieved with platelet transfusion prompted scientists to attempt granulocyte (white cell) replacement for treatment of infection in leukemia patients. Granulocyte transfusions can be given with beneficial effects to some patients with bacterial infections, but it has been diffi-cult to obtain these cells in adequate amounts from normal blood dona-tions.

To increase the availability of granulocytes, a special centrifuge can be used to separate granulocytes from the other blood elements, which are then returned to the donor. It is now possible, using this continuous-flow centrifuge, to obtain as many granulocytes from one normal donor at one sitting as are contained in 30 to 40 units of blood collected by standard methods. A suitable donor can effectively support the granulocyte levels of otherwise granulocytopenic patients (patients with a deficiency of granulocytes in the blood) for several weeks.

Another approach to controlling infection in leukemia patients is the use of relatively germ-free environments plus decontamination proce-dures, to reduce the degree of contact with bacteria and thus the risk of infection. Germ-free laminar air-flow rooms have been developed by the National Cancer Institute and are under study at the Institute and at several other major cancer centers assisted by Institute funds. The occurrence of severe infection has been diminished significantly by the use of these isolation systems.

Also, newly developed antibiotics have been of value in the treatment of bacterial infections. A search is under way for antibiotics more effective against certain resistant bacteria, fungi, and viruses.

Rehabilitation and other services

You should continue to have medical examinations regularly so that your doctor can check your progress. Staff at your hospital and other community organizations are ready to give you many kinds of help.

The social service department of the hospital can advise you about many local organizations that offer help for cancer patients and their families. The American Cancer Society and other organizations provide services that may include financial aid, transportation to and from the hospital for medical care, person-to-person assistance through group meetings, as well as other services.

In addition, the Cancer Information Service is a toll-free telephone inquiry system which supplies information about cancer and cancer-related resources to cancer patients, their families, and health professionals. Cancer Information Service Offices are based in major cancer programs around the country. Addresses and phone numbers for the national offices of the American Cancer Society and for the Cancer Information Service are given at the end of this article.

Emotional aspects

You may feel many different emotional reactions from the time cancer is diagnosed. "Why me?" is a question every patient asks. This is a normal reaction to the diagnosis of cancer. You also may have periods of anxiety or depression. You may need to go through these feelings before you can accept the diagnosis and learn to live with it.

Talking with your doctor, other health professionals, your family, and even other cancer patients can give you emotional support during and after treatment. Because your doctor knows your condition, he is in the best position to answer questions about your individual case. Making a list of questions before you see the doctor can help you remember to ask him everything you want to know. You may be assured that your doctor and other health professionals will continue to offer you the best care that medicine has to offer.

You and your family may be able to handle the emotional strain of cancer better by discussing your problems openly with each other and with your doctor. But you may need help. You should feel free to ask for counseling if your problems become too difficult to handle.

Questions you may want to ask your doctor

You or your family may find it difficult to know how to ask your doctor some of the questions you may have about cancer. This is understandable. Cancer and its treatment are complex. Even your doctor may not always be able to give definite answers. But he or she will be happy to discuss your questions with you. Some typical questions might include these:

What kind of cancer do I have?

Is the tumor benign or malignant?

If it is benign, can it be cured?

If it is cancer, has it spread?

Can you predict how successful an operation or radiation treatment would be?

What are the risks?

Should I get an opinion from another doctor?

If an operation is done, will I need other treatment?

How helpful will this be in resuming normal activities afterward?

If I take anticancer drugs, what will the side-effects be?

How often will I need medical checkups?

What should I tell my relatives and friends?

Research

The National Cancer Institute, a bureau in the U.S. Department of Health and Human Services, is the Federal Government's principal agency for cancer research. The Institute supports research in many of the nation's universities, medical centers and laboratories, and conducts research in its own laboratories and clinics.

The National Cancer Institute has developed PDQ (Physician Data Query), a computerized database designed to give doctors quick and easy access to the latest treatment information for most types of cancer; descriptions of clinical trials that are open for patient entry; and names of organizations and physicians involved in cancer care. To access PDQ, a doctor may use an office computer with a telephone hookup and a PDQ access code or the services of a medical library with online searching capability. Most Cancer Information Service offices provide a physician with one free PDQ search and can tell doctors how to get regular access. Patients may ask their doctor to use PDQ or may call 1-800-4-CANCER themselves.

Research has shown that some types of leukemia in animals may be caused by a virus. However, scientists have not shown that human leukemia can be caused by a virus. Leukemia, like all forms of cancer, is not contagious. No one can catch cancer from another person. Cancer is not transmitted by coughing or sneezing, nor by sexual intercourse or any other kind of physical contact.

Although the cause of cancer remains unknown, new research findings may suggest ways of preventing it. At the same time, the trend toward improved diagnosis and treatment provides hope that more patients with this disease will be treated effectively.

GLOSSARY

Acute Lymphocytic Leukemia   A disorder of blood cell production in which abnormal white blood cells accumulate in the blood and bone marrow. (Also called acute lymphatic leukemia and acute lymphoblastic leukemia.)

Antibody   A substance, probably made by lymphocytes and certain other specialized cells, which helps defend the body against infections due to viruses, bacteria, and other foreign organisms.

Antigens   Chemical structures in a cell which can be recognized by a patient as foreign and thus stimulate immune reactions.

Biopsy   The removal and microscopic examination of tissue from the living body for purposes of diagnosis.

Blast Cells   An immature stage in cellular development before appearance of mature cells.

Blood Typing and Cross-matching   The blood cells contain factors which are not the same in all people. Before a transfusion can be given, blood samples from the donor and recipient are typed, or classified (type A, B, AB, or O). Once the two blood samples have been typed, they are cross-matched to be absolutely sure that they are compatible. This is done by placing red cells of the donor in a sample of the recipient's serum, and red cells of the recipient in a sample of the donor's serum. If the blood does not "clump," or agglutinate, the two bloods are compatible. Techniques for typing white blood cells and platelets are similar, but more complex.

Bone Marrow   The marrow is the spongy material which fills the cavities of the bones and is the substance in which many of the blood elements are produced. In order to determine the condition of the marrow, a doctor may take a small sample from one of the bones in the chest, hip, spine, or leg. Such examinations are performed with the help of local anesthesia and are not extremely painful.

Cancer   A general term for about 100 diseases characterized by abnormal and uncontrolled growth of cells. The resulting mass, or tumor, can invade and destroy surrounding normal tissues. Cancer cells can spread through the blood or lymph to start new cancers in other parts of the body.

Central Nervous System   The brain and spinal cord together form the body's central nervous system. The brain controls body functions by receiving and transmitting messages along a network of nerves that extend throughout the body. The messages reach the brain through the spinal cord.

Chemotherapy   Treatment with anticancer drugs.

Erythrocytes   Red blood cells. They use their main component, hemoglobin, to carry oxygen as it is breathed in through the lungs to all parts of the body.

Granulocytes   One type of white blood cell that destroys invading bacteria.

Granulocytopenic   A term indicating a deficiency of granulocytes in the blood.

HL-A   Human histocompatibility antigens. These antigens appear on white blood cells as well as cells of almost all other tissues and are analogous to red blood cell antigens (A, B, etc.). By typing for HL-A antigens, donors and recipients of white blood cells, platelets, and organs can be "matched" to insure good performance and survival of transfused and transplanted cells.

Hemorrhage   A general term for loss of blood brought about by injury to the blood vessels or by a deficiency of certain necessary blood elements such as platelets.

Leukocytes   White blood cells.

Liver   An organ in the body which performs many complex functions necessary for life. These include processes related to digestion, production of certain blood proteins, and elimination of many of the body's waste products.

Lymph Nodes   Bean-shaped structures scattered along vessels of the lymphatic system. The nodes can act as filters, collecting bacteria or cancer cells that may travel through the lymph system.

Lymphocytes   White blood cells.

Neutrophils   A type of white blood cell that plays a major role in the body's defense against bacteria, viruses, and fungi.

Platelet   One of the main components of the blood. Forms clots that seal up injured areas and prevent hemorrhage.

Plateletpheresis   A process in which platelets are removed from normal whole blood by centrifugation.

Radiation Therapy   Treatment using high-energy radiation from X-ray machines, radium, cobalt, or other sources.

Red Blood Cells   Cells that carry oxygen to all the various organs and tissues of the body.

Remission   The decrease or disappearance of a cancer and its symptoms. Also the period during which this occurs.

Spleen   Abdominal organ which performs a function similar to that of lymph nodes in that it acts as a filter. It frequently becomes enlarged in leukemia.

White Blood Cells   Leukocyte. The two types of white blood cells are called granulocytes and lymphocytes.

X-rays   High-energy radiation used in high doses to treat cancer or in low doses to diagnose the disease.

For additional information, call the toll-free telephone number of the Cancer Information Service at

1-800-4-CANCER*

*In Alaska, call 1-800-638-6070; in Hawaii, on Oahu call 524-1234 (neighbor islands call collect). Spanish-speaking staff members are available to callers from the following areas (daytime hours only): California, Florida, Georgia, Illinois, northern New Jersey, New York, and Texas.

American Cancer Society
90 Park Avenue
New York, NY 10016
212-736-3030

See your telephone book for local units.

Leukemia Society of America
733 Third Avenue
New York, NY 10017
212-573-8484

For further information

The following printed materials may be helpful to cancer patients, their families, and others. They are available free of charge from:

Office of Cancer Communications
National Cancer Institute
Building 31, Room 10A18
Bethesda, Maryland 20892

Chemotherapy and You
Eating Hints
Taking Time
Fact Sheet: Control of Cancer Pain
Questions and Answers About Pain Control (also available from the American Cancer Society)
Services Available to People with Cancer—National and Regional Organization
When Cancer Recurs: Meeting the Challenge Again
Radiation Therapy and You
Research Report: Leukemia

U.S. Department of Health and Human Services, Public Health Service, National Institutes of Health, National Cancer Institute. NIH Publication No. 87–1572, reprinted November 1986.

Lou Gehrig's Disease

A.L.S. 'Lou Gehrig's Disease' Still Needs A Cure

Etiology is a doctor's word for the cause—or causes—of a disease. Some of the most dreaded are of unknown etiology, because the less known about the cause of an illness, the less likely that there is a cure for it, or some way to prevent it or avoid getting it.

Amyotrophic lateral sclerosis is that kind of disease, a devastating, disabling, eventually fatal ailment affecting the motor nerve cells that control the muscles, and for which, so far, no cure has been found. Not only are we in the dark about why it strikes, but we don't know whom, where, and when it may strike.

What we do know is that ALS (as it's often called) generally affects the nerves leading from the brain to the spinal cord and from the spinal cord and brain stem to the muscles, resulting in a progressive weakening and wasting of those muscles that have lost their nerve supply, as well as taut muscles and exaggerated muscular reflexes.

The name of the disease comes from *A*—lack of, *Myo*—muscle,

Trophic—nourishment, *Sclerosis*—hardening of areas in the *Lateral*—side (as well as the forward) portions of the spinal cord.

In time these progressive ravages, in the most common form, cause near or complete helplessness. The patient becomes a prisoner of his or her own body. At the same time the five senses (touch, taste, sight, smell, hearing) remain intact and the intellect is commonly unimpaired. As a victim commented, "It's like being given a ringside seat at one's own dissolution."

Ordinarily ALS does not directly affect the bladder, bowel or sexual function. Some patients may have a noticeable lack of control over emotions. The patient, even though conscious of behaving oddly, may cry easily or laugh loudly in situations where others normally exert more control.

ALS is sometimes referred to as "Lou Gehrig's disease." It was this ailment that cut short the career and the life, in 1941 at age 35, of the great major league baseball slugger whose batting record and years of performance (2,130 consecutive games played) won him the nickname, "The Iron Man." Other celebrities who have fallen to the disease include former heavyweight champion prizefighter Ezzard Charles and actor David Niven. Another ALS victim was former Senator Jacob Javits of New York.

ALS is relatively uncommon. Although estimates vary as to the number of ALS cases diagnosed each year, the recorded deaths from this disease are a good indicator of occurrence because of its incurability. The National Center for Health Statistics reports that 2,305 persons died of ALS in this country in 1978 and 2,635 in 1979, a rate of slightly more than 1 per 100,000 of population. It's estimated that at any given time there are five to seven living victims of ALS per 100,000 people.

Most ALS victims are 40 to 70 years old, although some are very rarely as young as 20 or as old as 80. ALS claims about two times more men than women. Race or nationality does not matter in who gets ALS, although the highest incidence worldwide has been among natives of the Mariana Islands in the western Pacific. About 5 to 10 percent of the cases occur in families where there already has been a victim. There is no basis, however, for predicting that any person in such a family is likely to get ALS.

Impaired speaking, swallowing (and subsequent choking from saliva accumulation) and cough reflexes, difficulty in breathing, and progressive weakness all result from degeneration of the nerve cells, or motor neurons, from the spinal cord to the muscles—the so-called lower motor neurons. Spasticity, or stiffness of the muscles, results from degeneration of the nerve cells that travel from the brain to the spinal cord—the upper motor neurons. ALS symptoms are a consequence of this as yet unexplained destruction of these two neuron systems, and can eventually result in total paralysis. About 50 percent of patients die within three years, and only 10 percent survive beyond 10 years. Generally the disease seems to progress steadily at a rapid or slow rate, and sometimes it seems to reach a plateau or standstill for varying periods, according to the Amyotrophic Lateral Sclerosis Society of America. The society reports that for some patients there appears to be a remission when the disease reaches a plateau, and some report improvements in varying degrees. No cause has been found for such variations.

In a paper on current research, the society says that patients don't die directly from ALS but from such secondary complications as malnutrition or choking caused by inability to swallow, pneumonia, or others, often equally treatable. The society notes that various respiratory aids can be used to help a patient to breathe; nutrition can be maintained by the use of various devices, some requiring surgery, and the use of foods that are softer and more nutritious. There are drugs to treat or control excess salivation, spasticity, cramps, and other problems. The steady improvement in effective treatment of some symptoms and complications seems to be extending the period of patient survival, the society reports, although no treatment has been found to alter the natural progression of the disease.

Communication is a critical element in therapy for an ALS patient who has become unable to speak. Since the disease does not noticeably affect the eye muscles, communication devices that use codes based on eye movements have been developed for transmitting messages between patient and medical people or family. There are others, including small computers with artificial speech articulation, available for patients who can use their hands.

There are three major signals that can warn of the possible onset of ALS. In about a third of cases the hands become clumsy; the person may drop objects or have trouble doing tasks that require fine coordination or manipulation of the hands and fingers, such as sewing or working with tools. Another third experience weakness or cramps in the legs, or involuntary jerks of the limbs. The patient may stumble or trip because of a slight foot drop. A third main sign is slowed speech or difficulty in swallowing, symptoms indicating involvement of nerves that emanate from a part of the brain stem. Weakness in speech can include slurring, thick speech, a monotonous tone, hoarseness, or reduced volume. Other difficulties are encountered in swallowing, shifting food in the mouth, and controlling saliva.

A person may have ALS for a long time before symptoms are noted or pronounced enough to seek medical help. Some doctors believe the disease may exist without being diagnosed for up to 10 years. This may be because nerve cells that are still functioning take over much of the work of those lost as the disease progresses. A tendency to tire easily may be an early symptom. There may also be stiffness and spasticity or involuntary jerking of the limbs.

Although generally the disease begins with effects on muscles more distant from the brain and spine, as in the limbs, its progression eventually results in complete paralysis. The muscles that control eye movements are affected very late in the course of the disease, if at all.

A suspected ALS victim is usually examined by a neurologist, who may set up a series of tests, no single test normally being adequate to confirm the disease. An electromyogram (EMG), in which needles are inserted into muscles to record their electrical activity, may be ordered. Other diseases, which may mimic ALS and which are treatable, may be identified by various studies. There may be X-ray checks for spinal column troubles. Or a myelogram may be done—injection of a dye into the spinal fluid to look for treatable problems of the spine that may affect the nerves.

For the spunky patient who wants to fight, there are many ways medical staffs and family can help, the society says. In the past, patients died unnecessarily from respiratory complications, but today many of these can be alleviated with portable respirators that help the patient to breathe. Adequate nutrition is possible by feeding the patient soft food through a tube, either by mouth or a surgical opening. For patients with muscular atrophy, good nutrition is essential because it keeps the body from burning up as fuel whatever muscle tissue remains.

Much can be done to help the patient endure ALS. The patient should continue normal daily activities as long as possible, but avoid fatigue. It's quite often left up to the patient to decide how and when to use his or her strength. Simple exercises within the patient's capabilities can be done, with or without family assistance. Devices that enable a patient to continue daily activities include braces to prevent foot drop, hand splints and limb supports, wheelchairs, and lift devices.

Bedridden patients need skin care and massages, and should be shifted frequently to help prevent bedsores. Devices such as wheelchair cushions, sheepskins, and water mattresses also are helpful. A patient whose movements are limited will need help with bowel and bladder functions. The ALS Society recommends drinking 10 glasses of water or other liquids daily, to assure adequate urinary elimination, if the patient does not have too much difficulty swallowing this amount. Medicines or stool softeners should be used, upon the advice of a physician. Elastic support hose and elevation of the legs may be needed to prevent swelling and to prevent possible formation of blood clots.

Methods to control the normal production of saliva when problems arise from difficulty in swallowing include suction devices, drugs to thicken saliva, or surgery to reduce the flow. Some patients are able to use a handkerchief to control drooling. Besides blow bottles and respirators, simple deep breathing exercises are used to enable the patient to maintain maximum lung capacity. Doctors can advise family members how to help a patient cope with coughing difficulties. The patient should not be exposed to persons with respiratory tract infections such as colds and flu.

There are several motor neuron diseases. Some are variants of classical ALS; these include spinal muscular atrophy, progressive bulbar palsy, primary lateral sclerosis, and benign focal amyotrophy. There are also two genetically determined childhood motor neuron diseases: infantile spinal muscular atrophy (appearing while the child is in the womb or during the first few months after birth) and juvenile spinal muscular atrophy, appearing at the age of 5 to 15, sometimes with multiple cases in one family.

Research into possible causes of ALS has looked into viruses and various toxic, immunological and metabolic factors, including possible environmental factors that may be common to all patients. Dr. Myron I. Varon, vice president and scientific director of the ALS Society, says he believes five areas will be important in solving the mystery of ALS:

- the identification, if it exists, of a protein that is needed to maintain the integrity of the motor neuron, and without which the neuron will die and the muscle atrophy;
- the nerve transport mechanism;
- relationship between male hormones (androgens) and motor neurons in males;
- drastic reduction (in the motor neurons of ALS patients) of ribonucleic acid (RNA), which helps manufacture vital proteins in the cell; and
- metabolic studies at the neuromuscular junctions, where the nerve meets the muscle.

Dr. Varon feels that if ALS is caused by failure of the skeletal muscle to produce nerve growth hormone, it may be possible to supply this hormone to patients as insulin is supplied to diabetics. "What we are hoping for, of course," he says, "is the discovery of the insulin for ALS. ALS is not an active virus infection, an autoimmune disease, or a peculiar toxic reaction. I believe it is a metabolic abnormality. . . ."

Harold Hopkins, FDA Consumer, December 1983–January 1984

Lungs

The Lungs Take In The Good, Expel The Bad

Oxygen is essential to life; deprive the body of this vital element for three to five minutes and its cells will die.

Carbon dioxide, on the other hand, is not. Except for a very small amount needed to regulate respiration, this waste product of the cells must be eliminated from the body. The lungs have the dual task of bringing oxygen in and removing carbon dioxide from the body. This process is called "gas exchange."

The lungs occupy the chest cavity, a space shared only with the heart. Although they look large, the lungs weigh only about two pounds. Air entering the respiratory system through the mouth and nose travels to the lungs via what's called the tracheobronchial tree. The main trunk, represented by the trachea or windpipe, divides into two branches, one for each lung. From these branches or bronchi, progressively smaller tubes divide into thousands of still smaller tubes. These in turn subdivide into millions of bronchioles, the smallest tubes in the system. The bronchioles end in tiny air sacs called alveoli, which constitute the bulk of the lung tissue. The lungs of the average-sized adult contain about 300 million of these tiny air sacs.

Blood, which conveys both oxygen and carbon dioxide, enters the lungs via the pulmonary arteries. These arteries, like the bronchioles, divide and subdivide into smaller and smaller vessels, following the path of the tiny air tubes. Finally, the blood vessels open out in a network of capillaries enmeshed in the alveoli walls.

As the blood reaches the alveoli, the carbon dioxide it has picked up from the cells passes through the thin capillary and alveoli walls into the air sacs. At the same time, hemoglobin in the red blood cells picks up oxygen from the air sacs. The carbon dioxide is transported through the respiratory system to be exhaled, while the newly oxygenated blood returns to the heart for distribution throughout the body. Although the two gases pass through the same membranes, they do not interfere with each other.

Oxygen is not the only thing that gets into the lungs. The respiratory system also is a port of entry for all manner of pollutants that abound in the environment. Many harmful particles that are breathed in are removed by the body's own cleaning system. Some never make it past the twisting passages in the nose; others are trapped by mucus or by finger-like cells called cilia that line the windpipe. These cells sweep the mucus with a wave-like motion, carrying trapped particles upward to the mouth where they can be expelled. Many do make it all the way to the lungs, where they can cause a variety of lung problems.

Some of these problems are related to specific occupations. The most serious are the pneumoconioses, caused by dust inhalation. Asbestosis, for one, results from inhalation of asbestos fibers. Silicosis, a fibrosis of the lungs, is caused by breathing silica, or quartz dust. Black lung disease, officially called Coal Worker's Pneumoconiosis, occurs in people who work in both underground and surface coal mines. The popular name is appropriate, for the fine coal dust particles inhaled over the years accumulate in the lungs and darken them to the color of coal itself.

Other mineral dusts that present occupational hazards of a lesser degree include beryllium, which can cause berylliosis; iron dust, which can cause siderosis or welder's disease; tin dust, which produces stanosis; and barium, the cause of baritosis.

Organic materials are linked to a number of lung diseases, known collectively as hypersensitivity pneumonitis. One such disease is byssinosis, resulting from inhalation of cotton lint. Grain fever comes from grain dust and bagassosis from moldy sugar cane.

Organisms that grow in moldy hay can cause a hypersensitivity pneumonitis in farmers called "farmer's lung." These same organisms can grow in air conditioners and humidifiers, and even in sauna baths, where they live in the wooden water barrel.

Inhalation of noxious gases such as chlorine, phosgene, nitrogen dioxide, and sulfur dioxide may lead to acute bronchitis, an inflammation of the bronchi. This condition also may be caused by viral or bacterial infections. A variety of viruses and some bacteria, with the tongue-twisting names pneumococcus, staphylococcus, and klebsiella, are often the cause of pneumonia.

Tuberculosis is another lung disease that is bacterial in origin, resulting from infection by the tubercle bacillus. Once a leading cause of death, TB has been largely brought under control in technologically advanced countries, although it remains a health problem worldwide.

Cigarette smoke probably is the worst offender among the environmental pollutants. Cigarette smoking is the main cause of lung cancer in men, and males die of lung cancer more often than any other type of cancer. While women don't develop lung cancer at quite the same rate, they are beginning to catch up—a definite result of an increase in smoking among women. Cancers in other areas of the respiratory tract—larynx, esophagus, and oral cavity—are also associated with smoking.

Smoking is a primary cause of chronic bronchitis and emphysema, which together make up the disease category called chronic obstructive lung disease. The two closely related conditions are characterized by severe obstruction of the flow of air in and out of the lungs.

Chronic lung diseases have become increasingly important causes of disability and death in the United States. They are the direct or contributory cause of approximately 100,000 deaths a year and account for approximately 10 percent of Social Security disability benefits. Work lost because of chronic lung diseases is estimated to be as high as a quarter of a million person-hours per year.

In the case of emphysema, the ultra-thin walls of the alveoli lose their elasticity and tear. Groups of ruptured air sacs combine to form larger sacs. These trap stale air, keeping the lungs partially inflated all the time. As more air is inhaled and trapped, the lungs are less able to carry on the exchange of oxygen and carbon dioxide. This makes the body work harder to get enough oxygen.

Bronchitis is a swelling or inflammation of the linings of the bronchial airways with excessive mucus and other fluids that block the passageways, leading to a persistent cough and expectoration (spitting) of mucus. A person is considered to have chronic bronchitis if cough and sputum are present on most days for a minimum of three months for at least two successive years or for six months during one year. Prolonged exposure to air pollution and recurrent respiratory infections, as well as cigarette smoking, are underlying causes of chronic bronchitis.

While the chronic obstructive lung diseases occur most often among older people, people of any age can have asthma, a condition marked by repeated attacks of wheezing and shortness of breath. About half of the people with asthma develop the disease before the age of 10 and another third develop it before they reach 30.

In an asthma attack the air passages, especially the bronchi, go into spasm, obstructing the flow of air. There are two types of asthma. ''Intrinsic'' asthma is triggered by respiratory infections, inhalation of fumes and cigarette smoke, dust, cold air, exercise, and sometimes the ingestion of aspirin. ''Extrinsic'' asthma is triggered by pollens, animal danders, dust, and molds.

Asthma attacks can last from a few minutes to several days. Some people may not have any symptoms between attacks, while others may have mild wheezing for long periods. In some cases the asthma is mild and does not progress; in others the condition may get much worse and be accompanied by more severe symptoms such as difficulty in breathing, cough, rapid heart beat, apprehension, chest distention, and tenacious sputum.

Coughing, wheezing, and excess mucus all can accompany a minor illness such as the common cold. Running up a flight of stairs can make a person short of breath. However, if respiratory symptoms persist and shortness of breath occurs during normal everyday activities, it could be a sign of a serious lung disease. Anyone who has such symptoms should see a doctor and have a thorough examination.

Such an examination probably would include taking a medical history, to find out what pollutants the patient's lungs may have been exposed to and whether there is a family history of respiratory diseases such as tuberculosis.

By listening to the patient's chest through a stethoscope, the doctor can hear what's going on in the lungs. For instance, coarse rumbling and wheezing chest sounds are a clue that the patient has bronchitis. A chest X-ray also can help the doctor pinpoint some lung problems.

Pulmonary function tests can indicate how efficiently the lungs are working. In one such test the patient breathes into a machine called a spirometer, and the rate of inhalation and exhalation is recorded. Another test measures the amount of oxygen and carbon dioxide in the blood during exercise. Unfortunately, these tests do not detect serious lung disease before the lungs have been damaged irreversibly. They only tell the doctor how bad the damage is.

Bronchoscopy is another technique for examining the lungs. A flexible tube is guided through the patient's nose into the tracheobronchial tree. Tiny glass fibers carry light through the tube, enabling the doctor to see the inside of the breathing structure. The bronchoscope also can be used to obtain samples of lung fluid and cells.

Once an accurate diagnosis has been made, appropriate treatment can be started. A variety of antibiotics are available to combat viral and bacterial infections; and drugs, such as amphotericin B, miconazole, and ketaconazole, are effective against some fungal diseases that affect the lungs.

Treatment for the pneumoconioses is difficult, for once the lungs have been damaged they cannot be repaired. Efforts can be made to see that the condition doesn't get worse by relieving shortness of breath and coughing. Complicating infections, such as tuberculosis, can be treated with such drugs as streptomycin, para-aminosalicylic acid, isoniazid, and rifampin.

The chronic obstructive lung diseases cannot be cured, but symptoms can be treated with drugs called bronchodilators, which act by relaxing contractions of the smooth muscle of the bronchioles. Bronchodilators include isoproterenol, metaproterenol, terbutaline, epinephrine and ephedrine. They can be injected subcutaneously or intravenously, taken orally, or inhaled as aerosol sprays. Another bronchodilator is theophylline, which can be given intravenously, orally or rectally. Antibiotics are frequently given at the first sign of a respiratory infection. Corticosteroids may be used if wheezing can't be controlled with bronchodilators.

Bronchodilators also are used in the treatment of asthma. A number of these drugs are available without prescription, including epinephrine and ephedrine. FDA recently recommended that metaproterenol be switched from prescription to nonprescription status. On the other hand, the agency also recommended that theophylline as a single ingredient not be allowed in nonprescription asthma drug products. Nonprescription bronchodilators should not be used unless a diagnosis of asthma has been made by a doctor.

The drug cromolyn can prevent the symptoms of asthma, but since it does not act like the bronchodilators and has no anti-inflammatory effects, it is not useful once an asthma attack has started.

Obviously, it is not always possible to avoid environmental pollution. Not too many people have the luxury of being able to pick and choose where they will live and work. But there is one thing that can be done to prevent many serious lung problems—if you don't smoke, don't start; and if you do, give up the habit.

Annabel Hecht, FDA Consumer, March 1983.

Motion Sickness

When Motion Sickness Goes Along for The Ride

If diseases were classified by how they affect the people who *don't* get them, motion sickness would fall into the same category as hemorrhoids and halitosis: They all strike the unafflicted right in the funny bone. A joke about an air traveler's queasy stomach and "little brown bag" brings an unsympathetic chortle just as surely as a wisecrack about "old buzzard breath" or some poor soul's inflated hemorrhoid cushion.

There's also an air of superiority on the part of many nonsufferers, who feel they are somehow of stouter stock than those who succumb to such embarrassing annoyances. This seems to be especially true for motion sickness. Mark Twain once observed that, "If there is one thing that will make a man peculiarly and insufferably self-conceited, it is to have his stomach behave itself the first day at sea, when nearly all his comrades are seasick."

Not much can cheer up someone on a trip whose stomach is reacting so miserably that he wishes he had left home without it. But if misery does love company, the distraught traveler can take some solace in knowing that no one, no matter how strong their intestinal fortitude, is immune to motion sickness. Surveys have found that about nine out of 10 people have experienced the disorder. And experts agree that, given a strong enough stimulus, everyone with a normal sense of balance will succumb. In fact, Dr. K. E. Money, a Canadian authority on motion sickness, has said that the disorder is so pervasive that it "might be described better as 'the *normal* vomiting response to motion.' "

Some people are susceptible only to certain types of motion or only under special circumstances. Individuals may feel no queasiness at all riding in a car or plane, but fall victim to seasickness because of the ship's combined motions of pitching from front to back and rolling from side to side. In fact, sea travel is considered the strongest natural stimulus for motion sickness. Few seafarers green about the gills, leaning over the ship's rail waiting for the worst, would be surprised to learn that the words "nausea" and "nautical" both have the same Greek root (*naus,* meaning "ship").

Even fish can get seasick. In one study, codfish lost their lunch when they were placed in a tank on a boat and transported over rough water an hour after being fed. And many a family vacationing by car can confirm the finding that dogs are as susceptible to motion sickness as humans.

Among humans, infants rarely get motion-sick. The greatest susceptibility is between the ages of 2 and 12. After that, it gradually decreases through adulthood and is reportedly uncommon after age 50.

Some researchers have claimed that women are more prone than men to motion sickness. But others doubt that conclusion, noting that, where carsickness is concerned, men traditionally have done most of the driving, leaving women in the passenger seat, where the susceptibility to sickness is greater.

Fear, anxiety, and other psychological factors can contribute to the onset of motion sickness. (This is why the drowsiness brought on by some motion sickness medications is not always considered a bad side effect. Unless, of course, the patient is the pilot.) Some people with a history of motion sickness can get sick just thinking about a coming trip or even at the mere sight of the ship or other conveyance they'll be taking.

You don't have to travel far to become motion-sick. Sometimes a trip to the local movie theater is enough, particularly if the picture has a "chase scene" filmed from the viewpoint of the chase car. And carnival rides can leave many fun-seekers with a taste in their mouths far less pleasant than that of the cotton candy or popcorn down on the midway.

Even those who travel by such four-legged conveyances as elephants and camels have become motion-sick, including Lawrence of Arabia. Lawrence may have done better on an Arabian stallion, since horses are not known to bring out the worst in their riders.

American and Soviet space travelers have fallen victim to a special zero-gravity form of motion sickness that the National Aeronautics and Space Administration has dubbed "Space Adaptation Syndrome." The syndrome was first reported among astronauts on the Apollo 8 moon voyage in 1968. Apparently the crews of earlier space flights were not afflicted because they were generally restricted to their seats in the small capsules. But in the roomier digs of Skylab and the space shuttles, where the astronauts can float weightlessly about the cabin as their spacecraft hurtles around the earth, about half of the crew members have reported nausea or vomiting. NASA is sponsoring much research to learn more about the causes and possible cures for Space Adaptation Syndrome, as it not only can bring misery to the affected crew but can also interfere with their performance. As ex-astronaut Russell Schweickart put it, getting spacesick simply "wasn't the right stuff."

While the symptoms of Space Adaptation Syndrome differ slightly from those experienced by earthbound travelers, motion sickness is by and large the same whether it comes on in a Chevy, a skiff, or a 747. Generally, the first symptom is unusual paleness of the skin. This may be followed by yawning, restlessness, and a cold sweat. As the symptoms progress, malaise and drowsiness may set in, sometimes accompanied by a slightly upset stomach, or "gastric awareness" as the experts euphemistically call it. By this time the victim usually realizes what's up and what's likely to follow: excessive salivation, nausea, and vomiting. The symptoms may progress rapidly in highly susceptible individuals. Those more resistant may experience a waxing and waning of symptoms and perhaps never actually vomit. But vomiting sometimes brings relief, if only for a time.

While motion sickness can ruin one's pride, one's suit, or an entire vacation, it seldom causes severe health complications. In extreme cases, though, prolonged vomiting can bring about severe headache, prostration, dehydration, and disturbed mineral balance in the body. Motion sickness is not a fatal disease, but that is not always taken as good news by those sufferers who'd pay any price for relief.

The reasons for the body's unpleasant reaction to movement other than by its own two feet are not fully known. Whatever the reason, the process by which motion sickness occurs in the body centers around the inner ear. (It is known that individuals whose inner ear apparatus is not functioning, such as deaf persons, are immune to motion sickness.) The inner ear is an organ not only of sound but also of balance. It contains three fluid-filled, hollow tubes called the semicircular canals. The canals work like a gyroscope. The shifting of the fluid as the body moves sends signals to the brain to let us know (even with our eyes closed) the direction our bodies are moving—forward or backward, up or down, or sideways. The inner ear also contains a number of calcium crystals called otoliths that are sensitive to the pull of gravity. Signals from the otoliths to the brain tell whether the head is erect, tilted, or upside down.

In some instances, motion sickness can be brought on simply by overstimulation of the inner ear. But more commonly, the sense of sight is involved in the process, too. According to one widely accepted theory, riding in a vehicle can cause a "mismatch" between the signals from the inner ear about the position of the body and the signals from the eyes. The "mismatch" affects the brain's chemoreceptor trigger zone, which sends a command to a part of the medulla oblongata ominously known as the vomiting center. It doesn't take a medical degree to guess what happens next.

Consider, for example, one of the most common situations in which motion sickness occurs—someone reading while riding in the back seat of a car. The semicircular canals of the inner ear register the movement of the car. But the eyes are fixed on the book or newspaper that is not moving in relation to the reader. Sensory conflict occurs and the sickness-inducing signals work their way from the vomiting center to the stomach, mouth, and other organs.

Prevention is easier than treating motion sickness once it has begun. While the best method of prevention is to limit one's travel to that which can be done by foot or by *National Geographic*, a number of precautions can provide some help:

- Place yourself where there is the least motion. In a car, sit in the front seat, looking ahead. In an airplane, choose a seat over the wing. On a ship, remain amidship (preferably on deck), rather than below.
- Lie on your back, in a semi-reclined position, and keep your head as still as possible.
- Look ahead, at the distant horizon. If that's not possible, it may be better to close your eyes rather than focus on fast-moving scenery or waves. Children especially can be helped by having them sit in the front seat of a car, in an elevated safety seat if appropriate. This enables them to see through the front windshield rather than looking at the inside of the car.
- Focus attention on something other than the motion of the vehicle. Even though reading is not recommended, occupying children with coloring books, for example, may be better than having them looking out the side window of a car or doing nothing.

- Although the length of time since eating has not been found to affect susceptibility to motion sickness, overindulging in food or drink, especially the night before a trip, can predispose an individual to nausea and promote the onset of other motion-sickness symptoms.
- Tobacco smoke and other odors, particularly from food, should be avoided, since they can push a traveler's queasy stomach over the brink. (Old salts in the Navy have been known to initiate new recruits who haven't found their sea legs yet by standing nearby on deck, chewing on a juicy piece of bacon, and letting the aroma of pork fat finish what the roll of the ocean had begun.)

Research done by NASA and others has found that the practice of biofeedback can lower susceptibility to motion sickness. By learning to control the early warning signs of impending sickness, such as faster breathing, heartbeat, and rate of perspiration, about two out of three research subjects were able to ward off the nausea and vomiting that normally affected them.

But for those not skilled in the practice of biofeedback and for whom reclining in a deck chair while gazing at the horizon is little help, medications are available. There are currently three nonprescription drugs for preventing or treating the nausea and vomiting of motion sickness. They are cyclizine hydrochloride (trade name Marezine), meclizine hydrochloride (Bonine), and dimenhydrinate (Dramamine). All three have been found to be safe and effective by the Food and Drug Administration for this use. The three are antihistamines, believed to work by blocking signals from the inner ear to the notorious vomiting center. Protection is best when the drugs are taken 30 minutes to an hour before traveling. If the drugs are taken only when the traveler begins to feel sick, it's usually too late to stop the progress of nausea and vomiting.

These drugs can cause drowsiness, so users are cautioned not to drive, operate machinery, or drink alcoholic beverages while taking them (because alcohol may add to the drug's depressant effects). None of these drugs should be taken by persons with asthma, glaucoma, or enlargement of the prostate, except with the advice and supervision of a physician. Children under 2 should not take dimenhydrinate, those under 6 should not take cyclizine, and those under 12 should not take meclizine without a doctor's OK.

A number of prescription anti-nausea and anti-vomiting drugs also are available to help ward off motion sickness. The most popular is scopolamine, which, like the nonprescription antihistamines, blocks nerve signals between the inner ear and the brain.

Scopolamine can produce a number of side effects, including drowsiness, dryness of the mouth, blurred vision, a sensitivity to light, and heart irregularities. To combat the drowsiness, NASA has given its space-

sick-prone astronauts the stimulant dextroamphetamine along with scopolamine, a combination the space agency calls ScopeDex. For earthbound
travelers, FDA approved in 1981 a novel form of scopolamine that reportedly reduces some of the drug's side effects because it is taken not in
pill form but through the skin, releasing the medication at a slower,
more constant rate. The product, Transderm-Scōp, was the first transder-
mal (through the skin) drug approved by FDA. It is a thumbnail-size
disk made up of an outer layer of polyester film, a reservoir to hold
the scopolamine, a membrane that controls release of the drug, and an
adhesive layer to hold the disk in place behind the ear. The disk provides
enough scopolamine for three days. It should be applied two to three
hours before traveling.

Even though the disk reduces some of scopolamine's side effects,
dry mouth, drowsiness and blurred vision may still occur, so users should
avoid driving or operating machinery. Because the very young and the
very old are particularly susceptible to scopolamine's side effects, Transderm-Scōp should not be used in children and should be used with
special caution by the elderly.

Another prescription anti-motion-sickness drug that warrants a special
warning to users is the antihistamine buclizine. This drug contains the
coloring FD&C Yellow No. 5 (tartrazine), which can cause allergic-
type reactions in susceptible individuals. Physicians should use extra
caution in prescribing buclizine to those who may be sensitive to the
coloring, such as asthma sufferers and those who have reactions to aspirin.

Some travelers have found ginger effective in preventing motion sickness. A report in 1982 in the British medical journal *Lancet* claimed
that research subjects who took two capsules containing powdered ginger
root were spared the ravages of motion sickness better than those who
took dimenhydrinate.

Once the stomach starts to churn, there's little to offer the suffering
traveler other than sympathy and, perhaps, fresh air. Since the effectiveness of motion-sickness pills would be lost along with the rest of the
stomach's contents in someone already in the throes of vomiting, certain
prescription drugs can be given by injection or suppository to try to
stem the symptoms.

Those who, despite their best efforts, continue vomiting several times
a day for more than two or three days should see a physician. Food
poisoning (always a possibility when traveling) or some other serious
disorder may be the real culprit.

As the nauseated globe-trotter tries to keep his spirits up and his
lunch down, he can cling to the hope that most sufferers do adapt to
the sickness-inducing motion. Usually after a couple of days, the nausea,
vomiting, and other embarrassing and distressful symptoms will disap-

pear. But though he may find relief, it's doubtful that the ex-motion-sickness-sufferer will ever again find the condition as amusing as, say, someone else's hemorrhoids.

Bill Rados, *FDA Consumer*, March 1985.

Multiple Sclerosis

Former Notre Dame football coach Ara Parseghian summed it up: "I spend my life working with beautiful young adults, the kids who play for me, but there are hundreds of thousands of other beautiful young adults in this country who are struck down in the prime of life by multiple sclerosis. They need our help." Ara Parseghian knows: his sister and daughter have multiple sclerosis (MS).

These men and women, and others like them throughout the world, have one of the more common disorders affecting the brain and spinal cord, which together comprise the central nervous system.

Yet, considerable confusion exists about multiple sclerosis. As one young woman with MS wrote, "Most people, I now realize, don't know what multiple sclerosis is—they often confuse it with muscular dystrophy. Ignorance of the disease, I had learned, compounds the patient's problem." (The muscular dystrophies are a major group of neuromuscular disorders which are distinctly different from MS, and occur primarily in children.)

However, there is no reason for people to remain uninformed. Knowledge of MS gained during the past two decades of research has expanded at a rate greater than occurred during the entire 100 years following the initial description of the disorder by the great French neurologist, Charcot. A better understanding of what we do know often can aid those with MS in learning to cope and live with it; and it can provide families and friends with important insights about ways to help and the value of their support.

But we do not stop here. Researchers throughout the world are committed to finding the cause of MS and to developing effective methods of treatment and prevention. In this country these efforts are spearheaded by the National Institute of Neurological and Communicative Disorders and Stroke (NINCDS), and the National Multiple Sclerosis Society which was a major force behind establishing the Institute. This research will continue until the answers are found.

The MS population

Most of the estimated 250,000 young American men and women diagnosed with MS are between the ages of 20 and 40. Usually their families have had little or no known familiarity with MS. Thus they are struck at the prime of life by an unexpected disorder and frequently have no prior knowledge or experience to guide them.

At the time of diagnosis, patients learn that since MS affects the central nervous system, both the sensory and motor (muscle) functions of the body may be impaired and that the symptoms may vary unpredictably, and last for differing amounts of time. Initially, symptoms usually will come and go (termed a ''relapsing'' course). Most often patients will find that symptoms improve after an attack; only rarely will symptoms initially get progressively worse.

Most patients also learn that MS is not a killer. In fact, the majority of persons with MS can expect to live their normal life span. Recent studies have indicated that at least half of those persons with MS can still engage in a majority of the activities they performed before developing MS, as long as 15 to 20 years after onset of the disorder. These MS patients have a relapsing course and some—who have mild or infrequent symptoms—may never know they have MS. In the remaining half of MS patients, the degree of severity varies. Some persons with chronic MS have a slowly progressive course, while a small percent develop a more rapid, severely incapacitating form. This variability and unpredictability stems from the very nature of the disorder.

The Nature of MS

The brain and spinal cord, where MS occurs, send out and receive signals from all parts of the body. Therefore, symptoms of MS can be experienced anywhere in the body, depending upon the specific site or sites in the brain or spinal cord which are affected.

Nerves, following orders from the brain, control functions within the human body. This mammoth task seems all the more impressive when you realize that each nerve is composed of individual cells, called ''neurons.'' Each nerve cell communicates with its neighbor by passing along the brain's messages, called impulses. Just as a chain's strength depends on its weakest link, a nerve is only as strong as its weakest cell in controlling the body's activities.

Nerve cells in the central nervous system (CNS)—which includes the brain and spinal cord—send out long fibers called axons. For example, nerve cells in the brain which control leg movement have axons which extend to the lower part of the spine. Many are normally surrounded by a fatty covering which insulates them, and speeds up the passage of messages along the nerve fibers. MS is a disease of this covering which is called "myelin." The disease process causes destruction of patches of myelin (demyelination) in an erratic and seemingly random fashion. Thus messages which ordinarily travel at 225 miles per hour are slowed to a fraction of that figure. Although we do not yet know whether destroyed myelin actually repairs itself in the human brain and spinal cord, there is some indication that initially myelin may be partially restored at these "demyelinated" areas which begin to dot the central nervous system. Messages may still get through, but they are slower and weaker. The nervous system can sustain a certain amount of demyelination. But eventually, at "multiple" sites throughout the brain and spinal cord—in the process for which multiple sclerosis was named—scar or "sclerosed" tissue forms in place of myelin. At these "multiple" sites impulses then are blocked or greatly slowed down and the message is lost. This causes the symptoms of MS.

Usually MS symptoms occur and disappear (or lessen) in varying and unpredictable episodes. The pattern can take many forms. Symptoms may occur only once and not return; or they may recur sporadically. In this case, symptom severity either will stay the same or become progressively worse. Finally, a small number of persons with MS experience symptoms which can become progressively more severe. Exacerbations (the occurrence and sometimes worsening of symptoms) are considered by many doctors to be a sign of demyelination, while remissions (periods of cessation or lessening of symptoms) are thought by some doctors to signify myelin repair, although this remains to be proved. Symptom type and severity are determined by the extent and location of myelin damage; by the type of function ordinarily performed by the nerve; and by whether that function is specific or general.

During periods of remission, symptoms will either lessen or disappear completely. Although scientists do not yet know what determines the extent of symptom improvement during remission, some have suggested that—if myelin repair indeed does occur—the extent of repair might influence the degree of symptom improvement. Because the course of MS is so dependent upon the course of demyelination—which varies with every person with MS—no two persons will have the identical experience. In fact, experiences can, and often do, differ completely.

MS symptoms

One of the most common initial manifestations of MS is optic neuritis, a fleeting disorder of the optic nerve which is involved in vision. Optic neuritis often produces "blind spots" in the center of vision and can cause blurriness or transient blindness. It also can affect color vision of one eye. These disturbances usually do not last for long periods of time, but they may recur in the same eye or affect the other eye. Very rarely are they permanent. The course of optic neuritis usually is benign, and vision returns to normal although some disturbances in color vision may remain. About half of the persons with optic neuritis never develop MS. But since the other half do eventually develop other MS symptoms, optic neuritis is strongly suspected to be related to—or actually a partial form of—MS. Occasionally after optic neuritis, blurred vision may occur following exercise or hot baths. Other visual disturbances such as double vision or the sensation of objects moving or shaking may occur.

Because nerves can be damaged anywhere in the body, any of a number of MS symptoms may occur. However, RARELY will any patient experience all or a majority of these. Moreover, many of these symptoms can be minimized by supportive treatment. In addition to the visual disturbances mentioned above, other possible sensory symptoms include dizziness and RARELY deafness. Occasionally sensory symptoms may be manifested as pain. Muscle symptoms may include impaired coordination, weakness, intention tremor (mild shaking when performing a muscular task), and spasticity (muscle rigidity), especially at night. Numbness or feelings of "pins and needles" may occur, but this rarely creates discomfort. Other symptoms may include: bladder problems (frequency or urgency of urination or incontinence), bowel difficulty (constipation), and sexual impotence (of either physical or psychological origin).

Depression also may be encountered in MS. Initially, a period of depression may set in after diagnosis, but this usually gives way to acceptance of the condition. In fact, some patients actually live with a degree of disease-produced euphoria. Nonetheless, some patients may experience depression while adjusting to the disease, or may actually consider it part of the disease process.

On the positive side, patients are spared any mental disability, except in rare instances. They remain as bright, alert and capable as they were before onset of MS. Patients sometimes worry that their memory is worsening, but this usually is a reflection of the normal aging process or a symptom of depression rather than loss of any mental ability. These symptoms, suggesting a diagnosis of MS, can be produced by a number of other disorders as well, not all of which involve demyelination. In fact approximately 250,000 Americans have other disorders which are closely related to MS. Thus patients experiencing symptoms similar to those which have been described should seek medical attention and advice to determine their cause.

MS diagnosis can be difficult to make

Patients with MS-like symptoms may be referred to a neurologist, a specialist in brain, spinal cord and muscle disorders, who is skilled in looking for clinical evidence of involvement of parts of the central nervous system. For only when various parts of the central nervous system become involved, producing symptoms in different parts of the body, can a clinical diagnosis of MS begin to be developed.

Currently a number of tests aid the diagnosis of MS, but none as yet yields an absolute answer. Diagnosis is based on the clinical determination that myelin damage has occurred in different parts of the central nervous system at different times. For when demyelination occurs in only one area of the central nervous system, doctors cannot rule out the possibility that some disorder other than MS may be responsible. This problem frequently is frustrating for physicians and patients alike. For example, when a patient has had only one episode, or a symptom occurring in only one part of the body, the most likely diagnosis may be MS. However, the physician cannot be sure, and must wait for additional signs to appear before making a positive diagnosis. Although realizing that obtaining a diagnosis is a source of great concern to the patient—anxious to pinpoint the cause of his or her difficulties—the physician in good conscience does not want to render a premature judgment.

Some laboratory tests may be useful diagnostic aids, particularly those involving removal of a sample of fluid which bathes the spinal cord. A spinal tap for removal of this fluid is a benign procedure which causes only minimal pain and NO further MS damage. Spinal fluid samples are used primarily to measure levels of certain proteins and white cells (used by the body to ward off infection). Of particular interest is immunoglobulin G (IgG), a protein fraction which is elevated in approximately 75 percent of patients with MS. However, elevated IgG is not specific for MS, and not everyone with higher than normal levels has MS; moreover, 22 percent of MS patients do not have elevated levels of IgG. Another diagnostic tool examines visual evoked potentials. This painless test measures the time it takes for an electrical impulse to travel from the eye to the brain. An electrode placed on the skin at the back of the head records signals as the patient watches an alternating white and black checkerboard. This test can detect trouble in the optic nerves even when vision seems entirely normal.

Other similar experimental diagnostic procedures called auditory (hearing) and sensory (touch) evoked potentials are aimed at providing evidence of multiple areas of demyelination.

But despite these procedures, MS remains difficult to diagnose. When evidence of trouble in only one part of the central nervous system can be found, it is often necessary to do special X-ray tests to rule out other causes, particularly tumors. Thus patients may be asked to participate in sophisticated X-ray tests using a CAT (computerized axial tomography) scan, or tests called myelograms or angiograms to be sure there are no other treatable causes of the symptoms.

The impact of diagnosis often is twofold. As expressed by one woman who was told she had MS, ''I felt completely alone. Why was this happening to me?'' But then, she wrote, ''It's oh so much better to know. Then you know how to cope with it and what you can and can't do.''

Once a diagnosis of MS can be established reliably, it often comes as a relief to the person with MS who has been struggling to find an explanation for the unpredictable and baffling appearance and disappearance of symptoms. For once the MS diagnosis is made, the work of understanding its nature and of learning how to accept and deal with it can begin in earnest.

Unpredictable course

The immediate question following diagnosis is how will it affect my life? How mild or serious will it be? And will it limit activity, and if so, by how much? Currently, there is no foolproof method for making a long-range prediction. Some doctors feel that the MS pattern established during the first three to five years may be indicative of the long-range course. For instance, the disorder may cause fewer problems in the future if initial symptoms occur in the sensory rather than in the motor system. Thus, if initial exacerbations are sporadic, occur infrequently and not too closely together, and leave little remaining impairment, there is good reason to expect that the overall course may follow this trend.

Treatment

The nature of MS renders treatment difficult to evaluate. For since remissions and exacerbations occur sporadically and unpredictably, it is difficult to prove that the experimental treatment—and not a naturally occurring remission—is responsible for improvement. Nonetheless, active research is pursuing means for developing effective methods for controlling MS.

To date no treatments have proven effective in stopping MS, although many have been suggested over the years. Suggestions have included diets, certain drugs, electrical (dorsal spinal column) stimulation, substances which suppress the immune (defense) system responses (immunosuppressants), and substances which stimulate the immune response. While many of these still are under investigation, including transfer factor (using donor immune white cells), none yet has been shown to alter the course of MS. And unless, or until, compelling evidence is discovered indicating that these proposed treatments are indeed helpful in MS, the reaction produced in many patients often is similar to that expressed by one woman with the disorder who wrote: "Other persons, well-meaning, but ill-informed, often plague patients with miraculous 'cures' of which they have read or heard. Inevitably, these tales produce guilt (I should be doing something more to help myself than I am already doing.) and frustration (the 'cures' by an odd coincidence, nearly always are hundreds, if not thousands of dollars and miles away)."

Now, exciting new research techniques (discussed later) which may permit objective assessment of a treatment's efficacy may partially alleviate that problem.

Until effective treatment is found, however, many MS symptoms *can* be helped. Doctors agree that maintaining good general health, following a balanced diet, avoiding excessive overweight or underweight, getting sufficient rest and relaxation, and appropriate daily exercise can help the person with MS feel better. During periods of exacerbation of symptoms, doctors may advise bed rest.

In addition, specific measures benefit several symptoms in many MS patients. (Since each person with MS is unique, the patient's doctor is in the best advisory position concerning use of these measures.) For instance, many patients with incontinence problems often benefit from drug treatment of urinary infections and from regulating the amount of fluids they consume during each day; moreover, urinary frequency and urgency often can be controlled with drugs, such as propantheline bromide and amitriptyline, which relax the bladder. In selected instances a bladder operation may be helpful. Many patients with muscle stiffness may be aided by physical therapy, as well as by moderate exercise. This keeps limbs supple, and although it cannot replace lost muscle strength, it can help the functioning of remaining muscular abilities. Electrical stimulation of the spinal cord to aid some muscle and bladder functions is being tried experimentally in a few centers. In addition, some patients have reported short-term benefit from steroids such as ACTH. This has been most useful in treating sudden worsening of symptoms.

Constipation can be helped by laxatives or bran. Spasticity or cramps often can be aided by muscle relaxants (such as diazepam, baclofen, and dantrolene sodium). However, spasticity can be helpful in some instances in compensating for lost muscle strength. Depression often can be helped by psychotherapy, antidepressant drugs, discussions with health professionals (including—in addition to the physician—nurses, social workers, occupational therapists, and psychologists). Often the patient's spouse and family members can be an invaluable resource of support and help.

Professional counseling can be a major help to both the patient and family in alleviating emotional concerns which actually may contribute to or result from the physical situation. Counseling referrals often are offered by the local chapters of the National MS Society. Sometimes referrals can be obtained from state or local health departments.

The patient's own physician is in the best position to offer advice on treatment for relief of symptoms and to coordinate management of the patient's problems. As medical research produces effective new methods of diagnosis or treatment, every effort will be made to see that the general medical community and the public are immediately informed. If questions arise concerning possible new methods of diagnosis or treatment or other MS research results, patients may wish, in addition to consulting their own physician, to contact either the NINCDS, the National Multiple Sclerosis Society, 205 East 42nd Street, New York, N.Y. 10017, or the Regional Health Administrator in one of the Department of Health and Human Services' 10 Regional Offices (see last page for a listing of these offices).

Furthermore, while demyelination is considered to be the primary cause of exacerbations, several factors which may accentuate MS symptoms can be effectively controlled. Among those considered to have a direct influence on symptoms are: heat, stress, emotional upset, anxiety, and fatigue. Of course, tolerance to these factors varies greatly among patients. But when these conditions worsen, symptoms, often their removal will lessen the symptoms' severity. Fevers and infections also can worsen symptoms.

Additional factors whose possible effects on MS symptoms are less well established include serious injury and mild physical trauma.

During pregnancy, patients may tend to have fewer MS attacks. However, following delivery, patients may experience an increase in attacks. Patients planning families should fully discuss the matter with their partner and should understand that physical limitations could attend raising children. Except in very severe instances, there are no contraindications to pregnancy, and no significant risk to the fetus. Moreover, MS is NOT a directly inherited disease, though there is a small percentage of familial incidence. These probably are due to similarities in environment and to inherited immune system characteristics. Consultation with the patient's physician regarding pregnancy can be particularly helpful in providing guidance and perhaps in allaying possible undue concern.

Many consider motivation to be the key in living with MS. One man with MS wrote, "Platitudes and encouraging words do little good for the MS patient until that patient has motivated himself.'' But family and friends can play an important part in encouraging self-motivation and determination to get on with life. In addition, sensitivity by family and friends to the needs and concerns of those with MS often can do much to enhance the quality of life. Professional counseling often can provide valuable guidance in this regard. As one woman with MS expressed, ''I want understanding or help friends can give in any way. But I don't want pity. I've always been a person that has done for herself.''

Research seeks the answers

MS research is devoted to finding the elusive cause of this disorder so that effective means of prevention can be developed and to finding improved methods of diagnosis and treatment.

The NINCDS conducts a vigorous MS research effort at its Bethesda, Maryland laboratories, and supports intensive MS studies at major medical centers throughout the country. In addition, the Institute also supports several clinical research centers involving participation by a limited number of patients in studies seeking the cause of MS. A list of these centers can be obtained from the NINCDS.

These efforts are joined by those of the National MS Society, and its more than 160 local chapters and branches which help to support more than 70 clinics, clinical programs and MS centers. The National MS Society has waged a tireless effort to support research and to maintain a valuable link between the scientists working on the problem and patients and their families, providing information on MS and on services available throughout the country.

Through the joint efforts of researchers, clinicians, patients, and their families—with government, voluntary, and private agencies—the reality of finding the answers to MS comes a bit closer every day.

In a disease of unknown cause, various scientific approaches are being pursued, some of which are diametrically opposed. For example, potential avenues of research include the possible role of either an underactive or overactive immune (defense) system response.

The most promising areas of research primarily center on viruses, the immune (defense) system, autoimmunity (a misdirected attack by the body against itself), the biochemistry of myelin, and population and genetic patterns of MS. Current scientific thought supports the possibility that MS may be caused by an interwoven combination of these factors or of others yet to be discovered.

The past several years have led to a tremendous advance in our knowledge of viruses and the body's defense system. Recent—though inconclusive and unconfirmed—studies of possible viral involvement in MS are accelerating increased interest in this approach.

This interest stems in part from demonstration by NINCDS Nobel Laureate Dr. D. Carleton Gajdusek and colleagues of the existence of at least two human neurological disorders caused by slow viruses which lie dormant in the body for years before some event triggers them into action. Since MS usually does not occur until early adulthood, the possibility of a slow viral infection is particularly intriguing. Supporting this theory are the population and geographical studies of MS which indicate that certain regions of the world with a temperate climate, such as the northern U.S., Canada, and Europe have a high prevalence of MS (and are thus called high-risk areas) compared with tropical regions (low-risk areas). Moreover, the age of 15 seems to be significant in terms of risk: well-documented studies indicate that a person moving from a high- to a low-risk area before the age of 15 tends to adopt the risk of the new area; while other studies (although less well documented) suggest that those moving after age 15 maintain the risk of their homeland. These findings encourage speculation that predisposing events for MS may occur sometime during the first 15 years of life.

Research on how the body defends itself against disease has leaped ahead in the past few years, through use of new scientific tools, and now is one of the most exciting and promising areas of MS research. Scientists can take an MS patient's antibodies (formed by the body to ward off a particular invader) and observe their action in a test tube.

Scientists are particularly interested in one type of antibody, IgG (mentioned in the "diagnosis" section) which is found in blood and spinal fluid. Since many patients with MS have elevated amounts of this antibody, scientists are working to determine the antibody's target. They are using a test which exposes the antibody to a variety of agents to see if the antibody, like a magnet, is drawn to one particular agent.

Some studies are concentrating on the possibility that the defense system is unable to differentiate an MS-causing factor from a naturally occurring substance in the patient's body. Thus a misdirected (autoimmune) attack by the body against itself may be taking place in persons with MS. This has been demonstrated in animals. For example, an NINCDS researcher, using a tadpole with a transparent optic nerve, has shown that spinal fluid from MS patients harms myelin surrounding the tadpole's nerve. Thus the search is intensified to determine what property of MS patients' spinal fluid causes this myelin destruction.

There is also some evidence to suggest that MS patients may have too little immune system activity. This has been found to occur in another disease affecting myelin. But if a defective defense system is involved in MS, neither increasing nor decreasing the MS patient's immune response has proved to be a successful treatment for MS. However, definite conclusions regarding these approaches cannot be made until additional studies are completed.

Research also is continuing on an MS-like animal disease called experimental allergic encephalomyelitis (EAE) which can be induced in animals using a part of myelin, called myelin basic protein, isolated from CNS tissue material. EAE in animals produces demyelination, scar tissue formation, and, under certain experimental conditions, a remitting course. Studies of the mechanism responsible for this disorder in laboratory animals may provide important clues to the cause, and possibly to the treatment of MS.

By using new laboratory techniques, scientists have identified myelin basic protein in the blood and cerebrospinal fluid samples of MS patients which, initial studies indicate, is not found in fluid of persons with other nervous system disorders. So this test has possible diagnostic potential. Furthermore, the test has implications for testing experimental MS treatment, for the scientists have found that levels of myelin basic protein in MS patients correlate with symptom levels. Patients experiencing an attack (and presumably demyelination) have higher levels of the protein than patients who are in a period of remission. Thus any treatment which decreases myelin basic protein levels might reasonably be expected to decrease symptoms, possibly by containing demyelination.

Each year the NINCDS prepares a summary of current research approaches and advances, which can be obtained by writing to the Institute. In addition, as mentioned earlier, information on a variety of topics is available through the National Multiple Sclerosis Society. No one knows where the breakthroughs will emerge. They may come from one of these scientific approaches, or they may come from studies of some other neurological disorder, or from some as yet unknown and unexplored avenue of research. Every year, advances in scientific research and technology are being made. With the continued dedication, imagination and hard work of scientists, and the continued cooperation, energy, and participation of patients, the answers to MS will be found.

In the meantime, it is often the courage and perseverance of the men and women with MS which can make the fight a winning one. As one patient wrote in an MS Society Award-winning article published in the *New York Sunday News:* "I live with MS. My family lives with MS. What is there to say? We have our moments. I and many other MS patients in my area have discovered that we are not alone . . . that there is practical assistance available now while work is going forward to find the cause and cure for this mysterious disease."

DHHS regional offices

Region I
Connecticut, Maine, Massachusetts, New Hampshire, Rhode Island, Vermont

> Regional Health Administrator
> John F. Kennedy Federal Building
> Government Center
> Boston, Massachusetts 02203
> (617) 223-6827

Region II
New York, New Jersey, Puerto Rico, Virgin Islands

> Regional Health Administrator
> Federal Building
> 26 Federal Plaza
> New York, New York 10007
> (212) 264-2561

Region III
Delaware, Maryland, Pennsylvania, Virginia, West Virginia and District of Columbia

> Regional Health Administrator
> 3535 Market Street
> P.O. Box 13716
> Philadelphia, Pennsylvania 19101
> (215) 596-6637

Region IV
Alabama, Florida, Georgia, Kentucky, Mississippi, North Carolina, South Carolina, Tennessee

> Regional Administrator
> 101 Marietta Tower
> Atlanta, Georgia 30323
> (404) 221-2398

Region V
Illinois, Indiana, Michigan, Minnesota, Ohio, Wisconsin

> Regional Health Administrator
> 300 South Wacker Drive

Chicago, Illinois 60606
(312) 353-1385

Region VI
Arkansas, Louisiana, New Mexico, Oklahoma, Texas

Regional Health Administrator
1200 Main Tower
Dallas, Texas 75202
(214) 767-3879

Region VII
Iowa, Kansas, Missouri, Nebraska

Regional Health Administrator
601 East 12th Street
Kansas City, Missouri 64106
(816) 374-3291

Region VIII
Colorado, Montana, North Dakota, South Dakota, Utah, Wyoming

Regional Health Administrator
19th and Stout Streets
Denver, Colorado 80294
(303) 837-4461

Region IX
Arizona, California, Hawaii, Nevada, Guam, Trust Territory of Pacific
Islands, American Samoa

Regional Health Administrator
Federal Office Building
50 United Nations Plaza
San Francisco, California 94102
(415) 556-5810

Region X
Alaska, Idaho, Oregon, Washington

Regional Health Administrator
Arcade Plaza Building
1321 Second Avenue

Seattle, Washington 98101
(206) 442-0430

Prepared by the Office of Scientific and Health Reports, National Institute of Neurological and Communicative Disorders and Stroke. National Institutes of Health, Bethesda, Maryland 20205. NIH Publication No. 81–75, Reprinted June 1981.

Osteoporosis
Cause, Treatment, Prevention

What is osteoporosis?

Osteoporosis literally means "porous bone." While the outer form of the bones does not change (unless there is a fracture), the bones have less substance and so are less dense. Osteoporosis is a common condition, affecting as many as 15 to 20 million individuals in the United States. It has been estimated to lead to 1.3 million bone fractures a year in people over 45 years of age, which is about 70 percent of all fractures occurring in this age group. Looked at in another way, each year about 1.7 percent of Americans between 45 and 64 years old and 2 percent of those age 65 and older break a bone because of osteoporosis.

In osteoporosis, bone mass decreases, causing bones to be more susceptible to fracture. A fall, blow, or lifting action that would not normally bruise or strain the average person can easily break one or more bones in someone with severe osteoporosis.

The spine, wrist, and hip are the most common sites of osteoporosis-related fractures, although the disease is generalized, that is, it can affect any bone of the body.

When the bones of the spinal column (the vertebrae) are weakened, a simple action like bending forward to make a bed or lifting a heavy roast pan out of the oven can be enough to cause a "crush fracture," or "spinal compression fracture." These vertebral crush fractures often cause back pain, decreased height, and a humped back or "dowager's hump."

The occurrence of osteoporosis of the spine increases with age. One recent study of a group of about 2,000 women showed X-ray evidence of osteoporosis in the spine in about 29 percent of those age 45 to 54 years, 61 percent of those age 55 to 64, and 79 percent of those age

65 and older. Vertebral crush fractures are more common in women than men and generally occur in women between 55 and 75 years of age.

Wrist fractures also occur commonly among people with this disorder. For example, an otherwise healthy, vigorous woman in her fifties or sixties slips on ice, falls, reaches out to catch herself, and is taken to the emergency room with a broken wrist.

Osteoporosis is often the underlying cause of the broken hips suffered by more than 200,000 Americans over age 45 each year. A fall from a standing position can fracture a hip weakened by osteoporosis. In cases of severe osteoporosis, a change of posture or weight distribution alone can actually break the hip, and the fracture then causes a fall.

People who have hip fractures due to osteoporosis are generally older than people who suffer spinal fractures. There is more even distribution between women and men than with vertebral fractures, the rates for hip fractures being two to three times higher in women than in men.

Who is at greatest risk?

A number of risk factors for osteoporosis have been identified. These include:

- *Being a woman.* Osteoporosis—as evidenced by vertebral fractures—is estimated to be six to eight times more common in women than in men, partly because women have less bone mass to begin with. Furthermore, for several years after menopause, women also lose bone much more rapidly than men do, due to a fall in their bodies' production of estrogen.
- *Early menopause.* This is one of the strong predictors for the development of osteoporosis, especially if menopause is induced by surgery or other means that remove both ovaries or cause a sufficient drop in estrogen. Many experts define ''early'' menopause as menopause occurring before the age of 45.
- *Being white, that is, Caucasian.* White women are at higher risk than black women, and white men are at higher risk than black men. Some experts estimate that by age 65 a quarter of all white women have had one or more fractures related to osteoporosis. Oriental women are also thought to be at greater risk for the disease, but there are not enough data to confirm this.
- *A chronically low calcium intake.*
- *Lack of physical activity.* However, exercising at an extreme level that halts menstruation in a young woman also may lead to bone loss.
- *Being underweight.* (This is *not* to suggest that being overweight is a

good idea. Both overweight and underweight people are better off trying to attain their desirable weight.*)

Other *possible* risk factors include:

- A family history of osteoporosis.
- Smoking cigarettes.
- Excessive use of alcohol. It is not known exactly how much alcohol is too much, in terms of osteoporosis, but alcoholics may be at risk for the disease.

Other factors often listed as increasing a person's risk of osteoporosis, although these are *not* well-established by scientific studies, include:

- High intake of caffeine-containing foods such as coffee.
- Extremely high protein intake (to the extent that the diet is almost entirely protein).
- Phosphorus. Some people suggest avoiding eating large amounts of foods high in phosphorus and low in calcium such as red meats, cola drinks, brewer's yeast that does not have added calcium, and certain processed foods. Animal studies suggest that increases in phosphorus intake might speed bone loss; however, studies in humans show dietary phosphorus either promotes a positive calcium balance in the bones or has no effect.

What causes osteoporosis?

Living bone contains a protein framework (the osteoid matrix) in which calcium salts are deposited. In fact, the bones and teeth contain about 99 percent of the calcium in the body. Calcium makes bone hard.

Bone, like many other tissues of the body, is constantly being rebuilt or "remodeled." Old bone is torn down, "resorbed," and replaced with new bone in much the same way that people remodel buildings by tearing out and replacing walls.

This process of bone resorption and remodeling serves two purposes: It keeps the skeleton well-tuned for its mechanical uses, and it helps to maintain the body's balance of certain essential minerals such as calcium. The body keeps a relatively constant level of calcium in the blood, because important biological activities such as contraction of muscles, beating of the heart, and clotting of blood require quite constant blood levels of calcium.

When the blood calcium level drops, more calcium is taken out of the bones to maintain the appropriate level. When the blood calcium

---

*The 1959 Metropolitan Life Insurance Desirable Weight Table can be used as a guide for determining this.

level returns to normal, increased amounts of calcium are no longer taken from the bones.

As a person grows during youth, bones are metabolically active, and calcium is deposited into bone faster than it is taken out. The deposition of calcium into bone peaks at about 35 years of age in men and women. At the time of "peak bone mass" the bones are most dense and strong.

Some experts believe that the level of bone mass at this age may help determine whether a person may later lose enough bone to fracture easily. If a young woman achieves a high peak bone mass—possibly through increased calcium intake, moderate weight-bearing exercise, and other lifestyle choices—she may be less likely to develop osteoporosis later.

During a person's late thirties, after peak bone mass is attained, calcium begins to be lost from bones faster than it is replaced, and bones become less dense. This occurs naturally and gradually in both men and women. In addition, in general, as both women and men age, their bodies begin to absorb less calcium from food. This begins at about age 45 for women and age 60 for men.

Summarizing then, several complex factors influence the quantity and quality of bone throughout life, particularly after the age of 40. These include: level of adult peak bone mass; rates of bone loss due to menopause and due to aging; certain systemic hormones (such as calcitriol, an active form of vitamin D; parathyroid hormone; and calcitonin); substances produced by the bones themselves; diet (especially calcium intake); intestinal and kidney function; and physical forces that act on the bones such as those caused by body weight and exercise.

Given the complexity of the factors that influence bone, there may be many ways in which osteoporosis can develop. Current data point to two strong contributing factors: a drop in estrogen levels in women due to menopause (technically known as "estrogen deficiency") and a chronically low intake of calcium ("calcium deficiency").

Menopause As a woman passes through menopause, her body's production of sex hormones declines and monthly bleeding—menstruation— gradually diminishes until it stops altogether. (If menopause occurs because of removal of the ovaries, the drop in estrogen is relatively sudden.) Hormones are chemical substances produced by glands to control activities of bodily organs. Estrogen, the female hormone, seems especially to influence bone substance by slowing or halting bone loss. It may also improve the absorption of dietary calcium by the intestine.

This role of estrogen makes biological sense. During the childbearing years, a woman needs a strong skeleton and a healthy reserve of calcium in case she becomes pregnant and later nurses children. After menopause, she no longer has the same need for this protective reserve of calcium. As her estrogen level drops, her bones start to contribute a larger share of calcium to meet the body's needs.

Too Little Calcium in the Diet Many scientists believe that a chronic shortage of dietary calcium is one important factor leading to osteoporosis. Each day, adults lose some calcium in the urine and feces and, to a lesser extent, through their skin. If these losses are not balanced by adequate amounts of calcium in the diet, "the body goes to the 'bank,' " as one expert put it, "and the bank, of course, is the skeleton." The bones begin to break down to supply the body's need for the mineral in maintaining the proper blood level of calcium.

Other Causes of Osteoporosis Certain diseases or drugs can lead to bone loss. A doctor can evaluate a person who has one of these disorders or is taking one of these drugs and work with her to avoid osteoporosis. These include:

- Medications such as corticosteroids and heparin (an anticoagulant)
- Diseases such as hyperthyroidism, hyperparathyroidism, kidney disease, and certain forms of cancer (lymphoma, leukemia, and multiple myeloma)
- Impaired ability to absorb calcium from the intestine caused by diseases of the small intestine, liver, or pancreas
- Excessive excretion of calcium in the urine (idiopathic hypercalciuria).

What are the symptoms?

In most cases, a patient is 50 to 70 years of age when osteoporosis is diagnosed. The disorder, however, can strike a woman as early as her mid-thirties. People with osteoporosis may have no symptoms until their bones become so weak that a sudden strain, bump, or fall causes a bone fracture. Then, of course, pain can be severe and can drastically curtail physical activity.

Crush fractures of the vertebrae can occur with or without causing pain. Thus, other clues to the presence of osteoporosis besides back pain are loss of height or curvature of the upper back. However, a chronic aching along the spine or, more often, pain from spasm in the muscles of the back may occur. With a partially collapsed spine, the muscles of the back must take a greater share of supporting the upper half of the body, so that these muscles may "complain" periodically.

Osteoporosis first may be discovered on an X-ray taken for some other purpose. In some cases, such X-rays may reveal that one or more weakened vertebrae have already been fractured. X-rays or other medical imaging methods can reveal that bones have weakened. A person has to lose about a quarter of his or her bone mass before the loss can be detected on a regular X-ray. Unfortunately, by the time this much bone loss has occurred the bones already may be susceptible to breaking.

Scientists have developed new techniques to measure bone density, which might detect early bone loss, before fractures are likely to occur. These techniques are not available to some doctors. In one technique, called "photon absorptiometry" or "photon densitometry," rays like X-rays are passed through the skeleton and a machine measures how much these rays penetrate the bone (and therefore how dense the bones are).

Another technique is computed tomography (CT) scanning. It uses X-rays to measure bone density. Researchers are now adapting this technique to CT equipment already available in some hospitals.

While no blood or urine tests specifically diagnose osteoporosis, these tests may eliminate secondary causes of bone loss such as the disorders and medications listed before.

How can osteoporosis be prevented and treated?

In recent years, scientists have identified several measures that may help reduce the toll of osteoporosis. These measures were described in the 1984 NIH Consensus Development Conference on Osteoporosis and are explained in the pages that follow. *Estrogen replacement is the only one of these measures in which there is well-documented evidence of its effectiveness in the prevention of fractures from osteoporosis.*

Although complete proof is lacking that the other measures—such as increased calcium intake—prevent bone loss leading to fractures, many believe that current data are sufficient to suggest that these measures be adopted.

Many of these measures can be taken throughout life to promote healthy bones. (Exceptions include estrogen replacement therapy for postmenopausal women and a newly approved drug, calcitonin, for the treatment of existing osteoporosis.) It is possible that young women could build a high peak bone mass to reduce the risk of developing osteoporosis. Middle-age and older women may be able to keep osteoporosis from occurring or progressing. Men too may lessen their risk of osteoporosis.

All of these measures are best undertaken with the advice of a doctor.

Estrogen Replacement Therapy For women at risk of osteoporosis, a doctor may prescribe estrogen when the body's production of the hormone drops, that is, during and after menopause. Menopause occurs naturally around the age of 50, although it can occur when a woman is in her late thirties or into her early sixties. Menopause also will occur if the ovaries are removed by surgery.

Many experts feel that, in terms of its effects against osteoporosis, the benefits of estrogen replacement outweigh its risks. The decision to use estrogen, however, is one that should be made carefully by a woman and her doctor.

On the side of benefits, there is good evidence that low-dose estrogen is highly effective for the prevention and possible treatment of osteoporosis in women. Estrogen reduces the amount of calcium taken out of bones and thus slows or halts postmenopausal bone loss. It cannot, however, restore bone mass to premenopausal levels. Studies have shown that women who have begun taking estrogen within a few years after the onset of menopause have fewer hip or wrist fractures and possibly fewer spinal fractures than women who do not take estrogen. Even when started as late as six years after menopause, estrogen therapy reduces further loss of bone.

There is also some scientific evidence that estrogen replacement therapy confers some protection against cardiovascular disease. It is thought to raise blood levels of a fraction of cholesterol known as "HDL" or high density lipoprotein and to lower blood levels of "LDL" or low density lipoprotein. Raised HDL levels and lowered LDL levels are associated with lower rates of heart and blood-vessel disease.

On the risk side of the ledger, estrogen replacement therapy is thought to increase the risk of a type of cancer of the uterus known as endometrial cancer from 1 per 1,000 women to about 4 per 1,000 women. Endometrial cancer, fortunately, is relatively easy to detect and treat and is rarely fatal. It is not a problem for a woman who has had her uterus removed, of course. Estrogen is not linked to breast cancer, according to most studies. The therapy may increase the risk of blood clot formation (thrombosis).

In women on estrogen replacement therapy, periodic bleeding may resume. (Because estrogen therapy may cause the lining of the uterus to build up, it is often prescribed on an on-and-off basis—for example, 20 days on the drug, then 10 without it—so that the uterus lining can be shed during the days off the hormone.)

Estrogen may be combined with another female hormone, progestin, also called progestogen. (Progesterone is one form of progestin.) Progestins may reduce the risk of endometrial cancer. There is preliminary evidence that they may reduce bone loss.

There is little information on the *long-term* risks or benefits of estrogen combined with progestin in postmenopausal women. Studies on *younger women* taking progestins in birth control pills have shown an increased risk of high blood pressure and of disorders of the heart and blood vessels. Moreover, some progestins may blunt or do away with estrogen's protective effects against heart disease.

Until more data on the risks and benefits of estrogen replacement are available, *doctors and patients may prefer to reserve estrogen (whether or not it is combined with a progestin), for situations in which there is a moderate to high risk of osteoporosis.* Premature menopause—especially through surgical removal of the ovaries several years before the time of natural menopause—places a woman at high risk of osteoporosis. *Postmenopausal women having risk factors other than an early menopause may also want to discuss estrogen therapy with their doctors.* (The section on risk gives these other factors as: being white, having a low calcium intake, being inactive, having a slight build, and possibly heredity, cigarette smoking, and excessive use of alcohol.)

The recommendations above apply mainly to Caucasian women. Women of other races and their doctors might consider estrogen on a case-by-case basis. There is no good evidence that elderly women should be started on estrogen therapy to prevent osteoporosis.

Increased Calcium Intake An intake of calcium of 1,000 to 1,500 mg (milligrams) per day—through diet or diet plus supplements—is thought to help protect against development of osteoporosis.

People, particularly women, should get plenty of calcium in their diets throughout life. Certainly children and teenagers need an adequate calcium intake as they are growing.

Studies show that the usual intake of calcium for adult women (ages 25 to 74) in the United States is 450 to 550 mg per day. This is well below the current Recommended Dietary Allowance (RDA) of 800 mg per day for women and men who are over 18 years old. Furthermore, studies cited by the 1984 NIH Consensus Development Conference on Osteoporosis led the conference panel to offer the opinion that the RDA for calcium is too low, especially for postmenopausal women, and may well be too low for elderly men.

The panel recommended that women consume the following amounts of calcium each day:

• Premenopausal and older women receiving estrogen need about 1,000 mg of calcium per day for calcium balance, that is, to keep the amount of calcium in the bones constant.

• Postmenopausal women (that is, all women past the age of menopause) who are not on estrogen need about 1,500 mg of calcium per day.

In addition, men who increase their calcium intake may prevent age-related bone loss as well.

Taking these recommendations into account, calcium requirements are summarized in the following table:

Table 1

Daily Calcium Requirements

For children:[*]

Age	Mg calcium per day
Birth–0.5 years	360
0.5–1	540
1–10	800
10–18	1,200

For adults,[**] except pregnant or nursing women:

Premenopausal women	1,000
Estrogen-treated women	1,000
Postmenopausal women	1,500
Men	1,000

For women who are pregnant or nursing:[*]

Women 19 years or older	400 above normal requirement[**] (a total of 1,400)
Women under 19	800 above normal requirement (a total of 2,000)

[*]Based on the most recently available RDA's (1980) developed by the National Academy of Sciences, National Research Council.
[**] Based on the 1984 NIH Consensus Development Conference Statement on Osteoporosis.

In essence, with the exception of pregnant and nursing women, the recommendations above mean that *adult women and probably men should have a total daily intake of 1,000 mg of calcium and women past menopause, not on estrogen therapy, need 1,500 mg daily.*

If the average American woman consumes an estimated 500 mg of calcium per day, based on her current eating habits, then an additional 500 to 1,000 mg are needed; that is roughly the amount of calcium in two to four servings of milk or several servings of other calcium-rich foods. It can be helpful to consult a doctor, registered dietitian or nutritionist who can estimate the amount of calcium in a person's usual diet. Then he or she can suggest ways to increase calcium in the diet and can recommend calcium supplements, if necessary, to bring the daily intake up to 1,000 to 1,500 mg. Some sources of calcium are discussed in the information that follows.

Milk, other dairy products, fish, and dark green vegetables are the major dietary sources of calcium in this country. One 8-ounce glass of milk contains about 300 mg of calcium and a quart contains about 1,200 mg. Skim milk or lowfat milk, which actually contain a little more calcium than whole milk, are preferred to minimize fat intake. (The American diet is generally high in fat and efforts should be made to reduce fat intake. Consumption of lowfat dairy products reduces both fat and calories in the diet.)

In addition to milk itself, other milk products such as lowfat yogurt and nonfat dry milk are also high in calcium. Other calcium-rich foods include fish and shellfish such as oysters, shrimp, and canned sardines and salmon (when the edible bones are also consumed); and dark green vegetables such as collard, turnip, and mustard greens, kale, and broccoli. Spinach is not a good source of calcium because, although it is high in calcium and other nutrients, it contains substances (oxalates) that diminish absorption of calcium.

Many other foods contain lesser amounts of calcium. A list of some foods especially high in calcium appears at the end of this article. Calorie counts are given as well so that a person may plan to increase his or her calcium intake without a substantial increase in calories. (An exercise program—also important in the prevention and treatment of osteoporosis—could also help to offset any increase in calories.)

People who have difficulty digesting milk (as in lactase deficiency or lactose intolerance) might try eating yogurt or drinking milk that has been treated with the enzyme lactase (known as LactAid®) so it can be digested. Some yogurts contain lactase naturally.

For some people, it may be difficult to reach the daily levels of calcium intake suggested previously without taking calcium supplements. As the list that follows indicates, different formulations of the supplements contain different amounts of elemental calcium, so it is important to read the product label.* For example, calcium carbonate is 40 percent calcium. That is, 100 mg of calcium carbonate contains 40 mg of calcium, or "elemental calcium." In the case of calcium lactate (at 13 percent calcium), 250 mg of the compound would contain about 34 mg of calcium. Calcium supplements are often in the form of tablets. Chewable tablets and powders may be available. One source of calcium carbonate is oyster shells, so this compound is sometimes called "oyster shell calcium." Certain antacids contain calcium carbonate; in fact, one popular brand is virtually 100 percent calcium carbonate with only added sweeteners and flavorings. Other antacids with calcium carbonate also contain alumi-

---

* See "Some Information for Label-Readers" given at the end.

Table 2

Calcium Supplement

Some Commonly Available Calcium Compounds	Percent Calcium
Calcium carbonate	40
Calcium lactate	13
Calcium gluconate	9

num, which can hamper the intestine's ability to absorb calcium from food.

It is wise to consult a doctor to determine how much calcium you currently consume, whether you should take calcium supplements, and if so, what type. The number of calcium preparations on the market is growing steadily, and there is no one supplement that can be uniformly recommended. If you cannot get enough calcium in your diet and you must take supplements, here is some information to keep in mind:

- There is recent evidence that taking supplements between meals promotes better absorption. Some believe that it is useful to take calcium at bedtime because of increased calcium loss during sleep. (So, for example, someone who takes calcium twice a day might take it mid-morning and at night.)
- A recent study found that absorption of calcium from calcium carbonate is impaired in people with little or no stomach acid, which is common in people over 60. However, the scientists found that in these people absorption improved if the compound was taken with meals.
- Bone meal and dolomite should *not* be taken regularly. Although they are both high in calcium, they also tend to contain high amounts of lead and other toxic metals.
- Be alert to calcium supplements that have vitamin D added to them. Most people get enough of this vitamin in their diet and through sun exposure. Vitamin D becomes toxic at high doses.
- Avoid taking aluminum-containing antacids as a regular source of calcium.
- Drink a full glass of water when taking a calcium supplement. (In general, it is a good idea to drink several glasses of water each day.)

Levels of calcium intake greater than those recommended previously (that is, 1,000 to 1,500 mg per day) can cause kidney stones in susceptible people. Thus, people with a history of kidney stones should take calcium supplements only with a doctor's guidance. These people should be especially careful to drink plenty of water.

Normal Levels of Vitamin D Vitamin D is required for optimal absorption of calcium in the intestine. People who get very little sunlight exposure are at risk of vitamin D deficiency. This particularly applies to older people who may be confined to a home or nursing facility.

Scientists recommend 400 I.U. (international units) of vitamin D each day. Most people get enough of this vitamin by being outside during the day and eating a normal diet. (Vitamin D is produced by the body naturally when a person is exposed to the sun.) Fifteen minutes to a hour of midday sunshine may meet the daily need for this vitamin. Food sources include vitamin D-fortified milk, vitamin-fortified cereals, egg yolks, saltwater fish, and liver.

The phrase "normal levels" is important here. Taking in *high* doses of vitamin D can have dangerous effects. No one needs to take more than the RDA per day without a doctor's guidance.

Moderate Weight-Bearing Exercise Exercise may be an important part of both prevention and treatment programs for osteoporosis. It is clear that inactivity leads to bone loss. Research studies have shown that normal, healthy people who are bedridden for periods of time lose bone mineral rapidly. Studies have also revealed that astronauts living in the weightlessness of space lose bone mass.

Scientists believe that activity involving the muscles working against gravity such as walking or jogging will help to reduce bone loss.

The best type and amount of physical activity to prevent osteoporosis have not yet been established. However, a modest program of weight-bearing exercise is recommended for people of all ages, including middle-age and older women who want strong bones, as well as young women who are working toward reaching a high "peak bone mass" in their mid-thirties. Possibilities for "weight-bearing" exercises include: walking, hiking, racewalking, jogging, running, jumping rope, aerobic dancing, ballroom dancing, gymnastics, tennis, racquetball, squash, handball, rowing, weight training, basketball, volleyball, cross-country skiing, and to some extent, bicycling. Swimming and yoga are healthy activities, but are not generally thought to be weight-bearing.

There are some cautions about exercise, of course. It is a good idea to consult a doctor before starting an exercise program, especially if there are heart, joint, or other problems or if a person has been sedentary for a long time. Exercise programs should also be started slowly and built up gradually. Exercising to the point of causing trauma to the bones should be avoided.

Some young women who do an exceptional amount of exercise (such as vigorous long-distance running) may stop menstruating. If so, recent evidence indicates that they may be at higher risk of osteoporosis.

Doctors encourage patients with osteoporosis to remain as physically active as possible. It is important to avoid sudden strains from jumping or twisting and situations where a person might fall. Walking, however, is highly recommended. The worst thing to do is to give in to the disorder and take to one's bed or chair. Lack of activity will almost certainly do harm—both physically and psychologically.

New Modes of Treatment Most of the measures described in this booklet are for the prevention, not the treatment, of osteoporosis. Treatment refers to methods of making more bone, rather than slowing down bone loss. The needs are great for drugs and techniques that can treat osteoporosis once it has occurred.

Several potential therapies for osteoporosis are being studied by researchers. In most cases, the effectiveness and safety of these therapies have not been fully established.

A new drug for osteoporosis was approved by the Federal Food and Drug Administration in December 1984. This drug is calcitonin. Calcitonin occurs naturally in the body, as it is a hormone produced by the thyroid gland. It slows bone breakdown. The form that is sold by prescription to patients is a synthetic form of calcitonin from salmon (also called calcitonin-salmon). As a treatment for osteoporosis, it is given by daily injection in conjunction with 1,500 mg of calcium and 400 I.U. per day of vitamin D.

Other agents under study include sodium fluoride; the hormone calcitriol (a form of vitamin D); anabolic steroids; thiazides (diuretics); biphosphonates; a biologically active fragment of parathyroid hormone; and "ADFR" (a complex series of drugs).

Sodium fluoride holds promise for treatment of severe osteoporosis but remains experimental. Sodium fluoride combined with calcium has been shown to increase bone mass. However, some patients have experienced side effects such as stomach pain, nausea, inflamed joints, and anemia caused by gastrointestinal bleeding. At high dosages of sodium fluoride, bone tends to become more crystalline, less elastic, and therefore more brittle than normal bone. Determining the role of sodium fluoride plus calcium awaits the results of ongoing clinical studies.

Calcitriol is also known as 1,25 dihydroxyvitamin D and 1,25 dihydroxycholcalciferol. Some researchers believe it can increase calcium absorption and decrease the rate of fracture in osteoporosis patients. However, ongoing clinical trials must be completed to determine its true effects on bone.

Prevention of Fractures There are ways that people can make fractures less likely to occur, especially if their bones are already fragile. Minimizing hazards in the home can help, such as avoiding slippery floors and loose throw rugs, removing objects that might cause a fall, providing adequate lighting, and adding handles or nonslip bottoms to bathtubs. Railings on stairways inside and outside of the home can help.

It is also a good idea to avoid actions that stress the bones unduly. In particular, do not lift while bending forward. Lifting this way creates an unusual and unnecessary strain on the vertebral column. A person should carry the weight close to the body, squatting and lifting straight up, using the legs and not the back. If the spine is weak, it is wise to avoid completely lifting heavy objects.

What is the research outlook?

Studies related to osteoporosis are being conducted by scientists at universities, medical centers, and other research institutions around the country. These scientists are supported by the National Institute of Arthritis and Musculoskeletal and Skin Diseases (NIAMS), by other Federal agencies such as the National Institute on Aging, and by private companies and organizations.

One important area of basic research is concerned with understanding the processes by which existing bone grows and new bone tissue is formed.

For example, it is already known that certain hormones that circulate throughout the body—such as glucocorticoids, insulin, parathyroid hormone, sex hormones, and growth hormone—affect bone "turnover," that is, the cycle of bone breakdown and rebuilding. Researchers are trying to define exactly how these hormones influence bone turnover. In addition, substances produced by the bone themselves are now known to affect bone turnover. Scientists believe that when the complex interaction of all of these substances is out of balance, the result can be osteoporosis or other bone disorders.

Basic research on the components of bone and the factors that influence bone metabolism can provide information important to understanding and managing osteoporosis. For example, scientists could determine markers for the early detection of the disease. In addition, new treatments could be based on replacing deficient or missing substances.

Some of the current clinical studies focus on improving ways to measure bone density such as the use of photon absorptiometry or CT scanning as described previously. Goals are to detect bone loss before the bones become likely to fracture and to be able to monitor the effects of a therapy on bone density.

Researchers are following selected groups of women over many years in order to determine those who are at highest risk and more precisely describe risk factors for the disease.

Other investigators are developing or evaluating new methods of treating or preventing osteoporosis. Several new agents such as calcitonin and sodium fluoride plus calcium were listed in the section on potential treatments. Researchers continue to assess the usefulness of various forms of estrogen and determine the risks and benefits of adding a progestin. Also being studied are the effects of exercise on bone density in young and older women.

Conclusion

Each year the cost of osteoporosis increases. The disease is estimated to cost a total of $6.1 billion per year, including direct costs for care such as hospitalization and nursing home services, plus indirect costs such as lost earnings. As the population ages, these costs will rise unless osteoporosis is effectively prevented and treated.

Many of the costs of osteoporosis for an individual, of course, cannot be measured in dollars. These costs can include pain, impaired mobility, disruption of daily activities, and reduced independence.

As this article has described, recent research shows that fractures from having fragile bones may *not* be an inevitable part of life for postmenopausal women or older Americans. Studies are yielding new information about bone biology and are providing new methods of diagnosis and treatment if osteoporosis develops. In the meantime, there are steps that can be taken—beginning immediately—to protect the bones. At the present stage of our knowledge, the greatest hopes for combating the pain and disability of osteoporosis are to identify and inform people at risk and initiate prevention programs promptly, before bone loss becomes too great.

Table 3

See your doctor about these measures:
- **Consider estrogen replacement therapy** if you are a woman going through or past menopause.
- **Get adequate vitamin D** if you get very little sunlight.

Make these a part of your lifestyle:
- **Consume plenty of calcium**—Aim for 1,000 mg per day in your diet (or 1,500 mg per day for postmenopausal women not on estrogen).
- **Exercise**—Get regular, moderate, weight-bearing exercise.
- **Prevent fractures**—Look out for your bones. Minimize hazards in the home and at work. Lift heavy objects carefully or not at all.

Appendix 1
Some Calcium-Rich Foods

Daily	Measure	Calories	Calcium (mg)
Cheese			
Blue	1 ounce	100	**150**
Cheddar, cut pieces	1 ounce	115	**204**
Feta	1 ounce	75	**140**
Mozzarella, made with whole milk	1 ounce	80	**147**
Mozzarella, made with part skim			
milk	1 ounce	80	**207**
Muenster	1 ounce	105	**203**
Parmesan	1 tbsp	25	**69**
Pasteurized process			
American	1 ounce	105	**174**
Swiss	1 ounce	95	**219**
Provolone	1 ounce	100	**214**
Swiss	1 ounce	105	**272**
Cottage Cheese			
Lowfat (2%)	1 cup	205	**155**
Creamed (4% fat)			
Large curd	1 cup	235	**135**
Small curd	1 cup	215	**126**
Milk			
Skim	1 cup	85	**302**
1% fat	1 cup	100	**300**
2% fat	1 cup	120	**297**
Whole (3.3% fat)	1 cup	150	**291**
Buttermilk	1 cup	100	**285**
Dry, nonfat, instant	¼ cup	61	**209**
Yogurt			
Plain, lowfat, with added milk			
solids	8 ounces	145	**415**
Fruit-flavored, lowfat, with added			
milk solids	8 ounces	230[*]	**345[*]**
Plain, whole milk	8 ounces	140	**274**
Dairy Desserts			
Custard, baked	1 cup	305	**297**
Ice cream, vanilla			
Regular (11% fat)			
Hardened	1 cup	270	**176**
Soft serve	1 cup	375	**236**

Appendix 1 *(Continued)*

Daily	Measure	Calories	Calcium (mg)
Ice milk, vanilla			
Hardened, 4% fat	1 cup	185	**176**
Soft serve, 3% fat	1 cup	225	**274**
Seafood			
Oysters, raw, meat only (13–19 medium)	1 cup	160	**226**
Salmon, pink, canned, *including the bones*	3 ounces	120	**167**[*]
Sardines, Atlantic, canned in oil, drained, *including the bones*	3 ounces	175	**371**[*]
Shrimp, canned, drained, solids	3 ounces	100	**98**
Vegetables			
Bok choy, raw, chopped	1 cup	9	**74**
Broccoli, raw	1 spear	40	**72**
Broccoli, cooked, drained, from raw, ½" pieces	1 cup	45	**177**
Broccoli, cooked, drained, from frozen, chopped	1 cup	50	**94**
Collards, cooked, drained, from frozen	1 cup	60	**357**
Dandelion greens, cooked, drained	1 cup	35	**147**
Kale, cooked, drained, from frozen	1 cup	40	**179**
Mustard greens, without stems and midribs, cooked, drained	1 cup	20	**104**
Turnip greens, chopped, cooked, drained, from frozen	1 cup	50	**249**
Dried Beans			
Cooked, drained			
Great Northern	1 cup	210	**90**
Navy	1 cup	225	**95**
Pinto	1 cup	265	**86**
Chickpeas (garbanzos), cooked, drained	1 cup	270	**80**
Red kidney, canned	1 cup	230	**74**
Refried beans, canned	1 cup	295	**141**
Soy beans, cooked, drained	1 cup	235	**131**
Miscellaneous			
Molasses, cane, blackstrap	2 tbsp	85	**274**
Tofu, 2½" x 2¾" x 1" (about 4 ounces)	1 piece	85[†]	**108**[†]

[*] These values may vary.

[**] If the bones are discarded, the amount of calcium is greatly reduced.

[†] Both of these values may vary, especially the calcium content, depending on how the tofu is made. Tofu processed with calcium salts can have as much as 300 mg calcium per 4 ounces. The label, your grocer, or the manufacturer can provide more specific information.

Source: Home and Garden Bulletin #72, Human Nutrition Information Service, U.S. Department of Agriculture, 1985.

Appendix 2
Some Information for Label-Readers

RDA's vs. US RDA's

There are really two RDA's. One stands for Recommended *Dietary* Allowances, and past versions such as the 1980 figures cited here have come from the National Academy of Sciences under contract from NIH. For calcium, several RDA's are given (see table in this booklet), depending on the age of the person or other factors such as pregnancy.

The other RDA's (always listed as "US RDA's") are the figures referred to on labeling of foods and supplements. The US RDA's are the Recommended *Daily* Allowances, and they come from the Food and Drug Administration. The US RDA's are based on the other RDA's, but generally only one or a few figures are given. The US RDA for adults for calcium is 1,000 mg, which makes it easier to figure out the amount of calcium from the label, as demonstrated below. (The US RDA for pregnant or lactating women is 1,400 mg.)

Food Labels

On a carton of milk, for example, you may see the following information given:

Nutrition Information Per Serving
    Serving Size   One Cup

    Percentage of US Recommended Daily Allowances (US RDA)

    Calcium   30

This means that one cup of milk contains 30 percent of the US RDA or 30 percent of 1,000 mg—which is 300 mg.

Or on a package of tofu, you may see this information:

    Serving Size   4 oz.

    % US RDA
    *Calcium   13**

which would indicate 130 mg calcium per serving or perhaps

    *Calcium   30**
which would indicate 300 mg calcium per serving.

---

* This number varies, depending on how the tofu is processed.

Calcium Supplement Labels

The information on calcium supplement labels varies widely. It may tell you exactly how many mg calcium, or simply how many mg of the compound, leaving you to figure out how much elemental calcium is provided. It may or may not be specific as to how and when to take the supplement. For assistance, consult your doctor or pharmacist or write to the manufacturer. Two examples of supplements from a drugstore are given below.

From a bottle of calcium carbonate tablets:

Front: *Calcium*
500 mg Supplement

Side: *Each tablet contains:*
1250 mg of calcium carbonate
Elemental calcium   500 mg
Directions: One tablet 2 or 3 times a day with meals or as
*   recommended by your physician.*

From a package of calcium lactate tablets:

Front: *Calcium Lactate Tablets*
USP 650 mg[*]

Side: *% US RDA for Adults and Children Over 4*
12 Tablets Contain: Calcium 1.014 grams[**]   *101*

Directions 3 tablets 4 times daily

---

[*] USP stands for *United States Pharmacopeia,* a legally recognized compendium of standards for drugs. The 650 mg refers to the total amount of calcium lactate in each tablet. Thus, since calcium lactate is 13 percent elemental calcium, each tablet contains 84.5 mg calcium.
[**] There are 1,000 mg in a gram, so this equals 1,014 mg of elemental calcium.

For more information, contact:

National Osteoporosis Foundation
1625 Eye St., NW, Suite 1011
Washington, DC 20006

The National Osteoporosis Foundation, a nonprofit voluntary health organization, was founded in late 1984 to provide nationwide programs of public and professional education and research on osteoporosis.

U.S. Department of Health and Human Services, Public Health Service, National Institutes of Health, National Institute of Arthritis and Musculoskeletal and Skin Diseases. NIH Publication No. 86–2226, revised May 1986.

Parkinson's Disease
Hope Through Research

Mary found she had Parkinson's disease when she was in her late fifties. For a while she continued to work as a housewife, but gradually her ability to walk and to do simple tasks decreased. By the time she was in her mid-sixties she was bedridden. Luckily her husband had reached retirement age by then, and he now takes care of her at home.

Jacob is in his late fifties and receiving drug therapy for Parkinson's disease. Most of the time the drugs—and the understanding of his students and the college administrators—enable him to teach in a Hebrew seminary. But increasingly he has to be helped to the classes, and sometimes in the middle of teaching he has problems speaking.

Tom, on the other hand, has received great benefit from taking standard antiparkinson drugs developed through scientific research. After 10 years of treatment his disease shows no sign of worsening.

Amy has also been greatly helped in living with her parkinsonism, but in her case the benefit came from joining a support group. "She was almost dead when I first saw her," says the nurse who directs the group. "Since she discovered other patients with Parkinson's, she swims every day and attends meetings regularly."

Four different people, four different courses of Parkinson's disease. Taken together, they emphasize several important facts about this neurological illness:

First, Parkinson's is a serious disease that, if left untreated, can disable the patient.

Second, treatment with drugs can help most parkinsonian patients to remain independent for many years. Some patients have been quite successful in maintaining the normal motor skills that we all take for granted. But current drug therapy does not cure the disease or even halt its progression. That is why scientists are continually looking for new medications to fight this debilitating illness. Several promising drugs are now being tested.

Third, the most effective therapy for Parkinson's disease includes, in addition to medications, an exercise program and a great deal of caring support from relatives and friends.

Research to improve treatment for Parkinson's disease and to find a cure is going on at many medical centers. Much of this work is supported by the National Institute of Neurological and Communicative Disorders and Stroke (NINCDS), a world leader in research on brain and central nervous system disorders and the focal point in the U.S. Government for the support of research in these areas.

In addition to a multimillion-dollar investment in research conducted through universities and medical institutions, the NINCDS also searches for answers to Parkinson's disease in its own laboratories and clinics at the National Institutes of Health in Bethesda, Maryland. Through this research, scientists hope to understand better the basis of Parkinson's disease, and ultimately to prevent the disorder's occurrence.

History

Before 1817, what we now know as Parkinson's disease was just one of a number of similar disorders of movement. Then a British doctor, James Parkinson, published a paper on what he called "shaking palsy." In it, he described the major symptoms of the disease that would later bear his name.

Dr. Parkinson's observations allowed the disease to be studied as a special illness for the first time. During the next century, scientists defined its distribution, symptoms and onset, and the prospects for recovery. But most important, in the early 1960's they identified the fundamental brain defect that is the hallmark of the disease. This information led to the first effective treatment for parkinsonism and suggested ways of devising new and more effective therapies.

A disease of later life

Very few persons with Parkinson's disease develop serious symptoms before age 40. The great majority of cases are diagnosed between ages 60 and 70, so that the average age of parkinsonian patients is 65 years. In one community studied, the frequency of the disease in those above 50 increased markedly with age. The increasing number of older persons in the U.S., therefore, would seem to foreshadow an increase in the number of people who will develop parkinsonism.

Both men and women appear to be equally affected. There are now perhaps 500,000 people with the disease in the United States, but this number is not exact since many cases are not severe enough to need treatment.

Among many populations in the world, there is wide variation in the occurrence of Parkinson's disease. Some scientists believe that high disease rates in certain populations might be due to an increased genetic susceptibility; but other research findings suggest that heredity may not play a major role in determining who gets the disease. An NINCDS study of over 40 Parkinson's disease patients who had an identical twin uncovered only one case in which the twin also had the disease. This and other findings lend support to the likelihood that an environmental factor, rather than heredity, causes parkinsonism—an idea that is now being investigated.

Early symptoms

The first signs of Parkinson's disease may appear to be simply part of the normal aging process: a little shakiness, some difficulty in rising from a deep, comfortable chair. This is especially true since most symptoms of Parkinson's are first noticed when persons are in their sixties.

But the signs very gradually become more pronounced and extensive. The shaking or *tremor* that affects about two-thirds of parkinsonian patients begins to interfere with daily activities. It may be more difficult to hold utensils steady when eating. A newspaper may shake enough to make it hard to read.

The shaking may become worse when the patient is relaxed. This is characteristic of Parkinson's. A few seconds after the hands are rested on a table, for instance, the shaking is most pronounced.

Although tremor is usually the most obvious early sign of Parkinson's disease, a more distressing problem to the patient is the symptom known as *bradykinesia*—the gradual loss of spontaneous movement. A person with Parkinson's may sit in one position for a long time without moving. Or the patient may find it difficult to start walking.

Bradykinesia may lead to the loss of facial expression. This is not a sign of an emotional problem, but a loss of activity in the nerves that control the facial muscles. The link between emotions and facial expressions is instinctive: expressions don't require conscious thought. In Parkinson's, a patient may have natural emotional responses, and not be aware that his or her face is not showing those feelings.

A parkinsonian patient may also have flat, expressionless speech. About half of Parkinson's disease patients experience such problems as loss of volume, difficulty beginning to speak, or inability to speak clearly. Again, these are not emotional problems, but a loss of normally spontaneous activity of the nerves and muscles.

A third characteristic of Parkinson's disease is *rigidity*. This symptom may not be as obvious to patients as is tremor. They may be aware only of a certain amount of stiffness when they move their arms or legs. But if another person tells a patient to relax and then tries to move the patient's arm, the movements will be ratchet-like: resistance, followed by a quick short movement, then rigidity again. The result is a series of short, jerky motions, as though the arm is being moved by a gear.

A major principle in the body is that all muscles have an opposing muscle. Movement is possible not just because one muscle becomes more active, but because the opposing muscle relaxes. It may be a disturbance of this dynamic balance that causes rigidity.

Parkinsonian patients may also experience other motor problems. For instance, the posture may become stooped with the shoulders bent forward. When the person is standing at rest, the arms may not hang down in the normal way, but may bend upward from the elbow.

Telltale signs

To an experienced neurologist the diagnosis of Parkinson's disease is usually obvious. Shakiness is part of several other diseases, but the special quality of the parkinsonian tremor—that it becomes worse after a few seconds of resting the hand—is very characteristic. By the time the patient has decided to seek medical help, other symptoms are usually also present. The neurologist can put the tremor together with the lack of spontaneous facial expression, flat speech, and the patient's unusual stillness while sitting, and arrive at a fairly certain diagnosis. Peculiar handwriting, which becomes smaller and more cramped after the first few written words, is also a strong clue.

The ability to make a diagnosis almost solely on the basis of clinical signs is fortunate, since there are no sophisticated tests for Parkinson's disease. In about 10 percent of the suspected cases of this illness, there may be some hesitation about making a diagnosis at the first visit. But with time the telltale signs of parkinsonism almost always appear.

As the disease worsens

Without treatment, Parkinson's disease becomes progressively more severe and disabling. But different patients experience different rates of disease progression. It is generally agreed, however, that with current treatments, many parkinsonian patients enjoy a normal life span.

The course of the disease is variable. With time, patients whose symptoms appeared only on one side of the body may have movement problems on the other side as well. On the other hand, cases of one-sided parkinsonism with no further development of movement problems are well known.

The patient may also begin to experience certain annoying problems, such as drooling. This comes from the difficulty in swallowing due to decreased function of the throat muscles. This swallowing problem can also make eating difficult, and can lead to choking if the patient is not careful. To some extent the patient can control this problem by eating slowly and swallowing often.

There may also be overproduction of the normal oily coating of the skin, a condition called seborrhea. Its cause is poorly understood. The condition is not dangerous, but does require extra care.

The more serious symptoms of advanced Parkinson's disease are aggravations of the movement problems, such as a severe loss of the sense of balance, sometimes compounded by loss of the normal armswing that we all use to maintain our walking rhythm. The short steps characteristic of a parkinsonian patient's walk are an attempt to compensate for lost stability.

With a failing sense of balance, the parkinsonian patient may develop a slight forward lean. This leaning causes a shift in the body's center of gravity, and the patient may take a series of quick, small steps forward to "catch up" with the changed gravity center. This stepping forward is the symptom called *festination*. Another problem—a backward lean—may also appear. When bumped from the front or when starting to walk, patients with this problem have a tendency to step backwards. This is known as *retropulsion*, and usually accompanies only fairly advanced disease. When either one of these symptoms appears, the use of lifts on shoes or a tripod cane can be helpful.

Late in the course of Parkinson's disease, the patient's loss of spontaneous movements may worsen. When severe, such bradykinesia results in periods when the person is completely unable to start movements. These "frozen states" are called *akinesia*. This loss of voluntary movement affects walking most dramatically.

A peculiar feature of these frozen states is that they may be triggered by situations or objects, such as an open doorway or a line drawn on the floor. Or patients may "freeze" when caught in crowds. Since this difficulty is partly psychological, personal support can be of considerable help. A hand or arm quietly offered to a parkinsonian patient experiencing akinesia can be all he or she needs to get going again. On the other hand, if a companion becomes agitated or obviously embarrassed by the patient's condition, the frozen state may get worse.

It is important to remember that most patients with Parkinson's disease continue to think clearly. Late in the course of the illness some patients do suffer loss of mental skills. They may become forgetful, have trouble calculating or counting money, and may lose their way when going between familiar places. These are symptoms of the disorder known as *dementia*. (Dementia does not mean wild behavior or emotional outbursts, as it is sometimes popularly understood, but only refers to loss of mental abilities.) How many parkinsonian patients undergo these losses is not clear, but it is interesting that James Parkinson did not include dementia in his original description of the disease.

Parkinsonian patients may also feel depressed. Some neurologists have suggested that depression is a result of the disease process, but this idea is still controversial. Another possibility is that the depression is simply "a realistic reaction to a progressive, crippling illness," as one clinician expressed it.

Parkinsonism symptoms themselves are not fatal. Patients most often die of an illness acquired while confined to bed during the latter stages of the disease. Loss of muscle tone makes coughing difficult, so the lungs are not effectively cleared and the patient becomes susceptible to pneumonia. Lying in bed also makes the patient susceptible to blood clots in the legs that can travel to the lungs and be fatal. Another problem is urinary tract infections, which can spread to the blood. Clearly, good nursing care of the bedridden parkinsonian patient is important.

Brain changes in Parkinson patients

In the early 1960's, research scientists were excited to discover several changes in specific areas of brains taken from deceased Parkinson's disease patients. These observations led to an important insight into the basis for Parkinson's disease: Parkinson patients cannot control their movements because of a deficiency in the part of the brain that produces smooth, directed muscle activity.

The scientists saw that certain pigmented nerve cells were lost from a region of the brain known as the basal ganglia, which appears to be responsible for the dynamic balance of opposing muscles mentioned earlier. This loss of nerve cells (or neurons) occurred in patients with longstanding Parkinson's disease, and was most evident in the substantia nigra ("black substance," so called because the cells in this area are dark), a part of the basal ganglia thought to adjust nerve signals passing to the muscles from the command centers of the brain.

In addition, all regions of the basal ganglia were deficient in a normal brain substance called dopamine, a chemical messenger that transmits signals from one nerve cell to another. Dopamine is made by the pigmented cells of the substantia nigra, the same neurons that are greatly reduced in parkinsonism. Since these cells send fibers throughout the basal ganglia, much like a tree sending out roots, loss of cells from the substantia nigra lowers the supply of dopamine in nearby areas as well.

Without dopamine, the nerve cells in the basal ganglia are like a team of astronauts with no radios in their spacesuits—they are ready for action but they can't communicate. As a result the nerve cells can't cooperate to fine-tune the signals flowing to the muscles.

This conclusion is supported by experiments in animals showing that dopamine loss in the brain leads to abnormal movement. An even more convincing observation is that the extent of loss of dopamine nerve cells found at autopsy is related to the severity of patients' symptoms, especially akinesia and tremor.

What causes Parkinson's disease?

In a small number of parkinsonism cases, a specific cause can be identified. Carbon monoxide and manganese poisoning may produce parkinsonism, as can certain drugs used to treat psychiatric illness. Parkinsonism caused by psychiatric drugs disappears when the drugs are withdrawn.

But the vast majority of cases of parkinsonism are "idiopathic," meaning that no cause is known. Even the finding that specific nerve cells are lost in the brains of parkinsonian patients has not led scientists to the cause of the disease.

Brain research has provided one important clue, however. Even persons who die early in the course of Parkinson's disease have advanced damage to their dopamine-containing nerve cells. This implies that the disease is the result of a gradual decay process that starts long before symptoms appear. So the search for the first event in the course of Parkinson's disease must involve persons in their forties, thirties, or earlier, when the unseen stages of the disease probably begin.

Treatment

Therapy of Parkinson's disease has involved both surgery and drug treatment. Many patients also benefit from exercises, which may provide added strength to help combat movement problems.

The only operation that has been of value for Parkinson's disease was a procedure called cryothalamotomy, or "destruction of the thalamus by cold." In the most successful form of this procedure, a probe cooled with liquid nitrogen was placed into a part of the brain called the thalamus. Guided by a framework around the patient's head, the probe touched only very specific areas of the brain. Nerve cells in these areas were destroyed by the supercooled metal tip of the probe.

This operation successfully stopped the tremor in many patients. Unfortunately, it did little to help the rigidity and loss of spontaneous movement that are the more disabling symptoms of Parkinson's disease.

Cryothalamotomy had another drawback. When performed on both sides of the thalamus (which was necessary to stop tremor on both sides of the body), the surgery itself could produce neurologic damage. Today, with the development of effective drug therapies, cryothalamotomy is seldom performed except in severe cases of unstoppable tremor or movement disorder.

Drug therapy

After James Parkinson clearly delineated the illness that bears his name, many chemicals were tested against it. These included fish-poison bark, strychnine, arsenic, and turpentine. It is not surprising that several classes of drugs were found that had at least some mild benefit for parkinsonian patients. Extracts from the belladonna plant, for example, were used against Parkinson's disease until the 1940's. But effective control of all symptoms was not possible until the drug levodopa was introduced in the 1960's.

The success of levodopa—sometimes called L-dopa—in treating the symptoms of Parkinson's disease has been one of the triumphs of modern research. After dopamine nerve pathways were shown to be depleted in persons with parkinsonian symptoms, several scientists tried to restore normal function by administering levodopa, a natural brain chemical that nerve cells can use to make dopamine. (Dopamine itself could not be given because it does not enter the brain.)

In initial studies, levodopa caused many patients to vomit. But in 1967 a New York neurologist showed that starting with small doses and slowly increasing the dosage overcame this problem. When doctors were able to gradually give higher doses of levodopa, their patients' conditions improved greatly.

Both rigidity and tremor were greatly reduced. But most important, levodopa reduced the most disabling symptom of the disease, bradykinesia, the difficulty in starting movements. No previous medication had controlled this problem.

Still, in the first few years of levodopa use little more than half of the patients improved. In the other patients, side effects made it impossible to give a high enough dose to reduce the symptoms. Besides nausea, patients experienced movements called *dyskinesias,* which are undirected involuntary movements. Some also suffered heart problems and others had dangerous drops in blood pressure.

The next major advance was the development of drugs that stopped levodopa from changing to dopamine before it reached the brain. These drugs, called "extracerebral decarboxylase inhibitors," include carbidopa and benserazide. When levodopa is kept from changing before it reaches the brain, nausea is reduced. Low blood pressure and heart problems are also avoided. With a decarboxylase inhibitor, many patients can reduce the number of levodopa pills they need, and full doses of levodopa can be reached in weeks instead of months. Carbidopa or benserazide is now combined with levodopa in most medicines.

With today's levodopa treatment, symptoms are reduced in about three of every four parkinsonian patients. The patients also remain independent longer, and many live out a normal life span.

In some cases, however, patients experience involuntary movements from the levodopa treatment, and others have mental symptoms. Reducing the dosage sometimes lowers these side effects. But this means that the doctor must be very skilled in adjusting the levodopa amount to improve symptoms while avoiding bad effects. The doctor must also be aware that certain drugs given for other illnesses can defeat the effect of levodopa.

Eventually, however, the benefits of levodopa may wear off. In about half of the patients with Parkinson's disease, several troubling problems are likely to appear suddenly after three to five years of successful levodopa control.

One of these problems is called the "on-off" reaction. The patient may alternate between dyskinesia (uncontrolled movements) and akinesia (lack of movement), switching back and forth between these states every few seconds or minutes.

A second problem is "end-of-dose akinesia," or the quick return of parkinsonian symptoms three to four hours after taking a dose of levodopa.

Some doctors think that these problems are due to the relentless advance of parkinsonism. But not all agree. One doctor who treats parkinsonian patients determined how long each benefited from levodopa therapy. If the reduced effectiveness of levodopa is due to progression of the disease, then the patients who had less severe symptoms at the start of treatment should have been helped by levodopa longer. But this was not so.

Instead, he found that patients who took the highest doses of levodopa lost the benefit of the drug soonest. The doctor suggested that giving high doses of levodopa may lower its effectiveness.

This theory is by no means proven. But it has led to two possible methods of prolonging the period of levodopa's effectiveness.

The first is to begin treatment with less powerful drugs, reserving levodopa for the more advanced stages of the disease. When levodopa is started, frequent small doses are given.

One class of drugs that is used first is called anticholinergic agents. These drugs were the main treatment for Parkinson's disease from the early 1940's until the introduction of levodopa. Some of the most common anticholinergic drugs are trihexyphenidyl (Artane®), benztropine mesylate (Cogentin®), and biperiden (Akineton®). They are helpful against tremor and rigidity, but do not affect bradykinesia. Antihistamines such as diphenhydramine (Benadryl®) are weaker anticholinergic agents.

Another drug that could be used for early parkinsonism is amantadine hydrochloride (Symmetrel®), which was first used to treat and prevent respiratory virus infections. Amantadine also produces modest improvement in tremor and rigidity, plus some reduction of bradykinesia.

A second method for coping with the problems of continued levodopa therapy is the so-called drug holiday. This is a period of three to seven days or more during which the patient is hospitalized and taken off levodopa completely. This hospitalization may be preceded by a period of gradually decreasing doses of levodopa at home. Hospitalized patients must be watched closely, especially if their disease has progressed to the point of affecting their breathing muscles. During the drug-free period, some patients participate in physical, occupational, and speech therapy programs to reduce the hazards of stopping the medication.

A number of doctors have had success with the drug holiday. They find that many patients can resume levodopa therapy without on-off problems or end-of-dose akinesia. Some patients can even benefit from lower doses than they were taking before the drug holiday. This method is still being tested.

Physical therapy

Besides drug treatment, many doctors prescribe muscle-strengthening exercises for their parkinsonian patients. These include exercises for speaking, swallowing, and overall muscle tone.

Exercise will not stop disease progression, but may provide a stronger body so that the patient may be less disabled by movement problems. Exercise can also improve the emotional well-being of parkinsonian patients.

As one doctor puts it, "I include physical therapy with a professional therapist as a standard part of my prescription. You are not doing anything fundamental to the disease, but you are bringing the patient's motor function to an optimal level."

Needed: support and understanding

One of the most damaging aspects of Parkinson's disease is its demoralizing effect. The patient's world is completely changed. Emotional support and understanding are needed to encourage the patient to remain as active as possible.

Parkinson's disease can also separate patients from their families. "This disease puts a terrible strain on families," says one neurologist who has treated many parkinsonian patients. One problem is that normal family relationships are changed and traditional expectations are turned upside-down.

A man used to supporting his family for years may find that he can no longer do his job. "I have to work two jobs to support us and pay for John's medical bills," said the wife of a parkinsonian patient. While the wife is working, the daughter must stay home to watch her partially disabled dad. These limitations and demands can create resentment in even the most closely knit families.

One older woman who lived alone after her husband died refused to accept the limitations of her Parkinson's disease. "I've had a terrible time with her," said her adult daughter. The patient refused to accept help even though her disease progressed and she fell and broke a hip.

After some time in a nursing home she is returning to her house, but still wants to live alone. Naturally this causes the daughter intense worry.

This situation may not be uncommon. One doctor believes that falling has replaced pneumonia as the greatest danger to parkinsonian patients. Levodopa therapy allows patients to walk around but does not completely reverse their impaired balance. If they are not cautious, they can easily fall.

For patients and their families, support groups can be a great help. At meetings, people learn ways of dealing with their problems. But, more important, they can talk to other people who understand the difficulties they are having.

Such an outlet can be important in relieving the frustrations that both patients and families feel. Parkinsonian patients can do many things for themselves, but they are often very slow. When a patient goes to a store or for a walk, the companion should not try to hurry the impaired person along. Even eating or speaking can be better managed if other people don't become impatient.

Another problem faced by families is the suspicion that a person with parkinsonism is "faking it." They may think, "Why is he so capable sometimes and so helpless at other times?" Talking with support groups will show them that this is a normal feature of the disease.

These groups can also help members learn about financial and support services. The parkinsonian patient with advanced disease may need custodial care, and support groups can help the family decide which options best suit its financial and personal situation.

Finding answers through research

Finding ways to treat, cure, and prevent Parkinson's disease requires carefully planned programs of scientific research. Subtle changes in parkinsonian brains must be uncovered, and new drugs to supplement or replace levodopa are needed.

One promising area of Parkinson's disease research involves studying the brain with a new imaging system called positron emission tomography (PET). PET produces pictures of chemical changes taking place in the brain or elsewhere in the body. For instance, PET can show how much sugar or oxygen various parts of the brain are using for energy, as a person performs an action like reading or listening to music.

According to Dr. Donald Tower, former director of the National Institute of Neurological and Communicative Disorders and Stroke, "With PET we will be able to see the development of brain lesions and look for functional differences in patients with neurological disorders." Such changes may be an early sign of the more obvious brain damage that shows up in the brains of Parkinson patients at autopsy.

Because the NINCDS believes so strongly in the research potential of this new technique, it established a national PET Research Program: major research centers around the country, including a center at its own research facility in Bethesda, Maryland, all working to perfect the technique and utilizing it to conquer neurological disease.

One group of NINCDS scientists is using PET to study parkinsonian patients who have symptoms only on one side of the body. The scientists hope to find differences between the two sides of the brain in these patients. This would further define which parts of the brain give rise to parkinsonism.

Studies like these may show other areas of the brain besides the basal ganglia that are not functioning correctly. This could provide new targets for drug therapy that can bring even greater benefit to parkinsonian patients.

Promising new drugs

Searching for new treatments for parkinsonism, NINCDS-supported scientists at the Illinois Institute of Technology have tried chemically attaching levodopa to the metals copper and zinc. In animal tests, these combinations sent more levodopa to the brain than the combination of levodopa with carbidopa or benserazide. If the same result is found in parkinsonian patients, the side effects of levodopa therapy could be reduced. It could also be possible to prolong the drug's period of effectiveness by allowing lower amounts to be used.

A second approach has been to combine levodopa with a specific type of drug that blocks the action of dopamine. Dopamine may act at several sites in the brain, perhaps reducing parkinsonian symptoms at the basal ganglia while causing dyskinesias at another site. One group of British doctors using the new L-dopa/dopamine ''blocker'' combination has reported improvements in parkinsonian symptoms and reduced dyskinesias.

Improved delivery of dopamine to the brain has also been tried by a radical new technique: implantation of a small number of cells from the adrenal gland into the brain. The adrenal gland, located on top of the kidney, contains some cells that make dopamine. A group of Swedish doctors recently placed some of these cells into the brain of a parkinsonian patient. According to one NINCDS scientist, this is ''a very exciting area,'' but the procedure is still experimental.

Perhaps the most promising group of new drugs is a class called dopamine agonists. Agonists are substances which produce effects similar to the effects of certain naturally occurring chemicals. Rather than increasing the amount of dopamine in the brain, as levodopa does, dopamine agonists mimic dopamine's activity in the brain. NINCDS scientists have taken the lead in selecting the dopamine agonists that are most promising for human trials and in evaluating the first treatment attempts. One of these drugs, bromocriptine, was introduced to clinical Parkinson's disease research in the United States in 1981. Several others, including pergolide and lisuride, are now being tested in parkinsonian patients.

Whether dopamine agonists should be used as a first treatment or after levodopa has lost its effectiveness has yet to be worked out. It is also possible that the best course will be to combine low doses of a dopamine agonist with low doses of levodopa. However they are used, it seems clear that one or two of this new class of agents will have a large role in future treatment of parkinsonian symptoms.

Another experimental substance soon to be tested in parkinsonian patients is called tetrahydrobiopterin. This chemical occurs naturally in the human brain and is necessary for nerve cells to make dopamine. NINCDS scientists have found that tetrahydrobiopterin is reduced in parkinsonian patients. These investigators plan to find out if giving the chemical to parkinsonian patients improves dopamine production and reduces symptoms.

NINCDS scientists are also testing the element lithium in parkinsonian patients who have developed on-off reactions after taking levodopa for a long time. On-off reactions are thought to be due to extreme sensitivity of the sites where dopamine acts. In animal experiments, lithium lowered this sensitivity. If lithium also lowers sensitivity to dopamine in the human brain, it could possibly eliminate on-off reactions while allowing levodopa to relieve symptoms.

Hope for the future

Research progress in drug treatment and improving technologies for exploring the brain are encouraging advances for thousands of Parkinson's disease patients. The promise of research and the support of generous families, friends, and volunteers sustain them in their fight against Parkinson's disease, and give them hope.

Human tissue banks

The study of brain tissue from persons with neurological disorders is invaluable in research, especially in conditions like Parkinson's disease where the cause is obscure. NINCDS supports two national specimen banks, one in Los Angeles and one near Boston. For information about tissue donation and collection write:

Dr. Wallace W. Tourtellotte, Director
Human Neurospecimen Bank
VA Wadsworth Hospital Center
Los Angeles, Calif. 90073

Dr. Edward D. Bird, Director
Brain Tissue Bank, Mailman Research Center
McLean Hospital
115 Mill Street
Belmont, Mass. 02178

Voluntary organizations

The following organizations are devoted to research, care, treatment, and ultimate prevention of Parkinson's disease. They also work to increase public awareness of the disorder, and to provide Parkinson's disease patients and families with assistance and support. For information write:

American Parkinson Disease Association
116 John Street
New York, N.Y. 10038
(212) 732-9550

National Parkinson Foundation, Inc.
1501 N.W. Ninth Avenue
Miami, Fla. 33136
(305) 547-6666

Parkinson's Disease Foundation
William Black Medical Research Building
640 West 168th Street
New York, N.Y. 10032
(212) 923-4700

United Parkinson Foundation
220 South State Street
Chicago, Ill. 60604
(312) 922-9734

Parkinson Support Groups of America
11376 Cherry Hill Road, Apt. 204
Beltsville, Md. 20705
(301) 937-1545

Bibliography

Other booklets on Parkinson's disease are available from the following sources:

American Parkinson Disease Association
A Manual for Patients with Parkinson's Disease

Home Exercises for Patients with Parkinson's Disease

Speech Problems and Swallowing Problems in Parkinson's Disease

Aids, Equipment and Suggestions to Help the Patients with Parkinson's Disease in the Activities of Daily Living

National Parkinson Foundation, Inc.
What the Patient Should Know About Parkinson's Disease

Psychological Factors in the Management of Parkinson's Disease

Parkinson's Disease Foundation
The Parkinson Patient at Home

Parkinson's Disease: Progress, Promise and Hope!

Exercises for the Parkinson Patient With Hints for Daily Living

United Parkinson Foundation
One Step at a Time (an exercise manual)

Other:
Bourke-White, Margaret (1963): *Portrait of Myself.* Simon and Schuster, New York, N.Y. (This now out-of-print book describes the famous photographer's life with parkinsonism.)

Dorros, Sidney (1982): *Parkinson's: A Patient's View.* Seven Locks Press, Inc., P.O. Box 72, Cabin John, Md. 20818. (A personal account of one man's 20-year struggle with Parkinson's Disease.)

Duvoisin, Roger C. (1978): *Parkinson's Disease: A Guide for Patient and Family.* Raven Press, 1140 Avenue of the Americas, New York, N.Y. 10036.

Stern, Gerald and Lees, Andrew (1982): *Parkinson's Disease: The Facts.* Oxford University Press, 200 Madison Avenue, New York, N.Y. 10016.

Prepared by the Office of Scientific and Health Reports, National Institute of Neurological and Communicative Disorders and Stroke. National Institutes of Health, Bethesda, Maryland 20205. NIH Publication No. 83–139, June 1983.

Prostate

Problems

The prostate is a small organ about the size of a walnut. It is located next to the bladder (where urine is stored) and surrounds the urethra (the canal through which urine passes out of the body). During sexual activity it secretes fluid which helps transport sperm.

Prostate problems are common in men over 50. Because it surrounds the urethra, an enlarged prostate can make urination difficult. Most problems can be treated effectively without harming sexual function.

Common prostate problems

Acute Prostatitis a bacterial infection of the prostate, is relatively uncommon but can occur in men at any age. Symptoms include fever, chills, painful or difficult urination, and pain in the lower back and between the legs. It can usually be treated successfully with antibiotics.

Chronic Prostatitis is a recurring prostate infection. The symptoms are similar to those of acute prostatitis but are usually milder. Fever is uncommon. Chronic prostatitis can be difficult to treat. Antibiotics, which may be used for up to three months, are often effective when the infection is due to bacteria. Sometimes no disease-causing bacteria can be found. In some of these cases, massaging the prostate to release fluids is helpful. Often the condition clears up by itself, but symptoms may last a long time.

Benign Prostatic Hypertrophy (BPH) is an enlargement of the prostate. It is caused by small noncancerous tumors which grow inside the prostate. It is not known what causes these growths, but they may be related to hormone changes with aging.

An enlarged prostate may eventually obstruct the urethra and cause difficulty urinating. Dribbling after urination and the urge to urinate frequently, even at night, are common symptoms. In rare cases, the patient is unable to urinate.

A doctor usually can detect an enlarged prostate by rectal exam. The doctor may also measure how much urine is left in the bladder after urination, since even small amounts can cause infections and possibly kidney damage. This is done by injecting a safe dye into a vein. The dye eventually appears in the urine remaining in the bladder and causes it to show up on an X-ray. The doctor may also examine the prostate and bladder by inserting an instrument called a cystoscope into the penis.

Drugs have not yet been successful in treating BPH. In severe cases surgery may be necessary to remove the overgrown portion of the prostate.

Prostate cancer

In the early stages of prostate cancer the disease stays localized (in the prostate) and does not endanger life. But without treatment the cancer can spread to other tissues and eventually cause death. Prostate cancer usually progresses very slowly.

Regular physical checkups that include a rectal exam increase the chances of detecting prostate cancer before symptoms appear and in its early, most curable stages. When symptoms do appear, they are usually similar to those caused by BPH.

A urologist (a specialist in diseases of the urinary system) is the best qualified doctor to diagnose and treat prostate cancer. If a suspicious area is found in the prostate, the urologist may recommend a biopsy (a simple surgical procedure in which a tiny piece of prostate tissue is removed with a needle and examined under a microscope). If the biopsy shows prostate cancer, other tests may be done to determine the type of treatment necessary. When the cancer is confined to the prostate, the cure rate is high. Even when the cancer is more advanced, it is still often possible to control it for long periods of time.[*]

Prostate surgery

Prostate surgery is often done to treat BPH and prostate cancer. Such surgery is generally safe and patients usually recover rapidly.

For BPH, it is common to remove only the portions of the prostate obstructing the urethra. This is sometimes called a simple prostatectomy. It does not damage the nerves which cause erection of the penis and men can usually resume normal sexual activity soon after the operation. However, a few men may experience problems, often psychological, that can lead to impotence. In these cases, counseling can help restore confidence and normal sexual functioning.

A transurethral resection of the prostate (TURP) is the most common procedure for slightly or moderately enlarged prostates. An instrument inserted in the penis trims away the excess tissue, which is flushed out through the penis. A catheter (tube) remains in the bladder for several days to drain out urine during healing. Since no incision is made through the skin, the patient usually recovers rapidly. After this operation, semen

---

[*] For more information about prostate cancer, write to the National Cancer Institute, Bldg. 31, Rm. 10A18, Bethesda, MD 20205.

released during sexual activity may flow into the bladder rather than out of the penis, but the sensation of orgasm will be the same.

When the prostate is very enlarged, an incision is made in the abdomen to remove the prostate growths. This surgery is somewhat more uncomfortable for the patient, but the long-term effects generally are the same as with TURP.

During surgery for prostate cancer the entire prostate and adjacent structures may be removed. This is called a radical prostatectomy. Many patients are impotent after this surgery, but special prosthetic devices inserted into the penis can restore the ability to have an erection. New surgical techniques are being developed to preserve the nerves going to the penis so that the patient will be able to have an erection after prostate removal.

Incontinence, the inability to hold urine, is a rare complication after surgery for BPH but is common just after radical surgery for cancer. Fortunately, most men regain urinary control within several weeks and only a few continue to have problems that require them to wear a device to collect urine.

Protecting yourself

The best protection against prostate problems is having regular medical checkups that include a careful prostate exam. See a doctor promptly if unusual symptoms occur, such as a frequent urge to urinate, difficulty in urinating, or dribbling. Waiting until severe symptoms appear may result in serious and sometimes life-threatening complications. Regular checkups are important for all men, even those who have had previous surgery for BPH. BPH surgery does not protect against prostate cancer since only part of the prostate is removed.

U.S. Department of Health and Human Services, Public Health Service, National Institutes of Health. U.S. Government Printing Office: 1983—418–428.

Rheumatic Fever
Down But Not Out

Just a few years ago rheumatic fever was described as a vanishing disease. Children's hospitals devoted solely to the care of rheumatic fever victims closed their doors forever because of lack of patients; registries maintained by some states to track the disease were allowed to languish. But sometimes you can't keep a bad disease down. Rheumatic fever—with its risk of serious heart complications—has reappeared in some parts of the country, and in a particularly virulent form.

Though this reemergence of a disease once thought to be mostly conquered worries physicians, the few hundred cases that have been reported in the current epidemic are still a small blip in the statistics compared to the incidence of rheumatic fever in days gone by. Up until the 1940s, an estimated 250,000 Americans developed rheumatic fever every year.

Much of the credit for eliminating this scourge goes to a team of medical researchers who conducted a clinical study at the end of World War II. Their efforts saved future generations of children and young adults, both here and throughout the rest of the world, from the effects of a sometimes savage disease.

The study took place at Fort Francis E. Warren, an Air Force technical training base in southeastern Wyoming. Its purpose was to determine whether acute rheumatic fever could be prevented by treating upper respiratory strep infections ("strep throat") with penicillin.

Rheumatic fever gets its name from two of its most common symptoms—joint pains and fever. When rheumatic fever develops, it appears a few weeks after a strep throat, usually when the patient seems to be fully recovered. In children, the illness often begins with a fever—sometimes as high as 104 degrees Fahrenheit in the first few days—that may last as long as two weeks. Rheumatism often follows.

In the 1940s, streptococcal disease was a major health problem both in the general population, where it was known as an "occupational disease of school children," and in the military. Over 7,000 servicemen developed rheumatic fever each year after such infections, spread by respiratory droplets and often reaching epidemic proportions in Army camps. In some cases, rheumatic fever led to the most feared complications—carditis (inflammation of the heart) and heart valve damage. Not only was the disease expensive to treat, but the armed services were compelled to discharge those who were left with serious disabilities.

The Air Force investigators were a group of enthusiastic physicians in charge of the streptococcal disease laboratory at Fort Warren. The subjects were over 1,600 Air Force trainees, divided into two groups; those whose serial numbers ended in an even digit were the treated group. When they reported to the hospital with strep throat or tonsillitis, they got an injection of penicillin—a drug that had been available for only a few years and whose effectiveness in treating strep throat for the prevention of rheumatic fever was not known.

Trainees with serial numbers ending in an odd number received treatment for their symptoms, but no antibiotic, because they constituted—in research language—the control group.

Of the 798 trainees who were treated with penicillin, only two developed rheumatic fever. Of the 804 men in the control group, 17 came down with the disease, a statistically significant difference. Thus, administering an adequate amount of penicillin resulted in over a 90 percent reduction in the occurrence of initial attacks of rheumatic fever. This proved to the researchers that penicillin therapy for strep throat infections would almost completely prevent the subsequent development of rheumatic fever. It also won for them the Lasker Award in medicine, one of the most prestigious awards for medical research.

The results of the study filtered over into civilian medicine and eventually changed the way doctors dealt with upper respiratory tract infections in children. Before the study, according to Dr. Milton Markowitz (writing in *The Journal of Pediatrics,* April 1985), doctors rarely took a throat culture to determine what was causing a sore throat unless diphtheria was suspected. Strep throats did not get special attention unless they were accompanied by a scarlet rash (scarlet fever). Drugs, such as sulfa and penicillin, were prescribed for these infections, but only for three or four days, not long enough to knock out the bacteria. But by 1970, says Dr. Markowitz, doctors throughout the country were routinely using throat cultures to diagnose strep infections. What's more, they were administering injections of long-acting penicillin or prescribing oral penicillin for a minimum of 10 days (or erythromycin for those allergic to penicillin), enough to cure the infection.

People, especially children, still get as many strep throats as they ever did, but because they're usually properly diagnosed and treated, acute rheumatic fever develops so infrequently now that many young U.S. doctors have never seen a case of it. Penicillin and throat cultures are not the only heroes of this public health triumph, however. Other factors undoubtedly contributed to this decline, because the incidence of rheumatic fever was decreasing even before the discovery of antibiotics. In the United States, Western Europe and Japan, a better standard of living—with less crowding in the home, better diets, better health care for low-income families—and possibly less virulent strains of streptococcal bacteria may have had an effect.

Dr. Helen Taussig, a renowned pediatric cardiologist, said in an interview in *Medical Times* in November 1978: "I don't think there's any question that penicillin controlled rheumatic fever. But when we learned not to put all of the children in one bed together, and with less poverty and more food—that too helped bring down the incidence of rheumatic fever. Getting the child who was infected and loaded with strep out of the household also helped."

As a result, in affluent societies such as ours, rheumatic fever has just about disappeared. In a *New England Journal of Medicine* editorial (Feb. 19, 1987), titled "Acute Rheumatic Fever: Forgotten but Not Gone," Alan Bisno, M.D., University of Tennessee College of Medicine, wrote: "The decline in the incidence of acute rheumatic fever in North America and Western Europe since the end of World War II has been truly phenomenal. Indeed in the past 20 years alone, the annual incidence rate among school-age children in major cities has dropped by more than 90 percent." New cases occur mostly among the poor or those who do not receive adequate medical attention. (It is difficult to estimate the number of cases that occur annually in the United States because the disease is not now required to be reported to public health officials, and it is often undiagnosed.)

But, obviously, while rheumatic fever is not the threat it used to be, it can't be counted out—not yet, anyway. A recent outbreak in Utah, as well as reports of new cases in Pennsylvania, Ohio, Texas, and other parts of the United States, attest to this fact.

The Utah epidemic is particularly serious. While, on average, only six cases a year were referred to physicians at Primary Children's Medical Center in Salt Lake City from 1975 to 1985, in the 18-month period from January 1985 to June 1986, 74 cases were referred. Since that time there have been almost as many more. Surprisingly, the children who developed rheumatic fever came not from poor, minority neighborhoods, but mostly from white families with above average incomes and good access to medical care. But crowding in the home may have been a factor in the epidemic. The children's families averaged twice as large (6.5 members) as other Utah families, and the majority of the children shared bedrooms with other family members.

Over 90 percent of the Utah children suffered from heart inflammation, a higher than normal rate for this complication. Thirteen children who had cardiac involvement suffered from congestive heart failure. Two of them needed artificial heart valve replacements. "We don't know why there was such a high incidence of heart damage in this sudden outbreak. It may be that particularly virulent strains of streptococci are being introduced into the population. This is of concern to biomedical scientists and clinicians, and we are looking into this possibility," says Edward L. Kaplan, M.D., head of the World Health Organization Collaborating Center for Reference and Research on Streptococci, Department of Pediatrics, University of Minnesota Medical School.

"The current outbreak is quite worrisome," Dr. Kaplan continues. "We have to rethink our current methods of control. Diseases are best controlled when we know exactly how they are caused. We know that rheumatic fever results from the strep infection, but we don't know how. This outbreak points out the need for additional intensive study and research of its epidemiology, microbiology, immunology, diagnosis, and therapy.''

While this rise in the number of cases alarms public health authorities, the incidence here is no match for that in developing countries, where about four-fifths of the world's population resides. There, rheumatic fever continues to rage unabated. Each year, rheumatic fever still "bites the heart and licks the joints" of 15 million to 20 million people, and is the leading cause of death from heart disease in those from 5 to 30 years of age. In Brazil, about 10 percent of school children have hearts damaged by rheumatic fever. In India, rheumatic heart disease accounts for 35 percent of all heart disease in a population of over 500 million.

As Dr. Kaplan noted, rheumatic fever is still not completely understood by physicians. It is not an infection in itself, but may follow an upper respiratory infection caused by certain strep bacteria—group A beta-hemolytic streptococci (*S. pyogenes*). Strep throats are contagious, but rheumatic fever is not. While antibiotics will usually prevent rheumatic fever from developing in the first place (as was conclusively demonstrated by the Air Force studies), they won't cure it.

The disease presents other paradoxes. A mild, untreated strep throat may lead to rheumatic fever, while a severe one may not. More than a third of patients with acute rheumatic fever don't remember having had a previous sore throat at all. (In the Utah epidemic, *two-thirds* of the children had no clear-cut history of a sore throat in the three months before the appearance of the disease.) Though some attacks of rheumatic fever can result in fatal heart damage—almost 13,000 deaths from rheumatic heart disease were reported in 1975—others produce no adverse effects. Also, unlike many other infectious diseases, in which one attack confers lifelong immunity, rheumatic fever can recur with subsequent strep throats.

Another insidious side of rheumatic fever is that some people can have an acute attack with heart damage and not be aware of it. The damage is discovered much later, sometimes by accident. In fact, many adults found to have rheumatic heart damage have no memory of a rheumatic fever attack. The disease wasn't detected in the first place because they didn't feel sick enough to go to the doctor. Some children have neither fever nor rheumatism, making diagnosis difficult. Also lacking is a specific lab test for the disease.

These problems have led physicians to rely on certain criteria set up by Harvard's Dr. T. Duckett Jones in the 1940s (and later revised by the American Heart Association) for differentiating between rheumatic fever and childhood rheumatoid arthritis, gout, acute appendicitis, sickle-cell anemia, and other diseases with similar symptoms.

Jones Criteria for Diagnosing Acute Rheumatic Fever

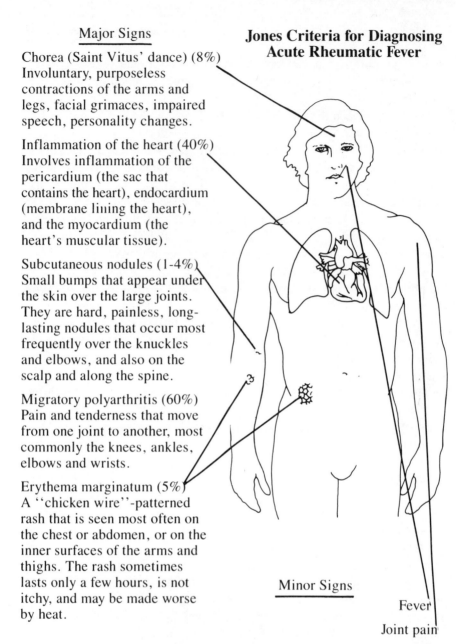

Major Signs

Chorea (Saint Vitus' dance) (8%) Involuntary, purposeless contractions of the arms and legs, facial grimaces, impaired speech, personality changes.

Inflammation of the heart (40%) Involves inflammation of the pericardium (the sac that contains the heart), endocardium (membrane lining the heart), and the myocardium (the heart's muscular tissue).

Subcutaneous nodules (1-4%) Small bumps that appear under the skin over the large joints. They are hard, painless, long-lasting nodules that occur most frequently over the knuckles and elbows, and also on the scalp and along the spine.

Migratory polyarthritis (60%) Pain and tenderness that move from one joint to another, most commonly the knees, ankles, elbows and wrists.

Erythema marginatum (5%) A "chicken wire"-patterned rash that is seen most often on the chest or abdomen, or on the inner surfaces of the arms and thighs. The rash sometimes lasts only a few hours, is not itchy, and may be made worse by heat.

Minor Signs

Fever

Joint pain

History of previous attacks of rheumatic fever.

Rheumatic fever can be suspected when painful arthritis follows a sore throat. When two major signs, or one major and two minor signs, are present, it is highly likely that the individual has rheumatic fever. (Percentages indicate the rate of occurrence of each sign among rheumatic fever patients.)

Adapted from Valvular Heart Disease of Rheumatic Origin, Neale D. Smith, M.D., and Jonathan Abrams, M.D., Hospital Medicine, October 1984.

Patients are likely to have rheumatic fever when two major symptoms, or one major and two minor, are present. The major symptoms are a painful form of arthritis, known as migrating polyarthritis, that travels from joint to joint (knee, ankle, elbow, wrist), and inflammation of the heart, which develops in about half of those who have the arthritis.

An unusual symptom called St. Vitus' dance, or Sydenham's chorea, may develop in about one out of 10 children up to six months after the initial attack and afflicts mostly girls who have not yet reached puberty. Facial grimaces, uncontrolled twitching of the arms and legs, clumsiness, and changes in personality are some of its features. Another uncommon major symptom is a fleeting, non-itchy, "chicken wire" rash, found on the chest and abdomen, that becomes more prominent when heat is applied to it. Painless, firm nodules that form under the skin over large joints can also develop in later stages of the illness, usually in conjunction with heart inflammation.

The minor manifestations are less specific and include fever, joint pains, and a history of previous attack of rheumatic fever. Symptoms such as evidence of prior strep infection—as shown by the strep antibody level in the blood, nosebleeds, and abdominal pain that resembles acute appendicitis—are also helpful in diagnosis. All symptoms disappear within weeks or months with no lasting ill effects, with the exception of heart valve damage.

Although what triggers rheumatic fever is known (the group A streptococcus), how strep damages the heart is still unclear. One explanation is that damage is done by toxins produced by the streptococci. Another is that an abnormal immune response by the body produces antibodies to strep bacteria that cross-react with heart tissue. These are theories that still need proof.

The heart damage takes various forms. During the acute stage of the illness, inflammation may occur in the heart's muscle tissue or in the sac that surrounds the heart, but more commonly in the heart's valves, particularly the mitral and aortic valves. When the valves heal, scar tissue makes the valves stiff, holding back the flow of blood, or preventing proper opening and closing. These irregularities in the heart's blood flow cause "murmurs" that the doctor can hear with a stethoscope.

Rheumatic fever is a double dealer. Even if the disease doesn't recur, the heart damage can get worse in time. If rheumatic fever *does* recur, the heart damage is likely to be more severe. Replacement of damaged heart valves with artificial valves is sometimes necessary.

Those who have had one attack of rheumatic fever are particularly susceptible to future ones. To prevent recurrent strep infections, doctors prescribe continuing antibiotics (mostly penicillin) for long periods— sometimes for life. It's especially important for those with rheumatic heart disease to have appropriate antibiotic prophylaxis (as suggested by the American Heart Association) before dental work or surgery, because bacteria entering the bloodstream during these procedures may infect the heart's valves or lining.

While the Air Force study proved one important point—that penicillin for strep throat is extremely effective in preventing the development of rheumatic fever—the disease continues to challenge researchers. Still to be discovered are how rheumatic fever develops, why it appears in some and not in others after a strep throat infection, how to recognize the disease when it has no symptoms, and how to identify susceptible individuals. Also waiting to be developed are drugs that will more adequately treat rheumatic fever's signs and symptoms.

Researchers are working on a vaccine to prevent streptococcal infections, but its development is hampered by the large number of different group A streptococci types. Another problem is that a vaccine must evoke protective immunity to group A streptococcal bacteria, but must be free of substances (antigens) that stimulate the production of antibodies that may cross-react with heart tissue.

Other researchers are taking another approach, as there's some preliminary evidence that susceptibility to rheumatic fever may be inherited. The goal of these scientists is to develop a blood test that would screen individuals for this genetic susceptibility, if it exists. High-risk individuals could then be identified and given priority treatment (or a vaccine, if one can be produced) when they develop strep infections.

Evelyn Zamula, *FDA Consumer*, July–August 1987.

Schizophrenia
Questions and Answers

What is it?

Schizophrenia is a term used to describe a complex, extremely puzzling condition—the most chronic and disabling of the major mental illnesses. Schizophrenia may be one disorder, or it may be many disorders, with different causes. Because of the disorder's complexity, few generalizations hold true for all people who are diagnosed as schizophrenic.

With the sudden onset of severe psychotic symptoms, the individual is said to be experiencing acute schizophrenia. "Psychotic" means out of touch with reality, or unable to separate real from unreal experiences. Some people have only one such psychotic episode; others have many episodes during a lifetime but lead relatively normal lives during the interim periods. The individual with chronic (continuous or recurring) schizophrenia often does not fully recover normal functioning and typically requires long-term treatment, generally including medication, to control the symptoms. Some chronic schizophrenic patients may never be able to function without assistance of one sort or another.

Approximately 1 percent of the population develop schizophrenia during their lives. This disorder affects men and women with equal frequency, and the information in this booklet is equally applicable to both. The first psychotic symptoms of schizophrenia are often seen in the teens or twenties in men and in the twenties or early thirties in women. Less obvious symptoms, such as social isolation or withdrawal or unusual speech, thinking, or behavior may precede and/or follow the psychotic symptoms.

Sometimes people have psychotic symptoms due to undetected medical disorders. For this reason, a medical history should be taken and a physical examination and laboratory tests should be done during hospitalization to rule out other causes of the symptoms before concluding that a person has schizophrenia.

The World of People with Schizophrenia

Unusual Realities Just as "normal" individuals view the world from their own perspectives, schizophrenic people, too, have their own perceptions of reality. Their view of the world, however, is often strikingly different from the usual reality seen and shared by those around them.

Living in a world that can appear distorted, changeable, and lacking the reliable landmarks we all use to anchor ourselves to reality, a person with schizophrenia may feel anxious and confused. This person may seem distant, detached, or preoccupied, and may even sit as rigidly as a stone, not moving for hours and not uttering a sound. Or he or she may move about constantly, always occupied, wide awake, vigilant, and alert. A schizophrenic person may exhibit very different kinds of behavior at different times.

Hallucinations The world of a schizophrenic individual may be filled with hallucinations; a person actually may sense things that in reality do not exist, such as hearing voices telling the person to do certain things, seeing people or objects that are not really there, or feeling invisible fingers touching his or her body. These hallucinations may be quite frightening. Hearing voices that other people don't hear is the most common type of hallucination in schizophrenia. Such voices may describe the patient's activities, carry on a conversation, warn of impending dangers, or tell the person what to do.

Delusions   Delusions are false personal beliefs that are not subject to reason or contradictory evidence and are not part of the person's culture. They are common symptoms of schizophrenia and can involve themes of persecution or grandeur, for example. Sometimes delusions in schizophrenia are quite bizarre—for instance, believing that a neighbor is controlling the schizophrenic individual's behavior with magnetic waves, or that people on television are directing special messages specifically at him or her, or are broadcasting the individual's thoughts aloud to other people. Delusions of persecution, which are common in paranoid schizophrenia, are false and irrational beliefs that a person is being cheated, harassed, poisoned, or conspired against. The patient may believe that he or she, or a member of the family or other group, is the focus of this imagined persecution.

Disordered Thinking   Often the schizophrenic person's thinking is affected by the disorder. The person may endure many hours of not being able to "think straight." Thoughts may come and go so rapidly that it is not possible to "catch them." The person may not be able to concentrate on one thought for very long and may be easily distracted, unable to focus attention.

The person with schizophrenia may not be able to sort out what is relevant and what is not relevant to a situation. The person may be unable to connect thoughts into logical sequences, as thoughts may become disorganized and fragmented. Jumping from topic to topic in a way that is totally confusing to others may result.

This lack of logical continuity of thought, termed "thought disorder," can make conversation very difficult and contribute to social isolation. If people cannot make sense of what an individual is saying, they are likely to become uncomfortable and tend to leave that person alone.

Emotional Expression   People with schizophrenia sometimes exhibit what is called "inappropriate affect." This means showing emotion that is inconsistent with the person's speech or thoughts. For example, a schizophrenic person may say that he or she is being persecuted by demons and then laugh. This should not be confused with the behavior of normal individuals when, for instance, they giggle nervously after a minor accident.

Often people with schizophrenia show "blunted" or "flat" affect. This refers to a severe reduction in emotional expressiveness. A schizophrenic person may not show the signs of normal emotion, perhaps using a monotonous tone of voice and diminished facial expression.

Some people with symptoms of schizophrenia also exhibit prolonged extremes of elation or depression, and it is important to determine whether such a patient is schizophrenic, or actually has a bipolar (manic-depressive) disorder or major depressive disorder. Persons who cannot be clearly categorized are sometimes diagnosed as having a schizoaffective disorder.

Normal Versus Abnormal   At times, normal individuals may feel, think, or act in ways that resemble schizophrenia. Often normal people are unable to think straight. They can be made extremely anxious, for example, speaking in front of groups so that they could feel confused, be unable to pull their thoughts together, and forget what they had intended to say.

Just as normal people may occasionally do strange things, many schizophrenic people often think, feel, and act in a normal fashion. Unless in the midst of an extremely disorganized state, a schizophrenic person will have some sense of common reality, for instance, knowing that most people eat three times each day and sleep at night. Being out of touch with reality (which is one way to describe the psychotic symptoms of schizophrenia) does not mean that an individual is living *totally* in another world. Rather, there are certain aspects of this individual's world that are not shared by others and that seem to have no real basis. Hearing a voice of warning that no one else can hear is not an experience shared by most people and is clearly a distortion of reality, but it is only a distortion of one part of reality. A schizophrenic person may, therefore, appear quite normal much of the time.

Schizophrenia Is Not "Split Personality"

There is a common notion that schizophrenia is the same as "split personality"—a Dr. Jekyll-Mr. Hyde switch in character. This is *not* an accurate description of schizophrenia. In fact, split or multiple personality is an entirely different disorder that is really quite rare.

Is Schizophrenia a New Disease?

Although the term "schizophrenia" was not used until the early 20th century, the disorder has existed for a great many years and has been found in all types of societies.

In Western society, "madness" or "insanity" was not generally regarded as a health problem until the early 19th century. At that time, a movement to offer more humane treatment to the mentally ill made it possible for them to receive more scientific, medical treatment. The mentally ill were unchained, released from prisons, and given more appropriate care. Several categories of mental disease were subsequently identified. By the early 20th century, schizophrenia had been distinguished from manic-depressive illness, and subcategories had been described. In 1911, Dr. Eugen Bleuler, a Swiss psychiatrist, first used the term, "the group of schizophrenias." Despite disagreement among scientists as to precisely what conditions should or should not be included in this group, the term has been commonly used since then.

Can Children Be Schizophrenic?

Children over the age of 5 can develop schizophrenia, but it is very rare before adolescence. Moreover, research is needed to clarify the relationship of schizophrenia occurring in childhood to that occurring in adolescence and adulthood. Although some people who later develop schizophrenia may have seemed different from other children at an early age, the psychotic symptoms of schizophrenia (for example, hallucinations, delusions, and incoherence) are rarely seen in children.

Are People With Schizophrenia Likely To Be Violent?

Although news and entertainment media tend to link mental illness and criminal violence, studies tell us that if we set aside those persons with a record of criminal violence before hospitalization, mentally ill persons as a whole are probably no more prone to criminal violence than the general public. Studies are underway to refine our understanding of the different forms of mental illness to learn whether some groups are more prone to violence than others.

Certainly most schizophrenic individuals are not violent; more typically, they prefer to withdraw and be left alone. Some acutely disturbed patients may become physically violent, but such outbursts have become relatively infrequent following the introduction of more effective treatment programs, including the use of antipsychotic medications. There is general agreement that most violent crimes are not committed by schizophrenic persons, and that most schizophrenic persons do not commit violent crimes.

What About Suicide?

Suicide is a potential danger in those who have schizophrenia. If an individual tries to commit suicide or expresses plans to do so, he or she should receive immediate professional help. People with schizophrenia appear to have a higher rate of suicide than the general population. Unfortunately, the prediction of suicide in schizophrenic patients may be especially difficult.

What causes schizophrenia?

There is no known single cause of schizophrenia. As discussed later, it appears that genetic factors produce a vulnerability to schizophrenia, with environmental factors contributing to different degrees in different individuals. Just as each individual's personality is the result of an interplay of cultural, psychological, biological, and genetic factors, a disorganization of the personality, as in schizophrenia, may result from an interplay of many factors. Scientists do not agree on a particular formula that is necessary to produce the disorder. No specific gene has yet been found; no biochemical defect has been proven responsible; and no specific stressful event seems sufficient, by itself, to produce schizophrenia.

Is Schizophrenia Inherited?

It has long been known that schizophrenia runs in families. The close relatives of schizophrenic patients are more likely to develop schizophrenia than those who are not related to someone with schizophrenia. The children of a schizophrenic parent, for example, each have about a 10 percent chance of developing schizophrenia. By comparison, the risk of schizophrenia in the general population is about 1 percent.

Over the past 25 years, two types of increasingly sophisticated studies have demonstrated the importance of a genetic factor in the development of schizophrenia. One group of studies examined the occurrence of schizophrenia in identical and fraternal twins; the other group compared adoptive and biological families.

Recent studies of twins have confirmed the basic findings of earlier, scientifically less rigorous studies. Identical twins (who are genetically alike) generally have a higher rate of "concordance" for schizophrenia than fraternal twins (who are no more genetically alike than ordinary siblings). "Concordance" occurs when both members of a twin pair develop schizophrenia. Although studies of twins provide convincing evidence of an inherited factor in schizophrenia, the fact that concordance for schizophrenia among identical twins is only 40 to 60 percent suggests that some type of environmental factor or factors also must be involved.

A second major group of studies looked at adopted children to examine the effects of heredity and environment. In Denmark, an exhaustive investigation of the mental health of adopted-away children of schizophrenic parents was conducted. These children were compared with adopted children whose biological parents had no history of mental illness. A comparison was also made of the rates of mental disorder among the biological relatives of two groups of adoptees—one known to be schizophrenic and the other without a history of mental illness. Findings of adoption studies have indicated that being biologically related to a schizophrenic person increased the risk for schizophrenia, even when the related individuals have had little or no personal contact.

These studies indicate that schizophrenia has some hereditary basis, but the exact extent of this genetic influence needs further exploration. Most scientists agree that what may be inherited is a vulnerability or predisposition to the disorder—an inherited potential that, given a certain set of factors, can lead to schizophrenia. This predisposition may be due to an enzyme defect or some other biochemical abnormality, a subtle neurological deficit, or some other factor or combination of factors.

We do not yet understand how the genetic predisposition is transmitted and cannot predict accurately whether a given person will or will not develop the disorder. In some people, a genetic factor may be crucial for the development of the disorder; in others, it may be relatively unimportant.

Are the Parents at Fault?

Most schizophrenia researchers now agree that parents do *not* cause schizophrenia. In past decades, there was a tendency for some mental health workers to blame parents for their children's disorder. Today, this attitude is generally seen as both inaccurate and counterproductive. Mental health workers now commonly try to enlist family members' aid in the therapeutic program and also show a heightened sensitivity to the very real feelings of burden and isolation many families experience in their attempts to care for a schizophrenic family member.

Is Schizophrenia Caused by a Chemical Defect?

Although no neurochemical cause has yet been firmly established for schizophrenia, basic knowledge about brain chemistry and its link to schizophrenia is expanding rapidly. Neurotransmitters—substances that allow communication between nerve cells—have long been thought to be involved in the development of schizophrenia. It is likely that the disorder is associated with some imbalance of the complex, interrelated chemical systems of the brain. Although we have no definite answers, this area of schizophrenia research is very active and exciting.

Is Schizophrenia Caused by a Physical Abnormality in the Brain?

Interest in this research question has been stimulated by the development of CAT scans (Computerized Axial Tomography)—a kind of X-ray technique for visualizing the structures of living brains. Some studies using this technique suggest that schizophrenic patients are more likely to have abnormal brain structures (for example, enlargement of the cavities in the interior of the brain) than are normal persons of the same age. It should be emphasized that some of the abnormalities reported are quite subtle. These abnormalities have been found neither to be characteristic of *all* schizophrenic patients nor to occur *only* in individuals with schizophrenia.

A more recent development is the PET (Positron Emission Tomography) scan. In contrast to the CAT scan, which produces images of brain structures, the PET scan is a way of measuring the metabolic activity of specific areas of the brain, including areas deep within the brain. Only very preliminary research has been done with the PET scan in schizophrenia, but this new technique, used in conjunction with other types of scans, promises to provide important information about the structure and function of the living brain.

Other special imaging studies that may increase our understanding of schizophrenia include MRI, rCBF, and computerized EEG measures. MRI stands for magnetic resonance imaging, a technique involving precise measurements of brain structures based on the effects of a magnetic field on different substances in the brain. This technique has sometimes been referred to as nuclear magnetic resonance (NMR) imaging. In rCBF, or regional cerebral blood flow, a radioactive gas is inhaled, and the rate of disappearance of this substance from different areas of the brain gives information about the relative activity of brain regions during various mental activities. The computerized EEG (electroencephalogram) is a kind of brain wave test that maps electrical responses of the brain as it reacts to different stimuli. All of these imaging techniques are being used for research. They are not new forms of treatment.

How is it treated?

Since schizophrenia may not be a single condition and its causes are not yet known, current treatment methods are based on both clinical research and experience. These approaches are chosen on the basis of their ability to reduce schizophrenic symptoms and lessen the chances that symptoms will return. A number of treatments and treatment combinations have been found to be helpful, and more are being developed.

What About Antipsychotic Drugs?

Antipsychotic medications (also called neuroleptics) have been available since the mid-1950's. They have greatly improved the outlook for individual patients. These medications reduce the psychotic symptoms of schizophrenia and usually allow the patient to function more effectively and appropriately. Antipsychotic drugs are the best treatment now available, but they do not "cure" schizophrenia or ensure that there will be no further psychotic episodes. The choice and dosage of medication can be made only by a qualified physician who is well trained in the medical treatment of mental disorders. The dosage of medication is individualized for each patient, since patients may vary a great deal in the amount of drug needed to reduce symptoms without producing troublesome side effects.

Antipsychotic drugs are very effective in treating certain schizophrenic symptoms (for example, hallucinations and delusions). A large majority of schizophrenic patients show substantial improvement. Some patients, however, are not helped very much by such medications and a few do not seem to need them. It is difficult to predict which patients will fall into these two groups and to distinguish them from the large majority of patients who *do* benefit from treatment with antipsychotic drugs.

Sometimes patients and families become worried about the antipsychotic medications used to treat schizophrenia. In addition to concern about side effects (discussed elsewhere in this pamphlet), there may be worries that such drugs may lead to addiction. Antipsychotic medications, however, do not produce a "high" (euphoria) or a strong physical dependence, as some other drugs do.

Another misconception about antipsychotic drugs is that they act as a kind of mind control. Antipsychotic drugs do not control a person's thoughts; instead, they often help the patient to tell the difference between psychotic symptoms and the real world. These medications may diminish hallucinations, agitation, confusion, distortions, and delusions, allowing the schizophrenic individual to make decisions more rationally. Schizophrenia itself may seem to take control of the patient's mind and personality, and antipsychotic drugs can help to free the patient from his or her symptoms and allow the patient to think more clearly and make better informed decisions. While some patients taking these medications may experience sedation or diminished expressiveness, antipsychotic medications used in appropriate dosage for the treatment of schizophrenia are not chemical restraints. Frequently, with careful monitoring, the dosage of the medication can be reduced to provide relief from undesirable effects. There is now a trend in psychiatry that favors finding and using the lowest dosage that allows the schizophrenic person to function without a return of psychosis.

How Long Should Schizophrenic Patients Take Antipsychotic Drugs?

Antipsychotic drugs also reduce the risk of future psychotic episodes in recovered patients. With continued drug treatment, about 40 percent of recovered patients will suffer relapses within two years of discharge from a hospital. Still, this figure compares favorably with the 80 percent relapse rate when medication is discontinued. In most cases, it would not be accurate to say that continued drug treatment *prevents* relapses; rather, it reduces their frequency. The treatment of severe psychotic symptoms generally requires higher dosages than those used for maintenance treatment. If symptoms reappear with a lower dosage, a temporary increase in dosage may prevent a full-blown relapse.

Some patients may deny that they need medication and may discontinue antipsychotic drugs on their own or based on someone else's advice.

This typically increases the risk of relapse (although symptoms may not reappear right away). It can be very difficult to convince certain schizophrenic people that they continue to need medication, particularly since some may feel better at first. For patients who are unreliable in taking antipsychotic drugs, a long-acting injectable form may be appropriate. *Schizophrenic patients should not discontinue antipsychotic drugs without medical advice and monitoring.*

What About Side Effects?
Antipsychotic drugs, like virtually all medications, have unwanted effects along with their beneficial effects. During the early phases of drug treatment, patients may be troubled by side effects such as drowsiness, restlessness, muscle spasms, tremor, dry mouth, or blurring of vision. Most of these can be corrected by lowering the dosage or can be controlled by other medications. Different patients have different treatment responses and side effects to various antipsychotic drugs. A patient may do better with one drug than another.

The long-term side effects of antipsychotic drugs may pose a considerably more serious problem. Tardive dyskinesia (TD) is a disorder characterized by involuntary movements most often affecting the mouth, lips, and tongue, and sometimes the trunk or other parts of the body. It generally occurs in about 15 to 20 percent of patients who have been receiving antipsychotic drugs for many years, but TD can occur in patients who have been treated with these drugs for shorter periods of time. In most cases, the symptoms of TD are mild, and the patient may be unaware of the movements.

The risk-benefit issue in any kind of treatment for schizophrenia is an extremely important consideration. In this context, the risk of TD—as frightening as it is—must be carefully weighed against the risk of repeated breakdowns that can terribly disrupt patients' efforts to reestablish themselves at school, at work, at home, and in the community. For patients who develop TD, the use of medications must be reevaluated. Recent research suggests, however, that TD, once considered irreversible, often improves even when patients continue to receive antipsychotic medications.

What About Psychosocial Treatments?
Antipsychotic drugs have proven to be crucial in relieving psychotic schizophrenic symptoms such as hallucinations, delusions, and incoherence, but do not consistently relieve *all* the symptoms of the disorder. Even when schizophrenic patients are relatively free of psychotic symptoms, many still have extraordinary difficulty establishing and maintaining relationships with others. Moreover, because schizophrenic patients fre-

quently become ill during the critical trade-learning or career-forming years of life (ages 18 to 35), they are less likely to complete the training required for skilled work. As a result, many schizophrenic patients not only suffer thinking and emotional difficulties, but they lack social and work skills as well.

It is with these psychological, social, and occupational problems that psychosocial treatments help most. In general, psychosocial approaches have limited value for acutely psychotic patients (those who are out of touch with reality or have prominent hallucinations or delusions), but may be useful for those with less severe symptoms or those whose psychotic symptoms are under control. Numerous forms of psychosocial therapy are available for patients with schizophrenia, and most focus on improving the patient's functioning as a social being—whether in the hospital or community, at home or on the job. Some of these approaches are described here. Unfortunately, the availability of different forms of treatment varies greatly from place to place.

Rehabilitation Broadly defined, rehabilitation includes a wide array of nonmedical interventions for those with schizophrenia. Rehabilitation programs emphasize social and vocational training to help patients and former patients overcome difficulties in these areas. Programs may include vocational counseling, job training, problem-solving and money management skills, use of public transportation, and social skills training. These approaches are important for the success of the community-centered treatment of schizophrenia, because they provide discharged patients with the skills necessary to lead productive lives outside the sheltered confines of a mental hospital.

Individual Psychotherapy Individual psychotherapy involves regularly scheduled talks between the patient and a mental health professional such as a psychiatrist, psychologist, psychiatric social worker, or nurse. These talks may focus on current or past problems, experiences, thoughts, feelings, or relationships. By sharing their experiences with a trained, empathic person and by talking about their world with someone outside it, schizophrenic individuals may gradually come to understand more about themselves and their problems. They can also learn to sort out the real from the unreal and distorted.

Recent studies tend to indicate that supportive, reality-oriented therapy is generally of more benefit to schizophrenic outpatients than more probing psychoanalytic or insight-oriented psychotherapy. In one large-scale study, patients given psychotherapy oriented toward reality adaptation and practical interpersonal skills generally did as well or better than patients given more frequent and intensive insight-oriented therapy.

Family Therapy As usually practiced, family therapy involves the patient, the parents or spouse, and a therapist. Brothers and sisters, children, and other relatives may also be included. The purposes vary. Meeting in a family group can enable various family members and the therapist to understand each others' viewpoints. It also can help with treatment planning (such as discharge from the hospital) and enlisting the aid of family members in the therapeutic program. Family therapy can also provide a way for the therapist to offer the family needed support and understanding in a time of crisis.

Very often, patients are discharged from the hospital to their families' care, so it is important that family members have a clear understanding of schizophrenia and are aware of the difficulties and problems associated with the illness. It is also helpful for family members to understand the ways of minimizing the chance of future breakdowns and to be aware of the different kinds of outpatient and family services that are available in the period after hospitalization.

Group Therapy   Group therapy sessions usually involve a small number of patients (for example, 6 to 12) and one or two trained therapists. Here, the focus is on learning from the experiences of others, testing out one person's perceptions against those of others, and correcting distortions and maladaptive interpersonal behavior by means of feedback from other members of the group. This form of therapy may be most helpful after symptoms have subsided somewhat and patients have emerged from the acute psychotic phase of the illness, since psychotic patients are often too disturbed or disorganized to participate. Later, when patients are beginning to recover, participation in group therapy will often be helpful in preparing them to cope with community life.

Self-Help Groups   Another kind of group that is becoming increasingly common is the self-help group. Although not led by a professional therapist, the groups are therapeutic because members—usually ex-patients or the family members of people with schizophrenia—provide continuing mutual support as well as comfort in knowing that they are not alone in the problems they face. These groups also serve other important functions. Families working together can more effectively serve as advocates for needed research and hospital and community treatment programs. Ex-patients as a group may be better able to dispel stigma and draw public attention to such abuses as discrimination against the formerly mentally ill.

Family and peer support and advocacy groups are now very active and provide useful information and assistance for patients and families of patients with schizophrenia and other mental disorders.

The National Alliance for the Mentally Ill is composed exclusively of family groups, with 550 of them as of the end of 1985 and adding about 150 to 200 new groups each year. The National Mental Health Association, the nation's oldest and largest nongovernmental citizen's voluntary organization, is concerned with all aspects of mental disorders and mental health. The National Mental Health Consumers' Association, a network of self-help organizations across the country, now has about 150 affiliates and operates a Self-Help Clearinghouse. These groups can be contacted at the following addresses:

The National Alliance for the Mentally Ill
1901 North Fort Myer Drive, Suite 500
Arlington, Virginia 22209
703/524-7600

National Mental Health Association
1021 Prince Street
Alexandria, Virginia 22314–2971
703/684-7722

The National Mental Health Consumers' Association
311 South Juniper Street, Room 902
Philadelphia, Pennsylvania 19107
215/735-2465

Residential Care

Prolonged hospitalization is now very much less common than it was 20 or 30 years ago, when approximately 300,000 schizophrenic patients were residents of State and county mental institutions. Despite this trend, a minority of patients still seem to require long-term inpatient care. For most patients, prolonged hospital stays are not recommended because they increase dependence on institutional care and result in a loss of social contacts with family, acquaintances, and the community. Short-term residential care in well-staffed facilities can give patients needed relief from stressful situations, provide a protective atmosphere for the troubled patient, allow restarting or adjustment of medication, and reduce pressure on the family.

Many schizophrenic persons can benefit from partial hospitalization (day care or night care), from outpatient treatment (going to a clinic or office regularly for individual, group, or occupational therapy), or from living in a halfway house (designed to aid patients in bridging the gap between 24-hour hospitalization and independent living in the community).

What About Other Forms of Treatment?

Electroconvulsive Therapy (ECT) and Insulin Coma These two forms of treatment are rarely used today in the treatment of schizophrenia.

In particular situations, however, electroconvulsive therapy may be useful. It can be of help, for example, if a severe depression occurs in the course of a schizophrenic episode. Insulin coma treatment is virtually never used now because of the availability of other effective treatment methods that have fewer potentially serious complications.

Psychosurgery Lobotomy, a brain operation formerly used in some patients with severe chronic schizophrenia, now is performed only under extremely rare circumstances. This is because of the serious, irreversible personality changes that the surgery may produce and the fact that far better results are generally attained from less drastic and hazardous procedures.

Large Doses of Vitamins Good physical hygiene, including a nourishing diet and proper exercise, is important to good health. Well-controlled studies have shown that the addition of large doses of vitamins to standard therapy regimens does *not* significantly improve the treatment of schizophrenia. Also, although vitamins have been thought to be relatively harmless, reports of side effects raise the possibility that these substances may have detrimental consequences when used in very high doses. Reliance on high-dose vitamins as a treatment for schizophrenia is not scientifically justified and does have risks.

Hemodialysis Preliminary reports that some schizophrenic patients appeared to improve following hemodialysis, a blood-cleansing treatment used in certain kidney disorders, attracted a great deal of attention. However, several more recent controlled scientific studies have reported that the procedure has no beneficial effect on the symptoms of schizophrenia. The weight of scientific evidence now indicates that hemodialysis is *not* useful in the treatment of schizophrenia.

How Can Other People Help?

A patient's support system may come from several sources, including the family, a professional residential or day program provider, shelter operators, friends or roommates, professional case managers, churches and synagogues, and others. Because the majority of patients live with their families, the following discussion frequently uses the term ''family.'' However, this should not be taken to imply that families ought to be the primary support system.

There are numerous situations in which patients with schizophrenia can be helped by people in their support systems. First of all, for patients who do not recognize that they are ill, family or friends may need to take an active role in having them seen and evaluated by a professional. Often, a schizophrenic person will resist treatment, believing that delusions or hallucinations are real and that psychiatric help is not needed.

Since laws regarding involuntary commitment have become very strict, families and community organizations may be frustrated in their attempts to see that a severely mentally ill individual gets needed help. These laws vary from State to State, but generally people who are dangerous to themselves or others due to a mental disorder can be taken by the police for emergency psychiatric evaluation and, if necessary, hospitalization. In some cases, a member of a local community mental health center can evaluate an individual's illness at home if he or she will not voluntarily go in for treatment.

Sometimes only the family or others close to the patient will be aware of strange behavior or ideas that the patient has expressed. Since schizophrenic patients may not volunteer such information during an examination, family members or friends should ask to speak with the person evaluating the patient so that all relevant information can be taken into account.

Seeing that a schizophrenic patient continues to get treatment after hospitalization is also important. Patients may discontinue medications or stop going for follow-up treatment—often leading to a return of psychotic symptoms. Encouraging and assisting the patient to continue treatment can be very important to recovery. Without treatment, some schizophrenic patients become so psychotic and disorganized that they cannot care for their basic needs, such as food, clothing, and shelter. All too often people with severe mental illnesses such as schizophrenia wind up on the streets or in jails, where they rarely receive the kinds of treatment they need.

Those close to people with schizophrenia are often unsure of how to respond when patients make statements that seem strange or are clearly false. The schizophrenic patient's bizarre beliefs or hallucinations seem quite real—they are not just "imaginary fantasies." Instead of going along with a patient's delusions, family members or friends can tell the patient that they do not see things the same way or do not agree with his or her conclusions, while acknowledging that things may seem that way to the patient.

It may also be useful for those who know the patient well to keep a record of what types of symptoms have appeared, what medications (including dosage) have been taken, and what effects various treatments have had. By knowing what symptoms have been present before, family members may know better what to look for in the future. Families may even be able to identify some "early warning signs" of potential relapses (such as increased withdrawal or changes in sleep patterns) better and earlier than the patients themselves. Return of the psychosis may thus be detected early and treatment may prevent a full-blown relapse. Also, by knowing which medications have helped and which have caused troublesome side effects in the past, the family can help those treating the patient to find the best treatment more quickly.

In addition to involvement in seeking help, family, friends, and peer groups can provide support and encourage the person with schizophrenia to regain his or her abilities. It is important that goals be attainable, since a patient who feels pressured and/or repeatedly criticized by others will probably experience this as a stress that may lead to a worsening of symptoms. Like anyone else, people with schizophrenia need to know when they are doing things right. A positive approach may be helpful and perhaps more effective in the long run than criticism, and this advice applies to all those who interact with the patient.

A common question raised by family and friends concerns "street drugs." Since some people who take street drugs may show symptoms similar to those typical of schizophrenia, people with schizophrenia may be accused of being "high on drugs." To help understand the cause of the patient's behavior, blood or urine samples can be tested for street drugs at many hospitals or physician's offices. While most researchers do not believe that schizophrenic patients develop their symptoms because of drug use, people who have schizophrenia often have particularly bad reactions to certain street drugs. Stimulants (such as amphetamines or cocaine) may cause major problems for schizophrenic patients, as may drugs like PCP or marijuana. In fact, some patients experience a worsening of their schizophrenic symptoms when they are taking such drugs. Schizophrenic patients may also abuse alcohol or other drugs for delusional reasons or in an attempt to lessen their symptoms. This can cause additional problems requiring multiple treatment approaches. Such patients may be helped by a combination of therapies such as medication, rehabilitation, psychotherapy, or Alcoholics Anonymous or other substance abuse programs.

What is the outlook?

The outlook for people with schizophrenia has improved over the last 25 years. Although no totally effective therapy has yet been devised, it is important to remember that many schizophrenic patients improve enough to lead independent, satisfying lives. As we learn more about the causes and treatment of schizophrenia, we should be able to help more schizophrenic patients achieve successful outcomes.

Studies that have followed schizophrenic patients for long periods, from the first breakdown to old age, reveal that a wide range of outcomes is possible. A review of almost 2,000 patients' life histories suggests that 25 percent achieve full recovery, 50 percent recover at least partially, and 25 percent require long-term care. When large groups of patients are studied, certain factors tend to be associated with a better outcome—for example, a pre-illness history of normal social, school, and work adjustment. Our current state of knowledge, however, does not allow for a sufficiently accurate prediction of long-term outcome.

The development of a variety of treatment methods and facilities is of crucial importance because schizophrenic patients vary greatly in their needs for treatment. In particular, better alternatives are needed to fill the gap between the relatively nonintensive treatment offered in outpatient clinics and the highly regulated treatment (including 24-hour supervision) provided in hospitals. With a wide variety of facilities available, mental health professionals will be better able to tailor treatment to the different needs of individual patients. Some patients require constant care and attention, while others need a place to learn how to function more independently without constant supervision.

Given the complexity of schizophrenia, the major questions about this disorder—its cause or causes, prevention, and treatment—are unlikely to be resolved in the near future. The public should beware of those offering "the cure" for (or "the cause" of) schizophrenia. Such claims can provoke unrealistic expectations that, when unfulfilled, lead to further disappointment. Although progress has been made toward a better understanding of schizophrenia, there is an urgent need for a more rigorous and broad-based program of basic and clinical research. Research on schizophrenia has benefited greatly from recent basic scientific discoveries, and we hope that a better understanding of neurobiological and psychosocial factors in schizophrenia will be achieved in the next decade.

Prepared by Schizophrenia Research Branch, David Shore, M.D., Editor, Division of Clinical Research, U.S. Department of Health and Human Services, Public Health Service, Alcohol, Drug Abuse, and Mental Health Administration, National Institute of Mental Health, 5600 Fishers Lane, Rockville, Maryland 20857, DHHS Publication No. (ADM) 86–1457, Library of Congress Catalog Card Number 86–600530, Printed 1986.

Sexually Transmitted Diseases

An Introduction

Sexually transmitted diseases (STD's), also called venereal diseases, are among the most common infectious diseases in the United States today. At least 20 STD's have now been identified, and they affect more than 10 million men and women in this country each year.

Understanding the basic facts about STD's—the ways in which they are spread, their common symptoms, and how they can be treated—is the first step toward prevention. The National Institute of Allergy and Infectious Diseases (NIAID), a part of the National Institutes of Health, has prepared a series of fact sheets about STD's to provide some of this important information. Research investigators supported by NIAID are looking for better methods of diagnosis and more effective treatments, as well as for vaccines that will one day ensure that STD's, like many other infectious diseases, no longer pose serious threats to health.

What are some of these basic facts? It is important to understand at least five key points about all STD's in this country today:

1. STD's affect men and women of all backgrounds and economic levels. They are, however, most prevalent among teenagers and young adults. Nearly one-third of all cases involve teenagers.

2. The incidence of STD's is rising, in part because in the last few decades, young people have become sexually active earlier; sexually active people today are more likely to have more than one sex partner or to change partners frequently. Anyone who has sexual relations is potentially at risk for developing STD's.

3. Many STD's initially cause no symptoms. When symptoms develop, they may be confused with those of other diseases not transmitted through sexual contact. However, even when an STD causes no symptoms, a person who is infected may be able to pass the disease on to a sex partner. That is why many doctors recommend periodic testing for people who have more than one sex partner.

4. Health problems caused by STD's tend to be more severe and more frequent for women than for men.

- Some STD's can cause pelvic inflammatory disease (PID), a major cause of both infertility and ectopic (tubal) pregnancy. The latter can be fatal to a pregnant woman.

- STD infections in women may also be associated with cervical cancer. One STD, genital warts, is caused by a virus associated with cervical and other cancers; the relationship between other STD's and cervical cancer is not yet known.

- STD's can be passed from a mother to her baby before or during birth; some of these congenital infections can be cured easily, but others may cause permanent disability or even death of the infant.

5. When diagnosed and treated early, almost all STD's can be treated effectively. Some organisms, such as certain forms of gonococci, have become resistant to the drugs used to treat them and now require higher doses or newer types of antibiotics. The most serious STD for which no effective treatment or cure now exists is acquired immunodeficiency syndrome (AIDS), a fatal viral infection of the immune system.

A brief description follows of the most common STD's in the United States today. More information about these STD's is contained in individual fact sheets available free from the NIAID Office of Communications (see address at the end of this fact sheet).

Acquired immunodeficiency syndrome

AIDS was first reported in the United States in 1981. It is caused by a virus that destroys the body's ability to fight off infection. People who have AIDS are therefore very susceptible to many diseases, called opportunistic infections, and to certain forms of cancer.

The virus is present in body fluids such as blood, semen, and vaginal secretions. It also has been found in saliva and tears. Transmission of the virus primarily occurs by intimate contact with semen during sexual activity and by sharing of needles used to inject intravenous drugs.

AIDS may be prevented by using condoms during sexual intercourse with an infected person and by not sharing needles to inject intravenous drugs. The U.S. Public Health Service has a toll-free hotline number for persons with questions about AIDS: 1-800-342-2437.

Chlamydial infections

These infections are now the most common of all STD's, with an estimated 3 to 4 million new cases occurring each year. Chlamydial infections often have no symptoms and are diagnosed only when complications develop. In men, chlamydiae can infect the urinary tract; in women, untreated chlamydial infection may lead to PID, one of the most common causes of infertility in women and of ectopic pregnancy. Many people with chlamydial infection have few or no symptoms at the early stage of the infection; when symptoms develop, they may include itching or burning in the genital area (especially during urination), a discharge from the vagina or penis, and pain in the abdomen (women) or testicles (men). Once diagnosed, chlamydial infections are treated with an antibiotic drug such as tetracycline.

Genital herpes

Genital herpes is a recurrent viral disease that affects an estimated 30 million Americans. Approximately 500,000 new cases of this incurable infection develop annually. The major symptoms of herpes infection are painful blisters or open sores in the genital area. These may be preceded by a tingling or burning sensation in the legs, buttocks, or genital region. The herpes sores usually disappear within two to three weeks, but the virus remains in the body and the lesions may recur from time to time. The recurring episodes are usually not as severe as the first episode. Genital herpes is now treated with acyclovir, an antiviral drug available by prescription; it helps control the symptoms but does not eliminate the herpes virus from the body.

Genital warts

Genital warts (also called venereal warts, or condylomata acuminata) are caused by a virus related to the virus that causes common skin warts. Genital warts usually first appear as small, hard, painless bumps in the vaginal area, on the penis, or around the anus; if untreated, they may grow and develop a fleshy, cauliflower-like appearance. Genital warts infect up to 3 million Americans each year. Scientists believe that the virus causing genital warts also causes several types of cancer. Genital warts are generally treated with a topical drug (applied to the skin), or by freezing. If the warts are very large, they may be removed by surgery.

Gonorrhea

Between 1½ and 2 million cases of gonorrhea occur each year in this country. The most common symptoms of gonorrhea are a discharge from the vagina or penis and painful or difficult urination. The most common and serious complications occur in women, and like those of chlamydial infections, these complications include PID, ectopic pregnancy, and infertility. Historically, penicillin has been used to treat gonorrhea, but penicillin-resistant forms of the bacteria have recently appeared. Other antibiotics or combinations of drugs must be used to treat these resistant strains.

Syphilis

Thanks to better methods of detection, treatment, and control, syphilis is now far less common than it once was. It remains a serious problem, however, with nearly 70,000 cases reported in 1986. The first symptoms of syphilis may go undetected because they are very mild. The classic first symptom of syphilis is the chancre (''shan-ker''), a painless open sore that usually appears on the penis, or around or in the vagina. If untreated, syphilis may go on to more advanced stages; the full course of the disease can take years. Penicillin remains the drug most commonly used to treat syphilis.

Other diseases that can be sexually transmitted include trichomoniasis, cytomegalovirus infections, hepatitis B, scabies, and pubic lice.

What can you do to prevent STD's?

Although there is no sure way for a sexually active person to avoid exposure to STD's, there are many things that he or she can do to reduce the risk.

A person who has decided to begin a sexual relationship should take the following steps to reduce the risk of developing an STD:
- Be direct and frank about asking a new sex partner whether he or she has an STD, has been exposed to one, or has any unexplained physical symptoms.
- Learn to recognize the physical signs of STD's and inspect a sex partner's body, especially the genital area, for sores, rashes, or discharges.
- Use a condom (rubber) during sexual intercourse and learn to use it correctly. Diaphragms or spermicides (particularly those containing nonoxynol-9), alone or in combination, also may reduce the risk of transmission of some STD's.

Anyone who is sexually active with someone other than a long-term monogamous partner should:
- Have regular checkups for STD's even in the absence of symptoms. These tests can be done during a routine visit to the doctor's office.
- Learn the common symptoms of STD's. Seek medical help immediately if any suspicious symptoms develop, even if they are mild.

Anyone diagnosed as having an STD should:

1. Notify all recent sex partners and urge them to get a checkup.
2. Follow the doctor's orders and complete the full course of medication prescribed. A follow-up test to ensure that the infection has been cured is often an important final step in treatment.
3. Avoid all sexual activity while being treated for an STD.

Sometimes people are too embarrassed or frightened to ask for help or information. Most STD's are readily treated, and the earlier a person seeks treatment and warns sex partners about the disease, the less likely that the disease will do irreparable physical damage, be spread to others or, in the case of a woman, be passed on to a newborn baby.

Private doctors, local health departments, and family planning clinics have information about STD's. In addition, the American Social Health Association (ASHA) provides free information and keeps lists of clinics and private doctors who provide treatment for people with STD's. ASHA has a national toll-free telephone number, 1-800-227-8922; in California, call 1-800-982-5883. Callers can get information from the ASHA hotline without leaving their names.

Research

STD's cause physical and emotional suffering to millions and are costly to individuals and to society as a whole. To help alleviate these burdens, the NIAID conducts and supports many research projects designed to improve methods of prevention and to find better ways to diagnose and treat these diseases. NIAID also supports several large university-based STD research centers.

Within the past few years, NIAID-supported research has resulted in new tests to diagnose some STD's faster and more accurately. New drug treatments for STD's are under investigation by NIAID researchers. In addition, vaccines are being developed or tested for effectiveness in preventing several STD's, including genital herpes, gonorrhea, and group B streptococcal infections.

It is up to each individual to learn more about STD's and then make choices about how to minimize the risk of acquiring these diseases and spreading them to others. Knowledge of STD's, as well as honesty and openness with sex partners and with one's doctor, can be very important in reducing the incidence and complications of sexually transmitted diseases.

Prepared by the Office of Communications, National Institute of Allergy and Infectious Diseases, National Institutes of Health, Bethesda, Maryland 20892. U.S. Department of Health and Human Services, Public Health Service, National Institutes of Health, NIH Publication No. 87–909A August 1987

Shingles
Hope Through Research

When the itchy red spots of childhood chickenpox disappear and the child goes back to school, the battle with infection seems won. But for all too many of us this triumph of the body's immune system over a virus is only temporary. The virus has not been destroyed, but lies low, ready to strike again later in life. This second eruption of the chickenpox virus is the disease called shingles.

"I was having exams at college and I got a rash in a band around my waist. I first thought it was chickenpox, but I'd had that years before and instead of itching, this time the spots were very painful," recalls a young woman who had shingles in her twenties.

The young woman's memory was correct. She *had* had chickenpox as a child. You cannot develop shingles unless you have had an earlier bout of chickenpox. The woman was also typical in her symptoms: Shingles is often more painful than it is itchy. Her age was unusual, however. While young people do develop shingles, the disease most often strikes in later years. About 10 percent of normal adults can be expected to get shingles during their lifetimes, usually after age 50. The incidence increases with age so that shingles is 10 times more likely to occur in adults over 60 than in children under 10.

The chances of developing shingles are greatest for individuals whose immune systems are weakened. That holds for children as well as adults. The child who is suffering from a disease which damages the immune system, or who is taking anticancer drugs that suppress the immune system, is a prime candidate for an attack of shingles. At present as many as 10 percent of children with leukemia and 52 percent of children with Hodgkin's disease develop shingles.

Still another group of children vulnerable to shingles are youngsters whose mothers had chickenpox late in pregnancy—5 to 21 days before giving birth. Sometimes these children are born with chickenpox or develop a typical case within a few days. In any case, as many as a third develop shingles during the first 5 years.

A "girdle" of pain

The first sign of shingles is often pain in or under the skin. The individual may also feel ill with fever or headache. After several days, a rash of small fluid-filled blisters appears on reddened skin.

The blisters, or lesions, are usually limited to a band spanning one side of the trunk or clustered on one side of the face. This striking pattern gives the disease its name: *Shingles* comes from *cingulum,* the Latin word for belt or girdle. Similarly, the medical term for the disease, *zoster,* is the Greek word for girdle.

More importantly, the distribution of the shingles spots is a telltale clue to where the chickenpox virus has been hiding for all the years following the initial infection. Scientists now know that the shingles lesions correspond to the area of skin supplied by one of the major nerves that exits from the brain or spinal cord.

The assumption is that the chickenpox viruses that weren't wiped out in the original battle were able to leave the skin blisters and travel in the nervous system. There the viruses settled down in an inactive form inside nerve cells (neurons) that lie in clusters adjacent to the spinal cord and brain. These neurons are called sensory cells because they relay information to the brain about what your body is sensing: whether your skin feels hot or cold, whether you've been touched or feel pain. Comparable nerve cell clusters in the head relay information about pain, temperature, or touch in that area, as well as information about what you're seeing, hearing, tasting, or smelling.

When the chickenpox virus reactivates, the virus moves down the long nerve fibers that extend from the sensory cell bodies to the skin. There the viruses multiply and the telltale rash erupts. Now the nervous system is deeply involved, however, and the symptoms are often more complex and severe than those of childhood chickenpox. People with "optical" shingles (where the virus has invaded an ophthalmic nerve) may suffer painful eye inflammations that leave them temporarily blind. Infections of facial nerves can lead to paralysis or excruciating pain.

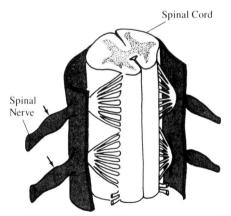

Spinal Cord

Spinal
Nerve

Shingles viruses hide inside nerve cells adjacent to the spinal cord and brain. The arrows point to the portion of the spinal nerve containing the sensory-cell bodies that house the virus.

People with lesions on the torso may feel spasms of pain at the gentlest touch or breeze.

Because of the nervous system involvement, the chickenpox/shingles virus is of great interest to the National Institute of Neurological and Communicative Disorders and Stroke (NINCDS), the principal Federal agency supporting research on the nervous system. The disease is of equal concern to the National Institute of Allergy and Infectious Diseases (NIAID). In addition, the National Cancer Institute and the National Institute on Aging support research on shingles because of the prevalence and severity of the disease among cancer patients and the elderly.

The aftermath

For the majority of normally healthy individuals, the second bout with the chickenpox virus is almost always a second triumph of the body's immune system. The shingles attack may last longer than chickenpox, and you may need medication for pain, but in most cases the body has the inner resources to fight back. The lesions heal and the pain subsides within three to five weeks.

There are exceptions. Sometimes, particularly in older people, the pain and other symptoms persist long after the rash is healed. It is important to realize that these individuals no longer have shingles: Their infection is over. Instead, they are suffering a neurological disorder, the result of damage to the nervous system.

Investigators think that the virus attack has led to scarring or other lesions affecting the sensory cells and associated nerves. If the eye is involved, the damage from shingles can lead to blindness.

In other cases, facial paralysis, headache, and persistent pain are the aftermath. Possibly because the nerve cells conveying pain sensations are hardest hit, or are exquisitely sensitized by the virus attack, pain is the principal complication of shingles. This pain, called *postherpetic neuralgia,* is among the most devastating known to mankind—the kind of pain that leads to insomnia, weight loss, depression, and that total preoccupation with unrelenting torment that characterizes the chronic pain sufferer.

Even in such severe cases, however, the paralysis, headaches, and pain generally subside, although it may take time. As one elderly sufferer recalls: "The worst thing was that the pain went on for months and months. Another bad part was reflecting on the 60 years since I had the chickenpox. Am I only a culture medium for viruses, for heaven's sake?"

Postherpetic neuralgia may be a nightmare, but it is not life-threatening. Doctors treating the pain currently employ a variety of medications. They generally avoid the powerful narcotic pain relievers in favor of newer nonaddictive but potent painkillers. Studies have also shown that some anticonvulsant drugs used to treat epilepsy, such as carbamazepine (Tegretol®) are sometimes effective in relieving postherpetic neuralgia. Antidepressants can help, also. In addition to their effects on mood, the antidepressants appear to relieve pain. Some doctors report that patients occasionally benefit from some of the more controversial treatments for pain, such as acupuncture and electrical stimulation of nerve endings.

Shingles *is* a serious threat to life in immunosuppressed patients. The child or adult with leukemia, Hodgkin's disease or other cancers is often treated by drugs or radiation to destroy cancerous tissue. Unfortunately these treatments also damage cells of the immune system that normally fight invading organisms. Patients with kidney or other organ diseases who receive organ transplants are also vulnerable to shingles. These patients are given drugs that suppress the immune system to prevent the body from rejecting the foreign tissue. Should any of these patients contract shingles, there is a real danger that the disease will spread throughout the body, reaching vital organs like the lungs. If unchecked, such disseminated shingles can lead to death from viral pneumonia or secondary bacterial infection.

Shingles in pregnancy

Many mothers-to-be are concerned about any infection contracted during pregnancy, and rightly so. It is well known that certain viruses can be transmitted across the mother's bloodstream to the fetus, or can be acquired by the baby during the birth process. What about shingles? The chief of the NINCDS Infectious Diseases Branch notes that there have been a few isolated reports of maternal shingles leading to birth defects, but the cases are poorly documented. "It is controversial," he says, "but I do not think shingles in the mother increases the risk for the baby."

In contrast, maternal *chickenpox* poses some risk to the unborn child, depending upon the stage of pregnancy when the mother contracts the disease. During the first 30 weeks, maternal chickenpox may, in some cases, lead to congenital malformations. Such cases are rare and experts differ in their opinion on how great is the risk.

If the mother gets chickenpox from 21 to 5 days before giving birth, the newborn may have chickenpox at birth or develop it within a few days, as noted earlier. But the time lapse between the start of the mother's illness and the birth of the baby generally allows the mother's immune system to react and produce antibodies to fight the virus. These antibodies can be transmitted to the unborn child and thus help fight the infection. Still, a third of the babies exposed to chickenpox in the 21-to-5 day period before birth develop shingles in the first 5 years.

Suppose the mother contracts chickenpox at precisely the time of birth, however. In that case the mother's immune system has not had a chance to mobilize its forces. The newborn may be infected at birth but will have precious little ability to fight off the attack because the baby's immunological system is immature. For these babies chickenpox can be fatal. They must be given "zoster immune globulin," a preparation made from the antibody-rich blood of adults who have recently recovered from chickenpox or shingles.

The clever culprit

The virus responsible for shingles and chickenpox belongs to the *herpes* group of viruses. The group includes the virus that causes cold sores, fever blisters, mononucleosis, and genital herpes—a sexually transmitted disease. Like the shingles-causing virus, many herpesviruses can take refuge in the nervous system after an individual has suffered an initial infection. The virus may remain latent for years, then travel down nerve cell fibers to cause a renewed infection.

Scientists call the chickenpox/shingles-causing agent the VZ virus, short for *varicella-zoster*. *Varicella* is a Latin word meaning "little pox" to distinguish the virus from smallpox, the scourge that once disfigured or killed its victims. (The word "chicken" conveys the same idea of weakness or mildness as in "chicken-hearted.") Like many viruses, the varicella-zoster virus looks as though it were designed by a mathematician. It is a microscopic sphere encasing a 20-sided geometric figure called an icosahedron. Inside the icosahedron is the genetic material of the virus, deoxyribonucleic acid (DNA). When activated, the virus reproduces inside the nucleus of an infected cell. It acquires its spherical wrapping as it buds through the nuclear membrane.

As early as 1909 a German scientist suspected that the viruses causing chickenpox and shingles were one and the same. In the 1920's and 1930's the case was strengthened. In an experiment, children were inoculated with fluid from the lesions of patients with shingles. Within 2 weeks about half the children came down with chickenpox. Finally in 1958 detailed analyses of the viruses taken from patients with either chickenpox or shingles confirmed that the viruses were identical.

Note what that means: A person with shingles can communicate chickenpox to a susceptible individual. But the opposite is not true: A person with chickenpox cannot communicate shingles to someone else. You must already harbor the virus in your nervous system before shingles can develop.

"It's a clever virus," notes the NINCDS virologist. "It doesn't kill its host, but lives for a long time in a suppressed state. And it can reactivate, given the opportunity," he adds.

Killing the opportunity

Shingles imposes two immediate challenges to medical research. The first is to develop drugs to fight the disease and to prevent complications. The second challenge is to understand the disease well enough to prevent it, especially in people known to be at high risk.

Only recently have scientists succeeded in developing antiviral drugs. In 1975 there were virtually no virus-fighting drugs available. Progress has been impressive since then and now there are several antiviral agents in clinical use, with more on the way. While no medications have yet been approved for treatment of shingles, several candidates are being tested:

- Vidarabine. One drug in limited use is vidarabine (also known as Ara-A®). Vidarabine interferes with the virus's ability to make new genetic material and thus prevents the virus from reproducing and spreading in the body. Early treatment with vidarabine decreased the duration of shingles in a group of 87 patients with deficient immune responses. The patients treated early also had more rapid pain relief and a shorter period of lesion formation compared to patients who received the drug later in the course of their disease. This trial was conducted by the NIAID Collaborative Antiviral Study.
- Acyclovir. Another drug being tested on zoster patients is called acyclovir. It is administered to the patient in an inactive form. When the drug reaches a VZ virus-infected cell, a chemical produced by the virus activates acyclovir. Once activated, acyclovir is able to destroy a vital chemical that the virus needs to reproduce. This oddly self-destructive behavior on the part of the virus—cooperating in its own demise—has led some investigators to label acyclovir a "suicide promoter." Acyclovir has appeared promising in preliminary tests on cancer patients with shingles.

    Newer, even more potent drugs are in earlier stages of testing. The chief of the Medical Virology Section of NIAID predicts that within a few years drugs taken by mouth or applied to the rash will effectively shut down VZ virus infections.
- Interferon. This disease-fighting substance is not a drug, but a compound naturally produced by body cells. It is currently being investigated as a cure for everything from the common cold to cancer—and shingles. In studies at Stanford University, some 150 immunosuppressed patients were given a particular type of interferon. The compound not only reduced the pain and extent of the shingles lesions, but also lessened complications. Currently, not enough interferon is available for clinical use. By using the newer genetic engineering techniques that enable interferon to be produced in specially treated bacteria (instead of having

to isolate interferon from human blood), scientists expect to have enough on hand for future treatment.

The goal of prevention

The second major challenge to investigators is to protect susceptible patients from a shingles attack. To do that, scientists will need to know much more about the VZ virus, especially how it remains latent in the body for so long, and what induces it to become active again.

While the virus is presumed to hide in the nervous system between bouts of chickenpox and shingles, it has never been recovered from nerve cells at autopsies unless the patient had shingles at the time of death. In contrast, herpes *simplex,* which causes recurrent infections of cold sores and fever blisters, has been identified in spinal nerve cells during its latent periods.

If the whole VZ virus does not remain intact in nerve cells, perhaps its core genetic material—the DNA—survives. Scientists suspect that the viral DNA may be inserted into one of the chromosomes of the nerve cell—the larger units that house the cell's own genetic material. The chief of the Virology Section at NIAID is using new gene-splicing techniques to produce copies of parts of the viral DNA. To find out if the viral DNA is built into a nerve cell's chromosomes, he plans to label the viral DNA with a radioactive substance. Such labeled DNA will bind to matching strands of DNA in a cell and the radioactivity given off will pin down its precise location. The virologist hopes by this method to locate viral genes in human nerve cells.

The technique is expected to show how many people carry latent VZ virus in their nerve cells. The number may be as high as 90 percent of the adult population—the people who have had chickenpox.

What keeps the VZ virus quiet during its long latency? Probably the immune system, scientists think. A healthy immune system protects against all kinds of diseases, but people with depressed immunity are vulnerable to many illnesses, and have a high incidence of shingles. Even among normal individuals, temporary depression of the immune system because of stress, a cold, and even sunburn, may be associated with an attack of shingles.

Antibodies, one of the immune system's major defense mechanisms against infection, are not very helpful against shingles. Studies have shown that patients with shingles produce VZ antibodies: They just don't check the infection. Similarly, injections of antibody-rich blood serum do not prevent the dissemination of shingles in cancer patients or others whose immune systems are depressed. (This is in contrast to the protection conferred by the serum when given to newborns with chickenpox.)

The components of the immune system that do appear to combat shingles are two types of white blood cell: the T lymphocyte, and a scavenger cell called a macrophage. Scientists are trying to find ways of boosting the activity of these cells—especially in patients at high risk for severe or disseminated shingles.

A human disease

The development of preventive measures and treatment for shingles has been hindered by scientists' difficulty in working with the VZ virus in the laboratory. The virus grows very poorly in laboratory cells and does not infect animals other than man. A leading investigator says that less is known about the biology of VZ virus than about any other herpesvirus.

Current research is aimed at finding better methods for growing the VZ virus and identifying animal models of the disease. So far, the best animal model is the patas monkey. NINCDS scientists working with these monkeys note that the animals succumb to a disease resembling chickenpox when injected with a virus very similar to the VZ virus. Indeed, the two viruses are so closely related that a vaccine made from the human virus can be used to protect the monkeys from their version of chickenpox.

But the monkey studies are aimed at learning more about the behavior of the VZ virus in the body, not at developing a shingles vaccine. A successful vaccine against shingles is considered unlikely because the disease typically develops in people who have naturally built up an immune response. Remember, if you have had chickenpox, you have developed the same antibodies against the VZ virus as a vaccine would induce—but those antibodies do not control shingles.

On the other hand, there is considerable interest and experimental work in developing a vaccine for chickenpox. Japanese investigators have produced a vaccine containing live VZ virus which has become inactivated by growing it in tissue culture in the laboratory. More than 2,000 healthy people and more than 500 hospitalized or chronically ill children have received the vaccine in Japan. There were few side effects, and most of the recipients not only developed antibodies to the virus, but also did not succumb to chickenpox when exposed to it under test conditions.

Whether the vaccine is truly protective will depend on continued experience with the vaccine in high-risk patients. If those vaccinated do not get chickenpox when exposed to the natural disease in the community, the vaccine may be of enormous benefit, a true lifesaver for many leukemic children and other high-risk patients.

There is a catch, however. If you inject a vaccine that contains an altered but still living VZ virus, might not the virus take refuge in the nervous system and later give rise to shingles? To resolve that question, the National Institute on Aging is currently supporting trials of chickenpox vaccine at New York University in New York City.

The NYU scientists plan to observe children with acute leukemia—a group that is particularly vulnerable to shingles. The investigators will note the incidence and severity of shingles occurring in children who have received the chickenpox vaccine in comparison with children who have had natural cases of chickenpox. The data from Japan suggest that shingles will not be a problem among the vaccinated.

Investigators at the University of Texas (San Antonio), as well as at Children's Hospital in Philadelphia, are also conducting vaccine experiments with leukemic children. In addition, the Philadelphia group thinks that a chickenpox vaccine might provide a general boost to the immune system for people who have had chickenpox, helping them ward off shingles. They plan to inoculate elderly volunteers who have had chickenpox and note if they have a lower than normal incidence of shingles for their age group. If that is so, the VZ virus vaccine might confer immunity to shingles as well as to chickenpox—double protection.

But maybe not. "In the long run, the VZ virus will be more difficult to eliminate than the smallpox virus," says the NINCDS Infectious Diseases Laboratory chief. "Because the virus is so widespread and because it can reactivate at any time, even an effective vaccine would need to be administered indefinitely." Currently, physicians are uncertain whether it will ever be desirable to vaccinate whole populations of normal children routinely against chickenpox.

So it looks as if shingles will continue to afflict people in the years to come. The greatest practical hope lies in the measures rapidly being developed to decrease the discomfort and risk of shingles. In the course of that work scientists expect to uncover important information to use against other diseases, learn more about the body's immune system and ultimately outwit the clever viruses that evade that system.

For further information

A number of institutes of the National Institutes of Health support research on shingles and related herpesviruses. For details on current programs or other inquiries write:

> Office of Scientific and Health Reports
> National Institute of Neurological and
> Communicative Disorders and Stroke
> Building 31, Room 8A06

National Institutes of Health
9000 Rockville Pike
Bethesda, MD 20205

or

Office of Research Reporting and Public Response
National Institute of Allergy and
Infectious Diseases
Building 31, Room 7A32
National Institutes of Health
9000 Rockville Pike
Bethesda, MD 20205

Prepared by the Office of Scientific and Health Reports, National Institute of Neurological and Communicative Disorders and Stroke. National Institutes of Health, Bethesda, Maryland 20205, NIH Publication No. 82–307, November 1981.

Sleep Apnea
Sounds Like Sleep Apnea

Sleep, even when accompanied by loud snores and snorts, has always been looked upon—almost without question—as a restorer of health. In fact, sleep was deemed so beneficial that until about 20 years ago medical experts didn't realize that some sleepers' snoring might be more a danger sign than a condition to be laughed at or complained about. Similarly, most doctors didn't stop to speculate that inadvertent snoozing during the day might be part of the same condition that caused troublous nighttime sleep.

These two conditions—daytime dozing and disturbed nighttime sleep—are the principal symptoms of a "new" disease called sleep apnea syndrome. Actually, the condition is not new at all, but was rediscovered 20 years ago in the wake of some genuinely new findings about what happens to humans while they sleep.

Sleep apnea syndrome is a disorder in which the victim, while sleeping away the night, stops breathing dozens or even hundreds of times for intervals lasting at least 10 seconds and then, during the next day, finds it next to impossible to stay awake.

Full medical recognition of sleep apnea as a serious, even life-threatening disease has been a long time coming. The first more or less complete clinical description of the condition was published in the 1890s, but most doctors at the time were reluctant to recognize a disease that didn't arise from physical changes or a tumor. Sleeping sickness, then newly discovered in Africa, got far more attention, along with another sleep disorder, narcolepsy, first described in 1880. In fact, some cases which were obviously sleep apnea were mistakenly referred to as narcolepsy—a condition characterized by sudden and uncontrollable attacks of deep sleep. (However, about 1 in 10 narcoleptics also has sleep apnea.) So sleep apnea did a kind of Rip Van Winkle, dropping out of sight until 1966, when it was again described in medical literature.

The rediscovery came in the wake of startling findings about the nature and structure of sleep itself. Researchers were able to tie sleep apnea to a condition then known as pickwickian syndrome, characterized by daytime sleepiness and associated with obesity. The newly described condition not only included daytime sleepiness, but also the nighttime sleep disturbances that had been found to threaten the victim's health and life.

Until its rediscovery, sleep apnea's nightly ordeals, which produced thundering snores, violent snorts, and desperate gaspings for breath, generally had been thought to be no more than a nuisance that robbed the household of sleep.

There are perhaps 30 million people of all ages in the United States who snore, according to *Guide to Better Sleep,* a book published by the American Medical Association. Most people snore lightly and intermittently and have no trouble obtaining the oxygen they need to supply body organs and tissues and get rid of carbon dioxide, a waste product. But, this book reports, 2.5 million Americans do experience seriously disturbed breathing at night from sleep apnea. Some other estimates of the total number of sleep apnea victims have ranged considerably higher than that.

The loudest snores come from those who experience seriously disturbed breathing during sleep. Some victims may not breathe at all for three-quarters of their time asleep. Breathing pauses have been recorded for as long as three minutes. Four minutes without oxygen can result in irreversible brain damage. Alcohol, sleeping pills, and tranquilizers can make sleep apnea worse.

The attention directed at last to the condition touched off a flurry of research. Medical experts have conducted scores of studies. Sleep disorders centers have been established in or near major hospitals or medical centers in practically every state. And doctors are now able to precisely evaluate and diagnose sleep apnea and other sleep disorders. These advances offered new hope for wrecked marriages and romances that couldn't survive the Big Snore, new horizons for those who formerly snoozed away valuable time during work or at public gatherings, household relief from the mighty rumbles of the night, and reduced numbers of auto accidents among those who had been subject to dozing off while tooling down a street or highway.

Ironically, the first person to aptly describe some of the symptoms of sleep apnea was an observant novelist, not a doctor. In 1836, Charles Dickens, in *The Pickwick Papers,* introduced a character called Joe, the red-faced Fat Boy. Fat Joe had constant difficulty performing his chores as a serving boy because of his greed for food and a tendency to fall asleep and snore at the drop of an eyelid.

Dickens' readers recognized these traits in people they knew. But nobody, not even Dickens, considered the symptoms significant, other than as a subject for humor and ridicule.

Later in the 19th century, doctors dubbed this daytime sleepiness, snoring, and obesity the "pickwickian syndrome" in tribute to Dickens' wickedly accurate pen. But no connection was made to nighttime sleep disorders.

There are three types of sleep apnea syndrome: central apnea; obstructive, or upper airway, apnea; and mixed apnea, which is a combination of the first two.

In central apnea, the victim undergoes episodes of "forgetting" to breathe during the night until the oxygen-starved brain sends out distress signals to activate the diaphragm and lungs. Central apnea is considered extremely rare. One pioneer doctor in the field says he has seen only three or four cases among the 2,000-odd sleep apnea victims he has treated.

In obstructive, or upper airway, apnea, the muscles of the sleeper's soft palate (the area at the rear of the tongue) and the uvula (the small, conical, fleshy tissue suspended from the center of the soft palate) become so flaccid from loss of muscle tone and so relaxed from sleep that the suction of indrawn air causes them to flop together and block the air from reaching the lungs. This is the predominant type of sleep apnea.

In mixed apnea, the victim experiences an episode of central apnea, promptly followed by another of obstructive apnea.

The onset of central apnea tends to come later in life than obstructive apnea, and it affects men and women in equal numbers. Of those with obstructive apnea, men outnumber premenopausal women 30 to 1; the frequency among women increases as they get older. Some patients may suffer from all three types of apnea in a single night.

Sleep apnea may occur in infancy or childhood. It's more common in overweight children, and more boys than girls are victims. Some children with sleep apnea complain of morning headaches, and some are sluggish and function poorly in school. Enlarged tonsils or adenoids may interfere with breathing during sleep, and surgical removal may be necessary. Autopsies suggest that sudden infant death syndrome may be caused by repeated periods of inadequate oxygen intake brought on by respiratory abnormalities such as sleep apnea, though other factors may also be involved.

An episode of obstructive apnea is normally preceded by loud snoring. This labored breathing is then interrupted when the airway is constricted and blocks the inflow of air. The episode ends when the muscles of the diaphragm and the chest, continuing to try to function, build up sufficient pressure to force the airway open again. The sleeper then partly awakens with a strangled snorting noise caused by gasping for air, then slips back into a slumber until the obstruction again develops and the cycle is repeated.

Arousal is so brief, so incomplete, that sleep is resumed immediately without full awakening, and there is no memory of the episode. Hypopneas also may occur; these are partial or incomplete blockages that reduce the amount of oxygen delivered to the lungs and thence to other body systems.

The loud snoring so characteristic of obstructive apnea results when indrawn or expelled air produces vibration of the muscles of the upper airway which have become flabby from one or more causes. The reduction in the muscle tone of the victim's palate, pharynx, and uvula can result from aging, but also may be caused by abnormalities of the part of the brain that sends signals to these muscles. The airway also is constricted by the reclining position of the body at night. In some cases, the tongue muscle may relax so that this organ falls back and obstructs air flow.

Obesity and a short, thick neck are physical attributes that contribute to breathing difficulty during sleep, although the exact way this works is not known. The upper airway also can be narrowed by enlarged tonsils or adenoids, a deviated nasal septum, nasal polyps, abnormal growths, and congenital or other defects.

Most researchers believe that daytime sleepiness results from the frequent sleep interruptions of the previous night and the aggregate sleep-time lost. But this daytime sleepiness could be to some extent a symptom of more ominous developments that result from inadequate oxygen in the system.

The entire pickwickian syndrome, obesity-sleepiness-snoring, occurs only in about one in 20 victims of obstructive sleep apnea. Thin and normal-weight persons have sleep apnea too. Some of these do have the short, thick neck associated with severe cases of sleep apnea.

In central apnea, the diaphragm and chest muscles simply stop functioning, and partial or full awakening occurs before breathing resumes. The

SOS signal that wakens the victim is believed to be set off when the blood's oxygen drops to a critical level, triggering a chemical warning mechanism in the brain. A victim who is fully awakened often enough may complain to a physician about insomnia. Unless the condition is correctly diagnosed, a sedative or tranquilizer may be prescribed inappropriately, with potentially disastrous, even fatal, results since these can impede the sleeper's awakening responses to the apnea episodes.

Severe sleep apnea can result in continuing or prolonged oxygen starvation in the brain and other parts of the body, which in turn causes general body deterioration. Death during sleep can result from failure to resume breathing or from heart arrhythmias during an episode. Some researchers believe sleep apnea may be implicated in many unexplained deaths that occur during sleep. This could someday cause new thinking among those who believe that dying in one's sleep, when the time comes, is the most beautiful way to go, especially if that time otherwise might have been postponed a matter of years.

Some common complications of obstructive sleep apnea, particularly over a prolonged period, are high blood pressure, disrupted heart rhythm and other heart complications, abnormal levels of oxygen and carbon dioxide in the blood, and peripheral edema (swelling of the extremities). All usually worsen unless the sleep apnea is treated.

Some other conditions that may appear as the disorder progresses: sleepwalking; blackouts or automatic (robot-like) behavior; intellectual deterioration—as evidenced by poor concentration, disorientation, senility, and mental retardation; hallucinations when fighting sleep; personality changes such as anxiety, irritability, aggressiveness, jealousy, suspicion, and irrational behavior; loss of interest in sex; morning headaches; and bed-wetting.

Elevating the head at night using two pillows, sleeping in a recliner chair, or setting the bed's headposts on six-inch to eight-inch blocks is recommended to let gravity help keep the victim's tongue from falling backward and blocking the upper airway. These practices help make breathing easier.

Some victims are diagnosed as having positional apnea. They experience fewer incidents or none when they sleep in a certain position, such as lying on the side. For them, the doctor may recommend sewing a tennis ball or other bulky object into the back of the sleeping garment to make sleeping on the back so uncomfortable that they turn over.

Obstructive sleep apnea is where most treatment developments have been concentrated. These include diet regimens, drugs, surgery, and devices. Sleep apnea can be reduced in severely overweight patients by weight loss, and this is encouraged in therapy.

Drugs used experimentally to treat obstructive sleep apnea include some that stimulate breathing and others that reduce REM (rapid eye movement) sleep, the sleep stage when the worst apnea episodes occur. Some drugs under study include theophylline, protriptyline, pemoline, thioridazine, clomipramine, and nicotine.

Surgical treatments include removal of enlarged tonsils or adenoids, nasal polyps or a deviated septum. Gastric bypass surgery—in which a portion of the stomach is closed off—has been performed on grossly obese victims of obstructive sleep apnea. This limits the amount of food that can be consumed at one time.

The most drastic surgery is tracheostomy. It is 100 percent effective for obstructive apnea, but is used only in life-threatening cases where less drastic methods are not effective. A T-shaped tube is inserted into the windpipe through a small incision just above the notch of the breastbone. The protruding end of the tube is closed off in the daytime, to allow speaking and normal breathing, and opened at night. A tracheostomy can be made temporary or permanent, depending on the severity of the case. There can be complications such as irritations and infections that the patient must take precautions to avoid. Many patients, and their spouses too, are bothered by its appearance.

A surgical technique developed in Japan in 1980 and used increasingly in this country is uvulo-palato-pharyngoplasty—called, for obvious reasons, UPPP. Droopy tissues are tightened in the back of the mouth and top of the throat, and excess tissues that block the airway in those areas are trimmed away. UPPP is helpful in 50 percent to 60 percent of the cases of obstructive sleep apnea.

One device, developed in the United States, is a mouthguard worn during sleep that pulls the tongue forward by suction, thus clearing the airway. Another method, developed in Sweden, is the insertion of tubes through the nose and into the windpipe at night. These two methods are not in wide use, one problem being a low level of patient tolerance.

One of the most promising devices, first tested in Australia, employs a system called Continuous Positive Airway Pressure, or CPAP. The device reportedly is completely effective in about 85 percent of sleep apnea cases. It has been embraced enthusiastically by sleep disorder experts everywhere, and a version is manufactured in this country.

At night the patient's nose (only) is covered by a mask, from which a tube runs to the device, about the size of a small TV set, placed on a bedside table. The bedside mechanism has a fan that forces air through the tube at low pressure, just sufficient to open the patient's upper airway and permit air to enter the lungs. It is designed not to harm the patient should it malfunction or the power fail. The pressure is set to fit the patient's own breathing pattern. It can be rented or purchased. It's portable, and can be bundled along to any place where the patient stays overnight.

The CPAP device is manufactured by Respironics Inc., Monroeville, Pa. Called SleepEasy, the current version sells for close to $1,100. It must be prescribed by a doctor.

Despite all the hurrahs, it has one shortcoming. The motor makes a noise all night somewhat like the sound of a vacuum cleaner or a window air conditioner. But those who praise it figure that the user will be doing what comes unnaturally—sleeping—and will never hear the whir, and that the sleeper's spouse or others in the household would be more than willing to put up with the new sound in preference to the old.

Harold Hopkins, *FDA Consumer*, December 1986–January 1987.

Sore Throat

Whatever the Cause, A Sore Throat Is Hard to Swallow

The sensation is a familiar one. It hurts to swallow and there's a scratchy sensation way in the back of the mouth. The whole area feels raw. All signs point to a sore throat, that universal complaint, usually associated with the winter months.

It's not surprising that the throat is the target of pain. It is, along with the nose, the body's first defense against invading organisms. Anything that comes in via the nose or mouth must pass through this area, known technically as the pharynx. Pharyngitis—i.e., throat inflammation—is one of the most common complaints that bring people to see a doctor. And it's the cause of 100 million days of absence from work each year.

A sore throat is a symptom of some underlying problem, the body's way of signaling that something is wrong. And there are a host of reasons why the throat becomes sore.

Infectious diseases caused by viruses, bacteria, and fungi have sore throat as a primary symptom. A sore throat may be an early sign of aplastic anemia (a serious form of anemia) and acute leukemia and is also a manifestation of pharyngeal gonorrhea and an advanced stage of syphilis.

Some throat problems come from eating irritating foods. In the June 1984 *American Family Physician,* two Canadian physicians told of a sore throat epidemic among students from Saudi Arabia. The illnesses were traced to their overzealous use of an unfamiliar hot sauce on their food.

A sore throat can also result from excessive nasal secretions (popularly called postnasal ''drip''), injury from a bone or sharp object unintentionally swallowed, inhaled noxious fumes, and allergies. Together with fever, a sore throat is also a rare side effect of some prescription drugs.

Dental and surgical procedures, such as tonsillectomy or biopsy, can leave the patient with varying degrees of throat pain.

Of the lot, viral and bacterial infections are the most frequent causes of acute sore throat.

Among the viruses that affect the throat are the coxsackieviruses, Group A. Any one of the 23 varieties of these viruses may cause herpangina, an illness that occurs mostly in the summer and mainly affects children. A fever that comes on suddenly, sore throat, headache, and loss of appetite are characteristic symptoms. There is no specific treatment for herpangina, which usually clears up on its own in a few days.

High fever, sore throat, and swollen glands are the mark of infectious mononucleosis, a familiar problem on college campuses. Caused by the Epstein-Barr virus, which is one of the herpesviruses, this illness is spread through close contact, mainly by the oral-respiratory route. Called the ''kissing disease,'' mononucleosis usually lasts one to four weeks, but it can drag on for as long as three months. Treatment of uncomplicated cases includes bed rest, aspirin or other analgesics for headache, and gargles for throat pain.

About 4 to 5 percent of upper respiratory infections are caused by the adenoviruses, named for the adenoids from which they were first isolated. Adenoviruses are responsible for a number of acute respiratory diseases seen primarily in children, including one that affects the throat and eyes. Rest in bed is the usual treatment.

Influenza is an all too familiar viral disease. The flu ranges from a barely noticeable infection to full-blown pneumonia, but the typical case is one accompanied by cough, headache, fever, malaise, loss of appetite and often nausea, vomiting and, of course, a sore throat.

The parainfluenza viruses are linked to a number of usually mild respiratory ills, including an influenza-like pneumonia, but the most common is a febrile (feverish) croup seen in young children. Initially, the child has a fever and cold-like symptoms. A moderate sore throat and dry cough develop early on. Hoarseness and a harsh cough often follow.

And then there is the most common cause of sore throat, the common cold, considered by many experts to be the greatest cause of sickness in the United States. Throat discomfort, sneezing, runny nose, and generalized aches and pains are the characteristic features of this aptly named illness. More prevalent during the winter months, colds can be blamed on hundreds of different viruses, including the influenza and parainfluenza varieties, adeno- and coxsackieviruses, and the rhino-, corona- and certain echoviruses. At this time, there is no cure for the common cold, which usually runs its course in four to 10 days.

Throat pain that is a symptom of a viral illness will disappear as the condition improves; the best treatment is simply bed rest, an analgesic for fever, and a warm saltwater gargle. (Children with viral illnesses such as flu or chicken pox should not be given aspirin because of its association with a rare but serious condition known as Reye syndrome.) Sore throats due to injuries or irritants also will heal by themselves with time.

But for those who can't wait, there are over-the-counter oral health-care products that may ease the pain until nature runs its course. A panel of experts, reviewing ingredients in OTC oral health-care products for the Food and Drug Administration, said relief can be found in anesthetic/analgesic lozenges and sprays containing ingredients such as benzocaine, dyclonine hydrochloride, hexylresorcinal, menthol, and phenol. Astringents containing alum and zinc chloride can provide a protective coating over the throat, the panel said, while urea peroxide, hydrogen peroxide, and sodium bicarbonate, in the form of a rinse or gargle, are useful in removing thick mucus or phlegm in the throat. Products containing elm bark, gelatin, glycerin, or pectin also can sooth irritated areas of a sore throat, according to the panel.

The effectiveness of gargles in relieving sore throat discomfort is questionable, however, the panel noted. In the act of gargling, the tongue rises and the sides of the throat draw together, preventing any fluid from reaching the area of inflammation.

Some sore throat sufferers who are not satisfied with the relief provided by these over-the-counter products feel that what they need is a good healthy dose of antibiotics. What they often don't realize is that these overused drugs are of no help against viral illnesses and should only be taken when a doctor has determined that the cause of the sore throat is a bacterial infection.

"Strep throat," or Group A beta hemolytic streptococcal infection, is the most common bacterial infection involving the throat. Although it is less prevalent than virus-caused varieties, strep throat is justly feared, for if it is not properly treated, it can lead to rheumatic fever, which in turn may lead to serious complications involving the joints, brain, heart, subcutaneous tissues, and skin.

The peak months for strep infections are November to May. Children between the ages of 5 and 15 are most susceptible to the infection.

Strep germs do their dirty work by invading healthy tissue, usually the pharynx. Typical symptoms include sore throat, fever, a beefy-red pharynx, and pus on the tonsils. A runny nose and cough are not part of a strep infection. However, in many strep cases the patient may have no symptoms at all, or just fever and sore throat, or some other nonspecific symptoms. A strep throat develops rapidly, in contrast to other types that are slow to make their presence known.

In order to distinguish a strep throat from other types of sore throats that sometimes produce a similar appearance, the doctor takes a swab of the inflamed area for laboratory examination. In the past, this procedure, called a throat culture, took 24 hours or more. Today there is a recently approved test being introduced that can produce results in the doctor's office in 10 minutes.

Strep throat, since it is a bacterial infection, is treated with antibiotics, usually penicillin. Treatment thwarts the development of complications and prevents spread of the infection, particularly among schoolmates. But it doesn't hurt to delay treatment for a day or two until the results of the throat culture are in, although some doctors prescribe antibiotics right away, just in case the infection is of the streptococcal variety.

Among other bacterial infections that cause sore throat are diphtheria and gonorrhea. Largely controlled by vaccination, diphtheria is still found in some parts of the United States, such as the Southwest and Northwest. Diphtheria is caused by an organism with the tongue-twisting name *Corynebacterium diphtheriae*. The organisms invade the tonsils or nasopharynx, and as they multiply, they produce toxins that damage surrounding cells.

The characteristic feature of diphtheria is a dirty-gray, tough pseudomembrane that forms in the area of the tonsils. The lymph glands in the neck may also be swollen. Complications can be severe if the disease is not treated promptly with antitoxin.

Gonorrhea, caused by the gonococcus bacterium *Neisseria gonorrhoeae*, is spread by sexual contact, and its symptoms usually appear on the genital organs. However, this organism can cause pharyngitis as a result of oral-genital contact, and the incidence of this type of illness is rising. As in other forms of gonorrhea, penicillin or other antibiotics are the preferred treatment.

The throat and mouth sometimes are affected by fungal diseases such as blastomycosis, sporotrichosis or actinomycosis. The most common, however, is thrush, caused by *Candida albicans*. Symptoms of thrush include white patches over the pharynx, tonsils and base of the tongue. Once seen almost exclusively in children and malnourished adults, thrush now occurs in people of all ages—thanks, surprisingly, to antibiotics. Prolonged use of these drugs destroys the organisms that normally live in the oral cavity, allowing the overgrowth of the everpresent *Candida*.

Annabel Hecht, *FDA Consumer*, Vol. 19, No. 2 March 1985.

Stroke

Fighting Back Against America's No. 3 Killer

Try discussing the subject of stroke with someone who's middle-aged, and the reaction is usually immediate. "If I have to have a stroke, I'd rather die than end up as a cripple or vegetable," he or she is likely to say.

The fear is understandable, because many in this age group are acquainted with the aftermath of strokes in aged parents or other relatives. They have witnessed firsthand the effects of stroke—the inability to speak, the distorted face and useless arm, the loss of control of bodily functions.

The statistics are not reassuring. Each year, about 400,000 Americans suffer from stroke. About 160,000 die immediately or shortly after the stroke's onset. Of every 100 who survive the acute illness, about 10 will be able to return to work virtually without impairment, 40 will be slightly disabled, 40 will be more seriously disabled and require special services, and 10 will need institutional care. Only about 16 percent of the 1.8 million Americans today who have survived stroke are completely independent. What's really discouraging is that after a stroke does its damage, in most cases it's difficult or impossible to reverse its effects. Stroke is the third leading cause of death in this country, behind heart disease and cancer.

Most people have heard about stroke and know it has something to do with the brain, but are not exactly sure what it is. A stroke occurs when an area of brain tissue dies because its blood supply has been cut off or decreased. As brain cells die, the functions they control—speech, muscle movement, understanding—die with them, or are impaired.

Although the brain represents only about 2 percent of the body's weight, it commands a lion's share of the body's oxygen supply—about 25 percent—and about 70 percent of the glucose consumed by the body.

It receives 15 percent of the blood pumped by the heart through the arteries. This disproportionate amount is necessary because the brain, unlike other organs, cannot store the energy that it makes from glucose and oxygen in the blood. Brain cells can live only for a few minutes if their blood supply stops, as when the heart stops beating in cardiac arrest. Once they die, they cannot be regenerated.

The old word for stroke—apoplexy—conjures up an image of someone who is felled suddenly by a blow, much as a tree is felled by lightning. Though a major stroke can occur quickly, just like a bolt of lightning, the factors leading to a stroke usually have been building up within the body for a long time.

About two-thirds of all strokes occur because of blockages that gradually form in the arteries that feed the brain. (Strokes from such blockages are called ischemic strokes or infarctions, just as the death of part of the heart muscle is called myocardial infarction.) The blockages are caused by a clot—called a thrombus or embolus, depending on where it's formed.

A thrombotic stroke occurs when an artery in the head or neck becomes either completely clogged or so narrowed that not enough blood reaches a particular area of the brain. This clogging is usually caused by atherosclerosis, also known as hardening of the arteries. Though this disease is associated with aging, atherosclerosis can begin as early as childhood. Through the years, plaque (consisting of fat-containing material and calcium) builds up on the inner linings of blood vessels, much as mineral deposits build up within a water pipe. The plaque may get so thick it shuts off the blood supply. Or clots may form on the rough surface of the plaque, plugging up the arteries.

Atherosclerosis is also a factor in embolic stroke, which occurs when a clot or piece of a clot breaks away from a diseased artery in another part of the body (in the heart or lungs, most frequently) and is carried along by the bloodstream until it ends up in a smaller artery in the brain.

A hemorrhagic stroke occurs when a blood vessel ruptures in or around the brain. Hemorrhagic strokes are more dangerous than those caused by blockages because not only does the part of the brain served by the blood vessel die, but blood may spurt out so forcefully that surrounding brain tissue is damaged. They occur primarily when a spot in an artery wall that has been weakened by disease—most often atherosclerosis or high blood pressure—breaks suddenly or begins to leak blood. Hemorrhagic stroke can also be caused by a defect called an aneurysm, a section of an artery wall that is so thin that it balloons out under normal blood pressure and may burst under high blood pressure. Hemorrhagic strokes account for about 15 percent of all strokes and are fatal in about 50 percent of cases.

About 10 percent of the time, there is advance warning of an impending stroke in the form of one or more transient ischemic attacks. A TIA is a kind of mini-stroke which signals that the blood flow to the brain has been temporarily interrupted (ischemia)—in most cases from tiny clots (emboli) that have broken loose from plaque in heart or neck arteries. Depending on the part of the brain affected, a TIA can cause blindness in one eye (a "blackout" or "whiteout" of vision, blurring, or something often described as if a shade were being pulled down over the eye), difficulty in speaking or writing, or numbness or weakness of the face, arm or leg on one side of the body. An attack usually lasts less than 30 minutes, with complete return to normal (thus the word transient).

A TIA is a strong predictor of stroke—about one-third of those who've had one can expect to have a stroke within five years. So it's important to report episodes of this type to a doctor. A doctor can often determine whether atherosclerosis is causing the problem by listening with the stethoscope to the sounds in the carotid arteries, which are located on each side of the neck. If either is partially obstructed, a swishing sound called a bruit (pronounced brew'ee) is sometimes heard as the blood is pushed through the narrowed segment of the artery with each heartbeat. (Sometimes people can hear their own bruits.)

When someone has many TIAs, a test called an arterial angiogram can be performed in the hospital to locate the narrowed blood vessel. A long, thin, flexible tube is inserted into an artery in the arm or leg and is threaded up into a neck artery. After dye is injected into the artery via the tube, X-ray pictures of the head and neck are taken in rapid succession, enabling a doctor to see the movement of blood through the arteries in the brain.

In cases where the blockage looks severe, the doctor may recommend an endarterectomy, in which a surgeon opens the artery and cleans out the blockage. (Texas surgeon Dr. Michael DeBakey performed the first successful carotid endarterectomy in 1953.) Since an endarterectomy carries risks (as does an angiogram), some doctors prefer to treat TIAs with blood-thinning drugs rather than surgery. Among the drugs used, FDA has approved aspirin—which prevents blood platelets from clumping together—to treat men who have had TIAs caused by emboli. Studies have not shown that aspirin is as effective in reducing TIAs in women.

When stroke finally does occur, it may be difficult to diagnose which type it is, because different areas of the brain are affected, producing a variety of symptoms. However, there are some clues.

In thrombotic strokes, symptoms often progress by steps: It may take minutes or even hours for the full damage to be felt. Typically, a victim may experience clumsiness upon getting up in the morning, soon followed by a headache. At breakfast, the right half of the field of vision in both eyes may disappear (sometimes the victim is not aware of this loss). Then, suddenly, the victim may find it difficult or impossible to speak, and ultimately may develop weakness or complete paralysis on the right side of the body, all in a matter of seconds or minutes.

In such cases, a diagnosis of damage to the left side of the brain caused by thrombosis can be made almost with certainty, especially if the victim has a history of one or more TIAs. (Each side of the brain controls the opposite side of the body, but speech and language are associated with areas in the left, or dominant, hemisphere.) High blood pressure is present in about 60 percent and diabetes in about 24 percent of patients. The peak age for thrombotic stroke is 70.

An embolus, in contrast, plugging one of the brain arteries at random, produces all its damage within a matter of seconds or minutes at the most. There is usually no warning or pain. Though this type of stroke can happen at any time, it comes more frequently during sleep than other strokes, which occur more often in the morning. The symptoms vary depending on the area of the brain involved, but are similar to those of thrombotic strokes.

A hemorrhagic stroke caused by a ruptured aneurysm of an artery to the brain often strikes while the victim is awake and active and produces a sudden, excruciating headache. The sufferer may then complain of a stiff neck, become nauseated, vomit, and finally lapse into unconsciousness. It is thought these aneurysms may be present at birth or may develop after birth at weak points in the arteries. Blood found in the spinal fluid or seen on a CT scan (computerized tomography—a form of X-ray exam) would confirm the diagnosis. This type of hemorrhage most commonly occurs between 35 and 65 years of age.

Hemorrhages within the brain (intracerebral) tend to come on abruptly, preceded in half of the victims by a headache. In most cases, the blood pressure is extremely high. Nausea and vomiting are also common. The damage done by this type of stroke progresses gradually over minutes or hours; it doesn't occur in steps as in thrombotic strokes. Since hemorrhagic strokes generally occur during the day when a person is active, victims may be alert when the stroke begins and quite aware that something terrible is happening to them. As a rule, they deteriorate quickly and often are in a coma upon arrival at the hospital. This type of stroke is fatal in about four of five cases. Those who survive are left with major disabilities.

Correct diagnosis of the type of stroke suffered is important because treatment varies. When strokes are caused by blockages, anticoagulants such as warfarin and heparin may be used to prevent clots from becoming larger. But that treatment could be fatal if the stroke was caused by an aneurysm, where the goal is to stop the hemorrhage and preserve the blood clot that forms where the blood vessels ruptured. Therapy, therefore, may involve drugs that prevent further bleeding. Reducing blood pressure and the brain swelling that develops at the injured site may also be part of this treatment.

Besides an angiogram (or arteriogram—the words are used interchangeably), physicians are helped in diagnosing strokes by a variety of techniques. CT scans, which have revolutionized stroke diagnosis, use computers to construct black-and-white pictures of the brain obtained from multiple X-rays beamed through the head. The scan can detect dead brain tissue or areas that are bleeding. The CT scan can be repeated more often than angiograms. That's also true for ultrasound, which is used to detect blockages in the neck arteries.

There are a few bright spots in all this gloom. Many people have made remarkable recoveries from severely disabling stroke. Walt Whitman, the famous American poet, had his first stroke at 40, then suffered from multiple strokes over many years. He made a satisfactory recovery after each. When he died at 72, it was from tuberculosis.

The body tries to repair stroke damage as quickly as possible. Small blood vessels around a blocked artery enlarge to allow more blood to get through to the affected area. Some damaged brain cells recover completely or in part. Also, in many cases other parts of the brain have the ability to take over the functions of a damaged area. This is especially true in very young children whose nervous systems are still developing. Hospital management of stroke victims has also improved, while better methods of rehabilitation have made life more bearable for those left with handicaps.

The best news is that fewer people are dying from strokes. Starting in the 1950s, a modest decline began in the number of stroke deaths. The decline accelerated in the 1960s, and picked up further speed in the 1970s. In the May-June 1985 issue of *Stroke,* Dr. Philip A. Wolf reported that stroke deaths had declined about 50 percent in a little over a decade in men and women, blacks and whites, and in all areas of the United States.

No one knows exactly why this has happened. Some researchers say it's because high blood pressure—even mildly elevated blood pressure—is being more aggressively treated. The treatment of rheumatic heart disease—which often produces clots that travel to other parts of the body—with antibiotics has also contributed to declining stroke deaths. Others say the increased attention that Americans have been giving to weight, exercise, diet and blood cholesterol levels in the last few decades is paying dividends. A Dutch researcher has postulated that the decreasing use of salt as a food preservative—with dependence instead on refrigeration and deep-freezing—might be playing a part in stroke decline through changes in dietary habits, since the sodium in salt has been linked in some people to high blood pressure.

Whatever the reasons, there is no room for complacency. Since the results of stroke can be devastating, it's preferable for those with multiple risk factors to do as much as possible—reducing blood pressure, not smoking, drinking only in moderation—to prevent stroke and avoid the consequences of this much-feared disease.

Evelyn Zamula.

What's Your Risk of Stroke?

A number of factors influence stroke risk:

Age Although stroke may occur at any age, even in newborns, the danger of stroke grows with age. Eighty percent of strokes occur in persons 65 and older.

High Blood Pressure Perhaps the greatest stroke risk factor. Strokes occur two to four times more frequently in people with high blood pressure—160/95 or greater—as in those with normal blood pressure. As blood pressure, especially systolic pressure (the first number), goes up, the chance of stroke goes up, too.

History of Stroke Those who have had one stroke and survived are at greater risk for another stroke. In the Framingham study—a study of 5,000 residents of a Massachusetts town that has been going on since 1949—it was found that of 198 men and 196 women who had initial strokes, 84 had second strokes and 27 had third strokes. Stroke survivors generally do not have as long a lifespan as the general population.

Heart Disease Clots, which can lead to stroke, don't form in normal hearts, but they may form occasionally in those with valve defects and after heart attacks and certain bacterial infections, such as rheumatic fever. Heart surgery also often causes emboli to form, as does the artificial heart.

Gender It helps to be a woman rather than a man, because stroke is more frequent in males until the age of 75. (After 75 the incidence is about the same for men and women.) Men have a 44 percent greater chance of having a first stroke, with a five-year recurrence rate almost double that of women. However, women who use oral contraceptives run a slightly higher chance of stroke than women who do not. Oral contraceptive users above 35 who also smoke and have high blood pressure have a 14 times higher risk of having a stroke than women with none of these risk factors.

Diabetes People who have too much sugar in the blood run almost double the risk of stroke. One possible explanation currently being explored by researchers is that the excessive blood sugar that results from diabetes not only damages blood vessels, but also appears to interfere with the normal breakdown of fibrin, a plasma protein that holds blood clots together.

Race Stroke mortality in blacks is almost double that of whites in the 35- to 74-year age group. The greater incidence of high blood pressure among blacks is definitely a factor in adult strokes, while sickle-cell anemia, which occurs almost exclusively in blacks, often causes atherothrombotic strokes, especially in children under 15.

"Thick" Blood In some diseases, such as polycythemia, too many red blood cells are manufactured, causing the blood to become thick and sludge-like. The flow of this "thick" blood to the brain is slowed and the tendency to form clots is increased, both of which may lead to brain infarcts. In people who have this problem, the age-old technique of bleeding (phlebotomy) is used to reduce the number of red blood cells.

Heredity Some people carry stroke risk in their genes. Stroke victims, more often than others, have a parent or parents who also had strokes. Several studies have shown that high blood pressure and diseases of the blood vessels in the brain are more frequent among identical twins than fraternal twins of the same sex, pointing further to a genetic risk factor, since identical twins have exactly the same genes, while fraternal twins don't.

Smoking In the Framingham study, cigarette smoking has been shown to be an apparent risk factor for stroke, but only in men under 65. Other studies have confirmed the relationship between cigarette smoking and stroke in younger age groups. In one study, male college students who smoked 10 or more cigarettes a day were at twice the risk for eventual fatal stroke than those who smoked less than 10 a day or didn't smoke at all. The evidence that smoking, by itself, is a risk factor for stroke in women is not strong. But smoking is related to other risk factors (alcohol consumption, use of oral contraceptives) and to diseases of other organs, particularly the heart. The good news is that the risk of stroke decreases if the person stops smoking.

Alcohol People who drink heavily, are obese, and lead sedentary lifestyles are also said to run a greater risk of stroke, but the evidence is strong only for alcohol. Though obesity and high blood pressure often go hand in hand, those who are obese but don't have high blood pressure or diabetes do not run a significantly greater risk of stroke.

Drug Abuse   Stroke can be caused by amphetamines, cocaine, and "Ts and Blues" (pentazocine and tripelennamine). Heroin and LSD are also implicated in stroke.

Reprinted from July/August 1986, *FDA Consumer*, HHS Publication No. (FDA) 86–1131. Department of Health and Human Services, Public Health Service, Food and Drug Administration, 5600 Fishers Lane, Rockville, Md. 20857, Office of Public Affairs. U.S. Government Printing Office 1986–491–341/40056.

Surgery

Thinking of Having Surgery? Think about getting a second opinion.

Every day we make decisions. Some are easy, like what to wear to work. Some are harder, like whether to buy a house. When you must make a difficult decision, it helps to know as much as possible about the pros and cons.

The same is true when a doctor advises you to have non-emergency surgery. There are risks with any surgery and you should know what these are. You should also know what the surgery will do and whether other medical treatment might be used instead of surgery.

When thinking about non-emergency surgery, one way you can help yourself to reach a decision is to seek the advice of another qualified doctor. This advice is called a second opinion.

There are differences of opinion about medical problems. One doctor may recommend surgery; another may tell you to wait a while; another may suggest another kind of treatment. When you ask the right questions, receive thorough information, and have the opinions of two doctors, you increase your chances of making the decision that is right for you.

A second opinion *should not* be used to delay or avoid having an emergency operation. When there is time, a second opinion should give you additional information to help you decide if surgery is the best thing for you. You have every right to that information.

Questions you should ask

Before agreeing to any non-emergency surgery, you should know the answers to these questions:

1. What does the doctor say is the matter with you?

2. What is the operation the doctor plans to do?

3. What are the likely benefits to you of the operation?

4. What are risks of the surgery and how likely are they to occur?

5. How long would the recovery period be and what is involved?

6. What are the costs of the operation? Will your insurance cover all of those costs?

7. What will happen if you don't have the operation?

8. Are there other ways to treat your condition that could be tried first?

Ask these and any other questions you might have. The more you know, the better prepared you'll be to make a decision about surgery.

When you should get a second opinion

Sometimes surgery is done on an emergency basis. It must be done right away, or within a few days, as in the case of acute appendicitis or injuries from an accident. *Because any delay could be life-threatening, second opinions are seldom possible for this kind of surgery.*

But much surgery is not an emergency. You have the time to choose when you want to have it, and even if you will have it. Some operations that are *usually* not emergencies are tonsillectomies, gall bladder operations, hysterectomies, hernia repairs and some cataract operations.

Anytime a doctor suggests non-emergency surgery, you should consider getting a second opinion.
- Make sure that a short delay will not be harmful.
- Make sure you have as much information as possible about the benefits and risks of the surgery.
- Find out if there are any other methods of treatment that you and your doctor can try first.
- Weigh the benefits and risks of having the operation against the benefits and risks of *not* having it.

Getting a second opinion is standard medical practice. Most doctors want their patients to be as informed as possible about their condition.

How to find a specialist to give you a second opinion

If your doctor recommends non-emergency surgery, there are several ways to find a surgeon or another specialist in the treatment of your medical problem:

1. Ask your doctor to give you the name of another doctor to see. Do not hesitate to ask; most physicians will encourage you to seek the second opinion.

2. If you would rather find another doctor on your own:
- You can contact your local medical society or medical schools in your area for the names of doctors who specialize in the field in which your illness falls.
- You can call the government's toll-free number, (800) 638-6833—in Maryland, call (800) 492-6603, to find out how to locate a specialist near you.
- If you're covered by Medicare, you can call your local Social Security Office (listed in your telephone directory under U.S. Government, Department of Health and Human Services).
- If you're eligible for Medicaid, you can call your local welfare office.

How to get a second opinion

Some people do not feel comfortable letting their doctor know that they are getting a second opinion. However, if you tell your doctor, you can ask that your records be sent to the second doctor. In this way, you may be able to avoid the time, costs and discomfort of having to repeat tests that have already been done.

When getting a second opinion, you should tell the second doctor:
- the name of the surgical procedure recommended, and
- any tests you know you have had.

If the second doctor agrees that surgery is the best way to treat your problems, he or she will usually send you back to the first doctor to do the surgery.

If the second doctor disagrees with the first, most people find that they have the facts they need to make their own decision. If you are confused by different opinions, you may wish to go back to the first doctor to further discuss your case. Or you may wish to talk to a third physician.

How to pay for the second opinion

Many private insurance companies pay for second opinions. You can contact your health insurance representatives for details.

Medicare will pay for the second opinion at the same rate it pays for other services. Most state Medicaid programs will also pay for second opinions.

Key points to remember about second opinions

- You can get a second opinion whenever non-emergency surgery is recommended. Most doctors approve of patients getting a second opinion and will assist you in doing so.
- Second opinions are a way for you to get additional expert advice from another doctor who knows a lot about treating medical problems like yours.
- Second opinions can reassure you—and your doctor—that the decision to have the surgery is the correct one.
- Second opinions are your right as a patient. They can help you make a better, informed decision about surgery.

The final decision regarding non-emergency surgery is up to you. After all, it's your body. Isn't your body worth a second opinion?

U.S. Department of Health and Human Services, Health Care Financing Administration, HCFA-02114

Toothache

Drugs Take The Bite Out of Toothache

A few people sometimes have throbbing toothaches. Others wake up in the morning with bad breath. Those with toothaches can get some temporary relief with non-prescription drugs containing oil of cloves (or eugenol). But for those who want to freshen their breath, medical ingredients in mouthwashes may not provide any health benefits and indeed may do some harm.

These are the conclusions reached by two expert advisory panels reviewing the ingredients in toothache remedies and oral health-care products respectively as part of FDA's massive study of the safety and effectiveness of non-prescription, or over-the-counter (OTC), drugs. The reports of the Advisory Review Panel on OTC Dentifrice and Dental Care Drug Products and of the panel on OTC Oral Cavity Drug Products were published by FDA in the May 25, 1982, *Federal Register* to elicit public comment. The recommendations are those of the panel members and are not binding on the agency. After the public comments have been reviewed, FDA will propose standards covering products promoted for non-prescription use for toothaches and for oral health care.

Here is more detail on what the two panels had to say.

There is a consumer population with occasional needs for non-prescription products to treat minor trauma or irritation of the teeth and gums, according to the expert panel on dentifrices and dental care products. Despite the need, the panel found only a few ingredients on the market that are safe and effective for use as (1) agents for the relief of toothache; (2) oral mucosal analgesics (pain-killers); (3) oral mucosal protectants; and (4) tooth desensitizers.

Of the 12 active ingredients in common toothache remedies, only clove oil, or a similar oil containing 85 to 87 percent eugenol (a derivative of cloves), is safe and effective for toothache. But, said the panel, this ingredient should be used only on a tooth with "persistent throbbing" pain. This kind of pain indicates the tooth pulp is already irreversibly damaged, so topical pain-killing products can't cause additional injury, the group reasoned. But if the pain is occasional or intermittent, a characteristic of reversible damage, such products could injure the pulp, perhaps causing irreversible damage, and should not be used.

Three of the 12 ingredients reviewed were not considered safe and effective toothache remedies. They are capsicum (from hot pods of pepper) when used on an open cavity, menthol and methyl salicylate. Further study is needed to determine the safety and effectiveness of nine ingredients, including benzocaine, creosote, phenol and thymol preparations, and capsicum as a counterirritant in a poultice that's applied to the gum near the toothache.

Labeling for toothache remedies should warn that the product is only for persistent, throbbing tooth pain. The user should see a dentist as soon as possible and not use the product for more than seven days, the panel recommended. Toothache products should not be promoted for rapid and effective relief of sore gums or for sore gums following tooth extractions, they said.

Benzocaine, butacaine sulfate, and phenol preparations (phenol and phenolate sodium) are all safe and effective as oral mucosal pain-killers, but camphor and methyl salicylate are not, according to the expert panel. Benzyl alcohol and cresol should be further tested.

Oral mucosal pain-killers can be labeled for the temporary relief of pain from minor irritation or injury of soft tissues of the mouth, minor dental work, or canker sores already diagnosed by the dentist, the panel said. Labels for products containing benzocaine or phenol can also claim to ease the discomfort of teething in infants and children 4 months of age and older. But, said the panel, these products cannot be labeled as quick acting or especially soothing after extractions or for temporary relief of pain from tooth cavities.

Only two ingredients were reviewed as oral mucosal protectants (substances that help protect irritated areas of the mouth from further irritation from chewing and swallowing). One of them, benzoin preparations (benzoin tincture and compound benzoin tincture), was found safe and effective by the panel, while the other, fluid extract of myrrh, was recommended for further study.

Approved labeling for protectants includes such claims as "forms a coating over a wound" and "protects against further irritation." Labels should warn consumers not to use the product for more than seven days. Unacceptable to the panel are claims such as "especially soothing after extractions or for minor gum boils" or "gives quick relief that lasts for hours."

As for desensitizers, the panel found no ingredients it considered safe and effective to treat hypersensitive teeth, that is, teeth that are extra sensitive to heat and cold. The combination of sodium fluoride, strontium chloride, and edetate disodium should not be marketed. Five ingredients, including fluoride preparations, formaldehyde solution, and potassium nitrate, should be subjected to additional testing to establish whether they are effective as tooth desensitizers.

Annabel Hecht, *FDA Consumer*. Vol. 16, No. 7, September 1982.

Tuberculosis

TB: Curable, Preventable, but Still a Killer

To many people in the United States, tuberculosis is an almost forgotten disease, one that is read about, but seldom encountered. But it wasn't too long ago when 126,000 cases of TB were being reported every year. That was the case in 1944 when the U.S. Public Health Service launched its tuberculosis control program. A little more than four decades later, in 1985, the number of cases had dropped to 22,201.

While this may seem to be a dramatic improvement, health authorities warn that tuberculosis is still a serious public health problem in the United States. Deaths from tuberculosis—about 2,000 annually—outnumber those for all other infectious diseases reported to the U.S. Centers for Disease Control (CDC). Only pneumonia and influenza, which are not required to be reported, take a greater toll. Worldwide, tuberculosis is a major problem, with as many as 4 million new cases and 3 million deaths every year.

Tuberculosis in humans is caused by two species of rod-shaped bacteria that are called mycobacteria. *M. tuberculosis* primarily causes pulmonary (lung) tuberculosis, the most prevalent form of the disease. *M. bovis* causes bovine tuberculosis, a disease of cattle that can be transmitted to humans through cow's milk, resulting in both pulmonary tuberculosis and disease of other body sites such as the cervical (neck) lymph nodes and the spine. Pasteurization of milk and testing of dairy herds for infected cows has virtually eliminated bovine tuberculosis in the United States.

Pulmonary tuberculosis is spread via contaminated droplets that are coughed, sneezed or otherwise put into the air by a person with active TB. Inhaled by a susceptible individual, the smallest droplets end up in the alveoli, minute air sacs in the lungs located at the tips of the bronchial tree. The bacteria (also called tubercle bacilli) may also infect the kidneys, bones, lymph nodes, and membranes surrounding the brain (meninges), or they may be spread throughout the body.

During the first stage of infection, white blood cells called phagocytes attack and may destroy any bacilli that have gotten into the lung. Those bacilli that escape this defense may continue to grow.

About two to 10 weeks after infection, the individual develops a hypersensitivity to the tubercle bacillus or its proteins, known as tuberculins. This heightened sensitivity persists for a very long time, and a small amount of the tuberculins subsequently injected into the skin will produce a hard, red, raised spot at the injection site. This is the basis for the skin test used to detect exposure to *M. tuberculosis*.

The response of sensitive lymphocytes (white blood cells) to tuberculin results in the activation of another type of white blood cell, called a macrophage, which engulfs and attempts to destroy the bacilli. The affected tissue becomes infiltrated with macrophages and layers of other cells to form the characteristic tubercle that gives the disease its name.

After this initial tubercle has healed, the lesion becomes calcified, in effect "walling off" the bacilli. There they may remain dormant for months, years or a lifetime.

If healing is imperfect, or if the person's immune capability is lowered, the bacilli may multiply more rapidly than the body's defenses can cope, the bacilli spill out, become engulfed by new macrophages, and start new tubercles in the lungs or throughout the body. In the process, macrophages and other tissue and blood cells that are killed form a soft, caseous (cheese-like) mass that eventually becomes liquified and is discharged into nearby air passages, leaving a cavity in the lung. As the disease becomes extensive and more cavities form, lung function is impaired. Blood in the sputum is usually from ulceration of the lining of the bronchi. Massive hemorrhage can occur if a pulmonary artery in a tuberculous cavity ruptures. In advanced cases, death may occur from loss of blood or obstruction of airflow.

Most persons exposed to the bacilli do not develop TB. In those people who do develop active TB, the disease may spread rapidly and produce a high fever. (This acute form of TB was once called "galloping consumption.") Or it may become a chronic, slowly progressive disease with low fever, weakness, and loss of weight. If left untreated, many patients eventually die of the disease.

The impact of tuberculosis is felt most by older and poorer people. Cases usually occur in individuals who were infected years ago, particularly the elderly. Many of these people grew up in the first decades of the century when 80 percent of the population had been infected (though not necessarily afflicted with an active case of the disease) by the time they were 30. By CDC estimates, currently 10 million people in this country are infected by the tubercle bacillus, carrying a small but lifelong risk of developing active TB.

Although most newly diagnosed tuberculosis patients in the United States are adults infected long ago, there were 1,200 new cases of tuberculosis in children in 1984. This means that TB is still being passed on by people with active infections. Also, every year thousands more children are infected, but do not get the disease, adding to the pool of those at risk of TB in the future.

By all rights, this disease—once the nation's leading cause of death—should have been eliminated. That was the hope some 40 years ago when the first effective anti-TB drug, streptomycin, was introduced. The number of cases has been going down steadily, but slowly—about 5 percent to 6 percent annually. At that rate, elimination of the disease could not be expected until after the year 2100, according to CDC Director James O. Mason, M.D. "This is unacceptable for a disease which today is considered curable and preventable," he told a 1985 national conference on tuberculosis research in Pittsfield, Mass.

Even more disturbing is that this decline in the number of cases seems to have come to a virtual halt. The number of reported cases in 1985 was only 54 less than that in the previous year.

TB experts believe the slowdown is related in part to the increasing occurrence of tuberculosis among patients with AIDS (acquired immunodeficiency syndrome). Their suspicions are based on the fact that patients with other disorders that affect the immune system—as AIDS does—also have an increased risk of developing active TB.

In addition, some of the areas with the largest number of TB cases are also the areas with the largest number of AIDS cases (New York City, California, Florida, and Texas). In New York City, matching AIDS and TB case registers has revealed an increasing number of AIDS patients with a history of tuberculosis. In Dade County, Fla., a substantial number of people with AIDS either had tuberculosis at the time that AIDS was diagnosed, or had it in the previous 18 months. Thus, tuberculosis may prove to be the first AIDS-related "opportunistic" infection that can be a threat to the general public. (An opportunistic infection is one that takes hold because the patient's immune system is weakened.)

Two other reasons for the persistence of TB are outbreaks of the disease among the homeless, and the growing number of immigrants and refugees from areas where there is a high prevalence of TB, such as Southeast Asia and Central and South America.

Tuberculosis can be reduced by finding and treating new cases, and giving preventive therapy to those who were in contact with TB patients and those who have positive reactions to tuberculin skin tests. Unfortunately, control efforts have been hampered by several factors, Dr. Mason told the Pittsfield conference. One of them is that health-care providers just don't think of tuberculosis as a major problem.

This perception has been fostered by past success in reducing the number of cases and deaths from tuberculosis, Dr. Mason said. Because the disease is less common than in the past, doctors are less likely to consider it as a possible diagnosis. The classic symptoms—cough, loss of appetite, and blood-tinged sputum—often don't appear in older patients or they may go unrecognized because they are masked by another illness or by the use of drugs such as antibiotics, steroids, and anticoagulants (blood-thinning drugs).

Despite the availability of an array of effective drugs to treat tuberculosis, health-care providers are not always up-to-date on the latest recommendations for their best use. And patients often don't take their medications correctly or stop taking them too soon. Until recently, tuberculosis patients had to take a number of drugs for a year or more. Unfortunately, the price of noncompliance can be the emergence of drug-resistant bacteria and continued transmission of the infection to others.

Today the length of treatment has been reduced in most instances to nine months. The primary drugs used are isoniazid and rifampin, both of which destroy the mycobacteria. During the initial phase of treatment, other drugs may be added: streptomycin, ethambutol or pyrazinamide. TB drugs must be taken in combinations to avoid the emergence of drug-resistant strains of the tubercle bacillus and to increase effectiveness. When a drug-resistant strain is suspected, the initial use of at least three drugs is necessary.

The regimen can be reduced to six months if three drugs—isoniazid, rifampin, and pyrazinamide (and perhaps ethambutol, if isoniazid-resistance is detected)—are given for two months, followed by an additional four months of isoniazid and rifampin, according to recently published recommendations by CDC and the American Thoracic Society, the medical section of the American Lung Association. Treatment lasting less than six months is not acceptable because of the risk of relapse.

Most patients have no problems with isoniazid and rifampin, although some may develop liver disorders. Ethambutol may cause reversible eye problems such as blurred vision, eye pain, red-green color blindness, or even temporary loss of vision. Streptomycin may permanently damage hearing. Pyrazinamide occasionally causes rash, hepatitis, and gastrointestinal disturbances.

TB drugs may also interact with other medications. Isoniazid, for instance, increases the blood concentration of phenytoin, used to treat epilepsy. Rifampin may lessen the expected effects of oral contraceptives, quinidine, corticosteroids, warfarin (a blood thinner), and oral hypoglycemics taken for diabetes. Patients being treated for TB should make sure their doctor knows what other medications they are taking.

While combinations of various drugs can cure active cases of TB, the eradication of tuberculosis from the population rests, in large part, on preventing the disease from developing in those already infected by the tubercle bacillus. The risk of disease is particularly high in infected infants, adolescents and patients on immunosuppressive therapy, such as organ transplant patients. Many years ago, the Public Health Service demonstrated that a year's treatment with isoniazid was very effective in preventing active TB in infected individuals.

Public health officials recommend that isoniazid preventive therapy be given to contacts of persons with active disease; people who have recently had a change from a negative to a positive tuberculin skin test; people with previously known tuberculosis, now inactive, who have not had adequate treatment; and other positive tuberculin reactors. This last group includes particularly those with abnormal findings on a chest X-ray or underlying medical conditions such as diabetes, leukemia or Hodgkin's disease (a form of cancer), and those under 35.

Lately, however, some experts have questioned the application of isoniazid preventive therapy to those under 35, who may be at greater risk of developing hepatitis from the drug than tuberculosis. In addition, the inconvenience of long-term drug taking and the lack of motivation on the part of apparently healthy individuals pose problems of compliance with the drug regimen.

Recently, a group of physicians and scientists involved in tuberculosis therapy met in Atlanta, under the auspices of CDC, to consider short-course alternatives to the long-term preventive approach. One suggestion by the group was that a six-month course of rifampin alone or a two-month multiple drug regimen with rifampin and pyrazinamide, with or without isoniazid, may prove as effective as the year-long treatment with isoniazid alone. Rifampin and pyrazinamide are particularly effective in eliminating the tuberculosis bacteria that persist in the bodies of infected individuals.

The group recommended evaluation of the short-course regimen in animals and pilot studies in humans, followed by full-scale human trials here and abroad.

CDC's Mason sees an end to the transmission of tuberculosis by the year 2000, if more effective use is made of existing diagnostic, treatment, and other control measures and new technologies are developed. Many of the tools now used to control tuberculosis—the tuberculin skin test, X-rays, and methods of culturing the bacillus—are adaptations of 19th-century discoveries, Mason said.

He also called for more effective drugs that need fewer doses to cure the disease, better ways to monitor and improve patient compliance, a better approach to preventing disease among infected persons, and a reliable, effective vaccine.

"Let us declare total, all-out war against a disease that should only be part of our history," Mason said.

If the campaign is successful, the disease the 17th-century English author John Bunyan called "The captain of all these men of death" can be demoted to the lowest rank of all.

Annabel Hecht, *FDA Consumer*, December 1986–January 1987.

Ulcer

When Digestive Juices Corrode, You've Got An Ulcer

The image sticks in the mind: A middle-aged executive grimacing over a pain in his stomach, gulping down a chalky tasting antacid and mournfully waving away pizza or chili because his doctor won't "let" him eat spicy food. The portrait of a man with an ulcer.

In truth, more than a third of ulcer sufferers are women, and they appear to be gaining on men. Children and teen-agers also develop ulcers. Antacids are still a popular treatment, but three new prescription drugs are now available. And, instead of giving up broad categories of food, ulcer sufferers need only avoid foods that bother them.

Peptic ulcers are small sores or lesions in the lining of the stomach or small intestine. The term "peptic" comes from pepsin, a digestive enzyme that acts in concert with hydrochloric acid to digest food in the stomach. The thought, sight, smell, and taste of food can cause even an empty stomach to secrete acid and pepsin. Normally the lining of the stomach and small intestine can resist corrosion from these digestive juices, but sometimes resistance breaks down and an ulcer develops. Why this happens is not completely understood.

An estimated 4 million Americans suffer from peptic ulcer disease at any given time. About 12 percent of U.S. males and 4 to 8 percent of females will develop one or more ulcers during their lifetimes.

Peptic ulcer disease can be painful and debilitating, but it is usually not life-threatening unless there are complications. In 1982, 176,000 men and 175,000 women were hospitalized with peptic ulcer, according to the most recent survey by the National Center for Health Statistics. About 6,000 people die each year from complications of peptic ulcer. The death rate increases with age, and in many cases the ulcer combines with another disease to cause death. The Stanford Research Institute has estimated that in the United States peptic ulcer disease costs nearly $3 billion annually in medical expenses and lost earnings (including earning losses due to death).

There are two main types of peptic ulcer: Duodenal ulcer occurs in the duodenum, the first few inches of the small intestine after it exits from the stomach. More than twice as many men as women have duodenal ulcers. They usually strike people during their most productive years and are four to eight times more common than gastric ulcers. Gastric ulcer occurs in the stomach, most commonly in older patients. It rarely develops before age 40, and the peak incidence is from 55 to 65. Incidence is the same for men and women.

Who is most likely to develop an ulcer? Smokers are, and their ulcers take longer to heal. They have more ulcer recurrences, more complications, and a higher ulcer-related death rate. The same does not appear to be true for alcohol users, except those with cirrhosis of the liver.

The tendency to have ulcers can run in families. The risk of developing a duodenal or gastric ulcer is three times greater in people who have close relatives with these ailments. Persons with group O blood are at greater risk of having duodenal ulcer disease. Blacks appear to have a higher ulcer rate than whites, including deaths from complications.

Several studies have shown more gastric ulcer disease among patients who take large quantities of aspirin than those who don't. Aspirin is known to cause lesions in the lining of the stomach. The same ulcer rate is shown for buffered aspirin as for plain aspirin, but the risk is much smaller with enteric-coated aspirin (which dissolves in the small intestine instead of the stomach). Other drugs for arthritis, the steroids and the non-steroidal anti-inflammatory drugs, also are suspected of contributing to stomach ulcers.

Stress may help cause some people's ulcers, but its importance has not been conclusively shown. Emotional stress is difficult to measure, and people do not react to stressful situations in the same manner. A pressured executive, for instance, may be less anxious than an assembly line worker or a 2-year-old's mother. There is no occupation or personality type that characterizes ulcer sufferers.

Some studies indicate that stressful events frequently precede the development of an ulcer, but other studies fail to implicate such events in ulcer cases. Air traffic controllers as a group experience tremendous occupational stress, but they develop no more ulcers than the general population. However, during the bombing of London in World War II there was a notable increase in the incidence of certain ulcer complications. Apparently, some people are more susceptible than others to the effects of stress on their gastrointestinal tracts.

Certain foods, beverages, and spices may bring on indigestion, but there is no convincing evidence that they cause or reactivate ulcers. Food buffers stomach acid and can temporarily relieve ulcer pain. However, some foods are particularly potent stimulators of stomach acid secretion. A few of the most common offenders are certain beverages, such as carbonated drinks, beer, tea and coffee (regular, decaffeinated, and acid-neutralized). To make matters worse, these buffer little acid, particularly if they travel rapidly through an empty stomach. Many ulcer sufferers drink milk because it neutralizes stomach acid, but unfortunately it has a "rebound" effect. That is, after a certain amount of acid has been buffered, the calcium and protein in milk stimulate the production of even more acid.

Several studies have shown that a bland "peptic ulcer" diet does not produce healing or relieve ulcer symptoms any better than regular or slightly modified diets. Current advice to ulcer sufferers is to eat several meals a day (to keep the stomach from being empty too long) and avoid foods that cause stomach distress. Coffee and other acid stimulators should be used in moderation, especially on an empty stomach. Milk should not be used as an antacid. Many ulcer patients take antacids or other medications at bedtime to control excess acidity; therefore, bedtime snacks, which stimulate acid secretion, are not recommended. If symptoms occur in the middle of the night, an antacid can provide relief.

Gastric ulcer patients are often advised to avoid or decrease alcohol use because alcohol in high concentrations can damage the lining of the stomach. The situation is different for duodenal ulcers because alcohol is partially absorbed or diluted in the stomach before it reaches the duodenum. The question of alcohol's impact on a duodenal ulcer remains to be answered.

"I don't diet, but through trial and error I've learned what food has an effect on me," says a 54-year-old former duodenal ulcer patient. "Some brands of beer, wine, and scotch really upset my stomach, but not others. Most foods are OK except cabbage, or sometimes highly acidic things like tomato sauce and pizza. And I've stopped skipping breakfast. The worst thing you can do for an ulcer is leave the stomach empty."

His ulcer experience was fairly typical. He learned he had an ulcer the way many people do. It told him.

"I was a guy who always took pride in having a cast-iron stomach. I had a job on a newspaper, and the greater the pressure the more I loved it. I started feeling this burning sensation in my gut, but I ignored it until I couldn't anymore and it was affecting my job. The soreness would persist for hours. It was never severe pain, just constant soreness, and it debilitated me. I couldn't think straight, couldn't concentrate. It drained me. I'd try different things—antacids, ice cream. Any relief would be temporary."

Following treatment with antacids his ulcer healed, and he is currently on medication to prevent a recurrence. "I've been lucky," he says.

Some people with an ulcer do not experience distinct symptoms and, ironically, many patients with symptoms do not have a detectable ulcer crater. Nevertheless, the most common sign of an ulcer is a steady gnawing or burning pain between the navel and the lower end of the breastbone. It usually starts when the stomach has emptied, and it can often be relieved by eating more food or by taking antacids. Pain may awaken the patient at night.

It is often difficult to distinguish between a gastric and duodenal ulcer from symptoms alone. However, with a duodenal ulcer it is not uncommon for symptoms to disappear and return repeatedly over several years, with intervening pain-free periods lasting a few months to a few years. One textbook noted that over half of duodenal ulcer patients have had symptoms for more than two years before seeking medical advice. Complications of gastric and duodenal ulcers may produce symptoms such as dark stool (a possible sign of internal bleeding), severe pain, nausea, vomiting and weight loss.

The traditional method of diagnosing an ulcer is a series of X-rays commonly known as an "upper GI (gastrointestinal) series." On an empty stomach, the patient swallows a chalky liquid containing barium, a metal that shows in X-rays. The stomach and duodenum are outlined on the film, and an ulcer crater may be seen filled with the barium.

In a newer technique called endoscopy, a long flexible tube (endoscope) made of optical fibers that transmit light is snaked down the sedated

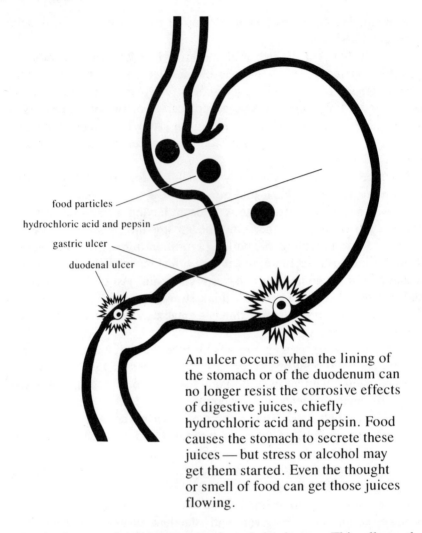

food particles
hydrochloric acid and pepsin
gastric ulcer
duodenal ulcer

An ulcer occurs when the lining of the stomach or of the duodenum can no longer resist the corrosive effects of digestive juices, chiefly hydrochloric acid and pepsin. Food causes the stomach to secrete these juices — but stress or alcohol may get them started. Even the thought or smell of food can get those juices flowing.

patient's throat and into the stomach and duodenum. This allows the physician to see the ulcer directly and to collect tissue for a biopsy if necessary. Endoscopy is more expensive, but it avoids exposing the patient to X-rays and offers somewhat greater accuracy in detecting ulcers.

The basic aim of ulcer treatment is to relieve pain and give the ulcer a chance to heal itself—either by reducing the amount of acid and irritants in the stomach or by coating and protecting the ulcerated area.

Antacids have been used for decades to neutralize hydrochloric acid in the stomach. They are still prescribed or recommended by many physicians for use alone or with other ulcer medications. (Antacids should not be taken at the same time as certain other ulcer drugs, since they can interfere with absorption.) Studies show that antacids compare favorably with newer drugs in ulcer healing, but the periods of relief are shorter, necessitating more frequent doses. Patients often become frustrated with the dosage schedule, the taste, and the side effects, and they neglect to follow the schedule.

The most common side effects are diarrhea from magnesium-based antacids, constipation from aluminum-based products, and acid rebound from calcium-type antacids. Some newer combination aluminum-magnesium preparations may reduce these bowel disturbances. Because of potential drug interactions, patients using antacids for prolonged periods should ask a doctor before taking other medications.

Since 1977 three new prescription drugs have been approved by the Food and Drug Administration for treatment of specific types of ulcers. Cimetidine (brand name Tagamet) entered the U.S. market in 1977 and is used to treat duodenal and gastric ulcers and to prevent recurrence of duodenal ulcers. Two other drugs—sucralfate (Carafate) and ranitidine (Zantac)—were approved in 1981 and 1983, respectively, for use in treating duodenal ulcers.

These drugs work in two very different ways. Cimetidine and ranitidine are powerful inhibitors of stomach acid and pepsin secretion, while sucralfate forms a protective coating over the ulcer to shield it from irritation as it heals. Various clinical studies do not show great differences between the three drugs in rates of duodenal ulcer healing. All three drugs have low incidences of side effects, but since some potential effects are serious, patients should be carefully monitored by a physician.

Several anticholinergic drugs are also occasionally used as adjuncts to other ulcer medications. They inhibit the action of a chemical called acetylcholine, which stimulates acid-producing cells in the stomach. Because anticholinergics are not as effective as the new acid blockers and often have unpleasant side effects, they are rarely prescribed by themselves. Several other drugs currently under study for treatment and prevention of ulcers include colloidal bismuth, pirenzepine, tricyclic antidepressants, and prostaglandins.

Many ulcers clear up without drug therapy or with only occasional use of antacids. Studies show, however, that a strict regimen of antacids or prescription drugs usually produces somewhat faster symptomatic relief and higher healing rates than placebos (inert substances). In duodenal ulcer studies, healing took place in about 70 to 85 percent of patients taking drugs, compared with 30 to 60 percent of those given a placebo.

After healing—with or without drugs—60 to 80 percent of duodenal ulcer patients will have an ulcer again. In about two-thirds of all cases, the disease seems to subside for good after about 10 or 15 years. One drug, cimetidine, is currently approved for use in preventing duodenal ulcer recurrence. It reduces the recurrence rate to less than 20 percent, but this protection disappears as soon as the drug is stopped. The consequences of long-term use of cimetidine—that is, beyond one year—are not known.

The pattern for gastric ulcer disease is different. Symptoms of a gastric ulcer are similar to those of stomach cancer, and it is therefore imperative to make sure the ulcer has healed (an indication it is benign). This finding may be made with an endoscope, which also can be used to remove tissue for biopsy. A patient with a persistent or recurrent gastric ulcer probably will have to undergo surgery to determine if the lesion is benign, as well as to relieve symptoms. In contrast, duodenal ulcers are rarely cancerous, and surgery is less often needed in recurrences.

Simple ulcers sometimes develop into more serious conditions that require hospitalization, and even surgery. The three main complications of peptic ulcers are hemorrhage, perforation and obstruction.

Internal bleeding or hemorrhage affects 10 to 20 percent of ulcer patients. As an ulcer burrows into a muscular portion of the intestinal wall, it can damage blood vessels and cause bleeding into the intestinal tract. One sign of slow internal bleeding is a dark, tarry stool. Eventually the patient may become anemic. If the ulcer damages a large blood vessel, there may be rapid hemorrhaging, vomiting of blood, faintness, and sudden collapse. Without prompt medical action, the patient may bleed to death.

Perforation—erosion by an ulcer all the way through the stomach or duodenal wall—occurs in about 5 percent of patients. It is often heralded by sudden, severe pain throughout the abdomen. Perforation may allow digested food and bacteria to spill into the abdominal cavity and cause infection, and it can be fatal if untreated.

Obstruction occurs when the narrow opening between the stomach and duodenum becomes blocked by swelling or scarring. This keeps food from passing out of the stomach, and the patient may vomit or constantly regurgitate stomach secretions. It affects about 2 percent of ulcer patients and often must be corrected surgically.

Each year about 50,000 Americans undergo surgery for peptic ulcers. Some surgery is to treat complications, but most often it is done to alleviate severe, incapacitating ulcers that won't heal or stay healed.

At one time, the most common ulcer operation consisted of cutting out two-thirds of the patient's stomach to reduce the amount of acid-secreting tissue. Now, there are less drastic techniques that produce fewer side effects.

One common operation involves severing the nerve that stimulates the stomach to secrete acid and empty food into the intestine (the vagus nerve). This is accompanied by a procedure that allows the stomach to empty its contents more rapidly into the intestine, or by removal of the small part of the stomach where a hormone is produced that stimulates acid secretion. These techniques drastically reduce ulcer recurrence, but some patients suffer severe digestive side effects and may need additional surgery.

The newest type of operation involves cutting selected branches of the vagus nerve instead of severing it entirely. This produces fewer side effects but is somewhat less effective in preventing ulcer recurrence.

Elective surgery for peptic ulcers is declining. Doctors are putting more patients on maintenance drug therapy and trying non-surgical methods for non-emergency complications. Lasers, electric probes, and balloon dilators now can be sent down to the stomach or duodenum through an endoscope. The first two "sizzle" tissue and stop an ulcer from bleeding, while the balloon helps open up obstructed passages.

For more information on peptic ulcer disease, write:

National Digestive Diseases Clearinghouse
1555 Wilson Boulevard
Suite 600 (FD)
Rosslyn, Va. 22209

Louise Fenner, Reprinted from July/August 1984, FDA Consumer, HHS Publication No. (FDA) 84–1113. Department of Health and Human Services, Public Health Service, Food and Drug Administration, 5600 Fishers Lane, Rockville, Md. 20857, U.S. Government Printing Office 1987—181–341/40087.

Urinary Infection
The Unwelcome Night Visitor

For sheer discomfort, it's hard to beat a full-blown urinary infection. This unwelcome visitor often comes after a day in which a woman— it's usually a woman—has not felt quite well. After going to bed, she is awakened during the night by an intense urge to urinate. But it hurts to do so, and it burns, too. Her urine smells different and looks cloudy and thicker than usual. She returns to bed, but soon has to urinate again, this time passing only a small amount. This can go on the whole night, each episode becoming more and more uncomfortable, until her body begins to bear down involuntarily while urinating, not too unlike labor. Frantic with pain and discomfort, she can hardly wait until morning to call the doctor.

Not all urinary tract infections (doctors call them UTIs) are so unpleasant, but most people get at least some of the usual symptoms, and sometimes fever, chills, and pain in the lower abdomen or kidney areas. One of the more frightening symptoms is blood in the urine. This needs the attention of a urologist.

Often UTIs are asymptomatic—they have no symptoms at all—and the only way a person knows is when the urine is checked during a physical examination. Statistics show, however, that if these "silent" infections go untreated, they will show up as a not-so-silent infection at a later date. To confuse the matter even further, sometimes dysuria (painful urination) can occur when there is no infection in the urinary tract. Testing a urine specimen is the only way to confirm whether the dysuria is due to bacterial infection or other causes.

Producing urine is such a normal function that we take the good health of our urinary tract for granted. But it is a complicated, fine-tuned system. Urine is formed in the kidneys, which remove waste products from the blood that passes through them at the rate of 18 gallons an hour. These large, bean-shaped organs are located below the ribs toward the middle of the back. From the kidneys, urine passes down to the urinary bladder via two tubes, called the ureters. Urine is stored in the bladder until it passes out of the body through the urethra. Depending on how much and what kinds of liquids and food are consumed, an average adult passes about a quart and a half of urine each day. Physical activity stimulates the kidneys to produce urine, so about twice as much urine is formed during the day as while sleeping.

The urinary system has its safeguards. Valve-like structures at the lower ends of the ureters prevent urine from backing up into the kidneys (called vesicoureteral reflux), where it could cause problems. Urination itself acts to flush out any bacteria that may enter the bladder. In ways still not completely understood, the whole urinary system is geared to rid itself of bacteria. When colonies of bacteria are deliberately inoculated into the bladders of experimental animals, frequently all traces of them are gone in 24 hours.

Normal urine contains water, waste products and salts. It can range in color from clear to deep yellow and has a faint odor. The less liquid a person has drunk, the darker and more concentrated the urine. Urine is normally sterile, though it does pick up some bacteria as it passes out of the urethra. When large numbers of bacteria are found in the urine, it means there is infection somewhere in the body, usually in the urinary tract.

Women visit their doctors about 5.7 million times a year with symptoms of cystitis—inflammation of the urinary bladder. (When both the bladder and the urethra are involved, as is frequently the case, it is called cystourethritis.) The symptoms are one of the most common causes of absentee-ism in working women, second only to upper respiratory infections.

One reason why women have more than their share of urinary infections lies in their anatomy. While the human body is wondrously fashioned, there are some flaws in the female design. The vaginal, urinary, and anal openings are too close together. Bacteria from the anal area can easily migrate across the perineum—a narrow band of flesh—to the urethra, the starting point for most UTIs. The female's short urethra provides a convenient pathway for ascending urinary infections, while the male's longer urethra serves as a barrier against this type of infection.

The proximity of the vaginal opening to the urethral opening is also a factor in infections. As far back as the 11th century, an Italian physician writing on women's diseases concluded that there was an association between UTIs and sex. A 1977 study reported that 83 percent of women had their first UTI after they had become sexually active.

It's not hard to understand why. During intercourse, bacteria from the vaginal area may be massaged into the urethra. The guilty bacterium in most cases is *E. coli,* normally a harmless resident of the bowels. When it is introduced into the bladder, however, it flourishes in the urine and irritates the tissue lining the bladder and the urethra. The presence of bacteria, often coupled with irritation of the tender urethral tissue during sex, opens the way to infection.

Although UTIs are uncommon in young males, men don't escape these troublesome infections entirely. As they grow older, their urinary problems increase. Frequently, the prostate, a gland in males that sur-rounds the neck of the bladder and the urethra, enlarges and obstructs the flow of urine, interfering with the normal emptying of the bladder. This disorder affects 50 percent of men by age 50 and more than 90 percent by age 80.

People can also run into trouble with UTIs as a result of sexually transmitted diseases. In males, urethritis follows infection with gonococ-cus, the bacterium that produces gonorrhea, or with other types of bacteria. Women get inflammation of the vagina from gonorrheal infections, and the proximity of the vagina to the urethra almost guarantees them a case of urethritis, too. The increasing resistance of gonococci to penicillin, the drug of choice for this infection, is making treatment of gonorrhea more difficult.

In the past, doctors often made a diagnosis of nonspecific urethritis when they couldn't pin down the cause of infections in patients who reported symptoms of cystourethritis, but whose urine showed no bacteria. It was found that the problem was often caused by *T. mycoplasma* or *Chlamydia trachomatis,* sexually transmitted organisms that are difficult to detect under the microscope and difficult to culture. Since these diseases are usually traded back and forth between sex partners, it's necessary that both persons be treated.

Children's urinary problems often arise from congenital (birth) defects in the urinary tract, such as strictures (narrowings) in the ureters or urethras, urethral valves (folds of the urethra that act as valves), or other defects. This is especially true for boys. *Pediatric Alert* (Oct. 11, 1984) reports that in one seven-year study, 75 percent of 83 boys between the ages of 2 weeks and 14 years with UTIs had anatomical abnormalities, most commonly those involving vesicoureteral reflux. Since it's better to detect and treat any kind of urinary obstruction early, before the kidneys are damaged by refluxing urine, it is essential that competent medical personnel observe the size and force of the urinary stream in newborn boys before they leave the hospital.

Because very young children cannot describe their symptoms, urinary infections should be suspected when a child is irritable or lethargic, does not grow at a normal rate, eats poorly, vomits, has diarrhea, urinates more frequently than normal, or fails to urinate at all. UTIs can also be present in older children who begin wetting after having been toilet-trained, or who complain of painful or frequent urination, or who have fever. It's important to seek medical help as soon as possible when these symptoms are present.

Fecal material that enters girls' urinary tracts (and women's, too) often causes UTIs. This is just one of the reasons why an infant's soiled diaper should be changed immediately and the contaminated area carefully cleansed. Female children should be taught to wipe themselves from front to back so that fecal material is not pushed into the urethra. A wise mother will also sponge the diaper area of either sex with water after changing a wet diaper. Urine left to dry on the skin can be irritating.

Although intestinal bacteria are the culprits in most lower urinary tract infections, any kind of blockage that prevents urine from flowing freely out of the body can set the stage for such an infection, too.

An improperly fitted diaphragm, some physicians say, may cause infection in women by pressing on the bladder and obstructing the flow of urine. Bacteria can also enter the urinary area during insertion and removal of the diaphragm, or may begin to grow in the vagina when the contraceptive is left in too long. When diaphragms cause urinary problems, doctors advise switching to a smaller size, or to another type of contraception.

Most UTIs are self-limiting, that is, they will clear up by themselves in a few days, providing the sufferer can stand the initial agony—which can last several hours or longer—and drinks plenty of water. But since an infection can ascend up through the ureters to the kidneys, where it can cause much more serious problems, it's important to see a doctor promptly when urinary symptoms are present.

Although a physician can guess what's wrong with a patient by merely listening to a description of the symptoms, for a firm diagnosis it's necessary to examine a urine sample under a microscope and have it cultured in a lab. The doctor can tell the patient how to take a "clean catch" specimen. (Some urologists prefer to take urine specimens from women directly from the bladder with a catheter to ensure that the sample is not contaminated by bacteria from the vagina or surrounding tissues.) When the bacteria are identified, the doctor can select the appropriate drug to clear up the infection.

Usually, either sulfa drugs or antibiotics are prescribed to fight the UTI. The patient is advised to drink plenty of water to flush bacteria out of the bladder. If pain is intense, the physician may prescribe a bladder analgesic to relieve the symptoms. (The most commonly used drugs for this purpose color the urine orange or blue.)

Most patients begin to feel better within 24 hours after treatment begins, but it is important to continue taking the medicine for the length of time the doctor has indicated. Drugs were formerly given for uncomplicated UTIs for a week or more, but doctors have changed their thinking about this course of treatment. Today they are more apt to give larger doses of drugs for two or three days or, in the case of recurrent infections due to sex, a preventive dose before and after intercourse is sometimes prescribed.

Doctors will want to do another urinalysis and urine culture after the patient has completed taking the medication. If the urine is free of bacteria and pus, no further treatment is necessary.

If the UTI recurs within a short time, doctors will reevaluate the patient to find out why. The recurrences could be due to infections descending from infected kidneys, bacteria in the bloodstream, stones in the urinary system, strictures or other causes. In women who have had several children, a condition called cystocele, a bladder hernia that protrudes through the vaginal wall, may be the troublemaker.

To track down the cause of recurrent infections, the urologist (a specialist in diseases of the urinary tract in both sexes and the genital organs in the male) will order a blood test and a complete urinalysis, and sometimes a procedure called a cystoscopy. After giving the patient anesthesia if necessary, the doctor inserts an instrument with a lighted lens into the urethra. This cystoscope enables the doctor to look into the bladder. Irritation, tumors, stones, ulcers or other pathology will be visible. With this instrument the urologist can also do a biopsy (remove a sample) of any suspicious growths that may be present.

Along with the cystoscopy, the doctor may order kidney X-rays, commonly called IVP (intravenous pyelogram). In this procedure, a radiologist injects into the veins an iodine-containing liquid dye. This dye concentrates in the kidneys and urine and flows through the ureters and bladder as X-ray pictures are being taken. The doctor can see any abnormalities in the X-rays.

These procedures, plus any other necessary tests, will most likely pinpoint the cause of the trouble. Surgery may be necessary to correct some abnormalities, but most cases of lower UTIs can be cleared up with antibacterial drugs and do not cause serious future problems.

Evelyn Zamula, *FDA Consumer,* March 1985.